HAIR REPLACEMENT

Surgical and Medical

HAIR REPLACEMENT

Surgical and Medical

EDITOR
Dow B. Stough, M.D.
Clinical Assistant Professor,
Department of Dermatology,
University of Arkansas Medical Science Campus,
Little Rock, Arkansas;
Department of Surgery,
St. Joseph's Regional Health Center,
Hot Springs, Arkansas

ASSOCIATE EDITOR
Robert S. Haber, M.D.
Assistant Professor of Dermatology,
Case Western Reserve University;
Assistant Director, Dermatologic Surgery,
University Hospitals of Cleveland,
Cleveland, Ohio

*with 759 illustrations
and 13 color plates*

Mosby

St. Louis Baltimore Boston Carlsbad Chicago Naples New York Philadelphia Portland
London Madrid Mexico City Singapore Sydney Tokyo Toronto Wiesbaden

Mosby
Dedicated to Publishing Excellence

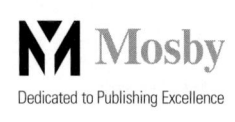

A Times Mirror Company

Publisher: Anne S. Patterson
Editor: Susie Baxter
Developmental Editor: Ellen Baker Geisel
Project Manager: Mark Spann
Manufacturing Supervisor: David Graybill
Editing and Production: Top Graphics
Designer: Judy Schmitt
Cover Design: Sheilah Barrett

Copyright © 1996 by Mosby–Year Book, Inc.

A NOTE TO THE READER
The editors, authors, and publisher have made every attempt to check dosages for accuracy. Because the science of pharmacology is continually advancing, our knowledge base continues to expand. Therefore we recommend that the reader always check product information for changes in dosage or administration before administering any medication. This is particularly important with new or rarely used drugs.

All rights reserved. No part of this publication may be reproduced, stored in a retrieval system, or transmitted, in any form or by any means, electronic, mechanical, photocopying, recording, or otherwise, without prior written permission from the publisher.

Permission to photocopy or reproduce solely for internal or personal use is permitted for libraries or other users registered with the Copyright Clearance Center, provided that the base fee of $4.00 per chapter plus $.10 per page is paid directly to the Copyright Clearance Center, 27 Congress Street, Salem, MA 01970. This consent does not extend to other kinds of copying, such as copying for general distribution, for advertising or promotional purposes, for creating new collected works, or for resale.

Printed in the United States of America
Composition by Top Graphics
Color separation by Color Dot
Printing/binding by Maple-Vail

Mosby–Year Book, Inc.
11830 Westline Industrial Drive
St. Louis, Missouri 63146

Library of Congress Cataloging-in-Publication Data

Hair replacement : surgical and medical / editor, Dow B. Stough;
   associate editor, Robert S. Haber.
       p. cm.
   Includes bibliographical references and index.
   ISBN 0-8151-7543-4
   1. Hair—Transplantation.   2. Hair growth stimulants.
   3. Baldness—Treatment.   I. Stough, Dow B.
   II. Haber, Robert S.
   [DNLM: 1. Alopecia—therapy.   2. Hair—transplantation.   3. Scalp—
surgery.   WR 460 H1534 1996]
RD121.5.H34   1996
617.4′779—dc20
DNLM/DLC
for Library of Congress   95-21443
                                                                     CIP

96 97 98 99 00 / 9 8 7 6 5 4 3 2 1

Contributors

James Arnold, M.D.
Lecturer of Dermatology, Stanford School of Medicine, Stanford University, Palo Alto, California; Senior Member, Department of Medicine, San Jose Medical Center, San Jose, California

Marc R. Avram, M.D.
Director, Hair Transplant Unit, New York University, New York, New York

Lydia A. Bazzano
Research Assistant, Department of Dermatology, Tulane University School of Medicine, New Orleans, Louisiana

William H. Beeson, M.D.
Associate Clinical Professor, Department of Otolaryngology/Head & Neck Surgery, Indiana University School of Medicine, Indianapolis, Indiana

Emil Bisaccia, M.D.
Associate Clinical Professor of Medicine & Dermatology, Columbia University, College of Physicians & Surgeons; Associate Attending Physician, The Presbyterian Hospital in the City of New York, Dermatology Services, New York, New York; Medical Director, Photopheresis Center, Department of Internal Medicine, Morristown Memorial Hospital, Morristown, New Jersey

Serge Jocelyn Boolauck, M.D.
Private Practitioner, Centre Medico Esthique Passy La Tour; Consultant of Plastic Surgery, Hôpital Tenon, Paris, France

Pascal Boudjema, M.D.
Private Practitioner, Centre Medico Esthique Passy La Tour, Paris, France; Consultant of Plastic Surgery, Hospital de Montreuil, Montreuil, France

Dominic A. Brandy, M.D.
Clinical Instructor, Department of Dermatology, University of Pittsburgh Medical Center; Attending Surgeon, St. Francis Central Hospital, Pittsburgh, Pennsylvania

Thomas F. Cash, Ph.D.
Professor of Psychology, Old Dominion University, Norfolk, Virginia

Yung-Chul Choi, M.D., Ph.D.
Togo Clinic, Seoul, Korea

William P. Coleman III, M.D.
Clinical Professor of Dermatology, Tulane University School of Medicine, New Orleans, Louisiana

Richard L. DeVillez, M.D.
Chief, Division of Dermatology, University of Texas Health Science Center, San Antonio, Texas

Zoe Kececioglu Draelos, M.D.
Clinical Assistant Professor, Department of Dermatology, Bowman Gray School of Medicine, Wake Forest University, Winston-Salem, North Carolina; Attending Physician, Central Carolina Dermatology, High Point, North Carolina

Leonard M. Dzubow, M.D.
Professor of Dermatology, University of Pennsylvania School of Medicine; Head, Dermatologic Surgery, Hospital of the University of Pennsylvania, Philadelphia, Pennsylvania

Jeffrey S. Epstein, M.D.
Clinical Instructor, Department of Otolaryngology-Head & Neck Surgery, University of Miami, Miami, Florida

Richard E. Fitzpatrick, M.D.
Assistant Clinical Professor, Department of Medicine, University of California, San Diego, San Diego, California; Consultant, Department of Dermatology, Scripps Memorial Hospital, La Jolla, California

Patrick Frechet, M.D.
Paris, France

Kouzo Fukuta, M.D., Ph.D.
Administrator, Kamiida First General Hospital; Chief Surgeon, Nido Institute, Nagoya, Aichi, Japan

Joseph Greco, PA-C, Ph.D.
Appearances Cosmetic Surgery, Venice, Florida

Edmond I. Griffin, M.D.
Assistant Professor of Dermatology, Emory University; Private Practice, St. Joseph's Hospital, Atlanta, Georgia

Robert S. Haber, M.D.
Assistant Professor of Dermatology, Case Western Reserve University; Assistant Director, Dermatologic Surgery, University Hospitals of Cleveland, Cleveland, Ohio

Ken N. Hashimoto, M.D.
Professor and Chairman, Department of Dermatology, Wayne State University; Dermatologist-in-Chief, Detroit Medical Center, Detroit, Michigan

Brian D. Jackson, M.D.
Staff Allergist/Immunologist, Department of Medicine, St. Joseph's Hospital, Hot Springs, Arkansas

Edward M. Jackson, Ph.D.
President, Jackson Research Associates, Inc., Sumner, Washington

Francisco Jimenez, M.D.
Fellow in Dermatologic Surgery, Duke University, Durham, North Carolina; Fellow in Hair Restoration Surgery, The Stough Clinic, Hot Springs, Arkansas

Sheldon S. Kabaker, M.D.
Associate Clinical Professor, Division of Facial Plastic and Reconstructive Surgery, Department of Otolaryngology, University of California, San Francisco, San Francisco, California

Sajjad Khan, M.D.
Director, Jinnah Cosmetic Surgery Center, Lahore, Pakistan; Private Practice, International Hair Transplantation Clinic, San Diego, California

Jung-Chul Kim, M.D., Ph.D.
Assistant Professor, Department of Immunology, School of Medicine, Kyungpook National University, Taegu, Korea

Russell Graham Knudsen, M.B.,B.S.
Edgecliff, New South Wales, Australia

Matt L. Leavitt, D.O.
Medical Director, Medical Hair Restoration; Medical Director, Advanced Dermatology and Surgery, Orlando, Florida

Robert Thomas Leonard, Jr., D.O.
Adjunct Clinical Professor, Departments of Family Practice and Dermatology, University of New England, College of Osteopathic Medicine, Biddeford, Maine; Medical Director, Leonard Hair Transplant Associates; Attending Physician, Department of Medicine, South County Hospital; Attending Physician, Roger Williams Hospital, Providence, Rhode Island

Marvin I. Lepaw, M.D.
Assistant Professor of Dermatology, State University of New York at Stony Brook, School of Medicine, Stony Brook, New York; Attending, Division of Dermatology, Department of Medicine, Nassau County Medical Center, East Meadow, New York

B.L. Limmer, M.D.
Clinical Professor, Department of Medicine, Division of Dermatology, University of Texas Health Science Center, San Antonio, Texas

Manfred Lucas, M.D.
Medical Superintendent, Meditra Institute, München, Graefelfing, Germany

Michael J. Mahoney
Founder, Past President, and Executive Director, American Hair Loss Council, Tyler, Texas

David J. Margolis, M.D.
Assistant Professor of Dermatology and Director, Cutaneous Ulcer Center, University of Pennsylvania Medical Center; Attending Physician, Department of Dermatology, Hospital of the University of Pennsylvania, Philadelphia, Pennsylvania

Emanuel Marritt, M.D.
Associate Clinical Professor, Department of Otolaryngology/Head & Neck Surgery, University of Colorado Health Sciences Center, Denver, Colorado

Hani S. Matloub, M.D.
Professor of Plastic Surgery and Hand Surgeon, Department of Plastic and Reconstructive Surgery, Medical College of Wisconsin, Milwaukee, Wisconsin

Douglass Mead
Sharplan Lasers, Inc., Allendale, New Jersey

Michael A. Meshkin, M.D.
Medical Director, Cosmetic Hair Replacement Surgery Institute, Newport Beach, California

Joseph Andrew Molnar, M.D., Ph.D.
Assistant Professor, Department of Plastic and Reconstructive Surgery, Bowman Gray School of Medicine, Wake Forest University; Assistant Professor, Department of Plastic and Reconstructive Surgery, North Carolina Baptist Hospital, Winston-Salem, North Carolina

O'Tar Norwood, M.D.
Assistant Clinical Professor of Dermatology, University of Oklahoma Health Sciences Center, Oklahoma City, Oklahoma

David S. Orentreich, M.D.
Assistant Clinical Professor, Department of Dermatology, Mount Sinai School of Medicine; Assistant Attending Physician, Department of Dermatology, The Mount Sinai Hospital, New York, New York

Damkerng Pathomvanich, M.D.
The Stough Clinic, Cosmetic Surgeon, Vichaiyuth Hospital, Bangkok, Thailand

Thomas Pruzinsky, Ph.D.
Associate Professor of Psychology, Quinnipac College, Hamden, Connecticut; Adjunct Faculty, Department of Plastic Surgery, New York University Medical Center, New York, New York

Patrick Quinlan, M.D.
Chairman, Division of Dermatology, and Chairman, Department of Specialty Medicine, Lovelace Medical Center, Albuquerque, New Mexico

John Karl Randall, R.Ph., M.D.
Director, Department of Dermatology and Hair Restoration, The Zollman Center for Plastic and Hand Surgery; Staff, Department of Dermatology, Methodist Hospital, Indianapolis, Indiana

William R. Rassman, M.D.
Private Practice, Los Angeles, California

Neil S. Sadick, M.D.
Assistant Clinical Professor, Department of Dermatology, Cornell University Medical College; Attending Physician, Department of Dermatology, New York Hospital, New York, New York

Gail Sansone-Bazzano, Ph.D.
Associate Professor of Applied Health and Dermatology, Tulane University, New Orleans, Louisiana

Dwight A. Scarborough, M.D.
Assistant Clinical Professor, Department of Medicine, Ohio State University Medical Center, Columbus, Ohio

David J. Seager, M.B.,B.S., L.R.C.P., M.R.C.S.
Active Staff, Centenary Health Center, Toronto, Ontario, Canada

Richard C. Shiell, M.B.,B.S.
Melbourne, Victoria, Australia

Stephen W. Shoultz, J.D.
Dallas, Texas

Michael Slatkine, Ph.D.
Vice-President for Market Development, Laser Industries Ltd., Tel Aviv, Israel

David M. Spencer, M.D.
Assistant Clinical Professor, Department of Dermatology, University of Arkansas, Little Rock, Arkansas; Staff, Department of Dermatology & Pediatrics, Forsyth Memorial Hospital, Winston-Salem, North Carolina

Dow B. Stough, M.D.
Clinical Assistant Professor, Department of Dermatology, University of Arkansas Medical Science Campus, Little Rock, Arkansas; Department of Surgery, St. Joseph's Regional Health Center, Hot Springs, Arkansas

Paul M. Straub, M.D.
President, International Society of Hair Restoration Surgery, Torrance, California

Bernd Strobele, M.D.
Sharplan Lasers GmbH, Freising, Germany

James M. Swinehart, M.D.
Assistant Clinical Professor, Department of Dermatology, University of Colorado Health Sciences Center; Director, Colorado Dermatology Center, Colorado Medical Research Center, Denver, Colorado

Nia Terezakis, M.D.
Clinical Professor of Dermatology, Tulane University Medical School, New Orleans, Louisiana

Carlos Oscar Uebel, M.D.
Assistant Professor of Surgery, University of Porto Alegre; Chief of the Clinique of Plastic Surgery, Porto Alegre Institute, Porto Alegre, Brazil

Malte M. Villnow, M.D.
General Surgeon, Transhair Institute of Hair Transplantation, Dusseldorf, Germany

James E. Vogel, M.D.
Attending Surgeon and Instructor, Division of Plastic Surgery, The Johns Hopkins School of Medicine and Hospital System, Baltimore, Maryland

Jeffrey C. Weidig, M.D.
Rockville, Maryland

David A. Whiting, M.D.
Clinical Professor, Department of Dermatology and Pediatrics, University of Texas Southwestern Medical Center; Medical Director, Baylor Hair Research and Treatment Center, Baylor University Medical Center, Dallas, Texas

Shiro Yamada, D.Sc.
Administrator, Nido Institute, Tokyo, Japan

To my loving wife and lifetime partner
Sara

To my children
Shannon, Burke, Bradley

DBS

———

To my wife
Gina
and my son
Max
for their love, patience, and understanding

RSH

———

To the surgeons
who share their knowledge

Foreword

In the past decade there has been a tremendous surge in interest in male pattern baldness and hair transplant surgery. There are a number of reasons for this:

- Commercialization of hair transplant surgery
- Improvement in the results of hair transplant surgery
- Increased communication between hair transplant surgeons
- Medical therapy of male pattern baldness with Rogaine, which has increased public awareness and stimulated the search for other medical approaches for male pattern baldness
- Dramatic changes in medicine with an exodus of physicians away from traditional medicine into the cosmetic fields

With all these changes and with new and more rapid means of transmitting information, is there a need for another book on hair restoration? The answer, of course, is a resounding yes. The purpose of a book is to pause, collect, organize, edit, and distill the available knowledge and present the information succinctly in one volume. Such a text provides a reference for the experienced surgeon and a foundation for the beginning surgeon. *Hair Replacement: Medical and Surgical* exceeds these expectations. Dr. Stough has brought together the world's leading experts in the field of hair replacement and has compiled their contributions in a book that should be essential reading for all who perform or plan to perform hair transplant surgery. This book offers cutting edge technology; readers will not find a rehash of old ideas and techniques.

Dowling B. Stough IV is one of the next generation of hair transplant surgeons and, like his father, D. Bluford Stough III, is destined to be a leader in the field. This book will fulfill that destiny.

O'Tar Norwood, M.D.
Editor, *Hair Transplant Forum International;*
Assistant Clinical Professor of Dermatology,
University of Oklahoma Health Sciences Center,
Oklahoma City, Oklahoma

Preface

We, being human, can only approach perfection by concentrating or specializing.

RICHARD C. WEBSTER, M.D.*

There is something about surgeons that I cannot explain but believe to be true. As a group, we tend to bond strongly with the first technique that we learn. Often this technique is demonstrated by those with considerable reputation and skills in the field. There is a natural desire to emulate and copy their techniques with the hope of producing similar results. Later, when confronted with new techniques and concepts, the listener first tends to disbelieve and resist. Change is difficult. However, for those who take the time to read, have a willingness to explore, and maintain an open mind, the burden of change is eased.

This book is about new versions, new ways, new philosophies, and new techniques. At the first meeting of the International Society of Hair Restoration Surgery, a memorable comment was made by one of the participants: "Don't you love this field," he said. "It's like the wild, wild West; everything is new and exciting." In the last decade we have experienced an explosive growth in techniques of hair restoration surgery. The field is unique in every way, from each individual patient to pioneering surgeons. Hair restoration surgery is in a state of flux.

Any book that presents only one view on hair transplantation, scalp reduction, scalp-lifting, and scalp expansion does a disservice to the readers. This book reflects the varied philosophies that exist today on hair transplantation. The controversial topics were not omitted but are embraced as true reflections of the current state of the specialty.

Perhaps more important than the technical achievements that have evolved in the last ten years is the widespread recognition of hair restoration surgery as a true specialty. Hair restoration physicians have now gained the respect of their colleagues involved in mainstream medicine. A factor responsible for stimulating advances in this field is the cooperative effort forged among various specialties involved in hair transplantation. A partial list of these specialties includes dermatology, otolaryngology, plastic surgery, family practice, psychiatry, and general surgery. No specialty owns this field, nor should they. Physicians who would like to relegate the field of hair transplantation to only those with operating room privileges are destined to fail. The combined knowledge and experience of hair restoration surgeons around the world has allowed for the rapid integration and exchange of new ideas that can have only a positive effect on patient care.

Although this book will give the novice a firm background in hair restoration surgery, its primary audience is those most experienced in hair restoration surgery. I am confident that no matter what level of expertise and degree of knowledge one has gained in this field, the information contained herein will serve to advance the reader's understanding of this rapidly changing specialty.

New instrumentation has now equipped the hair restoration surgeon with the tools needed to achieve the goal of extensive micrografting. New drugs offer hope for the future. If the advances in the next ten years keep pace with those of the last decade, one can only imagine the benefits offered by hair restoration surgery.

My thoughts again return to the comments likening this field to the wild, wild West. To that I reply happy reading and "ride 'em, cowboy!"

Dow B. Stough, M.D.

---

*Webster RC: The hair transplant story, *Am J Cosmet Surg* 11(1):9, 1994.

Acknowledgments

A few words of acknowledgment seem insufficient to recognize those responsible for bringing this book to fruition. My loving wife provided me with much encouragement for this task. My secretary, Carolyn Nagel, and my staff deserve ample credit.

As the preparation and editing of this book progressed, my reliance on the advice of Dr. Robert S. Haber increased exponentially. His methodical approach to problems, editing ability, and unselfishness enabled the timely completion of this text. I am privileged to share the honor of editor with a great friend and surgeon. Dr. Sajjad Khan has given his time and attention to developing new instruments and new ideas presented in this book. Dr. Francisco Jimenez, Dr. Mark R. Avram, and Dr. Tom Potter also deserve credit for their meticulous reviews of each chapter. In addition, I am most grateful for the help that Ellen Baker Geisel at Mosby and Linda Kocher at Top Graphics have provided.

I thank Dr. Jere D. Guin for setting the highest academic standards.

The true authors of this book are those whose names do not appear on the cover but who have contributed individual sections. They have sacrificed their time and shared their knowledge freely, for which I am grateful.

Dow B. Stough, M.D.

Contents

FOREWORD xi
PREFACE xiii
HOW TO USE THIS BOOK xxv

1 General Considerations for Hair Replacement 1

2 Preoperative Stages 59

3 Anesthesia 81

4 Instrumentation 111

5 The Donor Site 131

6 Technique—Small-Graft Hair Transplantation 151

7 Special Categories 201

8 Wound Healing 219

9 Scalp Reductions and Scalp-Lifting 229

10 Complications 299

11 Selected Topics in Hair Replacement 345

12 Drug Therapy 375

13 Hair Care Products 387

14 Nonsurgical Hair Replacement 399

APPENDIXES

A Trademark and Service Mark Laws Relating to Hair Transplantation 413

B Surgical Products for Hair Transplantation 417

C Scalp Debridement Unit 423

D Determination of Hairline Placement 425

E Overview of the Surgical Procedure 431

F Medical Questionnaire for Hair Replacement Surgery 433

G Consent for Hair Transplantation 435

H Patient Instructions for Hair Replacement Surgery 437

I Hair Transplant Forum International 439

COLOR PLATES I THROUGH XIII 134

Detailed Contents

FOREWORD   xi
PREFACE   xiii
HOW TO USE THIS BOOK   xxv

1 General Considerations for Hair Replacement

  A. The psychosocial effects of androgenic alopecia and their implications for patient care   1
     Thomas F. Cash
     Thomas Pruzinsky

  B. Pathophysiology of androgenic alopecia   8
     Richard L. DeVillez

  C. Alopecia: classification and incidence   13
     O'Tar Norwood

  D. Anatomy of the scalp   20
     Hani S. Matloub
     Joseph Andrew Molnar

  E. The consultation   26
     Patrick Quinlan

  F. Reassessment of male pattern baldness: a reevaluation of the treatment   30
     Emanuel Marritt
     Leonard M. Dzubow

  G. Standardized photography for hair restoration   41
     Robert S. Haber

  H. Medicolegal issues in hair replacement   54
     Robert Thomas Leonard, Jr.

2 Preoperative Stages

  A. The history of hair restoration surgery   59
     David S. Orentreich

  B. An approach to the younger patient   62
     Jeffrey C. Weidig

  C. Surgical microbiology and antibiotic prophylaxis for hair restoration surgery   68
     John Karl Randall

  D. Standard terminology of graft sizes   76
     Russell Graham Knudsen

  E. The surgical suite   78
     Dow B. Stough

3 Anesthesia

- A. Local anesthesia in hair transplantation   81
  David J. Seager

- B. Nerve block anesthesia of the scalp   89
  Robert S. Haber
  Sajjad Khan
  Dow B. Stough

- C. Tumescent anesthesia for surgery of the scalp   93
  William P. Coleman III

- D. Buffered lidocaine and postoperative edema   96
  Paul M. Straub

- E. The use of monitored anesthesia care as an adjunct to local anesthesia for scalp surgery   97
  Dwight A. Scarborough
  Emil Bisaccia

- F. Nitrous oxide in hair restoration surgery   104
  Neil S. Sadick
  Dow B. Stough

- G. Pain control and management of the postoperative period   105
  David J. Seager

4 Instrumentation

- A. Instrumentation for hair transplantation and scalp reduction   111
  James M. Swinehart

- B. The multibladed knife for donor harvesting   117
  Emil Bisaccia
  Dwight A. Scarborough

- C. NoKor microslit grafting technique   122
  Michael A. Meshkin

- D. Single-hair and bundled-hair transplantation using the Choi hair transplanter   125
  Yung-Chul Choi
  Jung-Chul Kim

- E. Retraction-sectioning   127
  Joseph Greco

5 The Donor Site

- A. The donor area   131
  Dow B. Stough
  Robert S. Haber

- B. Accurate estimation of graft requirements when using multibladed knives   138
  Robert S. Haber
  Dow B. Stough

- C. Elliptical donor harvesting   142
  B.L. Limmer

- D. Micrograft survival   147
  B.L. Limmer

6 Technique—Small-Graft Hair Transplantation

- A. The art and science of small-graft hair transplantation   151
  William R. Rassman

B. Aspects of artistic craftsmanship when performing small-graft hair transplantation 162
Manfred Lucas

C. Hairline placement 170
Dow B. Stough

D. The punctiform technique with the 1000-graft session 172
Carlos Oscar Uebel

E. Combination micrografting with strip harvesting for male pattern baldness 177
Edmond I. Griffin

F. The origins of single-hair grafting 187
Dow B. Stough
Shiro Yamada

G. The single-hair graft technique for advanced male pattern alopecia 187
Dow B. Stough

H. Vertical strip dissection for graft production 195
James Arnold

7 Special Categories

A. Hua Laan Chon Kan 201
Damkerng Pathomvanich
Dow B. Stough

B. Hair transplantation in the Asian population 201
Damkerng Pathomvanich

C. Hair restoration in blacks 205
John Karl Randall
Dow B. Stough

D. Hair transplantation in the genetically male transsexual 207
Richard C. Shiell

E. The treatment of female pattern alopecia by hair transplantation 210
Edmond I. Griffin

F. Hair transplantation of the eyelashes and eyebrows 216
Jung-Chul Kim
Yung-Chul Choi

8 Wound Healing

A. Wound healing in hair restoration surgery 219
David J. Margolis

B. Postoperative dressings 224
Robert S. Haber
Dow B. Stough

9 Scalp Reductions and Scalp-Lifting

A. Scalp reductions 229
Paul M. Straub

B. The Frechet flap 243
Patrick Frechet
Richard C. Shiell

C. Expansion terminology 245
Dow B. Stough

D. Prolonged scalp extension 246
Patrick Frechet

E. Intraoperative scalp extension   249
David M. Spencer
Dow B. Stough

F. The biology of skin stretch and tissue expansion in hair restoration surgery   251
James E. Vogel

G. Rapid intraoperative tissue expansion created by tension clamps   259
James Arnold

H. The integration of scalp-lifting with small-graft hair restoration surgery   266
Dominic A. Brandy

I. Scalp-lifting   283
James M. Swinehart

10 Complications

A. The overwhelming responsibility   299
Emanuel Marritt

B. Adverse consequences in hair restoration surgery   299
Dow B. Stough
Francisco Jimenez

C. Corrective hair restoration   306
Matt L. Leavitt

D. Poor hair growth after hair transplantation: the X factor   314
Richard C. Shiell

E. Anatomical hair shaft sequelae of hair transplantation   316
Neil S. Sadick
Ken N. Hashimoto

F. Posttransplant epidermoid cysts secondary to small-graft hair transplantation   320
David A. Whiting
Dow B. Stough

G. Scarring and keloid development after alopecia correction surgery   323
John Karl Randall
Dow B. Stough

H. Arteriovenous malformation after hair transplantation   326
Jeffrey C. Weidig

I. Long-term problems associated with hair-bearing flaps for male pattern baldness   327
Sheldon S. Kabaker
Jeffrey S. Epstein

J. Hiccups following surgery of the scalp   332
James Arnold

K. Emergency situations in hair transplantation   334
William H. Beeson

L. Hereditary angioedema and hair restoration surgery   340
Brian D. Jackson
Dow B. Stough

M. Von Willebrand's disease and hair restoration surgery   342
Dow B. Stough
Marc R. Avram

11 Selected Topics in Hair Replacement

A. Synthetic hair grafting   345
Shiro Yamada
Kouzo Fukuta

  Critique
  Marvin I. Lepaw

B. Hair follicle regeneration after horizontal resectioning—implications for hair transplantation   358
Jung-Chul Kim
Yung-Chul Choi

C. Laser hair transplantation   363
  1. Principles
  Richard E. Fitzpatrick

  2. Laser-assisted hair transplantation
  Malte M. Villnow
  Michael Slatkine
  Bernd Strobele
  Douglass Mead

D. Automated hair transplant system: the Boudjema technique   370
Pascal Boudjema
Serge Jocelyn Boolauck

12 Drug Therapy

A. Drug therapy for pattern baldness   375
Richard L. DeVillez

B. Topical treatment of pattern baldness with a minoxidil/13-*cis*-retinoic acid solution   382
Nia Terezakis
Lydia A. Bazzano
Gail Sansone-Bazzano

13 Hair Care Products

A. The scientific basis and use of hair care products related to hair transplantation   387
Zoe Kececioglu Draelos

B. Camouflage products for hair loss   396
Edward M. Jackson

14 Nonsurgical Hair Replacement   399
Michael J. Mahoney

APPENDIXES

A Trademark and Service Mark Laws Relating to Hair Transplantation   413
Stephen W. Shoultz

B Surgical Products for Hair Transplantation   417
Marc R. Avram
Francisco Jimenez
Dow B. Stough

C Scalp Debridement Unit   423
Dow B. Stough

D Determination of Hairline Placement   425
Sajjad Khan
Dow B. Stough

E Overview of the Surgical Procedure   431
Marc R. Avram
Francisco Jimenez

F Medical Questionnaire for Hair Replacement Surgery   433

G Consent for Hair Transplantation   435

H Patient Instructions for Hair Replacement Surgery   437

I Hair Transplant Forum International   439
Dow B. Stough

COLOR PLATES I THROUGH XIII   134

How to Use This Book

This book represents the views and techniques of the international community of hair transplant surgeons. Those entering this field may search for a single, well-defined, cohesive approach that satisfies all short- and long-term concerns over hair loss. Unfortunately, such an approach does not exist.

There are several chapters that should be studied and reflected upon by all in this field. It is essential to understand the psychology of the patients we treat. Drs. Cash and Pruzinsky's contribution (Chapter 1, Part A) presents data obtained by extensive research that elucidate and explain the forces that compel men and women to seek treatment.* They suggest nonsurgical treatment alternatives that can be offered to patients not suited for surgical intervention. Counseling and support from those experienced in psychology may at times be recommended for such patients.

At what age should hair transplantation be undertaken? All surgeons struggle to address this important question, which can be answered only on an individual basis. The chapter by Dr. Weidig (Chapter 2, Part B) will no doubt assist you in your own decisions. Sensible recommendations in dealing with the younger patient are provided.

What constitutes informed consent? This difficult question is skillfully addressed by Dr. Quinlan (Chapter 1, Part E) and Dr. Leonard (Chapter 1, Part H). There is ample practical knowledge in their words. Experienced hair transplant surgeons will be surprised at their insights. The novice will obtain a grasp of the issues involved in informed consent of hair restoration surgery.

The issue of scalp reductions is a paradox—should we or shouldn't we? Drs. Marritt and Dzubow present persuasive, elegant arguments against scalp reductions in the younger patient (Chapter 1, Part F). From the opposing perspective, Dr. Paul Straub skillfully details the key technical elements for achieving maximum benefits of scalp reductions (Chapter 9, Part A). His criteria for patient selection and his precise descriptive surgical approach offer practical solutions to this perplexing problem. Adoption of his techniques would greatly reduce the problems now experienced with male pattern scalp reductions.

As a group, hair transplant surgeons have welcomed the departure of the large and "traditional" autografts and embraced the transplantation of small grafts that simulate the natural state. Although the techniques of the authors in Chapter 6 differ from one another, the theme of artistically distributed large numbers of small grafts is shared by all.

Will there one day be a medical cure for baldness? Perhaps. But until then, we must educate ourselves on the benefits of the most recent medications for alopecia. In this regard the chapter by Dr. DeVillez (Chapter 12, Part A) is most informative.

The practice of synthetic hair grafting is being revived and the complication rate associated with this technique appears to be decreasing. A scientific scrutiny of the safety of this modality is presented by Drs. Yamada and Fukuta in Chapter 11, Part A.

Despite a myriad of techniques and philosophies, this book offers a basic education and background in the field of hair restoration surgery. A foundation is laid for preoperative and postoperative care, rational use of antibiotics, local anesthesia, scalp anatomy, and complications that may arise as a result of medical or surgical intervention.

I have gleaned more knowledge from the composition of this text than I would have ever imagined. I am confident that the readers will benefit likewise. Those with open minds will find it an oasis of knowledge.

Dow B. Stough, M.D.

---

*It is important to note that although a small number of patients who seek treatment of alopecia are women, male pronouns are used throughout the text when referring to the patient to avoid awkward wording and to reflect the high percentage of male patients.

1

General Considerations for Hair Replacement

A. The Psychosocial Effects of Androgenic Alopecia and Their Implications for Patient Care

Thomas F. Cash and Thomas Pruzinsky

From birth to death what people look like is an integral part of their identity, both in how other people see them and in how they see themselves. The psychology of physical appearance may be neatly divided into two perspectives.[1,2] The first is the "view from the outside," the social view of an individual. This social-image perspective concerns how aspects of appearance affect interpersonal perceptions and social relations. The second vantage point is the "view from the inside," a person's subjective evaluation of his own physical attributes and aesthetics. Psychologists use the term *body image*—a core aspect of self-concept—to refer to these personal attitudes and perceptions concerning one's own appearance. A comprehensive psychology of physical appearance takes into account both views, especially because measures of body image often have only a modest correspondence with socially perceived reality.[2] Put simply, beauty does not ensure a satisfying body image nor does homeliness dictate that one loathe one's looks.

This chapter applies each perspective to elucidate the psychosocial effects of androgenic alopecia—first from the social-image viewpoint followed by an in-depth consideration of the effects of alopecia on body image and quality of life. Our discussion articulates the scientific evidence and its implications, with the aim of enhancing physicians' understanding and care of men and women with androgenic hair loss.

SOCIAL IMAGES AND ANDROGENIC HAIR LOSS

Behavioral scientists have amassed hundreds of controlled studies confirming that physical traits, such as physical attractiveness, weight, height, facial features, and grooming, can systematically shape social attitudes, attributions, and actions.[2-9] Physical appearance indeed provides the most readily available information about a person and conveys basic facts such as a person's gender, approximate age, race, and possibly even socioeconomic status or occupation. As a result of socialization by peers, parents, and society in general, we develop attitudes about physical attributes and aesthetics and, based on these assumptions, classify people into a variety of cognitive categories, often unconsciously. Our implicit stereotypes about appearance can influence who, among the many people we encounter in our daily lives, will remain strangers or mere acquaintances and who will become our close friends or loved ones. Beyond its obvious impact on dating and mating, physical attractiveness shapes the reactions of both sexes. Physical traits can influence social decisions and behaviors in any situation—in the workplace, classroom, courtroom, or bedroom.

The bottom-line scientific conclusion is that people who possess the physical qualities that our culture deems attractive are sometimes, albeit not always, viewed and treated more favorably than less attractive people. Homely persons, especially those who are obese or physically disfigured, encounter significant social prejudice and discrimination.[2,3] What are the implications for the social-image perspective of persons with androgenic alopecia? How are people with visible androgenic hair loss regarded by their fellow human beings?

Behavioral scientists have targeted numerous physical attributes for study, yet one nearly ignored area of inquiry has been hair loss. This oversight is certainly surprising given the prevalence of this socially visible condition and the enormity of hair care and hair restoration product and service industries. The dearth of research is also surprising considering that history evinces long-standing cultural symbolism associated with hair—its length as well as its loss.[10-12] Hair is one of the few body parts over which we have immediate control to express our individuality or chosen identity. Hair is deemed our "crowning glory." With rare exception, leading male and female screen stars have a full head of hair, even if they wear a hairpiece to appear so (e.g., John Wayne, Burt Reynolds, Ted Danson, and Sean Connery as James Bond). Baldness or the loss of hair is linked with powerlessness—consider infants, the elderly, and the biblical Samson. The heads of subjugated prisoners and soldiers are shaved to obfuscate their individualism and power. In contemporary western society, self-shaven skinheads are adamant racists. The average bald guy—"baldy," "cue ball," or "chrome dome" in the media—is commonly a comedic character or the butt of a joke.

Bald or Balding Men

Such observations suggest that alopecia may have a deleterious impact on the initial "view from the outside." The evidence of such a negative effect from studies that used either verbal descriptors or graphic sketches of men with and without hair loss is unclear.[13-15] In the one study of people's perceptions of men with alopecia, Cash[16] investigated the initial impact of visible alopecia in men on the social perceptions of subjects of both sexes. Subjects viewed color slides of balding and nonbalding men who were pair-matched based on actual age, race, and other attributes. Subjects rated these men on several key first-impression dimensions. Results revealed that balding men created generally less favorable impressions, including lower ratings of physical attractiveness, assumptions of less desirable personal and interpersonal characteristics, and overestimations of age. The influence of the subjects' sex and age on their perceptions was largely inconsequential. Relative to their true ages, balding men under 35 years of age were seen as older and nonbalding men over 35 years of age were perceived as younger. Thus, perhaps due to social expectations about age-normativeness, hair loss "matures" the younger man, whereas a full head of hair causes the older man to appear more youthful. The statistical control of judged physical attractiveness substantially attenuated the other perceived differences. This finding suggests that the social-image effects of male pattern baldness stem mostly from baldness lessening men's attractiveness rather from some distinct "baldness stereotype."

Although these experimental results do reveal consistently less positive first impressions of balding men than those of nonbalding men, several points must be made about the findings. First, less favorable impressions do not mean negative impressions. On a 10-point attractiveness scale, the average balding man in this study had only a half-point disadvantage; hair loss is no "prince-to-frog" phenomenon. Second, initial impressions are not necessarily etched in stone, and people who already know and like someone are not apt to withdraw their affection because of a person's hair loss. Third, other personal qualities may be pivotal in determining the influence of hair loss in initial social impressions. For example, warm and interesting people probably transcend most unfavorable social perceptions that might stem from hair loss. On the other hand, for people whose self-absorbed or antagonistic personalities already put them at a social disadvantage, baldness may intensify the social apathy or antipathy they receive.

Women with Alopecia

Women's hair length and hair color have been studied and found to affect social impressions,[12,17] yet no studies have examined how people view women with androgenic alopecia. In fact, most people probably fail to realize that the condition even exists among women, in part because the pattern of alopecia in women is one of diffuse thinning rather than baldness per se and therefore can be more readily concealed by hairstyling.

However, to the extent that a woman's hair loss is socially noticeable, it is not improbable that alopecia would detract from her perceived attractiveness. The general population associates female hair loss with advanced age, which in the double standard of our youth-is-beauty culture may unfairly diminish a woman's perceived attractiveness. Unfortunately, neither graying nor balding in a woman promotes positive perceptions or is thought to make a woman look "distinguished." Although this theory is unstudied, another factor that might come into play is the social inference that a woman's visible alopecia is the symptom of some dread disease or the side effect of disease treatment. Thus the fact that male pattern hair loss is considered a more normative, "to-be-expected" state may mitigate the social-image impact of alopecia for men but not for women.

SELF-IMAGE AND ANDROGENIC HAIR LOSS

Whereas visible hair loss can detrimentally influence social judgments, the more important consideration concerns how people with androgenic alopecia perceive and deal with their own hair loss. Several recent controlled investigations elucidate the effects of this condition on the quality of men's and women's lives in terms of psychosocial sequelae such as stress and distress, body-image experiences, and personality functioning.

Psychological Impact on Men

Using the Norwood classification system for reliable pictorial classification of the extent of male pattern baldness, Cash[18] studied three groups of randomly sampled men: 63 with modestly visible male pattern baldness, 40 with extensive male pattern baldness, and 42 nonbalding control subjects. No subject had received any medical or surgical treatment for hair loss; none wore hair additions. Subjects completed the Hair Loss Effects Questionnaire (HLEQ) by rating 70 possible effects of alopecia including emotional, cognitive, social, and behavioral effects. They also completed standardized tests measuring body image, self-esteem, social anxiety, sexual confidence, public self-consciousness, and locus of control.

Compared to men with modest male pattern baldness, men with extensive hair loss reported a more adverse impact. Of the 70 possible effects listed on the HLEQ, men with modest male pattern baldness reported that their baldness had a statistically significant impact on 60% of the effects, and men with extensive male pattern baldness reported such an impact on 79% of the items. The latter group experienced significantly more negative socioemotional effects, greater worry and preoccupation with their baldness, and marginally stronger behavioral efforts to conceal, compensate for, and cope with hair loss. Table 1-1 delineates how men reported that male pattern baldness specifically affected them and their lives.

These data confirm that androgenic alopecia is an unwelcome, stressful experience for most men. In fact, when the nonbalding control subjects were asked to imagine their reactions should they begin to experience gradual male pattern baldness, a mere 8% said they would *not* be bothered if they began losing hair. To determine whether the stress of alopecia might impair men's psychosocial functioning, nonbalding and balding men were compared further in terms of body image and personality. Results indicated that it is improbable that male pattern baldness dramatically damages psychosocial functioning in most men. Differences in psychosocial adjustment due to male pattern baldness were not significant with one important exception: men with androgenic alopecia had more negative body-image attitudes, meaning less satisfaction with their hair *and* with their overall physical appearance.

Correlations did reveal that the men who were most upset by hair loss had less adaptive psychoso-

TABLE 1-1 Reports by Men of Specific Effects Attributed to Androgenic Alopecia

	PERCENTAGE (%) REPORTING SPECIFIC BEHAVIOR	
EFFECTS ATTRIBUTED TO HAIR LOSS	MEN WITH MODEST HAIR LOSS	MEN WITH EXTENSIVE HAIR LOSS
Cognitive Preoccupation		
Wish for more hair	52	84
Notice bald/balding men	54	82
Spend time looking in mirror at hair/head	54	69
Wonder what others think	47	67
Negative Socioemotional Events		
Get teased by peers	45	79
Feel self-conscious	42	78
Look older than actual age	40	55
Worry that others will notice	39	56
Feel helpless about male pattern baldness	37	56
Worry about aging	37	46
Feel less attractive	31	51
Envy good-looking men	33	34
Behavioral Coping		
Try to improve hairstyle	63	66
Try to improve physique	41	36
Dress more nicely	26	45
Wear hats or caps	23	41
Seek reassurance about looks	23	39
Grow a beard or mustache	18	36

Modified from Cash TF: *J Am Acad Dermatol* 26:926, 1992.

cial functioning. Perhaps in instances in which alopecia causes considerable distress, psychosocial adjustment suffers. An alternative interpretation, of course, is that men with the poorest premorbid psychosocial adjustment may be less resilient to the stressful effects of hair loss. Analyses identified several other characteristics related to a more psychological impact of alopecia. Among those most distressed by hair loss were younger men with an early onset of hair loss, men who expected their noticeable balding to progress, and men who were single and not dating. Although causality cannot be inferred from a nonprospective study, the data collectively suggest that a positive self-concept and a sense of success in social or romantic attachments may buffer alopecia's psychological impact. Men who are insecure about their personal and social worth may view balding as a threat to their already vulnerable sense of acceptability.

Although the handful of published studies of the possible psychological impact of male pattern baldness provides a mixture of findings,[19] Franzoi, Anderson, and Frommelt[20] offer evidence consistent with Cash's results.[5] They too found that balding men may have a less positive body image than nonbalding men and that self-conscious men may be at greater risk for distress about ensuing hair loss than men who have a positive self-image.

Psychological Impact on Women

As upsetting as androgenic alopecia is for many men, there are several reasons as mentioned earlier (e.g., cultural and personal significance of hair, perceived normality or abnormality of hair loss) to expect alopecia to be more stressful, if not psychologically debilitating, for women. Cash, Price, and Savin[21] examined this question by studying newly referred patients with androgenic alopecia (96 women and 60 men). Included was a female control group of 56 nonalopecia patients seeking treatment for cutaneous conditions not publicly visible. The researchers used the HLEQ to assess specific effects experienced by the alopecia patients, and they administered tests to measure body image, personality, and psychosocial adjustment similar to those in the previous study.[18]

The findings indicated that although alopecia was clearly a distressing experience for both sexes, its effects were much more problematic for women. Compared to balding men, women with androgenic alopecia reported significantly more socioemotional stress and efforts to cope. Whereas about one fourth of the men were very or extremely upset by their alopecia, 70% and 52% of the women, respectively, expressed these high levels of past and current distress. Table 1-2 describes the specific effects that patients attributed to the experience of hair loss.

This research revealed that the majority of women with androgenic alopecia experienced considerable anxious preoccupation, helplessness, self-consciousness, and feelings of unattractiveness. To cope with this stress, most sought information and selective social support, struggled to control their intrusive negative thoughts and emotions about their condition, tried to camouflage the hair loss with hairstyling, and engaged in compensatory grooming activities to try to restore their body-image integrity. Androgenic alopecia was much more disturbing to these women than the inconspicuous skin conditions of the control group.

Further evidence of the psychological impact of androgenic alopecia on women appears in the differences between these women and the female control patients in body image and psychosocial adjustment. Compared to the control subjects, women with alopecia not only were much more unhappy about their condition but also experienced more negative overall body-image feelings as well. In addition, the women with hair loss also reported more social anxiety, poorer self-esteem and psychosocial well-being, and less of a sense of control over and satisfaction with their lives than the control subjects.

Statistical regression analyses indicated that the women most distressed by hair loss were the more poorly adjusted women who had considerable investment in their appearance and expected the alopecia to progress. Replicating Cash's previous findings,[18] the men affected most unfavorably were more publicly self-conscious, poorly adjusted, strongly dissatisfied with their hair, and invested in their appearance. Although these correlates cannot be assigned a causal role in people's psychological reactions to hair loss, the findings are unequivocal on a practical, clinical level: women who seek medical consultation for androgenic alopecia are more psychologically distressed than typical patients as represented by the control sample and men suffering from alopecia.

The study's findings of a moderately negative impact of androgenic alopecia on men reinforce Cash's earlier conclusions[18] based on a sample of balding men from the general population, none of whom were seeking treatment. A comparison of men's reactions in the two studies clearly reveals that distress was higher in the treatment-seeking sample than in the random sample of balding men. Understandably, it is psychological discomfort that in great part motivates patients to seek effective remedies for alopecia and associated anguish.

IMPLICATIONS FOR PATIENT CARE

Patients with androgenic alopecia present significant challenges for hair restoration professionals.

TABLE 1-2 Reports by Female and Male Androgenic Alopecia Patients of Specific Effects Attributed to Hair Loss

EFFECTS ATTRIBUTED TO HAIR LOSS	PERCENTAGE (%) REPORTING SPECIFIC BEHAVIOR	
	WOMEN	MEN
Adverse Effects		
Wish that I had more hair	98	90
Think about my hair loss	97	93
Try to figure out if I am losing more hair (by inspecting my head, brush, sink, etc.)	95	87
Feel frustrated/helpless about my hair loss	93	88
Spend time looking at my hair/head in the mirror	92	92
Worry about my looks	92	85
Feel self-conscious about my looks	92	78
Have negative thoughts about my hair/head	91	85
Worry about whether others will notice my hair loss	90	82
Worry about how much hair I am going to lose	89	93
Notice people who are balding	83	90
Think about how I used to look	78	77
Notice what other people look like	78	73
Have the thought "Why me?"	75	68
Think that I am not as attractive as I used to be	72	73
Wonder what other people think about my looks	71	65
Have thoughts that I am unattractive	68	53
Try to imagine what I would look like with more hair loss	67	80
Feel sexy looking	−65	−35
Feel depressed or despondent	63	38
Worry about getting older	62	62
Worry that my spouse or partner will find me less attractive	60	52
Feel embarrassment	55	53
Feel envious of good-looking people of my own sex	53	47
Feel physically attractive	−53	−35
Feel sensitive to personal criticism	50	53
Am conscious of how others react to me	42	50
Feel I look older than I am	42	70
Receive comments about my hair loss	36	65
Get friendly teasing or kidding from others	20	60
Behavioral Coping		
Try to figure out what to do about my hair loss	98	90
Try to hide my hair loss	94	63
Talk to my hairstylist/barber about my hair loss	82	58
Try to improve my hairstyle	79	63
Do things to improve my looks	75	55
Talk to friends of my own sex about my hair loss	71	52
Spend time on my appearance	70	55
Talk to my partner about my hair loss	64	57
Seek reassurance about my looks	62	57
Try to improve my figure or physique	44	52

Modified from Cash TF, Price VH, Savin RC: *J Am Acad Dermatol* 29:568, 1993.
NOTE: Positive percentages refer to the percentage of each group who reported an increase in the effect. Negative percentages reflect reported decreases in effects. Of the 69-item HLEQ, only those items endorsed by a majority of female and/or male patients are listed.

These patients struggle to cope with their condition and worry that it and their own physical acceptability will worsen. They search for ways to halt or reverse the course of their hair loss and to restore their body-image integrity. Neither sex escapes the difficulties caused by hair loss. But for women hair loss is more stressful and disruptive to their sense of well-being since alopecia comes as an unfamiliar and uncertain plight. Physicians must recognize that the effects of androgenic alopecia extend well beyond the mere physical parameters of hair loss and growth. As has been observed for other appearance-altering conditions,[22,23] patients' psychological reactions are less related to the actual ex-

ages: development, deviance, and change, New York, 1990, Guilford, pp 217-236.
24. Piepkorn MW, Weidner M: Comparable efficacy of 2% minoxidil gel and solution formulations in the treatment of male pattern alopecia, J Am Acad Dermatol 18:1059-1062, 1988.
25. Resnik HL: Psychiatric observations on patients who seek and undergo hair transplantation, J Dermatol Surg Oncol 6:1023-1025, 1980.
26. American Psychiatric Association: Diagnostic and statistical manual of mental disorders, ed 4, Washington, D.C., 1994, American Psychiatric Association.
27. Phillips KA: Body dysmorphic disorder: the distress of imagined ugliness, Am J Psychiatry 148:1138-1149, 1991.
28. Pruzinsky T: Psychopathology of body experience. In Cash TF, Pruzinsky T, editors: Body images: development, deviance, and change, New York, 1990, Guilford, pp 170-189.
29. Goin JM, Goin MK: Changing the body: psychological effects of plastic surgery, Baltimore, 1986, Williams & Wilkins.
30. Butters JW, Cash TF: Cognitive-behavioral treatment of women's body-image dissatisfaction, J Consult Clin Psychol 55:889-897, 1987.
31. Grant JR, Cash TF: Cognitive-behavioral body-image therapy: comparative efficacy of group and modest-contact treatments, Behav Ther (in press).
32. Rosen JC, Saltzberg E, Srebnik D: Cognitive behavior therapy for negative body image, Behav Ther 20:393-404, 1989.
33. Pruzinsky T: Collaboration of plastic surgeon and medical psychotherapist: elective cosmetic surgery, Med Psychother 1:1-13, 1988.
34. Marks I, Mishan J: Dysmorphophobic avoidance with disturbed bodily perception: a pilot study of exposure therapy, Br J Psychiatry 152:674-678, 1988.
35. Neziroglu FA, Yaryura-Tobias JA: Exposure, response prevention, and cognitive therapy in the treatment of body dysmorphic disorder, Behav Ther 24:431-438, 1993.
36. Rosen JC, Reiter J, Orosan P: Cognitive behavioral body-image therapy for body dysmorphic disorder, J Consult Clin Psychol (in press).
37. Hollander E and others: Treatment of body dysmorphic disorder with serotonin reuptake blockers, Am J Psychiatry 146:768-770, 1989.
38. Passchier J and others: Psychological characteristics of men with alopecia androgenetica and effects of treatment with topical minoxidil, Int J Dermatol 27:441-446, 1988.

B. Pathophysiology of Androgenic Alopecia

Richard L. DeVillez

Hair loss occurs in men and women, with the amount of loss increasing with age and varying greatly from one individual to another and one sex to the other.[1-4] In men the initial loss usually occurs in the frontotemporal region, producing a recessed hairline (Fig. 1-1). As the hair loss progresses, men notice episodes of increased hair shedding.[1,5] The hair on the vertex and frontoparietal area becomes shorter, lighter, and finer. At the same time the texture of the hair in the preauricular and postauricular areas changes to a consistency resembling that of beard hair (whisker hair).[6] The crown hair in some men develops short vellus hairs (fuzz), whereas in others the alopecia progresses, leaving only a horseshoe-shaped rim of hair around the scalp.[7] On the other hand, women retain a relatively normal frontal hairline and develop an obvious diffuse thinning on the frontoparietal area of the scalp.[8,9] The most striking change is a widened center part[10] (Fig. 1-2). The diffuse loss may become extensive, although a few fine vellus hairs may be found.[11] Despite differences in the way the hair is lost, rapidly or progressively, consistently or intermittently, the end result in both genders is a pattern hair loss.[12] Male pattern hair loss is usually more extensive and is classified according to the Hamilton pattern as modified by Norwood[13] (see

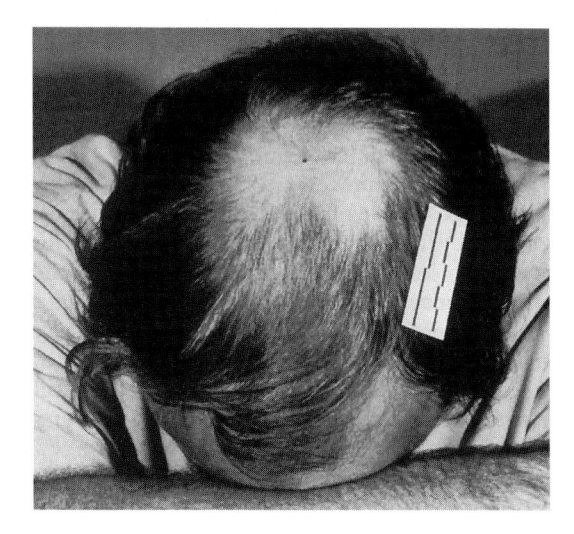

FIG. 1-1 Male pattern androgenic alopecia with frontotemporal and vertex hair loss.

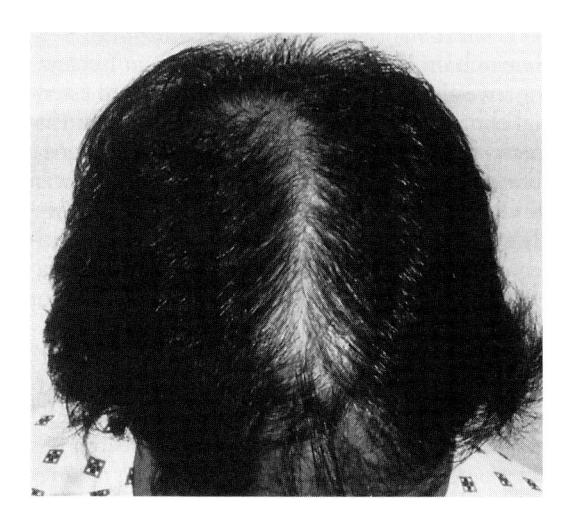

FIG. 1-2 Female pattern androgenic alopecia with a widened center part.

Fig. 1-7). Female pattern hair loss, as classified by Ludwig,[14] is usually less severe (Fig. 1-3).

The cause of pattern balding has not been established, but researchers generally agree that this trait is transmitted via a multifactorial or polygenic form of inheritance, which suggests that baldness is the result of an interaction of several genes combined with environmental factors.[1,15] Although increased virility has been touted by bald men, bald men father the same number and sex ratio of children as men with full heads of hair.[16,17] Hair loss in women generally provokes anxiety and depression (see Chapter 1, Part A); Eckert[18] believes that undue attention by women to their hair loss may be a symbolic way to obtain help for underlying anxiety and marital problems. Men regard hair loss as distressing but actively cope and are likely to retain the integrity of their personality.[19] Men under the age of 55 with pattern vertex baldness seem to have an increased incidence of coronary artery disease.[20-22]

It is presumed that pattern baldness in both sexes is an androgen-mediated miniaturization process that affects genetically susceptible hair follicles. The follicles become progressively smaller in size and have shorter periods of growth. Over time the coarse terminal hairs become thinner, more lightly pigmented indeterminate hairs and then become vellus hairs (Fig. 1-4). In the woman, this process is modified as reflected by the usual lack of vellus hairs on the balding scalp. In women with advanced male pattern balding, an underlying hyperandrogen cause for the advanced hair loss should be considered.[23]

In both sexes the balding scalp appears more greasy than the nonbalding scalp. This observation

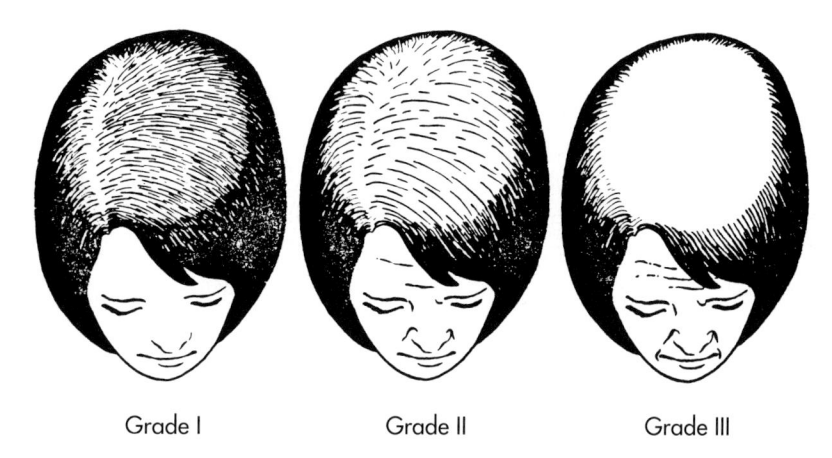

FIG. 1-3 Classification of female pattern hair loss by Ludwig. (From Montagna W, Parakkal PF: *The structure and function of skin,* ed 3, New York, 1974, Academic Press.)

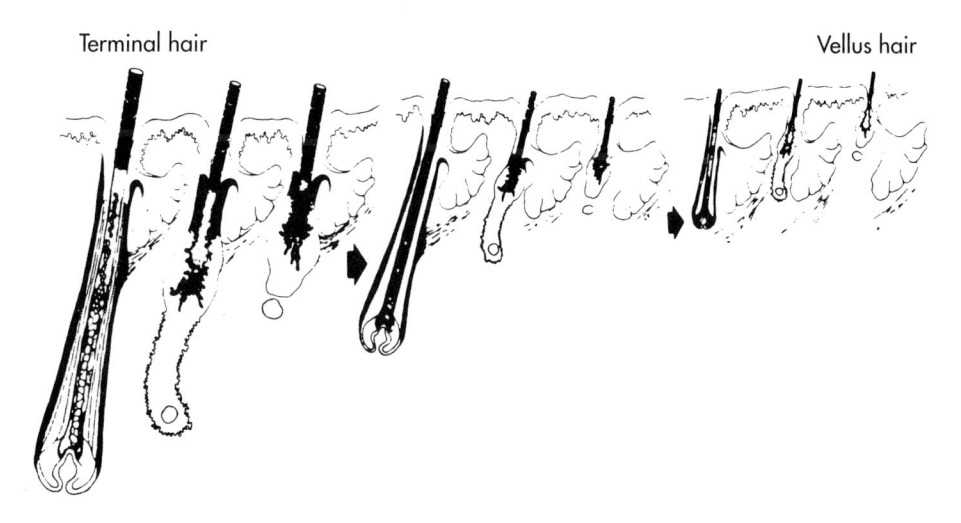

FIG. 1-4 Miniaturization of the hair follicle in pattern hair loss. Hair grows for shorter periods of time and becomes smaller, finer, and lighter as it approaches the vellus stage.

has led to the suggestion that microorganisms, altered sebum lipids, and oxidants cause and enhance the baldness.[24,25] Gravimetric studies of sebum levels and the hourly production of scalp sebum in bald and nonbalding male scalps showed no differences between the groups.[26] Washing the scalp does reduce hair loss for the next 24 hours, an observation readily explained by the fact that hair washing removes the hairs nearing the end of normal telogen, thus reducing physiological hair loss for a few days.

The altered cycle of scalp hairs in a balding area is demonstrated by the reduced number of hairs in anagen and a shortened anagen phase.[27] In a balding area more hairs are in telogen for a longer period of time and are more easily lost with daily grooming than in a nonbalding area. The shortened cycle results in shorter, finer, miniaturized hairs. It has been demonstrated in rodents that potential mitotic cells distributed in the follicular sheath and bulb can add to the diameter and length of the hair follicle. This noncyclic transformation of either gradual thickening or thinning of female scalp hairs may explain the usual lack of short vellus hairs with female pattern hair loss.[27]

PATHOLOGY

The principal finding in pattern baldness is the presence of vellus follicles; they are found in greatest numbers in the most advanced stages of alopecia.[28,29] At the base of the anagen follicles a basophilic smudging appears, which represents clumps of Arao-Perkins elastin-like bodies.[30] With shorter anagen hairs, these clumps of elastic fibers are retained in the fibrillary connective tissue sheath like rungs on a ladder.[30] Inflammatory infiltrates have recently been noted around the lower portions of the follicular infundibulum and the region of the follicular bulge.[31] Those patients with significant inflammation are less responsive to therapy.[32] Injury to the follicular stem cell epithelium and a thickening of the adventitial sheath may impair normal hair cycling or limit anagen growth, resulting in a miniaturized hair.[31] In one study, in about one third of the biopsies, multinucleated giant cells were found surrounding the hair follicles.[33] Other researchers noted that moderate chronic inflammatory infiltrate surrounded capillaries and adnexal structures in 50% of the specimens.[34] Furthermore, direct immunofluorescent studies have revealed third component of complement (C3) around the basement membrane zone of hair follicles in 20% to 90% of the biopsies.[35,36] It is not yet certain whether these findings confirm that inflammation contributes to the development of androgenic alopecia.

In the bald scalp the layers of epidermis, dermis, and subcutaneous fat are thinner than those of the nonbald scalp and thus thinning progresses with age.[37] As women near their 80s, the scalp becomes thicker, approaching the scalp thickness of middle-aged women.[37] There is no explanation for this phenomenon. Subcutaneous blood flow, as measured by xenon-133 washout method, is diminished in the early male pattern balding scalp compared to controls.[38] Whether diminished blood flow is a primary or secondary phenomenon is unclear. The hair shaft from the early male pattern balding scalp shows no abnormality on electronmicroscopy or in terms of chemical composition.

ANDROGENS

Androgens have been established as the initiating factor in pattern baldness; their mechanism of action has been the focus of much research. Their role in pattern baldness has been demonstrated in autograft studies. Full-thickness, hair-bearing autografts from the occipital scalp were successfully transplanted to the bald frontal scalp, demonstrating that each hair follicle is genetically predisposed to respond or be immune to androgenic factors that inhibit its growth.[39] Androgens variably affect different regions of hair growth, stimulating growth of pubic, axillary, beard, and chest hair while retarding growth of scalp hair in genetically susceptible people.[40] Not all androgen-sensitive hair growth is controlled by the same hormone; testosterone effects axillary and pubic hair growth, whereas dihydrotestosterone (DHT) effects beard growth and pattern baldness.[40] Pattern baldness is dependent on androgen receptors, 5α-reductase enzyme, and DHT.

When cultured dermal papilla cells from balding and nonbalding scalps were examined, specific, high-affinity androgen receptors were detected in both.[41] Androgen receptors have not been found in the matrix cells or external root sheath cells of the hair follicle.[41,42] The DHT–androgen receptor complex has a high affinity for receptors in the nuclear chromatin, which initiates the down-regulation of hair follicle growth and miniaturization of the hair follicle.[43-45] DHT metabolized from testosterone by the 5α-reductase enzyme affects the genetically receptive follicles, causing hair loss[46,47] (Fig. 1-5).

The 5α-reductase enzyme is responsible for the metabolism of testosterone to DHT; the aromatase enzyme metabolizes androstenedione to estrone and testosterone to estradiol[48] (Fig. 1-6). Both enzymes play a role in pattern baldness. Regional differences in androgen metabolism are present in the balding and nonbalding scalp, with 5α-reductase activity higher in the balding area.[49,50] Men were found to have twofold greater 5α-reductase enzyme activity

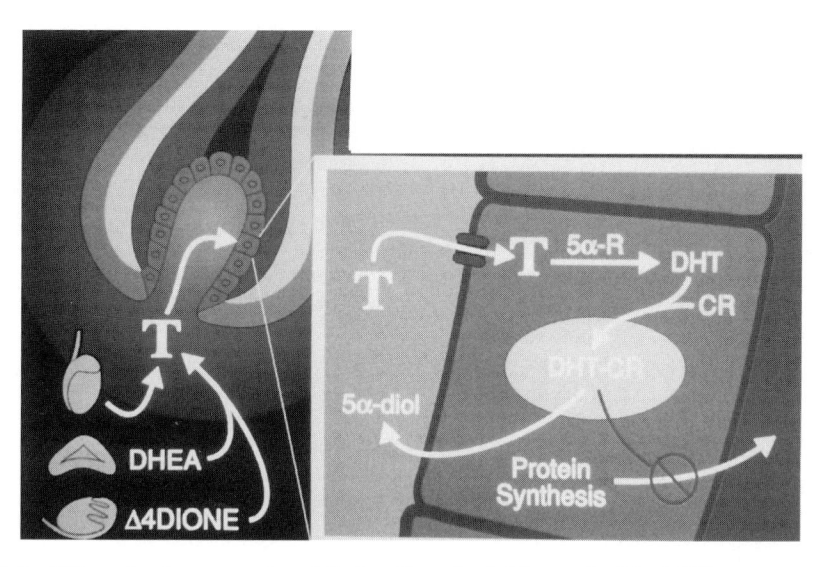

FIG. 1-5 Effect of androgens on hair follicle cells in the balding scalp. The DHT-receptor–nuclear chromatic complex down-regulates the cell metabolic activity. *T*, testosterone; *DHEA*, dehydroepiandrosterone; *Δ4dione*, androstenedione; *5α-R*, 5α-reductase; *DHT*, dihydrotestosterone; *CR*, cytosol receptor; *5α-diol*, 5α-androstenediol.

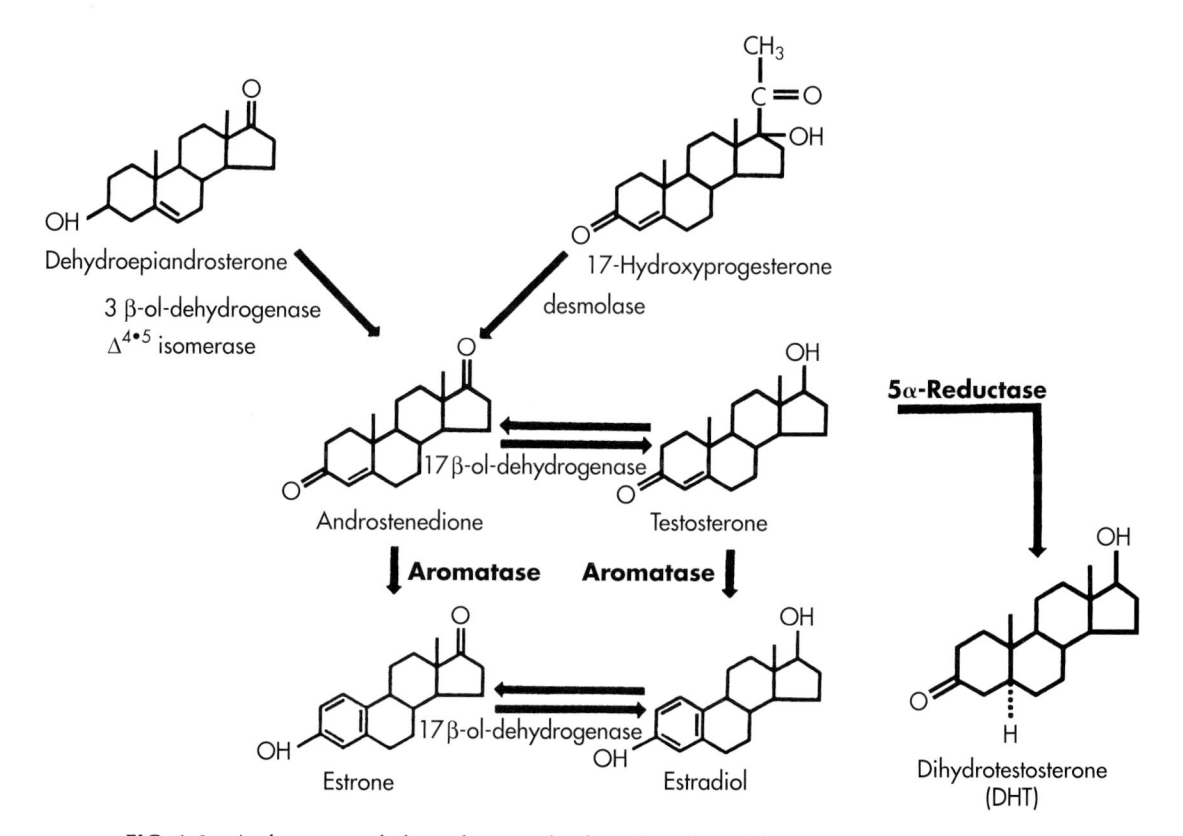

FIG. 1-6 Androgen metabolic pathway in the skin. The effect of the aromatase enzyme system vs. the 5α-reductase enzyme system on androgen metabolism is shown.

in the frontal scalp compared with that in the occipital area; minimal aromatase enzyme was present in both areas.[51] Women had twofold greater 5α-reductase enzyme activity in the frontoparietal area of the scalp compared with that in the vertex, yet women had only half the amount of 5α-reductase enzyme as men; however, aromatase enzyme activity was higher in both areas in women.[51] Sparing of the frontal hairline in most female alopecia patients may be due to the increase in aromatase enzyme, limiting the formation of DHT and converting the circulating androgen to estrogens.[51] Extensive hair loss in men may be due to the lack of aromatase enzyme, which thus increases the formation of DHT.[51] Several steroid enzymes such as 3α-, 3β-, and 17β-hydroxysteroid are capable of converting weak androgens such as dehydroepiandrosterone (DHEA) into more potent target tissue androgens.[52,53] The concentrations of each enzyme present in the bald and nonbald scalp tissue are the same; however, the level of specific activity varies greatly in the frontal vs. the occipital area. The levels of activity are elevated in the frontal area of both men and women with pattern baldness, with men having a greater level than their female counterparts.[51]

In addition, the effects of growth factors such as epidermal growth factor (EGF), platelet-derived growth factor (PDGF), and transforming growth factor–α and transforming growth factor–β (TGF-α and TGF-β) need to be considered.[54] Inflammation, present in nearly 50% of scalp biopsies,[34] may stimulate cytokine and growth factors. In cultured isolated human hair follicles, EGF and TGF-α promote the formation of club hair–like structures.[55] In sheep and mice these growth factors cause a depilatory effect. TGF-β inhibits hair growth in vitro.[55] These growth factors are expressed on human hair follicles from the balding and nonbalding sites, but their role in the miniaturization process has yet to be established.

CONCLUSION

Androgenic alopecia is considered to be a condition with a multifactorial or polygenic form of inheritance, meaning that for the trait to be manifested there is an interaction of several genes combined with environmental factors. It is androgen dependent, mediated by DHT through the 5α-reductase enzyme system. Weaker androgens are introduced to the hair loss process through the hydroxysteroid enzymes. Inflammation may play a role in some individuals by stimulating cytokines and growth factors, which retard hair growth. The end result is a miniaturized hair that has a shorter anagen phase; is shorter, finer, and lighter; and is less able to cover the scalp. The end result is pattern hair loss that progresses with age.

REFERENCES

1. Ebling FJ: The biology of hair, *Dermatol Clin* 5(3):467-481, 1987.
2. Cerviam Rebora A: Age-related severity of male-pattern alopecia, *Dermatologica* 166(2):81-83, 1983.
3. Rosenblum M, Leider M: Alopecia, *Br J Dermatol* 79(10):568-569, 1967.
4. Eckert J and others: Hair loss in women, *Br J Dermatol* 79(10):543-548, 1967.
5. Braun-Falco O: Dynamics of normal and pathological hair growth, *Arch Klin Exp Dermatol* 227(1):419-452, 1966.
6. Norwood OT: Whisker hair, *Arch Dermatol* 115(8):930-931, 1979.
7. Hamilton JB: Patterned loss of hair in man: types and incidence, *Ann N Y Acad Sci* 53:708-728, 1951.
8. Alexander S: Diffuse alopecia in women, *Trans St. Johns Hosp Dermatol Soc* 51(1):99-102, 1965.
9. Arlook TD: Diffuse scalp hairfall in women, *J Indiana St Med Assoc* 59(9):1009-1012, 1966.
10. Jacobs JP, DeVillez RL: Androgenetic alopecia, *Arch Dermatol* 126(10):1371-1372, 1990.
11. Jackson D, Church RE, Ebling FJ: Hair diameter in female baldness, *Br J Dermatol* 87(4):361-367, 1972.
12. Dawber RP: Common baldness in women, *Int J Dermatol* 20(10)647-650, 1981.
13. Norwood OT: Male pattern baldness: classification and incidence, *South Med J* 68(11):1359-1365, 1975.
14. Ludwig E: Classification of the types of androgenetic alopecia (common baldness) occurring in the female sex, *Br J Dermatol* 97(3):247-254, 1977.
15. Bergfeld WF, Redmond GP: Androgenic alopecia, *Dermatol Clin* 5(3):491-500, 1987.
16. Damon A, Burr WA, Gerson DE: Baldness of fathers and number and sex ratio of children, *Hum Biol* 37(4):366-370, 1965.
17. Burton JL and others: Male-pattern alopecia and masculinity, *Br J Dermatol* 100(5):567-571, 1979.
18. Eckert J: Diffuse hair loss in women: the psychopathology of those who complain, *Acta Psychiatr Scand* 53(5):321-327, 1976.
19. Cash TF: The psychological effects of androgenetic alopecia in men, *J Am Acad Dermatol* 26(6):926-931, 1992.
20. Cooke NT: Male pattern alopecia and coronary artery disease in men, *Br J Dermatol* 101(4):455-458, 1979.
21. Herrera CR, Lynch C: Is baldness a risk factor for coronary artery disease? *J Clin Epidemiol* 43(11):1255-1260, 1990.
22. Lesko SM, Rosenberg L, Shapiro S: A case-control study of baldness in relation to myocardial infarction in men, *JAMA* 269(8):998-1003, 1993.
23. Kuhn BH: Male pattern alopecia and or androgenic hirsutism in females, *J Am Med Wom Assoc* 27(7):357-364, 1972.
24. Silvestri U: Physical study of the hair in cases of alopecia on a seborrheic base, *Arch Ital Dermatol* 34(6):405-409, 1966.
25. Noguer-More S: From seborrheica alopecia to male pattern alopecia, [editorial], *Acta Derm Sifiliograf* 67(1-2):1-4, 1976.
26. Maibach HI and others: Scalp and forehead sebum production in male pattern alopecia. In Baccaradda-Bay A, Moratti G, Fray JR, editors: *Biopathology of Pattern Alopecias*, Basel, Karger, p 171.
27. Uno H, Kurata S: Chemical agents and peptides affect hair growth, *J Invest Dermatol* 101:143S-147S, 1993.
28. Bergfeld WF: Alopecia: histologic changes, *Adv Dermatol* 4:301-320, 1989.
29. Mian EU: Histangic patterns in seborrheic alopecia, *Angiologica* 7(2):109-116, 1970.
30. Pinkus H: Alopecia. Clinicopathologic correlations, *Int J Dermatol* 19(5):245-253, 1980.
31. Jaworsky C, Kligman AM, Murphy GF: Characterization of

inflammatory infiltrates in male pattern alopecia: implications for pathogenesis, *Br J Dermatol* 127(3):239-246, 1992.
32. Whiting DA: Diagnostic and predictive value of horizontal sections of scalp biopsy specimens in male pattern androgenetic alopecia, *J Am Acad Dermatol* 28(5 pt 1):755-763, 1993.
33. Domnitz JM, Silvers DN: Giant cells in male pattern alopecia: a histologic marker and pathogenetic clue, *J Cutan Pathol* 6(2):108-112, 1979.
34. Lattanand A, Johnson WC: Male pattern alopecia: a histopathologic and histochemical study, *J Cutan Pathol* 2(2):58-70, 1975.
35. Bystryn JC, Orentreich N, Stengel F: Direct immunofluorescence studies in alopecia areata and male pattern alopecia, *J Invest Dermatol* 73(5):317-320, 1979.
36. Young JW and others: Cutaneous immunopathology of androgenetic alopecia, *J Am Osteopath Assoc* 91(8):765-771, 1991.
37. Hori H and others: The thickness of human scalp: normal and bald, *J Invest Dermatol* 58(6):396-399, 1972.
38. Klemp P, Peters K, Hansted B: Subcutaneous blood flow in early male pattern baldness, *J Invest Dermatol* 92(5):725-726, 1989.
39. Orentreich N: Autografts in alopecias and other selected dermatological conditions, *Ann N Y Acad Sci* 83:463-479, 1959.
40. Price VH: Hormonal control of baldness, *Int J Dermatol* 15:742-744, 1976.
41. Randall VA and others: Androgens and the hair follicle cultured human dermal papilla cells as a model system, *Ann N Y Acad Sci* 642:355-375, 1991.
42. Hodgins MB and others: Androgen receptors in dermal papilla cells of scalp hair follicles in male pattern baldness, *Ann N Y Acad Sci* 642:448-451, 1991.
43. Itami S and others: Mechanism of action of androgen in dermal papilla cells, *Ann N Y Acad Sci* 642:385-395, 1991.
44. Schmidt JB: Nuclear and cytosol androgen receptor in androgen-dependent dermatoses in female patients, *Exp Clin Endocrinol* 90(1):107-112, 1987.
45. Bassas E, Pinto B: Experimental study on the male pattern alopecia. I. Differences between the testosterone transport protein in bald and hairy areas, *Arch Dermatol Forschung* 284(4):339-346, 1974.
46. Price VH: Testosterone metabolism in the skin. A review of its function in androgenetic alopecia, acne vulgaris, and idiopathic hirsutism including recent studies with antiandrogens, *Arch Dermatol* 111(11):1496-1502, 1975.
47. Dijkstra AC and others: Is increased 5 alpha-reductase activity a primary phenomenon in androgen-dependent skin disorders? *J Invest Dermatol* 89(1):87-92, 1987.
48. Sawaya ME, Hordinsky MK: The antiandrogens: when and how they should be used, *Dermatol Clin* 11(1):65-72, 1993.
49. Puerto AM, Mallol J: Regional scalp differences of the androgenic metabolic pattern in subjects affected by male pattern baldness, *Rev Esp Fisiol* 46(3):289-296, 1990.
50. Thigpen AE and others: Tissue distribution and ontogeny of steroid 5 alpha-reductase isozyme expression, *J Clin Invest* 92(2):903-910, 1993.
51. Sawaya ME: Steroid chemistry and hormone controls during the hair follicle cycle, *Ann N Y Acad Sci* 642:376-384, 1991.
52. Sawaya ME and others: Delta 5-3 beta-hydroxysteroid dehydrogenase activity in sebaceous glands of scalp in male-pattern baldness, *J Invest Dermatol* 91(2):101-105, 1988.
53. Crovato F, Moretti G, Bertamino R: 17-Hydroxy-steroid-dehydrogenases in hair follicles of normal and bald scalp: a histochemical study, *J Invest Dermatol* 60(3):126-133, 1973.
54. King LE, Jr and others: Growth factor receptors and hair loss, *J Invest Dermatol* 96(5):79S, 1991.
55. Philpott MP, Westgate GE, Kealey T: An in vitro model for the study of human hair growth, *Ann N Y Acad Sci* 642:148-166, 1991.

C. Alopecia: Classification and Incidence*

O'Tar Norwood

HISTORICAL NOTE

In 400 BC, Hippocrates observed in the *Hippocratic Corpus* that "eunuchs are not subject to gout nor do they become bald."[1] Aristotle, who suffered from baldness himself, was also interested in the fact that eunuchs did not experience baldness and were unable to grow hair on their chests.[2] These observations were either forgotten or overlooked for the next 25 centuries, and medical science remained baffled by male pattern baldness until 1949 when James B. Hamilton, an anatomist, made the observation that eunuchs did not become bald. He suggested that androgens are a prerequisite for male pattern hair loss.[3] He later classified the patterns and grades of male pattern baldness in a landmark study.[4] Time and subsequent investigations of hair loss[5] have confirmed the significance of androgens in male pattern baldness.

Many facts regarding baldness that we take for granted were proven by Hamilton in some brilliant and remarkably simple experiments and observations. He demonstrated conclusively that the extent and development of male pattern baldness were dependent on the interaction of three factors: androgens, genetic predisposition, and age.

In the course of studying 312 normal men and 104 eunuchs and eunuchoid men, Hamilton[3] noted the following findings:

1. Men who failed to develop sexually never developed baldness, even if they had a strong family history of baldness. This occurrence cannot be explained on the basis of fortuitous lack of genetic predisposition in view of the fact that some degree of baldness occurs in over one half of all adult men.
2. Certain men rapidly developed baldness on receiving androgen therapy. Progress of the baldness coincided with androgen therapy and stopped immediately with its discontinuance.
3. The amount of androgen had no relationship to the development and extent of male pattern baldness. Men who were not bald did not differ significantly from men who were bald with regard to urinary ketosteroid levels.
4. Androgens can induce male pattern baldness in women as shown by some cases of androblastoma and adrenal virilism. This male pattern hair loss in women ceases when the masculinity is treated.

---

*This text is revised and partially reprinted from *South Med J* 68(11):1359-1365, 1975.

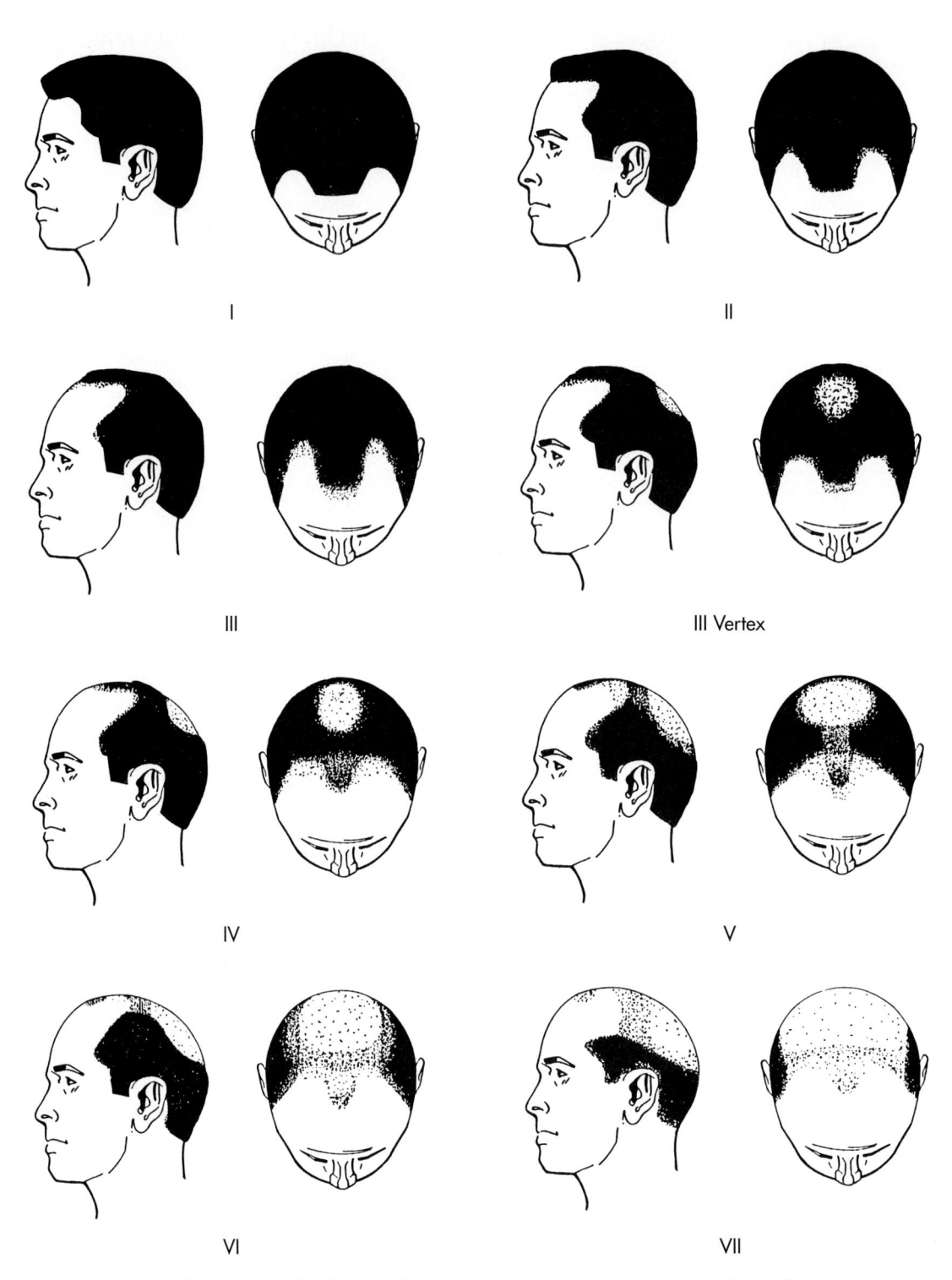

FIG. 1-7 Standards for classification of most common types of male pattern baldness. (From Norwood OT: *South Med J* 68(11)1359-1365, 1975.)

Alopecia: Classification and Incidence **15**

5. The role of genetic predisposition is demonstrated by the occurrence of alopecia with androgenic therapy in only those men with familial tendency to baldness and by the fact that alopecia did not occur with intensive androgen treatment of eunuchs whose family history indicated no predisposition to baldness.
6. Aging is shown to be a contributing factor in that in normal men, advancing age is accompanied by increased incidence and extent of baldness. In eunuchs castrated prepubertally and given androgen treatment in their 20s, hair was lost slowly over a period of years, resulting in hair loss similar to that experienced by noncastrated men of the same age. In contrast, eunuchs who were in their 60s before receiving androgens lost hair within a few months after beginning androgen treatment. Evidently susceptibility to alopecia increases with age but alopecia is not expressed in the absence of inciting agents such as androgens.

In summary, genetic, endocrine, and aging factors are interdependent. No matter how strong the inherited predisposition, male pattern alopecia will not result if androgens are lacking. In addition, androgens will not induce baldness in individuals who are not genetically predisposed to baldness. The influence of aging on alopecia is demonstrated by the immediate loss of hair in eunuchs in their 60s when exposed to androgens, whereas young eunuchs exposed to androgens tend to lose their hair at a much slower rate.

CLASSIFICATION OF MALE PATTERN ANDROGENIC ALOPECIA
Norwood Classification System

Classification has provided a useful standard for screening candidates for hair restoration, recording results of examination, discussing patients with colleagues, and documenting case reports.

The standards depicted in Figs. 1-7 and 1-8 categorize the typical sequences in the development of male pattern baldness. There are varied patterns of male pattern baldness and no single sequence is followed uniformly by all men. Some individuals fall between sequences at the time of examination, but most subjects can be classified quite closely. This classification system is easier to use than Hamilton's system. The Norwood classification system has been used for over 15 years and has become the standard of classification for hair restoration physicians[6] (Table 1-3).

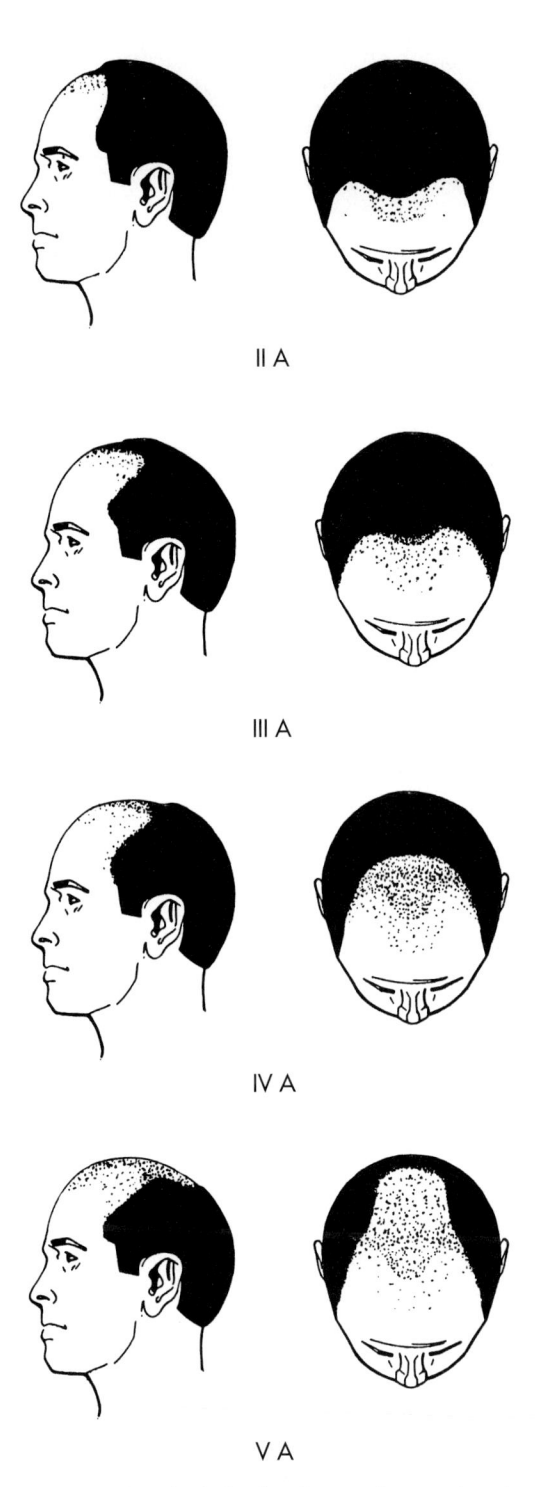

FIG. 1-8 Standards for classification for type A variant male pattern baldness. (From Norwood OT: *South Med J* 68(11):1359-1365, 1975.)

TABLE 1-3 Incidence of Male Pattern Baldness in 1000 Men by Type and Age

TYPE	18-29 YR	30-39 YR	40-49 YR	50-59 YR	60-69 YR	70-79 YR	80+ YR
I	110 (60%)	60 (36%)	55 (33%)	45 (28%)	29 (19%)	18 (17%)	12 (16%)
II	52 (28%)	43 (26%)	38 (22%)	32 (20%)	24 (16%)	20 (19%)	11 (14%)
III	14 (6%)	30 (18%)	37 (20%)	34 (23%)	22 (15%)	16 (16%)	12 (16%)
		(3V)*	(15V)*	(15V)*	(10V)*	(7V)*	(8V)*
IV	4 (3%)	16 (10%)	15 (10%)	21 (9%)	17 (12%)	13 (13%)	9 (12%)
V	3 (2%)	10 (6%)	13 (8%)	15 (10%)	22 (15%)	13 (13%)	9 (12%)
VI	2 (1%)	4 (3%)	7 (4%)	10 (7%)	19 (13%)	11 (11%)	10 (13%)
VII	0	2 (1%)	5 (3%)	4 (3%)	16 (10%)	11 (11%)	14 (17%)
TOTAL	185 (100%)	165 (100%)	165 (100%)	156 (100%)	149 (100%)	102 (100%)	77 (100%)

From Norwood OT: *South Med J* 68(11):1359-1365, 1975.
*Numbers in parentheses under type III represent type III vertex individuals.

STANDARDS FOR CLASSIFICATION OF MALE PATTERN BALDNESS

Type I. The essential feature of type I is no recession or very minimal recession along the anterior border of the hairline in the frontotemporal region.

Type II. The anterior border of the hair in the frontotemporal region has triangular areas of recession, which tend to be symmetrical. These areas of denudation extend no further posteriorly than approximately 2 cm anterior to a line drawn in a coronal plane between the external auditory meatus. Hair also is lost or is sparse along the midfrontal border of the scalp, but the depth of the affected area is much less than that in the frontotemporal region.

Type III. This classification represents the minimal extent of hair loss considered sufficient to represent baldness. Most type III scalps have deep frontotemporal recessions, which are usually symmetrical and are either bare or very sparsely covered by hair. These recessions extend farther posteriorly than a point that lies approximately 2 cm anterior to a line drawn in a coronal plane between the external auditory meatus.

Type III Vertex. In this type the hair is lost chiefly in the vertex. There may be some frontal recession, but it does not exceed that seen in type III. This type of baldness is most common with advancing age.

Type IV. The frontal and frontotemporal recession is more severe than that in type III. In addition, there is a sparseness or absence of hair in the vertex area. These bald areas are extensive but separated from each other by a band of moderately dense hair that extends across the top. This band joins the fully haired fringe on each side of the head. Type IV should not be confused with type III vertex in which the loss is primarily on the vertex.

Type V. The vertex region of alopecia remains separated from the frontotemporal region of alopecia. The separation is not as distinct as that in type IV because the band of hair across the crown is narrower and sparser. Both the vertex and frontotemporal areas of alopecia are larger than those in type IV. Viewed from above, types V, VI, and VII are all characterized by areas of alopecia that are outlined by hair on the sides and back of the scalp, forming the shape of a horseshoe.

Type VI. The bridge of hair that crossed the crown in the type V is absent. The frontotemporal and vertex regions of alopecia are confluent, and the entire area of alopecia is greater laterally and posteriorly than that in type V.

Type VII. This type is the most severe form of male pattern baldness. All that remains is a narrow horseshoe-shaped band of hair that begins laterally just anterior to the ear and extends posteriorly on the sides and quite low on the occiput. This hair is usually not dense and frequently is fine. The hair is also extremely sparse on the nape of the neck and in a semicircle over both ears. It should be noted that the anterior border of this band on each side of the head is receded posteriorly to just in front of the ears.

STANDARDS FOR CLASSIFICATION OF TYPE A VARIANT MALE PATTERN BALDNESS

Type A variant classification of male pattern baldness constituted approximately 3% of individuals studied. It is distinguished by two major features and two minor features. The major features *must* be present for the pattern to be designated as a type A variant (see box). The minor features are not necessary for this classification but frequently are present.

Type II A. The entire anterior border of the hairline lies high on the forehead. The usual midfrontal peninsula or island of hair is represented by only a

> **CHARACTERISTICS OF TYPE A VARIANT MALE PATTERN BALDNESS**
>
> *Major Features*
> 1. The entire anterior border of the hairline progresses posteriorly without the usual island or peninsula of hair in the midfrontal region.
> 2. There is no simultaneous development of a bald area on the vertex. Instead the anterior recession just advances posteriorly to the vertex.
>
> *Minor Features*
> 1. Scattered sparse hairs frequently persist throughout the entire area of denudation.
> 2. The horseshoe-shaped fringe of hair that remains on the sides and back of the head tends to be wider and reach higher on the head than that seen in types V, VI, and VII.

few sparse hairs. The area of denudation extends no farther than 2 cm from the midfrontal line.

Type III A. The area of denudation approaches or may actually reach the midcoronal line.

Type IV A. The area of alopecia extends beyond the midcoronal line. There may be a considerable amount of thinning posterior to the actual hairline.

Type V A. This classification is the most advanced degree of alopecia described with this variant. If the alopecia becomes more extensive, it cannot be distinguished from the usual types V and VI. The area of alopecia does not reach the vertex.

Other Types of Androgenic Alopecia

The possible variations of androgenic alopecia are infinite. Designation of all minor types would not only be impossible but also reduce the usefulness of the classification systems. However, there are several reasonably well-defined variations that deserve special mention. Generally, to qualify for these designations, the hair should be sparse enough that the scalp is plainly visible on casual inspection.

DIFFUSE, UNPATTERNED ALOPECIA. In this type there is a general decrease in hair density without any definite pattern, although hair loss is usually more marked over the top and front. This type is common in women.[7]

DIFFUSE, PATTERNED ALOPECIA. The patterns in this type of hair loss are essentially the same as those in the more common types of male pattern baldness, but the areas involved do not become totally bald; the hair only decreases in density. This type of alopecia also occurs in women.

MALE PATTERN BALDNESS WITH PERSISTENT MIDFRONTAL FORELOCK. This variant can be of any degree of severity and is essentially the same as male pattern baldness except that a midfrontal forelock persists.

SENILE ALOPECIA. This pattern of baldness occurs in all scalps, male and female, with age. The role of androgens is uncertain. The decrease in hair density involves not just the top and sides of the head but the entire scalp.

• • •

Because of the infinite variations of male pattern baldness, a considerable amount of judgment is required in classifying individuals with any standard. Subjects seldom fit a category exactly and usually must be placed in the category they come closest to fitting. The results of my previous studies along with research by others confirm that male pattern baldness affects at least 70% of the male population. The progressive nature of this condition should be appreciated by all hair restoration physicians (Figs. 1-9 and 1-10).

Comparison of Male Pattern Baldness in Whites, Blacks, and Orientals

The Norwood study[6] examined only white men. Hamilton,[4] in addition to the 240 whites, studied 77 Chinese and examined the results separately. Takashima, Iju, and Sudo[8] and Kakizo[9] studied male pattern baldness in Japanese, and Setty[10] evaluated male pattern baldness in blacks. There are significant differences between the races, but male pattern baldness is more common in whites than in other races. In blacks, the incidence of male pattern baldness is about one-fourth that in whites. In Japanese, the incidence of male pattern baldness is about one-fourth that in whites in early age but increases to one-third the incidence in whites in later years. In Chinese, male pattern baldness is minimal before the age of 40 years and although the incidence increases later in life, it always remains well below the levels of whites (Fig. 1-11).

Discussion

Unfortunately, over the past 25 years, most hair restoration physicians, including myself, have not paid too much attention to the results in Fig. 1-12. It is important to note that both studies show that the incidence of male pattern baldness progresses with age. Hamilton's study in fact showed an 85% incidence of significant male pattern baldness in men 65 years of age. The incidence in my original study was 20% to 30% less but still demonstrated a steady progression with age. Judging from observations over the past 25 years, I believe that the true incidence lies somewhere between the Norwood study and Hamilton's study.

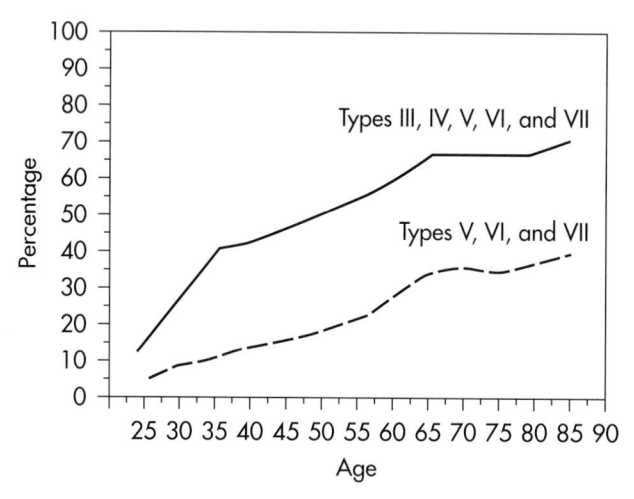

18 General Considerations for Hair Replacement

FIG. 1-9 The incidence of cosmetically significant male pattern baldness (types III, IV, V, VI, and VII) increases steadily with age (*solid line*). The incidence of male pattern baldness characterized by only a horseshoe fringe of hair (types V, VI, and VII) remains relatively low until men reach their 70s (*dotted line*). (From Norwood OT: *South Med J* 68(11):1369-1365, 1975.)

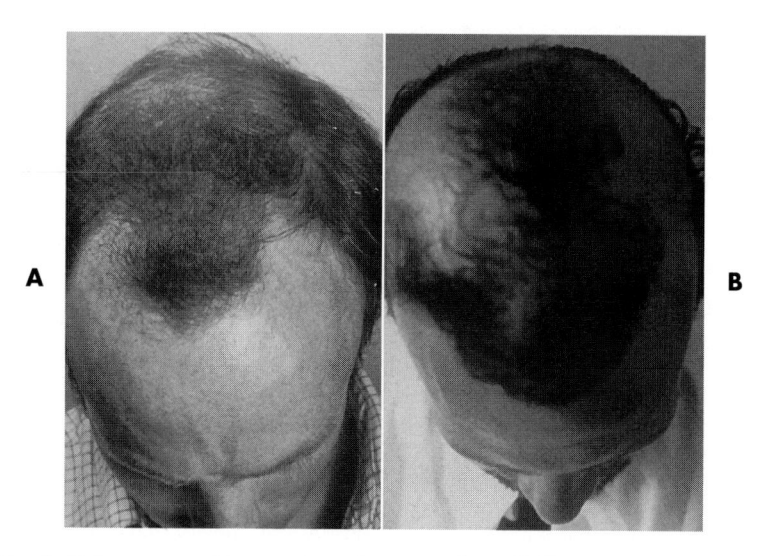

FIG. 1-10 A, Eighteen-year-old man prior to hair transplants. **B,** Twenty-year postoperative result after 232 grafts. Grafts were transplanted at the vertex.

Because we are now seeing the long-term results of surgery we performed 25 to 30 years ago, we are becoming painfully aware that male pattern baldness indeed progresses throughout life.

CLASSIFICATION OF FEMALE PATTERN ANDROGENIC ALOPECIA

In 1977, Ludwig[11] classified female androgenic alopecia, which consists of a diffuse thinning in an oval area on top of the scalp. Usually there is a narrow band of slightly more dense hair that remains at the hairline. There is no recession of the hairline. Rarification of hair becomes more pronounced with age. This type of alopecia is *not* associated with high levels of testosterone.

Onset occurs just prior to or around menopause but is not uncommon in the late 20s and early 30s. The earlier the onset, the more severe alopecia will be. The genetics involved with female pattern androgenic alopecia are unclear. Typical male pattern baldness can occur in women, but its manifestation is associated with high levels of testosterone.

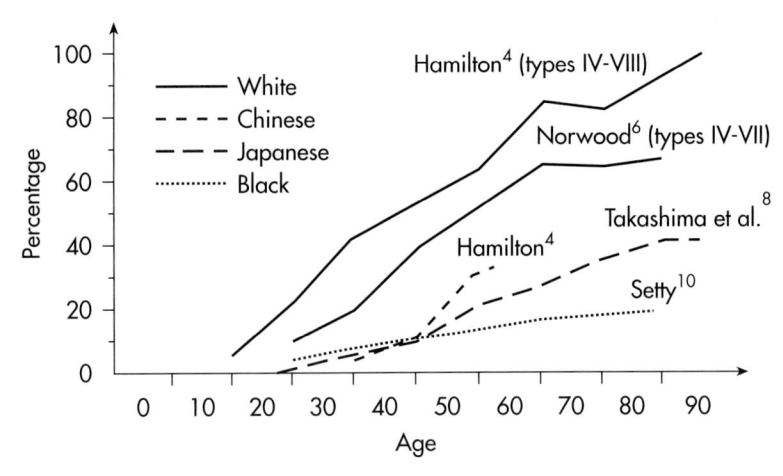

FIG. 1-11 Age-specific incidence of advanced baldness in whites, blacks, Chinese, and Japanese. (From Norwood OT: *South Med J* 68(11):1359-1365, 1975.)

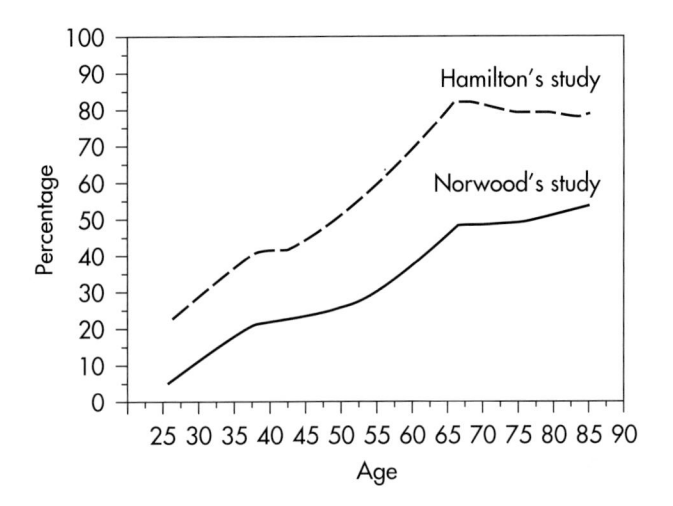

FIG. 1-12 Comparison of the incidence of types IV, V, VI, and VII of male pattern baldness between the Norwood study and the Hamilton study. The progression in incidence in both studies is remarkably similar except that Hamilton's findings range 20% to 30% higher than Norwood's. (From Norwood OT: *South Med J* 68(11):1359-1365, 1975.)

The development of androgenic alopecia in women is classified in three stages (see Fig. 1-3):

Grade I: Perceptible thinning of the hair on the crown. A thin band of higher density hair is retained at the hairline.
Grade II: More pronounced rarification of the hair within the crown area as seen in grade I.
Grade III: Total or almost total denudation within the crown area defined in grades I and II. Ludwig indicated that there was always a more dense area of hair at the hairline from 1 to 3 cm in width. This is true, but this hair at the hairline also thins with time.

Discussion

Hair transplant surgery can achieve reasonably good results in the treatment of female pattern androgenic alopecia, but there are three problems that should be explained to patients:

1. Limited donor hair. Usually the only hair dense enough for transplants is located on a small area at the occiput. The temples and

parietal areas do not provide dense enough hair.
2. The temporary telogen that occurs following hair transplant surgery can sometimes be more severe in women than in men. Telogen hairs that are near the end of their life cycle may not regrow. Patients should be made aware of this fact.
3. Women are frequently not satisfied with the density that transplants provide. They must understand that the transplanted hair will not be dense and will require considerable styling to appear "normal."

Female pattern androgenic alopecia is more common than generally believed and its incidence seems to be increasing in recent years. It responds better than typical male pattern baldness to antiandrogens and minoxidil treatment and may benefit from the continual search for a medical cure for male pattern baldness.

REFERENCES

1. Chadwick J, Mann WN (trans): *The Medical Works of Hippocrates*, London, 1950, Blackwell, p 171.
2. Rothman S: Introduction. In Montagne E, Ellis RA: *The Biology of Hair Growth*, New York, 1958, Academic Press.
3. Hamilton JB: Male hormone stimulation is prerequisite and an incitant in common baldness, *Am J Anat* 71:451-480, 1942.
4. Hamilton JB: Patterned loss of hair in man: types and incidence, *Ann N Y Acad Sci* 53:708-728, 1951.
5. Montagne W, Ellis RA: Aging of the human male scalp. In *The Biology of Hair Growth*, New York, 1958, Academic Press, pp 469-484.
6. Norwood OT: Male pattern baldness: classification and incidence, *South Med J* 68(11):1359-1365, 1975.
7. Rook A, Wilkinson DS, Ebling FJG: *Textbook of Dermatology*, vol 2, London, 1968, Blackwell, p 1383.
8. Takashima M, Iju, Sudo M: Alopecia androgenetica—its incidence in Japanese and associated conditions. In Orfanos CE, Montagna W, Stutgen G, editors: *Hair research status and future aspects*. Berlin, 1981, Springer-Verlag, pp 287-293.
9. Kakizo K: Correlation between cancer of the stomach and alopecia, *Kurume Med J* 32:1540-1565, 1969.
10. Setty LR: Hair patterns of the scalp of white and negro male. *Am J Phys Anthropol* 33:49-56, 1970.
11. Ludwig E: Classification of the types of androgenetic alopecia (common baldness) occurring in the female sex, *Br J Dermatol* 97(3):247-254, 1977.

D. Anatomy of the Scalp

Hani S. Matloub and Joseph Andrew Molnar

Efforts to develop new methods of hair restoration and scalp reconstruction have resulted in continued investigations of the anatomy of the scalp. Although these studies have added to our knowledge, they have also generated confusion when different terms are used to describe the same structures or when new findings are not reconciled with existing information. This discussion reviews these studies in an effort to minimize confusion in terminology and provide a comprehensive understanding of the contiguous structures of the scalp.

SUPERFICIAL LANDMARKS

Certain landmarks of the scalp topography are commonly referred to. The *frontotemporal recession*, or "gulf" region, is the area of receding hairline at the frontotemporal region. *Crown* may be used to describe the middle of the scalp or vertex but more often refers to the site of early balding at the back of the head. *Donor area* refers to the temporal and occipital regions, which contain hair that does not fall out with alopecia. These areas are separated by the *posterior inferior triangle* region, which usually contains thinner hair that does not grow long. *Frontal tuft* refers to the hair in the frontal midline between the two areas of frontotemporal recession. *Fringe hair* is located between the balding area and the donor area and represents fine, thin hair of little cosmetic value.

LAYERS OF THE SCALP

The scalp is usually described as having five layers, the first letters of which form the acronym SCALP: Skin, subCutaneous tissue, Aponeurosis, Loose areolar layer, and Pericranium. The boundaries of the scalp are best understood in terms of the musculoaponeurotic layer. Anteriorly the musculoaponeurosis begins at the supraorbital margin and extends along the frontal process of the zygoma and upper border of the zygomatic arch. It continues laterally along the upper border of the external auditory meatus, extends along the mastoid process, and wraps around posteriorly above the insertion of the sternocleidomastoid muscle and the origin of the trapezius muscle. The musculoaponeurosis ends posteriorly at the superior nuchal line.[1-4]

The *skin* is the most superficial layer of the scalp. It is thickest over the occiput and thinnest over the vertex, ranging from 3 to 8 mm in depth. The skin of the scalp is the thickest of the body, making it a good donor site for split-thickness skin grafting. This layer includes hair, sebaceous glands, and sweat glands, structures that may also involve the subcutaneous layer (Fig. 1-13).

The *subcutaneous layer* of the scalp is a fatty layer like elsewhere in the body. The amount of fat is unaffected by weight changes but may decrease with age. Unlike subcutaneous layers in other parts of the body, this layer in the scalp is dense and tough because of a substantial network of fibrous septa

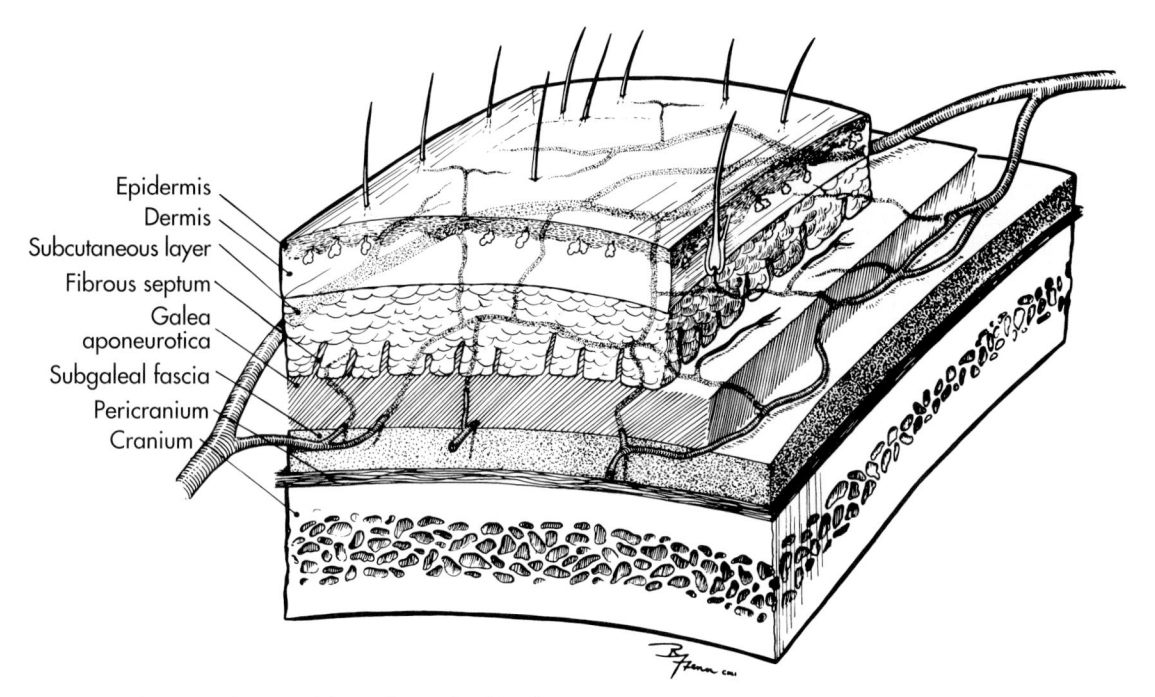

FIG. 1-13 Layers of the scalp. Each of five layers of the scalp has a different histological structure to allow for combined function. Although the major blood vessels course just superficial to the galea, there is a complex network of vessels connecting all levels.

that reach from the skin across the subcutaneous tissue to the deeper aponeurotic layer (Fig. 1-13). This network creates skin stability analogous to the linkage of the skin of the palms and soles to palmar and plantar fascias. In the case of the scalp, however, the top three layers move together as a unit over the pericranium via the mobility allowed by the loose areolar layer below the aponeurotic layer. The major vessels of the scalp traverse the deeper portion of the subcutaneous tissue resting on the galea (Fig. 1-13). This pattern of vasculature makes the subcutaneous layer a particularly poor plane of dissection because not only are the vessels large but also the fibrous septa interfere with blood vessel constriction. In addition, major sensory nerves traverse this layer; thus infection or hematoma in this layer causes pain.

The third layer of the scalp is not just an aponeurotic sheet as the acronym might suggest but it is really the musculoaponeurotic layer of the epicranius or occipitofrontalis muscle. The epicranius muscle consists of two muscle bodies, the frontalis and occipitalis, which are joined over the vertex by the galea aponeurotica or galea.[1-3] Laterally there is a close association with the temporalis and auricular muscles.

The frontalis portion of the epicranius muscle is a paired, quadrilateral-shaped muscle with its muscle bodies separated by a narrow, triangular-shaped fascia. The origin includes the supraciliary ridge of the frontal bone and the procerus, corrugator supercilii, and orbicularis oculi muscles, with attachments interdigitated with the subcutaneous tissue over the eyebrows and nose. The frontalis portion inserts into the galea aponeurotica at a variable level near the coronal suture. The motor nerve supply is the temporal branch of the facial nerve. The sensory nerve supply to this region is the supraorbital and supratrochlear nerves, which are branches of the ophthalmic division of the trigeminal nerve.

The occipitalis portion of the epicranius muscle is a similarly paired structure with its origin from the external occipital protuberance and superior nuchal line of the occipital bone as well as the mastoid portion of the temporal bone. The occipitalis inserts into the galea aponeurotica at a variable level approaching the lambdoidal suture, with a central extension of the galea aponeurotica separating the muscle bodies at the occipital protuberance. The motor nerve to the occipitalis is the posterior auricular branch of the facial nerve.

The term *galea* is derived from the Latin term meaning "helmet" and refers to the helmet-like covering over the vertex of the scalp. Strictly speaking, this term applies only to the central aponeurotic (hence, the term *galea aponeurotica*) portion of this layer and not to the associated muscle bellies of the occipitalis and frontalis. If these structures are also being referred to, the term *epicranius muscle* should be used for precision. The galea is a dense layer of collagen that provides most of the tensile strength of the scalp. Harvey Cushing was so adamant about the surgical importance of this layer that he reportedly said that he would most like to be remembered as the first to suture the galea. Although the strength of the galea can be used to surgical advantage, it represents a surgical obstacle in situations of scalp defects. This layer is the slowest to respond to tissue expansion and must be incised to release the scalp to close scalp flaps without tension.[4,5]

The *loose areolar layer* lies under the epicranius muscle (Fig. 1-13) and as such has been referred to as the *subgaleal fascia*.[4] As its name implies, the subgaleal fascia is a layer of fine connective tissue that is thinnest over the vertex but thicker laterally in the temporal region as it approaches its limit at the zygoma (Fig. 1-14). Anteriorly it is continuous with the loose areolar layer deep to the orbicularis oculi muscle; posteriorly it continues under the galea to the superior nuchal line. The flexibility of this fine layer allows the three more superficial layers to move as a unit. The subgaleal fascia represents an ideal level for surgical dissection and is a common level for scalp avulsion as well as subaponeurotic hematoma or abscess. Carstens, Greco, and Hurwitz[6] suggest that this layer has its own plexus of vessels including small arteries and emissary veins connecting the intracranial venous sinuses to the superficial veins of the scalp (Figs. 1-13 and 1-14). This plexus of vessels makes it possible to transfer this layer as a separate unit for surgical reconstruction.[4,6,7] However, the existence of true axial pattern vessels has been questioned by Tremolada and associates.[8]

The deepest layer of the scalp is the *pericranium*, which is the periosteum of the skull. Like periosteum of other bones, it is tightly adherent to its underlying bone. In the region of the cranial sutures it is particularly tenacious since it maintains fibrous connections to the dura mater at the time of suture closure.

The anatomy of the scalp in the lateral regions of the skull has been the subject of confusing terminology, but recent studies have brought a greater understanding of this area.[4,9-11] The skin and subcutaneous tissues are contiguous with the same layers in the rest of the scalp (Fig. 1-14). The confusion arises in the fascial layers over the temporalis muscle. The term *superficial temporal fascia* is syn-

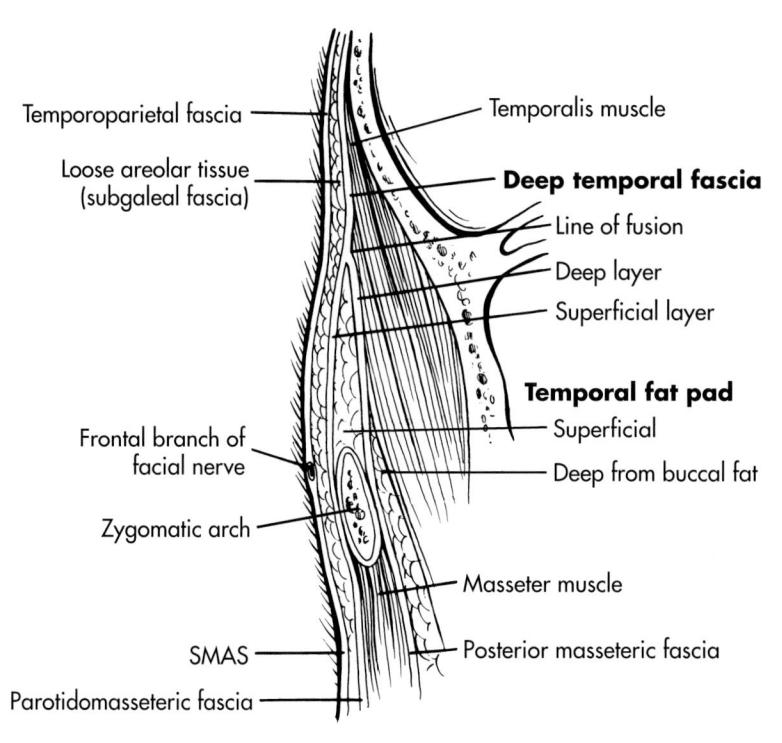

FIG. 1-14 Scalp in the temporal region. Confusion exists regarding the relationships between the scalp layers in the temporal region. Special attention must be given to the relationships of the deep and superficial temporal fascias and fat pads (see text).

onymous with the term *temporoparietal fascia*. This fascia is a continuation of the galea above and the superficial musculoaponeurotic system (SMAS) below. In the same way the major vessels of the scalp lie on the galea, the superficial temporal artery lies adherent to the superficial temporal fascia. The loose areolar layer (subgaleal fascia) lies deep to this fascia as in the rest of the scalp. Dissection deep to the subgaleal fascia above the temporal fascia provides an avascular plane.[9,11] The frontal branch of the facial nerve passes through this layer[10,12,13] at the level of the zygomatic arch and must be avoided in surgical dissection. Deep to the subgaleal fascia lies the deep temporal fascia, which is the well-defined muscular fascia of the temporalis muscle. Superiorly the deep temporal fascia fuses with the pericranium, but in the temporal region it splits around the superficial temporal fat pad, ending on the zygomatic arch.[10,11] The deep temporal fat pad lies under the deep temporal fascia and is continuous with the buccal fat pad.[4,7,10]

The auricular region includes the anterior, posterior, and superior auricular muscles. The anterior and superior auricular muscles arise from between the layers of the galea and therefore lie superficial to the temporalis muscle before inserting on the cranial surface of the ear.[8] The posterior auricular muscle lies in a similar plane, with its origin being the mastoid portion of the temporal bone. Superiorly in the retroauricular region, distinct fascial layers exist as described for the temporal region. However, these fascial layers fuse more caudally, making dissection difficult and creating a pad of heavy fibrous, fascial, muscular tissue.[14,15]

VASCULAR ANATOMY

The blood supply to the scalp consists of five paired arteries originating from the internal and external carotid systems (Fig. 1-15). Anteriorly the supraorbital and supratrochlear arteries exit the orbit from their respective foramina as terminal branches of

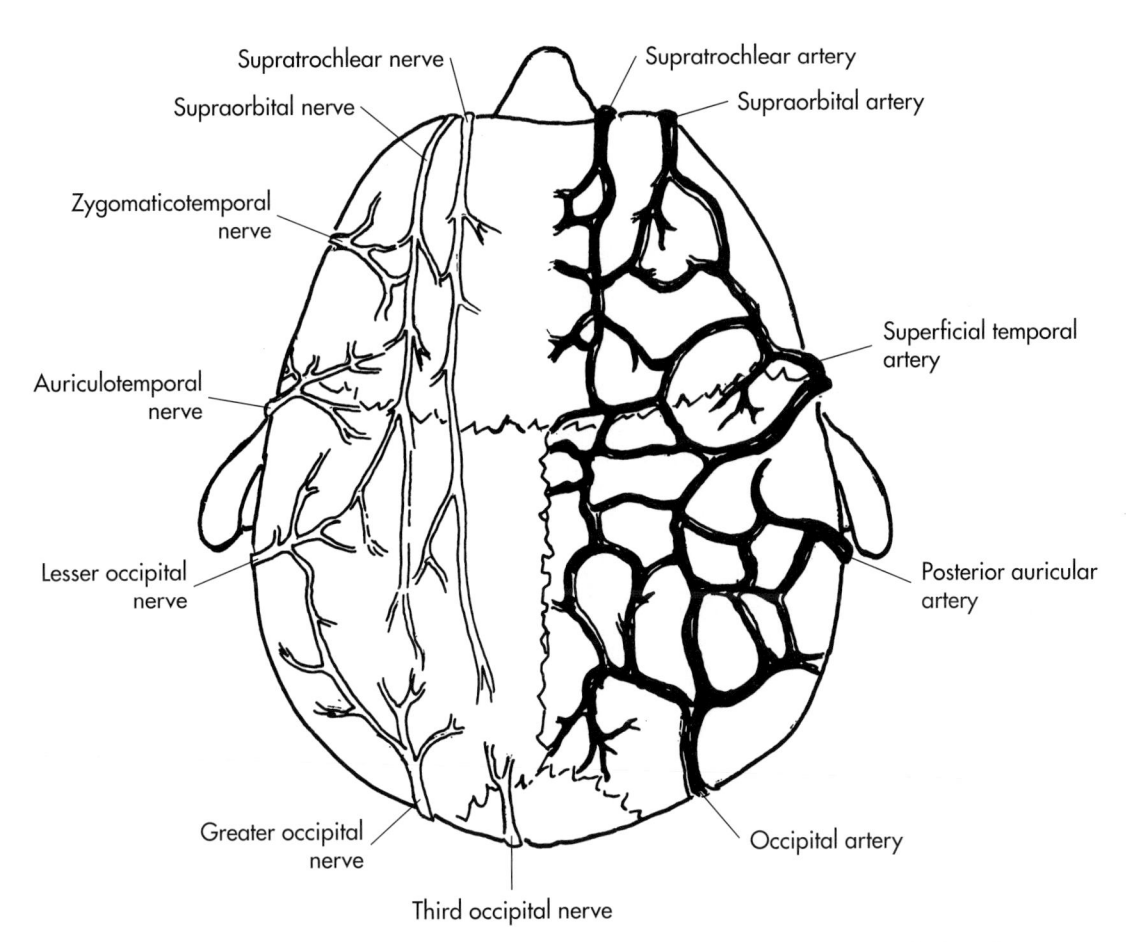

FIG. 1-15 Neurovascular supply of the scalp. The blood supply to the scalp primarily depends on five paired arteries. Common locations of sensory nerves are indicated.

the ophthalmic branch of the internal carotid artery. The supratrochlear artery arises at a point roughly corresponding to the medial portion of the eyebrow 1.7 to 2.2 cm from the midline.[16] It ascends almost directly vertically, piercing the orbicularis oculi and frontalis muscles at the level of the brow and ascending in a subcutaneous plane superiorly. The supraorbital artery exits the orbit lateral to the supratrochlear artery and ascends in a similar subcutaneous plane.[17] These vessels undergo multiple anastomoses with each other as well as with the auricular and superficial temporal arteries. Together or individually the supraorbital and supratrochlear arteries can serve as the pedicle for midline forehead flaps as well as for local pericranial flaps.[16-18]

In the temporal region the superficial temporal artery represents a terminal branch of the external carotid artery. Below the tragus nerve this vessel courses within the parotid gland until it emerges in a plane superficial to the galea in the temporal region and the subcutaneous fat plane superiorly.[4,9,19] Here the artery is palpable and more readily dissected. Near the zygoma the superficial temporal artery gives off the transverse facial artery and the middle temporal artery.[4,9,20] The middle temporal artery rapidly enters the deep temporal fascia.[8,9] It then joins the subcutaneous plexus 10 to 14 cm above the zygoma. The most common bifurcation into a dominant frontal branch and a smaller parietal branch occurs above a line drawn from the external auditory meatus to the supraorbital rim.[20,21] The artery in this region ranges from 1.8 to 2.7 mm in diameter.[9,20] The accompanying vein is usually located anterior to the artery and is of a similar diameter.[20] Considerable variation exists in the branching pattern of the superficial temporal artery (Fig. 1-16). Anastomoses include those to the supraorbital and supratrochlear arteries as well as to the retroauricular, occipital, and contralateral vessels over the vertex.[21,22]

The posterior auricular artery arises from the external carotid artery above the digastric and stylohyoid muscles, runs between the parotid gland and styloid process, and continues its course in the retroauricular groove adherent to the periosteum of the mastoid process.[23,24] In this groove between the external auditory canal, mastoid auditory canal, and mastoid process, the posterior auricular artery gives off the occipital branch, which passes laterally across the mastoid process. Superiorly the

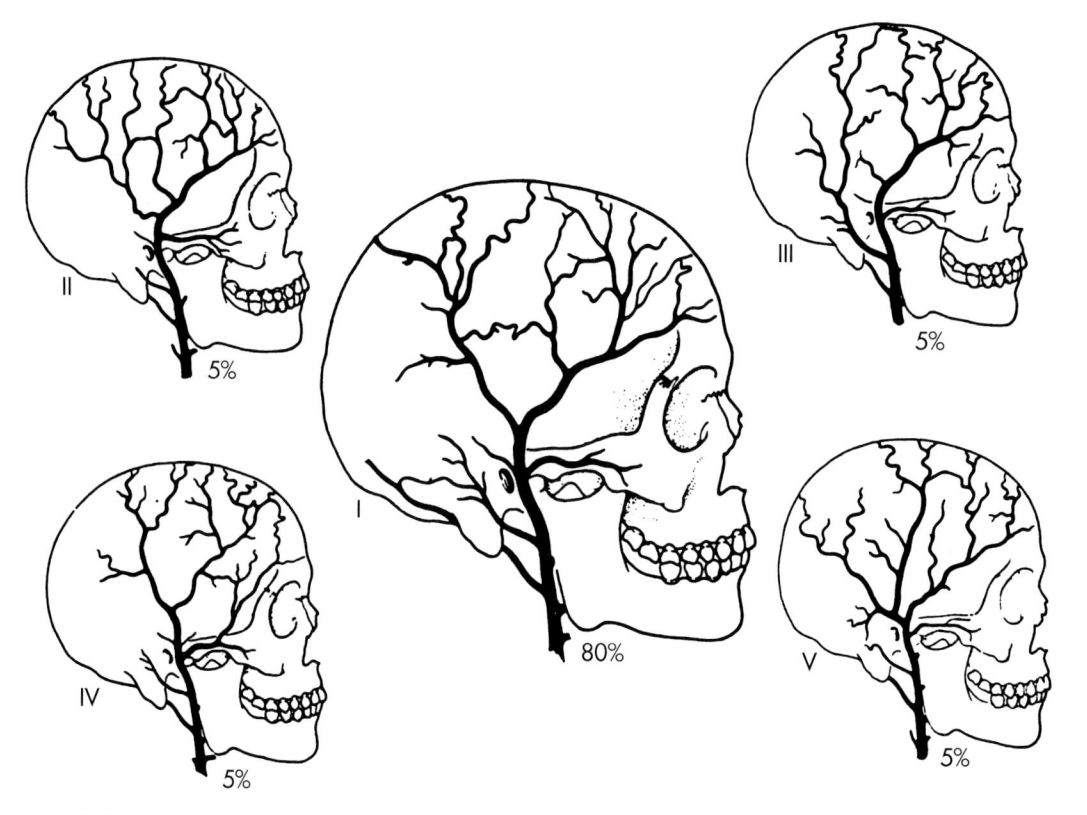

FIG. 1-16 Variability of the branching pattern of the superficial temporal artery based on 14 cadaver dissections and 14 clinical cases. Whereas 80% demonstrated type I bifurcation above the zygoma, the remaining 20% were divided equally among the remaining patterns. The transverse facial artery was consistent.

posterior auricular artery continues as the auricular artery deep to the posterior auricular muscle. Superiorly the vessel gives off branches to the cranial surface of the ear before terminating in the temporal region of the scalp, where it anastomoses with the superficial temporal artery. These anastomoses are those on which the Washio retroauricular flap is based.[25] Considerable variation exists in the number, origins, and distribution of the retroauricular vessel.[14,15,23,24]

The final artery of the scalp is the occipital artery. It originates from the external carotid artery at the lower margin of the posterior belly of the digastric muscle and then runs superiorly and posteriorly under the splenius capitis and the sternocleidomastoid muscles.[4,26] At the medial border of the splenius capitis and sternocleidomastoid attachments, the vessel becomes more superficial and takes an irregular, meandering course in the scalp (Fig. 1-15). At this point the vessel divides into an ascending or vertical branch, a descending branch, and a transverse branch (see Plate I). The descending branch supplies the superior portion of the trapezius, splenius capitis, and sternocleidomastoid muscles and overlying skin. The transverse branch runs horizontally in a region 2 cm below to 4 cm above the occipital protuberance (inion). It crosses the midline, making robust connections to the same branch of the contralateral occipital artery. The vertical branch ascends along the parietal region, anastomosing with the posterior auricular, superficial temporal, and supraorbital arteries. The anatomical territory served by these three branches includes the lateral half of the posterior scalp. However, throughout the numerous connections with vessels on both the ipsilateral and contralateral sides, the dynamic territory can encompass the entire posterior scalp. Conversely, these rich anastomoses with the occipital artery may be used to the surgeon's advantage to harvest parietooccipital hair-bearing scalp based on anastomoses with the temporal artery.

Recent studies suggest that the vascularity of the subgaleal tissue may be similar to that of the subcutaneous tissue.[8,27] Tremolada and associates[8] have demonstrated that the temporal vessels not only develop a subcutaneous plexus 10 to 14 cm above the zygoma but also send perforators to the subgaleal fascia at this level. In the frontoparietooccipital region these perforant vessels enter every 5 to 10 mm, creating a robust plexus. However, the axial blood supply of the galeal fascia in the temporal region reaches to within 1 cm of the sagittal suture.[27]

INNERVATION

The innervation of the scalp is both sensory and motor. Sensory branches have a distribution similar to that of the vascular anatomy (see Fig. 1-15). Anteriorly the supraorbital and supratrochlear nerves are the terminal sensory branches of the ophthalmic division of the trigeminal nerve. They exit the orbit to supply the forehead and anterior scalp. The auriculotemporal nerve from the mandibular division of the trigeminal nerve enters the scalp with the superficial temporal artery and vein. The small branches from the maxillary division of the trigeminal nerve also contribute to the scalp via zygomaticofacial nerves, between the supraorbital and auriculotemporal nerves. The greater cervical plexus innervates the retroauricular region of the scalp via the greater auricular and lesser occipital nerves. Dorsal rami of cervical nerves supply the posterior scalp via the greater occipital nerve.

The facial and trigeminal nerves provide motor nerve supply to the scalp. The anterior portion of the epicranius muscle is supplied by the frontal branch of the facial nerve as it enters the muscle above the level of the supraorbital rim. Its course in relation to the temporal structures is described earlier in the discussion on the layers of the scalp (see Fig. 1-14). The temporalis muscle receives its innervation from the anterior and posterior deep temporal branches of the mandibular division of the trigeminal nerve. The anterior and superior auricular muscles receive their innervation from the temporal branch of the facial nerve, whereas the posterior auricular muscle is innervated by the posterior auricular branch. The occipital portion of the epicranius muscle is supplied by the posterior auricular branch of the facial nerve.

REFERENCES

1. Gray H, Peck TP, Howden R: *Anatomy, descriptive and surgical*, ed 15, New York, Gramercy Books.
2. Woodburne RT: *Essentials of human anatomy*, ed 5, New York, 1973, Oxford University Press.
3. Grant JCB: *An atlas of anatomy*, ed 6, Baltimore, 1972, Williams and Wilkins.
4. Tolhurst DE, Carstens MH, Greco RJ: The surgical anatomy of the scalp, *Plast Reconstr Surg* 87:603-614, 1991.
5. Corso PF: Variations of the arterial, venous and capillary circulation of the soft tissues of the head by decades as demonstrated by the methyl methacrolate injection technique, and their application to the construction of flaps and pedicles, *Plast Reconstr Surg* 27:160-184, 1961.
6. Carstens MH, Greco RJ, Hurwitz DJ: Clinical applications of the subgaleal fascia, *Plast Reconstr Surg* 87:615-626, 1991.
7. Kaplan IB, Gilbert DA, Terzis JK: The vascularized fascia of the scalp, *J Reconstr Microsurg* 5:7-15, 1989.
8. Tremolada C, Candiani P, Signorini M: The surgical anatomy of the subcutaneous fascial system of the scalp, *Ann Plast Surg* 32:8-13, 1994.
9. Abul-Hassan HS and others: Surgical anatomy and blood supply of the fascial layers of the temporal region, *Plast Reconstr Surg* 77:17-28, 1986.
10. Stuzin JM, Wagstroni L, Kawamoto HK: Anatomy of the frontal branch of the facial nerve: the significance of the temporal fat pad, *Plast Reconstr Surg* 83:265-327, 1989.

11. Stuzin JM, Baker TJ, Gordon HL: The relationship of the superficial and deep facial fascias: relevance to rhytidectomy and aging, *Plast Reconstr Surg* 89:441-451, 1992.
12. Baker DC, Conley J: Avoiding facial nerve injuries in rhytidectomy, *Plast Reconstr Surg* 64:781-795, 1979.
13. Ishikawa Y: An anatomical study on the distribution of the temporal branch of the facial nerve, *J Craniomaxillofac Surg* 18:287-292, 1990.
14. Park C, Jong Lee T, Shun Shin K: A single-stage two-flap method of total ear reconstruction, *Plast Reconstr Surg* 88:404-412, 1991.
15. Park C, Shun Shin K, Suck Hang H: A new arterial flap from the postauricular surface: its anatomic basis and clinical application, *Plast Reconstr Surg* 82:498-505, 1988.
16. Shumrick KA, Smith TL: The anatomic basis for the design of forehead flaps in nasal reconstruction, *Arch Otolaryngol Head Neck Surg* 118:373-379, 1992.
17. McCarthy JG, Lorenc ZP, Cutting C: The median forehead flap revisited: the blood supply, *Plast Reconstr Surg* 76:866-869, 1985.
18. Horowitz JH, Persing JA, Nichter LS: Galeal-pericranial flaps in head and neck reconstruction, *Am J Surg* 148:489-497, 1984.
19. Whetzel TP, Mathes SJ: Arterial anatomy of the face: an analysis of vascular territories and perforating cutaneous vessels, *Plast Reconstr Surg* 89:591-605, 1991.
20. Abul-Hassan HS, Drasek Ascher G, Acland RD: Surgical anatomy and blood supply of the fascial layers of the temporal region, *Plast Reconstr Surg* 77:25-28, 1986.
21. Dingman RO, Argenta LC: The surgical repair of traumatic defects of the scalp, *Clin Plast Surg* 9:131-144, 1982.
22. Galvao M: A postauricular flap based on the contralateral superficial temporal vessels, *Plast Reconstr Surg* 68:891-897, 1981.
23. Park C: The chondrocutaneous postauricular free flap, *Plast Reconstr Surg* 84:761-771, 1989.
24. Kolhe PS, Leonard AG: The posterior auricular flap: anatomical studies, *Br J Plast Surg* 40:562-569, 1987.
25. Washio H: Retroauricular-temporal flap, *Plast Reconstr Surg* 43:162-166, 1969.
26. Matloub HS, Yousif NJ, Zhong YE: The occipital artery flap for transfer of hair-bearing tissue, *Ann Plast Surg* 29:491-495, 1992.
27. Har-Shai Y, Fukuta K, Collares MV: The vascular anatomy of the galeal flap in the interparietal and midline regions, *Plast Reconstr Surg* 89:64-76, 1992.

E. The Consultation

Patrick Quinlan

The consultation is about communication. The patient learns about hair restoration. The physician learns about the needs of the patient. The goal is simple—together they decide if a procedure or treatment will meet the needs of the patient.

Although the goal is easy to understand, it can be difficult to achieve. Basically the highly subjective needs of the patient must be met by the objective results created by the physician. It is incumbent upon the physician to identify the patient's spoken and unspoken needs and to make very clear what kind of results the patient can expect. Together they search for an agreement. A meeting of the minds is the foundation of successful hair restoration. With the help of the physician, the patient will understand and articulate his own desires. With the help of the physician, the patient will understand what can be objectively expected. With the help of the physician, the patient will decide if this procedure or treatment will meet his needs.

THE PATIENT

All potential hair restoration patients share one trait: they are uncomfortable with their appearance. This fact is the most important for the physician to realize about the patient and is the crux of the patient's problem. If this trait is defined well and remedied, the physician will have a satisfied patient. Failure to do either could result in disappointment.

Comfort is a very subjective term. Its definition is vague and very personal. To learn what comfort means to the patient requires candid yet sensitive probing by the physician. This process is an exploration in which it is helpful to record certain findings. It is useful for the physician to arrange these findings on one side of the page. Later the physician can address each finding when reviewing technique or treatment options. The physician should discuss with the patient how the procedure or treatment may or may not remedy his concerns. This discussion begins the transformation of ill-defined hope into concrete expectations. It is best to always underpromise and overdeliver. The following example shows a list of patient concerns and the adjacent notes of the physician regarding how hair restoration might address those concerns.

Discomforts (Subjective)	Goals (Objective)
High forehead	Reframe face
Shiny scalp	Reduce reflected light
I feel old	Reframe face
I don't look like myself	Reframe face
My spouse…	Subjective. Should spouse be included in the consultation?
My job requires…	Subjective. Unable to comment
I am embarrassed when I swim	Natural in use
I am uncomfortable in certain social situations	Natural in use, conventional in appearance
My situation is hopeless	Permanent hairline: positive action
My friends tease me	Natural in appearance

Comfort with appearance is in a sense the product of self-image. Tradition holds that a "normal," well-adjusted patient is one who has an objectively accurate perception of self. Recent research suggests that this is not the case. In fact, some researchers contend that illusions are a central part of normal human thought and that normal individuals tend to have an exaggerated sense of self-worth, control, and optimism. In addition, the authors assert that these illusions promote other conventional criteria of mental health, including happiness and well-being. They further contend that positive illusions stem from a mental filter through which experiences are skewed positively and negative experiences are isolated and thereby minimized.

Perhaps when hair loss is sufficient to overcome the positive cognitive filter, the patient can no longer maintain a positive illusion. Perhaps, with hair restoration, physicians can tip the balance back toward the positive and allow a positive illusion to develop. Regardless of these contentions, clearly the patient's personality is central to the consultative process.

To understand the patient, the physician must understand the processes by which needs arise and expectations develop. One such process is pattern recognition. Pattern recognition can work both for and against the patient. It can be detrimental because familiar visual patterns are so ingrained that any significant change engenders discomfort in the patient: "It's not so much that I look bad, it's just that it's simply not me."

However, pattern recognition can be a powerful ally as well. The visual system has many filters through which images are continuously screened and only items of interest are brought to conscious attention. With experience we develop a fund of familiar images that we then, in general, tend to ignore. This useful mechanism allows the mind to focus with less distraction. The relative disadvantage of this process is that we tend to become less observant. Witness the difference between children and adults: children have fewer experiences and much is novel to them. As a result, they are often keen observers of the mundane. An unfamiliar pattern will then generate the query "What's wrong with this picture?" to the consciousness. Therefore the challenge is to create a painfully ordinary hairline of common shape and location that will be ignored by others. The eye is easily bored—keep it that way. The goal is to have the hair become a nonissue. However, if a hairline that is unique in some way is created, the eye will be engaged and the "What's wrong with this picture?" question will be triggered, thus failing the patient.

THE PROCESS

The process of consultation is really the sum of the physician's knowledge applied to the unique needs of each patient. However, at its core in our practice is the clear delineation of specific goals in writing. These goals, in the most simple and broad terms, describe what can be done for a patient and how techniques or treatments can be applied to the specific needs of the patient. It is important that you develop your own approach based on your philosophy and resources.

We stress the following goals:

1. *Frame the face.* Artists have long recognized that typical ratios of the face and facial features exist. A prominent landmark of the face is the scalp and hairline. The scalp in any shape is not only significant in and of itself but also important in how it influences our perceptions of nearby features. Our perception of color and shape are dependent on the surroundings of the object in question. Thus the color of the hair affects our perception of adjacent colors such as the color of the eyes and skin. The shape, texture, and proportions of the scalp influence our perception of the shape, prominence, and location of all other facial features. The mind is very adept at pattern recognition and the hair/face ratio is a powerful pattern. One might suppose that the growth of a beard is an attempt to restore the hair/face ratio, albeit in an inverted form.

   It is not surprising then that hair loss often has a profound effect on an individual. We tend to be most comfortable with the most familiar. What is more familiar than one's face? Hair restoration seeks to restore a familiar appearance, in effect shortening the face and returning the focus to the center.

2. *Natural appearance and use.* Baldness is a natural condition. Any treatment of hair loss should be natural in appearance. The greatest concern of patients is that hair restoration will look odd or artificial. We stress that hair restoration cannot duplicate nature.

   When surgical options are chosen, we believe that smaller is better. This approach especially applies to the concept of "natural in use." Many individuals are satisfied with their hair transplantations when in a static environment—that is, there is no wind and the hair is combed and sprayed. In a dynamic environment, however—one in which wind, water, and sun are at work—they are uncomfortable with their appearance. The hair no longer looks natural. The goal is hair transplantation that is both natural in appearance and function. We generally believe that small grafts and conservative design best accomplish these goals.

3. *Permanent hairline.* The seemingly relentless nature of hair loss is a prominent patient concern. Many are more concerned about the future than the current status of their hair. Hair transplan-

tation can address this problem. The creation of a permanent hairline visually arrests the progressive change in appearance that many patients find so distressing. Positive action gives patients a sense of control over a situation about which many privately feel helpless. A permanent framing of the face creates a stable image that, over time, becomes familiar and comfortable. Predictability and hope are good antidotes for the uncertainty of change.

• • •

People learn in different ways. Some people receive information best verbally whereas others learn best with a visual presentation; some are ready to learn, whereas others are not. As a teacher, you must determine if the patient is ready to learn and choose the best method by which to instruct that patient during the consultation.

Hair restoration is the product of a number of techniques. Like an artist, the more techniques you possess and the greater facility you develop with them, the more likely you are to create a result that meets the patient's needs. Unlike most artists, your palette and your work surface are given to you by the patient, for better or worse. The patient has certain attributes: hair quality, hair density, hair color, hereditary hair growth/loss pattern, financial resources, and determination. With these resources, you have to create the effect necessary to meet the patient's needs. Share your evaluation of these attributes with the patient and lay them out clearly, just as you would arrange pigment, brush, and canvas, so that the patient understands what you see that he has to offer, how you can use these attributes, and what he realistically can expect. Explain clearly that the same procedure yields different results in different patients. The same procedure performed on an individual with white skin and fine, limp, jet black hair and on an individual with multicolored skin and dense, wavy, silver hair will have very different results. Most people can accept bad news, but no one likes unpleasant surprises.

In summary, we stress our concrete goals to the patient: "We will create a permanent hairline to arrest the hair loss process visually. The effect will be natural both in appearance and in use but will *not* be the equivalent of nature. It is an artificial attempt to mask a natural process." We then return to the central issue and ask the patient: "Will these alterations improve your comfort with your appearance?"

THE PITFALLS

The patient arrives for consultation with a given personality, certain spoken and unspoken expectations, and a finite knowledge base. Those elements must be understood in order to prevent you and your patient from falling into a pit or trap for the unwary—a pitfall.

Most problems with hair restoration stem from expectation, not technique. You must remember that satisfaction is a moving target. Hair is not unique in this regard. How often have you painted one room in the house only to notice how dull the rest of the house now seems? How often do you hear, "If only I had a certain job, a raise, a new car," only to find that after that goal is achieved, a new, higher standard develops. You need to clearly establish realistic expectations prior to the first procedure or treatment. Later, when the objective goals have been met but somehow the hair is not quite dense enough to the patient, remind the patient of the trap of the "moving target." There will never be enough hair. One can always find room for more hair, more time, more money. Return to the goals: does the hair frame the face, is it natural in appearance, and is it natural in its use? Reasonable people understand this concept. If forewarned, the patient can be gently reminded and expectations can be realigned with reality. However, it is very difficult, if not impossible, to establish this concept after the fact.

Unreasonable people are a different story. To the inexperienced or unwary, such patients may be difficult to detect. If, after consultation, the physician senses an unreasonable patient, the physician should *not* accept the case. Some unrealistic expectations are mild and may at first be overlooked by the physician. If the posttreatment patient says "My scalp feels thin," interrupt politely and state clearly, "It will always be thin. Remember, we try to fool the eyes of others, not your fingers. To be more precise, we fool the eyes of others, but not yours. With close examination, you could probably find your grafts as well." Some patients are merely focused on the past rather than on the future. Others, however, suffer from a profoundly altered sense of reality—body dysmorphic disorder.

Body Dysmorphic Disorder

As with most psychological disorders, the manifestations of this condition range over an entire spectrum and might be found in limited expression in the "normal" individual. When a trait or behavior becomes exaggerated and interferes with the patient's life, it is labeled a disorder. Body dysmorphic disorder is a psychiatric condition in which the patient has a profound negative distortion of body image. We are all familiar with the patient suffering from anorexia nervosa. This skin-and-bones patient sees a fat person when looking in the mirror. Such an individual suffers from body dysmorphic disorder. Something similar perhaps happens with hair loss: instead of fat, the patient sees bald. To a certain degree, such a patient may be generally normal and, given proper education, can in part be satisfied with the results. However, some patients, no matter how much hair they get, will always see the scalp and not the hair. How many times have you consulted with a patient with a virtual mop of hair who wants a hair transplant? The patient will probably never be satisfied. Proceed at your own risk. Decide early in your own mind where in the spectrum of reality-based judgment the patient lies. The closer the patient is to the fringe of body dysmorphic disorder, the more demanding and impossible to satisfy he is. Written, concrete goals become the anchor in such a storm.

Language

The patient appears to talk about hair, but the issue is really not about hair—it is about self-image. It is critical that you and the patient agree on the central issues; otherwise, you create the potential for persistent miscommunication. It is helpful to remember the difference between a verbal argument and a debate. In a verbal argument there is an unrealized misunderstanding concerning the disputed issues. Ostensibly the opposing parties discuss the same issues, but in fact they clash over similar-sounding—but different—issues. That is to say, they use the same words but these words have different, private meanings. Because they unknowingly discuss similar-sounding but fundamentally different issues, they can never achieve true agreement. Because the issues are unknowingly different, the discussions frequently escalate, and a solution never is developed. In contrast, in a debate the central issue is both clearly defined and mutually understood. In a debate resolution is possible; in a verbal argument not only is an agreement unlikely but also conflict at some level is almost a certainty.

Language presents a problem and an opportunity. The challenge is to establish clear communication that will create the opportunity to identify needs and to meet those needs. The cartoon illustrates this point at the most basic level (Fig. 1-17). The physician and the patient both are familiar with the words "hair transplant" and "full head of hair," but each has a fundamentally different understanding of the terms. A thorough consultation eliminates misunderstanding and allows for true informed consent. Does a "natural hairline" mean a low juvenile hairline to the patient but a high recessed one to you? Similar challenges exist for many terms such as "normal," "useful," "mature," "satisfied," "painless," "fair," "inexpensive," "unnoticeable," "permanent," and "safe." These terms, then, become critical in the physician's vocabulary. Be careful in your use of language and be attentive to the language used by the patient. Typically in medicine the "blind spot," the unforeseen complication, is often the most difficult problem.

Hairline

The hairline is a common source of contention. In general, patients want the hairline too low and too round. The younger the patient, the greater this problem tends to become. Remember that aging is a dynamic process. The trick is to establish a static hairline that, by its shape and location, will appear natural over the course of decades. Patients must be reminded that the hairline must look natural in old age as well as in youth, and at no time is any-

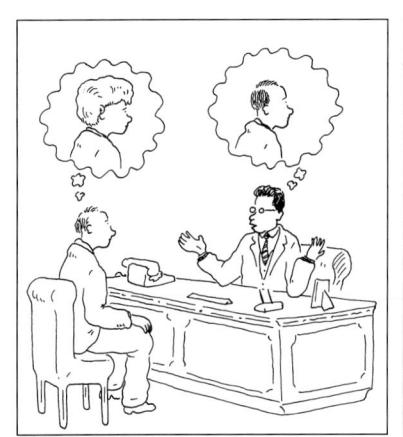

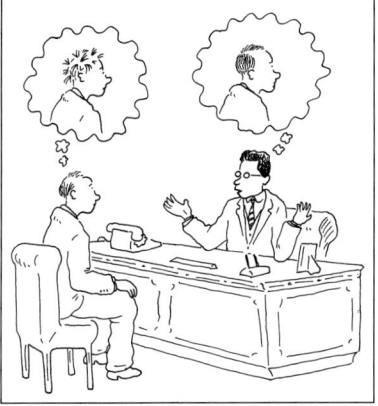

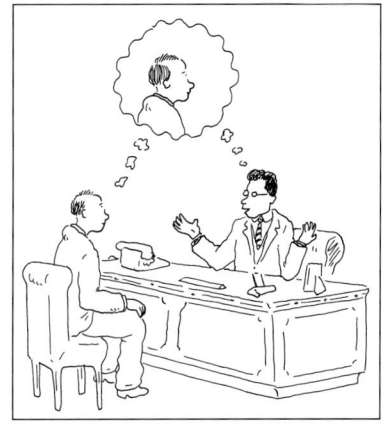

FIG. 1-17 The careful definition of terms and a thorough consultation will help to avoid miscommunication.

one willing to accept an odd appearance. A high hairline with recessions generally achieves this result. There are many advantages to this pattern. The higher the hairline and the greater the recessions, the lesser the amount of hair required to cover a given area. This pattern gives greater density and a more natural appearance than a low, round hairline. This hairline pattern is especially critical for patients with minimal donor area. Deeper recessions guard against temporal loss beyond the edge of the transplanted hairline. The lateral hair can retreat both posteriorly and inferiorly. With age an overly blunt hairline can be left isolated from the lateral scalp and result in a most unnatural appearance. In general, we must focus on the future, not on the past; we must not consider what the patient had but what he will have in the future with and without treatment. As physicians, we must provide the patient what he needs, not necessarily what he wants. We must be certain that the patient's wants are realistic and that fulfilling these wants would truly meet his needs. In summary, the patient may want the hairline of his youth, but what is really needed is a hairline that will age well and meet the constraints of donor hair volume and quality. It is better to do a small job well than a large job poorly.

THE PHYSICIAN

Consultants must clearly understand the range of their skills and the basis of their judgment. A safe physician knows these personal limits. Clinical acumen develops slowly; be patient. Become keenly aware of what you can do and when you can do it. The operating suite can be a cruel teacher for the unwary. Obtain the best training possible, join a society, learn from a mentor, and expand your skills but do so in a planned, conservative manner. You may be able to forget a disaster, but the patient who wears one forever will not. We need to examine our motives. We all want to satisfy our patients. Resist the persuasive patient, and do not promise more than you can deliver. Sometimes "tough love" is required. To truly serve a patient, often you must tell the patient what he does not want to hear. It is essential to work out differences in a consultation room before the procedure or treatment rather than in another "forum" afterward. Learn to trust your instincts. If you feel that something is a bad idea, it probably is.

Time can be your ally or your enemy. The greater the doubt, the better the reason for delay. With time you will be able to better judge and shape the needs and expectations of the patient. Give the patient time to "grow into" the condition and time to move into the acceptance phase. There is always time for good results. Haste may rush the patient into a bad one. Delay could cause you to lose a patient, but it will never cause you to lose your reputation, professional standing, or self-respect.

F. Reassessment of Male Pattern Baldness: A Reevaluation of the Treatment

Emanuel Marritt and Leonard M. Dzubow

The field of hair restoration is couched in illusion, a truth often little appreciated by both patient and physician. Sadly, hair restoration has nothing at all to do with the restorative process. Hair cannot be restored or resuscitated, only rearranged. The patient may appear to have more hair following a hair restoration procedure, but the alteration is only an optical illusion, not a net gain. This genetic limitation of raw material places a significant restriction on the final outcome of the process.

For most individuals, especially most young people, the balding process displays a callous disregard for stability and predictability. Therefore the process of hair rearrangement must be designed to undetectably accommodate the possibility of an ever-increasing bald area with an uncertain supply of permanent hair that is certain to be smaller than initially perceived. It is precisely this dynamic and capricious nature of male pattern baldness that may in future years frustrate almost all solutions that approach the patient as if the hair loss is a stable and predictable entity.

The purpose of this discussion therefore is to define (or, more accurately, redefine) the scope of the hair loss drama from patients' perceptions to physicians' goals. We suggest a new remedy that fulfills the criteria for a successful cosmetic treatment of hair loss. Successful cosmetic treatment is defined as the creation of a final result that (1) is perceived as a significant and positive change in appearance, (2) does not create detectability or deformity either in the present or with the progression of time and possible future loss, and (3) remains forever both natural and undetectable with minimal daily cosmetic maintenance.

It is crucial that the reader appreciate that every manipulation used to create the illusion of more hair *must* have a corresponding reciprocal consequence, often one that has serious negative implications, either immediately after the procedure or at some indefinite time in the future. Contrary to current popular thinking, there really is no "follicular free lunch." Rather the truth is simply that very careful and mature judgment must be rendered to decide which maneuvers are ultimately in the best interest of the patient throughout his life. Conversely, that same judgment must be used to evaluate those procedures that may create future dilemmas that are more serious, debilitating, and permanent than the originally perceived problem.

The first sequence of the hair replacement process begins with the patient's perceptions and desires: what he believes is happening to his head and how he wants it remedied. Unfortunately, the patient, especially the younger patient, is often misguided and misinformed on both counts. He frequently requires exhaustive and sobering counseling regarding these issues. Although the patient may view the problem as "fixed and frozen" in the present, it is the obligation of the physician to expand and maximize the very concerns that the patient struggles to suppress and minimize. The patient must be made to understand the relentless and unpredictable chronological progression of male pattern baldness.

A man with 3 inches of crown vertex baldness in his 30s may well become the man with 6 or 7 inches of baldness in his 50s. A youthful 5-inch donor fringe might in actuality become a middle-aged 3-inch fringe of permanent hair. Rather than minimizing and soothing the current concerns of the patient, the physician must instead amplify these facts by extrapolating the future progression of alopecia. The physician must therefore further reaffirm the moral obligation to treat the final possible or probable hair loss pattern, however remote that eventuality may seem right now.

The immutable law of reciprocal supply and demand dictates that greater baldness than anticipated must always mean less hair to remedy the baldness than anticipated. The patient almost always enters the consultation seeking relief from his dihydrotestosterone-induced depression and almost always leaves the consultation more deeply depressed than when he arrived (a sign that the ethical physician has done his/her job correctly). Significant time, energy, and above all empathy are required to convey this information to the patient (especially the younger patient) in a way that gains understanding and finally acceptance. Many patients begin the consultation with a euphoric attitude built on the scores of promotional brochures and infomercial videos that promise precisely what the patient seeks: total elimination of baldness, total restoration of lost youth, and total excision of follicular reality from his consciousness.

A sobering and deliberate discussion of the possible relentlessness and unpredictability of male pattern alopecia, unless carefully and sympathetically undertaken, might be misinterpreted as an elaborate rationalization for inadequate surgical skills or, even worse, downright incompetence! The physician then who advises and cautions against the complete removal of all baldness, can become, in the patient's mind, the physician who does not really know how to remove all the baldness. The patient is continually faced with the unenviable choice of an exciting, but possibly illusory, image of total scalp coverage or a disheartening but realistic image of more limited hair rearrangement.

The physician must lead this unhappy patient through the confusing morass of possibilities and carefully expose the array of permanent interconnected consequences that might result should impulsive and incorrect choices be made. The patient usually enters the consultation with the guiding motto that "baldness is bad" and therefore "less baldness" (or, better yet, "no baldness") is good." The patient must exit the consultation with the guiding principle that unnaturalness and detectability are the only true evils. Hair rearrangement is successful only if naturalness and undetectability are achieved in the present and preserved as the patient ages. In short, baldness may well be bad, but a lifetime of unwanted sidelong glances and pointed fingers is worse.

THE PHYSICIAN

Most physicians involved in hair restoration act from sympathetic and empathetic intentions. Patients desire total elimination of baldness, and physicians desire to satisfy that wish. Unfortunate misjudgments regarding the applications of techniques used in the pursuit of this goal result from the physician's misunderstanding, unconscious or otherwise, of three fundamental but pivotal phenomena: (1) predictability, (2) progression, and (3) Peter/Paul pilferage.

Predictability

Historically hair replacement surgery literature and lectures suggest that the end point of male pattern baldness may be reasonably predicted by the weight of genetic analysis (family history) coupled with a careful examination of the wetted scalp. Unfortunately, genetics supplies information about possible trends but fails to supply the concrete information so vital for the specific individual. Wet hair will certainly amplify the distinction between thick (terminal) and thinning (vellus) hair but for what may be only a fixed point in time. Examination of the wetted scalp of a 15-year-old teenager would lead to the erroneous conclusion that no adult would ever bald. Predictability therefore is statistically faulty at best. The only helpful and safe prediction is one that statistically forecasts the most pessimistic scenario; then plans can be made accordingly.

Progression

Predictability is further compounded (and confounded) by a lack of appreciation of the possible linear nature of alopecia progression over time. Traditionally hair loss has been depicted as biphasic: rapid from young adulthood to middle age and then significantly slower thereafter. Results following treatments based on this theory of alopecia diminution in and after the fourth decade often deconstruct as hair loss continues at the same or even greater pace throughout the 50s and 60s.

Pilferage

Misconceptions about predictability and progression often lead physicians with good and ethical intentions to attempt what they should not in many individuals with current or future extensive, significant baldness: total elimination of all baldness. All such attempts, both transplantation and reduction, share the common denominator of pilfering from Peter (donor area) to pay Paul (recipient area).

ALOPECIA REDUCTION FROM CONCEPTION TO MISCONCEPTION

Throughout the brief history of surgical hair rearrangement (1960 to present) there has been an overwhelming consensus among almost all practitioners about the aesthetic prominence of the frontal region or frontal zone (the anterior one third of the recipient area). Little controversy has ever existed regarding the primary cosmetic importance of the frontal region or the need to prioritize the transfer of the majority of available donor hair to this critical area. However, problems quickly emerged when the focus of treatment shifted to the area of remaining alopecia posterior to the frontal zone: the midscalp and crown/vertex. The aesthetic imperative of the frontal region and the limited, nonrenewable nature of the donor fringe almost always imposed the onus of incomplete transplantation on the middle and posterior scalp. In those patients with less than optimal hair/skin color camouflaging combinations, this situation translated surgically into grafts spaced at intervals that then revealed tufting under a variety of environmental situations. These frustrating and unsatisfactory cosmetic solutions to middle and posterior scalp baldness imposed by the heretofore immutable limitations of increasing recipient demand and decreasing donor supply suddenly seemed obsolescent in 1975 by the emergence of a procedure that seemed capable of permanently decreasing the vexatious bald skin posterior to the frontal area: the standard scalp reduction.[1-7]

The standard scalp reduction was conceived and designed to permanently alter the unfavorable and perhaps not so immutable ratio of supply and demand. Although the supply of donor hair could not be increased, perhaps the bald area requiring the donor hair could be decreased. The standard scalp reduction would become the process that would "juggle the numbers" and achieve a new, exciting, and permanently altered ratio! The theoretical implications were indeed impressive and led to the decade of "reduction euphoria" from 1975 to 1984.

Regardless of the degree of baldness, it seemed possible to decrease the amount of alopecia so that the remaining bald area could be successfully managed by the transfer of whatever donor supply was available. Large bald areas, of course, would require greater scalp reductions than small bald areas, but the procedure could be repeated indefinitely with impunity until middle and posterior scalp baldness was either completely eliminated or dramatically "downsized." Unfortunately, theory never translated into a successful reality in men with extensive baldness. To understand the ultimate limitations of the classic standard scalp reduction, the reader must now endure a brief but required course in the dynamics of skin stretch.

When a force is applied continuously to a segment of skin and maintained at a fixed tension, the length of skin will elongate. This process is called *creep*. If the force is applied and not maintained as the skin stretches, the tension on the skin will decrease. This phenomenon is termed *stress relaxation*.[8] A standard scalp reduction is performed so that the maximum tension vector is at the point of closure, which is at the zone of remaining bald skin; unfortunately the minimum tension vector is in the zone of hairy skin, the very zone requiring elongation. Stress relaxation will occur when the skin under tension stretches.

This process has been given the aptly descriptive clinical designation of *stretchback*. Not surprisingly, skin that is stretched will therefore stretch back! The phenomenon of stretchback is well recognized by both physician[9,10] and patient.

Despite sequential scalp reductions in which enough bald skin was removed to mean the quantitative removal of all or most midscalp baldness, oftentimes nearly the same area of alopecia remained (Fig. 1-18). Astute observers correctly attributed this frustrating complication of stretchback to the closing tension. They reasoned, again correctly, that if the closing tension on the suture line were

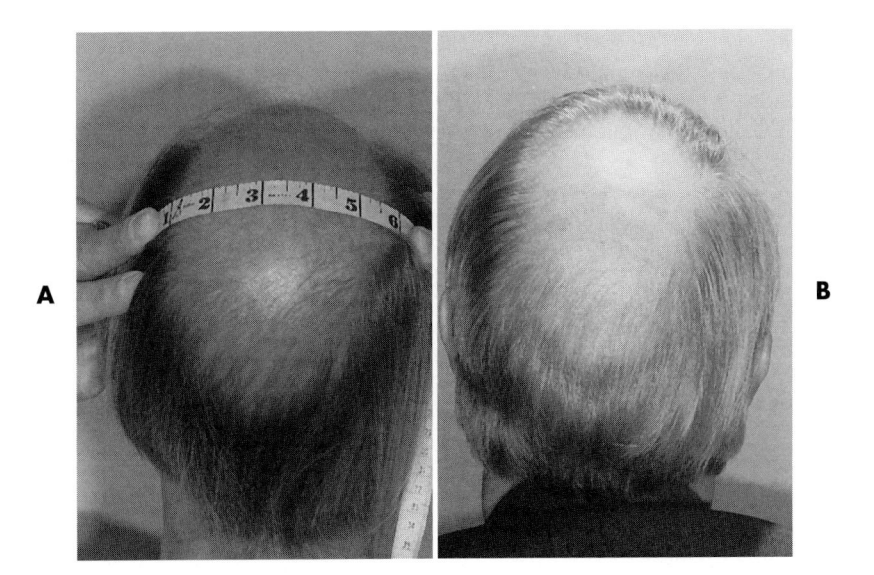

FIG. 1-18 A, Preoperative view of 44-year-old patient with approximately 5 inches of midscalp baldness prior to standard scalp reduction procedures. **B,** Postoperative result following punch grafting in frontal region and three standard inverted-Y scalp reductions. The first scalp reduction removed 1½ inches of bald scalp. The second scalp reduction removed 1¼ inches of bald scalp. The third scalp reduction removed 1 inch of bald scalp. Although a total of 3¾ inches of bald scalp was removed, the patient still has approximately 4 inches of bald midscalp remaining. Note that an almost undetectable scar is still a detectable scar.

minimized, stretchback would be minimized proportionately. If closing tension were insignificant, stretchback would be insignificant.

Although this approach was logically valid, it made the goal of the process—the elimination or significant reduction of baldness—unattainable for the vast majority of patients. Unless the scalp was loose and redundant, low-tension scalp reduction could not remove enough alopecic scalp to justify the surgery. If the surgeon exerted any significant physical effort to force the scalp closed, it stretched back, and the alopecia remained. If no force was exerted, it was rare that a significant area of baldness could be removed and again the alopecia remained.

TECHNOLOGY TO THE RESCUE

Although the recurrent reality of these surgical limitations threatened the survival of the standard scalp reduction, the recurrent dream of eliminating baldness by simply cutting it out did not expire. Rather this reverie was resuscitated and given new life by the second-generation "new and improved" models of alopecia-reducing procedures. These new techniques—extensive undermining (e.g., scalp-lifting), expanders, and extenders—all incorporated innovative modifications designed to slay the dragon of standard scalp reductions: stretchback. And all succeeded!

Scalp-lifting emerged as an alternative procedure that employed the rapid, dramatic, and extensive undermining of the entire donor scalp, for the first time well *below* the level of the inferior hairline and into the skin of the neck.[11-13] The primary forces restraining donor fringe movement were released by the radical undermining employed by this procedure, using the thinner, more resilient neck skin. This release permitted more movement with less closure tension on the remaining bald skin, which cleverly and correctly was never undermined and therefore not subject to stretch. Reduced closure tension coupled with the absence of recipient site undermining translated immediately into the absence or reduction of stretchback and consequently the dramatic diminution of the bald recipient area.

Another "heroic" approach was to elevate the superior margin of the donor fringe by slowly transferring the point of maximal tension away from the bald scalp and placing it squarely in the hairy, donor fringe where it also belonged! This approach permitted the hair-bearing skin to stretch and eliminated midscalp/crown alopecia, again with insignificant or no tension on the closure point. The absence of tension on the closure point logically translated into no stretchback. Scalp expansion used implanted inflatable, saline-filled bags,[14-18] whereas scalp extension used implanted linear, stretchable bands.[19]

34 General Considerations for Hair Replacement

All three procedures correctly identified the impediment to permanently reducing alopecic scalp and all three succeeded where standard scalp reduction had failed. Unfortunately these heroic, high-tech procedures also often failed in the correction of extensive baldness. The failure was aesthetic. These aesthetic liabilities, previously rarely seen in men with significant and extensive baldness, were (1) misdirected hair, (2) severely decreased donor density, (3) elevated inferior hairline, (4) detectable surgical scars, and (5) detectable halos—the strange island of hair that floated in the middle of the sea of bald scalp. Ironically, the deformity of halo formation was the direct consequence of the surgical solution to the problem of scar formation, namely hair transplantation, coupled with the passage of time and the loss of "permanent" donor hair. With time, it then appeared that the more we tried to make things better, the more we sometimes made things worse. What had first appeared to be the solutions to problems themselves became problems with no solutions.

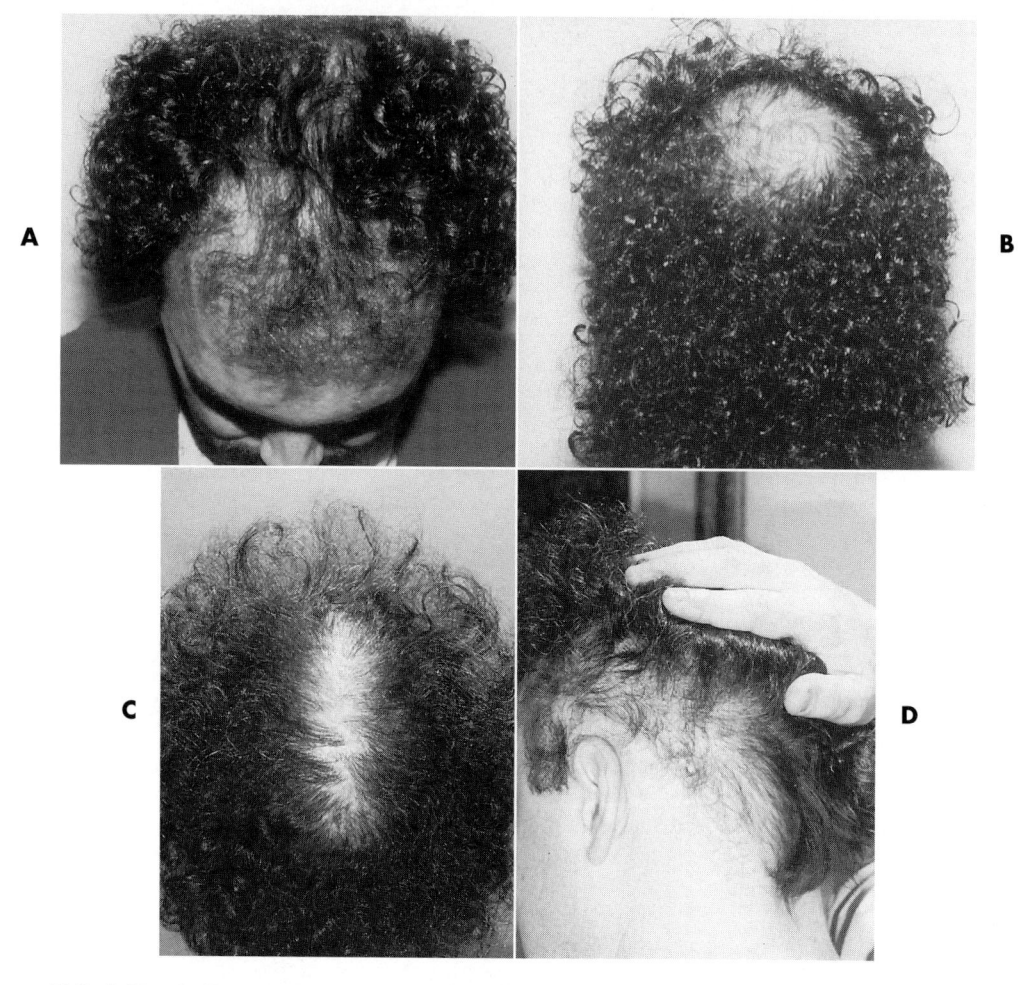

FIG. 1-19 A, Preoperative top view of 38-year-old patient demonstrating approximately 5 to 6 inches of midscalp baldness. **B,** Preoperative posterior view. Note that if this view were not considered in the context of the preoperative anterior view, it would incorrectly appear as if this patient had only 3½ to 4 inches of midscalp baldness. **C,** Postoperative result of the patient at 42 years of age. A combination of expansion and scalp-lifting procedures was performed to join both fringes in the midline and "remove all the baldness." Note "parting of the Red Sea syndrome": the hairs are unnaturally directed 180 degrees in the opposite direction on either side of the midline scar. Even if the obvious scar were only 1 mm in width, the patient would still have the deformity of permanently misdirected hair. **D,** Postoperative postauricular view demonstrates severe temporal thinning and an elevated inferior hairline. This unavoidable physical deformity is the consequence of expanding and stretching the fringe in men with significant baldness in an attempt to remove "all the bald area."

The Problem: Parting of the Red Sea Syndrome

The object of all second-generation alopecia-reducing procedures was initially to approximate superior fringe to superior fringe and thereby eliminate (or drastically reduce) midscalp baldness. Temporoparietal hair points directly down toward the ears and exits the scalp at an acute, rather flat angle. Midscalp hair, however, as previously noted, points in a *frontal* direction (a 90-degree shift) and has more elevation from the plane of the head. Touching or closely approximating both superior aspects of the fringe at or near the midline created a divergence of hair known as the "parting of the Red Sea syndrome." Hair that appeared perfectly natural in its old parietotemporal location suddenly appeared perfectly unnatural in its new midscalp location, 180 degrees divergent from its mirror-image twin just across the midline (Fig. 1-19).

The unhappy conclusion then was that total alopecia reduction for the middle and posterior scalp would result in a natural outcome only in older patients with minimal to moderate baldness. Ironically, many of this subset of patients have long since ceased to worry about an area they can no longer see.

In truth, the "Red Sea" dilemma had actually been recognized much earlier by practitioners of the standard scalp reduction. However, unless the patient had an unusually lax scalp, the "complication" of stretchback had prevented this occurrence in the vast majority of patients with 5 to 6 inches of midscalp baldness. Ironically, yet again, stretchback was working undercover to prevent a more serious complication, namely the "Red Sea" syndrome, and therefore grossly misdirected hair was only sporadically encountered and reported. Second-generation alopecia-reducing procedures, however, the savior for the extensively bald scalp, could produce this syndrome in all patients.

The Solution: Partial Scalp Reduction and Midline Transplantation

The proposed solution was to reduce the scalp only partially and subsequently transplant the vacant strip that was deliberately left in midline bald scalp with hair that pointed in the aesthetically appropriate direction. Again an answer that permitted the total elimination of baldness for almost all individuals appeared to be at hand. Again the solution was flawed. The frustrating factor in this instance was the unpredictable and often relentless progression of male pattern baldness.

Further Dilemmas: Halo Formation

Unless the patient was late middle aged or elderly, the viability of the superior fringe hair might be far from stable, that is, the so-called terminal hair might actually be terminal! As the superior border

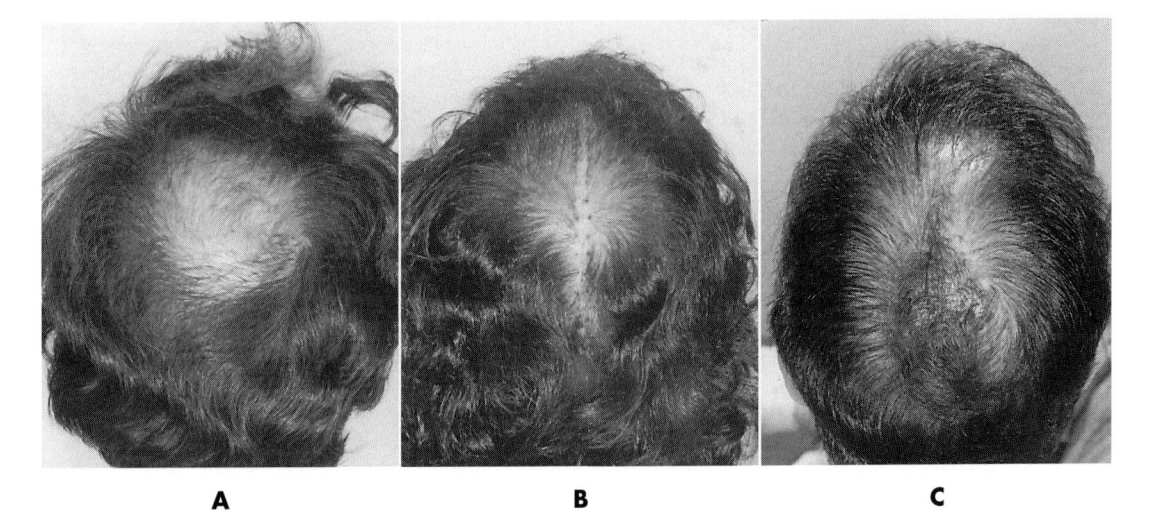

A **B** **C**

FIG. 1-20 **A,** Preoperative view of 41-year-old patient with approximately 4 inches of crown/vertex baldness prior to standard scalp reduction procedures. **B,** Postoperative view of the patient at 43 years of age following two standard scalp reductions with approximately 70% reduction of the bald area. Grafts were then transplanted into the scar and remaining bald area, resulting in the total elimination of crown/vertex baldness. **C,** Postoperative view of patient at 48 years of age demonstrating "halo" formation: a corona of new bald skin surrounds the previously transplanted vertex. The bald "halo" area represents the progression of male pattern baldness between the ages of 43 and 48 years, clearly demonstrating that what appears to be terminal hair at age 43 could become vellus hair by age 48.

of the fringe migrated southward, a perimeter or "halo" of new bald skin appeared between the fringe and transplanted hair (Fig. 1-20). Obviously a "Hare Krishna ponytail" of transplanted hair surrounded by a corona of bald skin is unnatural. The solution had with the passage of time become the problem.

Advocates of scalp-lifting correctly point out that extensive undermining permits the fringe to be elevated with less disturbance of donor density than expansion. Advocates of expansion point out, again correctly, that gradual inflation permits the fringe to be elevated with less disturbance of the inferior hairline than scalp-lifting. The patient and physician must simply decide which inevitable complication (deformity) is less objectionable. If total baldness removal has been accomplished with minimal disturbance of donor density, then the fringe must have suffered a disturbance of inferior hairline elevation. Conversely, if scalp reduction was accomplished with minimal inferior hairline elevation, then the fringe must have suffered a corresponding maximum disturbance of donor density. There is simply no escape from the physical laws that govern the reciprocal interlocking relationships among these various factors.

The Compromise

Second-generation attempts to achieve a statistically successful result that would remain stable over time continued to suffer the same frustrating consequences. A final effort to salvage the dream that refused to die led to the consideration of reducing some but not all of the baldness. The fringe margins would not be opposed and therefore misdirected hair divergence would not occur—one problem solved! The remaining bald area would not be transplanted so that halos would not cast their disturbing light in future years—another problem solved! There would be no inflated expectations of complete alopecic scalp elimination but simply the more modest expectations of a bald area still visible but now smaller—yet another problem solved!

The Solution: Careful Patient Selection

Of course, there is one solution to the vexatious dilemma of surgical scars that truly guarantees undetectability and total freedom from unnatural sequelae. That solution is to think very long and very carefully before ever making such a scar, especially on the scalps of patients in their 20s and early 30s on whose heads incidentally the majority of such "surgical signatures" are indelibly written.

During consultation, surgeons should go beyond the traditional seductively simple concept of alopecia reduction: "making the bald area smaller." What is often neglected is the fact that the description is purely relative: namely a procedure seen from the point of view of the alopecia reduction. But what if the surgeon were to describe to the significantly and extensively bald patient the same procedure but this time in terms of the fringe? What if the surgeon were to say, "I'm going to perform this fringe-stretching, hair-misdirecting, donor density–decreasing, inferior hairline–elevating, potentially detectable scarring procedure to treat an area that will probably be of little or no cosmetic consequence to you in a few years?" The procedure is the same, but the viewpoint is different.

At this point it might be incorrectly inferred that we are anti–alopecia reduction and pro–midscalp vertex baldness. Nothing could be further from the truth. But whenever a new position is suggested

---

FIG. 1-21 A, Preoperative frontal view of 43-year-old patient. **B,** Preoperative oblique view demonstrates a more revealing and accurate view of the eventual superior fringe loss than cannot be appreciated by **A** alone. **C,** Postoperative closeup view of hairline with comb following first minigraft session to demonstrate slight temporary "plugginess" that resulted when patient and physician decided to use large minigrafts. This "process" detectability is the price to be paid for eventual "product" density (see **E**). The second minigraft session was performed immediately after this photograph was taken. **D,** Result 6 months after a second session in which 200 quadrisected 5 mm minigrafts and 50 micrografts were transplanted into the frontal zone. Note the gradually increasing density and diminution of "plugginess." The third minigraft session was performed immediately after this photograph was taken. **E,** Postoperative frontal view 7 months after a third session in which 200 quadrisected 5 mm minigrafts were transplanted into 2 mm recipient sites and 50 micrografts were transplanted on the part side of the hairline. Note the dramatic alteration in appearance from **A** because of the deliberate decision *not* to achieve "see-through hair" over a larger bald area with the "1000-graft session." Product must *always* be a priority over process. **F,** Postoperative oblique view demonstrates the absence of transplants in the crown/vertex. The density of frontal region is a direct consequence of *not* covering the posterior area. In patients with dark hair/light skin, the area is left bald or covered with a nonsurgical hair addition. Micrografts could be used posteriorly and the result would appear natural but the patient might question the very marginal increase in density after hundreds of micrografts and thousands of dollars. **G,** Intraoperative view during fourth minigraft session. Note that no grafts are placed inferiorly in an attempt to connect the forelock to the fringe but rather the grafts are angled superiorly to mirror the eventual inferior migration of the temporoparietal fringe. In later years bald "lateral alleys" may develop as the fringe separates from the forelock due to male pattern baldness progression. The alternative, however, is to "chase" the fringe indefinitely with dwindling donor resources.

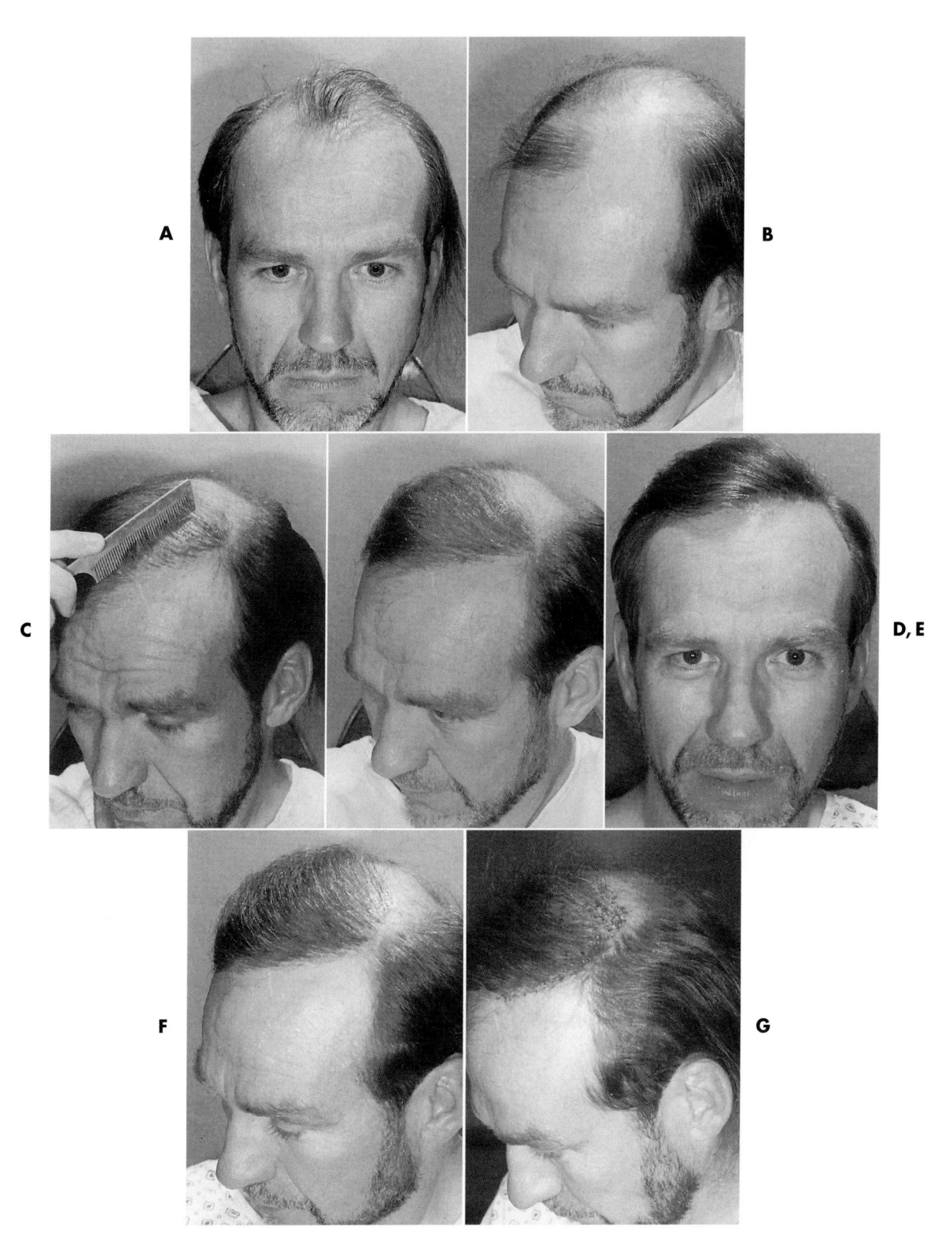

Reassessment of Male Pattern Baldness: A Reevaluation of the Treatment   37

FIG. 1-21 For legend see opposite page.

that appears to question or challenge any time-honored tradition in *any* field of endeavor, heightened emotions often produce confusion and misunderstanding. It is illogical to be either "for" or "against" alopecia reductions. They are merely surgical procedures with indications and contraindications. Indeed, if we are anti-anything, we are anti–male pattern baldness itself and not against the surgeon or the surgical technique employed to vanquish it.

Therefore, if the logic of this discussion is solid, then the conclusion is obvious. Unless the superior fringe has anterior- or anterolateral-pointing hair and is stable in position, any surgical reduction exposes the patient to risks of some combination of stretchback, divergent hairs, visible scars, decreased donor-site density, elevated inferior hairlines, and future halo formation depending on the type of procedure employed and the extent of current and future baldness.

Responsibility for the Risk of Adverse Long-Term Effects

Perhaps the patient should be allowed to assume these risks after a full disclosure of potential adverse consequences. Some physicians would permit the patient to participate in the decision of attempting to achieve total baldness elimination "today" with the possibility of a totally deconstructed, bizarre, and uncorrectable hair configuration "tomorrow." Other physicians recognize that a 20- or 30-year-old patient, although medicolegally responsible, may not be emotionally responsible when he asserts, "I just don't want to be bald at 30, and I don't care what I look like when I'm 50." If the surgeon is 50 years old, he/she knows only too well the logical fallacy behind such a viscerally vulnerable viewpoint and would find the downside risk unacceptable for a purely cosmetic endeavor. In short, the surgeon cares

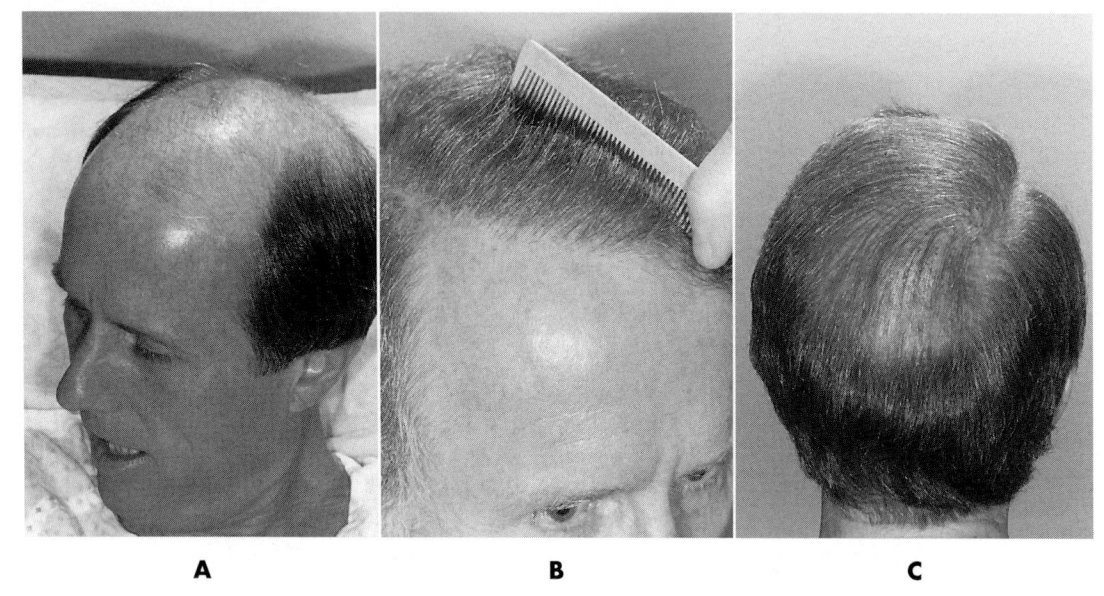

FIG. 1-22 A, Preoperative view of 51-year-old patient. **B,** Postoperative view. Note that the serendipitous combination of red-gray hair and ruddy complexion permits the illusion of maximum density after only four sessions and allows the surgeon to proceed farther posteriorly more quickly than would be possible if this patient had dark, straight hair and light skin. **C,** Postoperative posterior view after additional 400 quadrisected 5 mm minigrafts were placed into 2 mm recipient holes (in two sessions of 200 minigrafts per session) to create a thinning crown/vertex whorl. Note the placement of the whorl's center in the lateral aspect of the right upper quadrant. This design allows the hair to naturally cascade downward and cover the inferior bald vertex without wasting grafts in the lower region. Placing the center of the whorl in either lower quadrant forces the hair upward and does not permit maximum graft conservation. Note the excellent coverage achieved despite the fact that no scalp reduction has been performed to distort hair direction or leave possible unsightly scars. It is most important to note that these gratifying results are more attributable to this patient's fortuitous hair/skin combination than the skill of the surgeon. If this patient's hair were suddenly dyed black, the vertex would appear unacceptably "pluggy" and unnatural. In patients with dark, dense hair and light skin, *no* surgery or transplants should be performed in the vertex. If such a patient would accept "see-through" sparseness, then only micrografts should be performed. See the patient in Fig. 1-24 with this dark hair/light skin combination.

very much indeed how the surgeon looks at 50, and he/she knows that, despite the patient's protestations to the contrary, so will the patient when he arrives at the midcentury mark. The alternative viewpoint—that a cosmetic procedure should be considered ethically viable even if it might deteriorate into a noncorrectable deformity with the passage of time—is one that both surgeon and patient must carefully and leisurely explore. Male pattern baldness is after all still only a progressive condition; although unwanted, it is not a progressive disease.

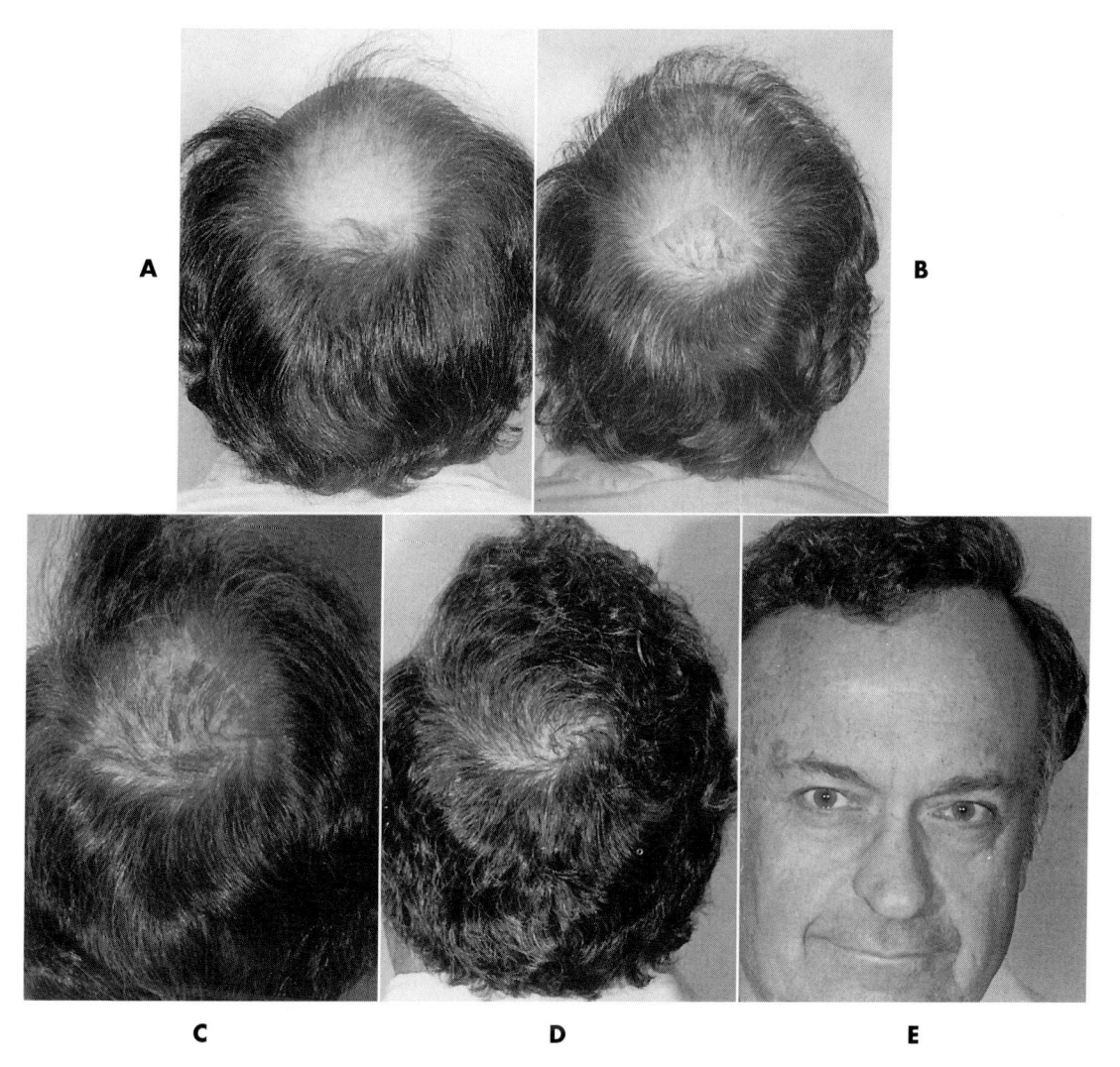

FIG. 1-23 A, Preoperative view of 58-year-old patient with moderate vertex alopecia. Note the cosmetically appropriate anterolateral direction of the hair at the superior border of "permanent" (permanent only because the patient is 58 years old) fringe. **B,** Postoperative result following one standard inverted-Y scalp reduction, two sessions of punch grafts anteriorly, and one session of punch grafts in the inferior bald vertex that begins the creation of the whorl. **C,** Postoperative result following second standard inverted-Y scalp reduction and second session of vertex punch grafting. Two small additional sessions of punch grafts were then performed in the crown/vertex to remove the reduction scar and to complete the whorl. **D,** Postoperative result following a total of two scalp reductions and four sessions of vertex transplanting. The patient is now 60 years old. Note that "all of the bald area" has been removed posteriorly and that the patient's hair appears naturally dense and properly directed. **E,** Postoperative frontal view demonstrating the "unconditional surrender" of male pattern baldness. Density and undetectability have been achieved both anteriorly and posteriorly not only because of surgical skill but also, and more important, because of the patient's hair color, pattern, and age. In real estate it is location, location, location. In hair replacement surgery it is selection, selection, selection!

The Solution: Frontal Forelock

Another approach is to do what can be done in a safe, conservative, and consistently natural manner. Unfortunately, this approach often requires patients to accept less than what they want and settle for partial, not total, correction. They experience "the thrill of victory" anteriorly and "the agony of defeat" posteriorly. If the full availability of an uncertain donor supply (the only certainty being that it will probably diminish with time) is exploited, a frontal forelock can be created that has excellent density, dramatically alters the appearance, and successfully frames the face (Fig. 1-21).

The forelock is constructed so that it will maintain a natural appearance whether it connects to the lateral fringes or is isolated from the fringes at the completion of surgery or in future years. It extends on its lateral aspects posteriorly toward the midscalp (not downward, chasing an unstable drifting fringe) in an upward slope that mirrors the

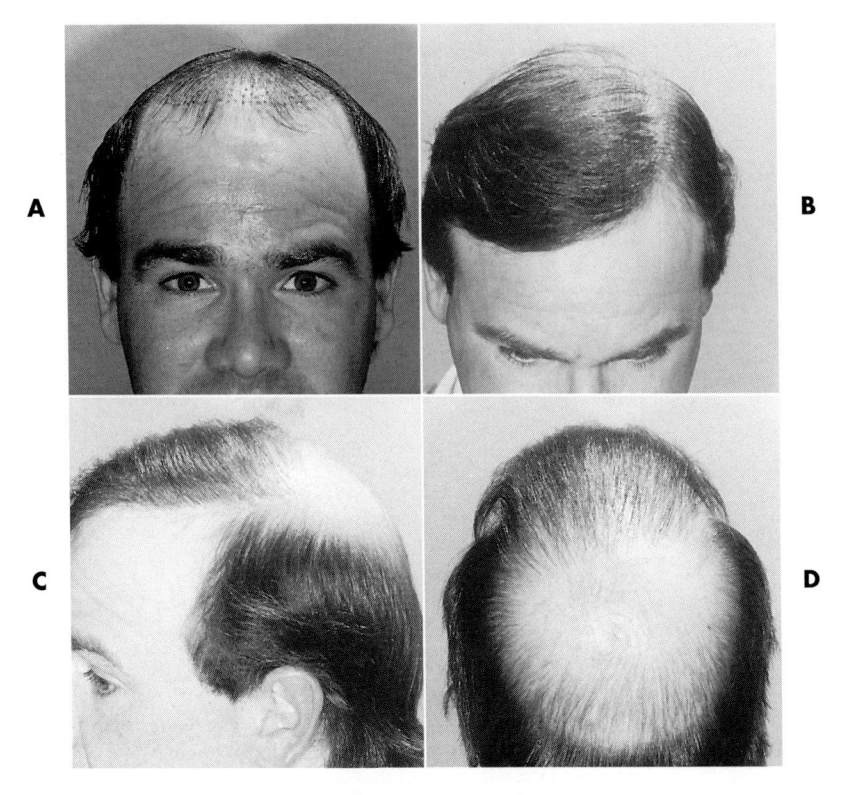

FIG. 1-24 A, Postoperative view of 26-year-old patient with dark hair and light skin 1 week after first transplant session in which 200 quadrisected 5 mm minigrafts were placed into 2 mm recipient holes and 50 micrografts were placed at the hairline anterior to minigrafts on the part side. **B,** Postoperative view after four transplant sessions in which 800 quadrisected 5, 4.5, and 4.25 mm minigrafts were placed in the anterior one half of the bald scalp. To soften the abruptness of the minigrafts, 200 micrografts were placed anterior to the minigrafts. Note the dramatic change in appearance afforded by the concentration of the grafts in the forelock area, thus deliberately avoiding the "1000 graft" squandering of precious donor seeds over the entire expanse of hairless acreage. Note that the density achieved is comparable to four-session standard 4 mm graft density. Whether a large number of small grafts are placed into a large number of small holes or a small number of large grafts are placed into a small number of large holes, the end result of density is similar. **C,** Postoperative lateral view. Note that the excellent four-session density achieved anteriorly always translates into a large bald area posteriorly. Note the resultant lateral bald alleys because no attempt was made to connect the frontal forelock to the inferiorly migrating fringe. Additional micrografts will be needed at the lateroposterior margin of forelock to mirror the thinning appearance of the superior border of the fringe directly below it. **D,** Postoperative posterior view. Note the density gradient of dense to thin to bald. If the appearance posteriorly appears "pluggy," the surgeon may quadrisect 4 mm grafts or ultimately use micrografts to soften the "posterior" hairline of forelock. Note that no further grafting is planned for the crown/vertex. The patient's options are to wear a hairpiece, be bald, or possibly undergo micrografting if he believes the cost/benefit ratio is acceptable to him.

downward angulation of the remaining fringe. The greatest density of the forelock is concentrated centrally, with a transition to extremely low-density, dispersed hairs on the perimeters laterally that mirrors exactly the gradient from thin to thick expressed by the hairs of the superior border of the existing fringe. This configuration is often created using large minigrafts centrally with small minigrafts peripherally, terminating in micrografts laterally. The worst scenario with this plan is the development of a naturally occurring variant of baldness: the isolated frontal forelock.

CONCLUSION

In the end the process of hair replacement (i.e., rearrangement) involves an unavoidable process of concessions and risks. The "pot of gold" is the total elimination of baldness, but the ride on the rainbow can be slippery and fraught with danger; if the surgeon and the patient fall off, it is a long way down! In an unpredictable way statistical probability dictates that some fortunate men with extensive baldness who attempt the journey will achieve a full head of hair that is natural in appearance, undetectable in terms of procedures required, and does not deconstruct with time because he ceases to bald significantly, and he begins the journey with a fringe of exceptional density, color, and texture (Figs. 1-22 and 1-23).

The same statistical probability also dictates that many more will face some degree of current or future deformity that will cause regrets and pain as the patient realizes, much to his surprise, that he actually does care how he looks at 50, and 60, and 70. Male pattern baldness is statistically progressive and statistically unpredictable (Fig. 1-24). Do we risk "shooting for the moon" or instead take the admittedly less than celestial course, the earthly path to reliable, but certainly not heavenly, results. Perhaps it is wisest to leave the moon just where it is—in the sky—and in the back of the head! Perhaps it is wisest for us, as surgeons, to approach each patient as if he were a member of our own family.

The answer might best be found with the principle that guides all of medicine and, incontrovertibly, cosmetic medicine: "above all else, first do no harm."

REFERENCES

1. Alt TH: Scalp reduction as an adjunct to hair transplantation. Review of relevant literature and presentation of an improved technique, *J Dermatol Surg Oncol* 6(12):1011-1018, 1980.
2. Alt TH: Advantages of the paramedian scalp reduction, *J Dermatol Surg Oncol* 14(3):257-264, 1988.
3. Bell ML: Scalp reduction, *Clin Plast Surg* 9(2):269-278, 1982.
4. Bell ML: Role of scalp reduction in the treatment of male pattern baldness, *Plast Reconstr Surg* 69(2):272-277, 1982.
5. Norwood OT: Scalp reduction in the treatment of androgenic alopecia, *Dermatol Clin* 5(3):531-544, 1987.
6. Unger MG: Scalp reduction, *Clin Dermatol* 10(3):345-355, 1992.
7. Unger MG: The modified major scalp reduction, *J Dermatol Surg Oncol* 14(1):80-84, 1988.
8. Manders EK, Au VK, Wong RK: Scalp expansion for male pattern baldness, *Clin Plast Surg* 14(3):469-475, 1987.
9. Nordstrom RE: "Stretch-back" in scalp reductions for male pattern baldness, *Plast Reconstr Surg* 73(3):422-426, 1984.
10. Norwood OT, Shiell RC, Morrison ID: Complications of scalp reductions, *J Dermatol Surg Oncol* 9(10):828-835, 1983.
11. Brandy DA: The bilateral occipito-parietal flap, *J Dermatol Surg Oncol* 12(10):1062-1066, 1986.
12. Brandy DA: Extensive scalp-lifting [letter], *J Dermatol Surg Oncol* 15(5):563-564, 1989.
13. Brandy DA: The modified bitemporal flap for the treatment of bitemporal recessions, *Aesthetic Plast Surg* 13(3):203-207, 1989.
14. Kabaker SS and others: Tissue expansion in the treatment of alopecia, *Arch Otolaryngol Head Neck Surg* 112(7):720-725, 1986.
15. Adson MH, Anderson RD, Argenta LC: Scalp expansion in the treatment of male pattern baldness, *Plast Reconstr Surg* 79(6):906-914, 1987.
16. Anderson RD: Expansion-assisted treatment of male pattern baldness, *Clin Plast Surg* 14(3):477-490, 1987.
17. Nordstrom RE, Pietila JP, Rintala AE: Clinical experience with tissue expansion, *Facial Plast Surg* 5(4):317-327, 1988.
18. Nordstrom RE: Continuous versus conventional tissue expansion [letter; comment], *Plast Reconstr Surg* 88(6):1108-1109, 1991.
19. Frechet P: Scalp extension. *J Dermatol Surg Oncol* 19(7):616-622, 1993.

G. Standardized Photography for Hair Restoration

Robert S. Haber

An effective presentation at a scientific meeting or for a high-quality journal article relies greatly on high-quality photographs. Unfortunately, at the time of a patient visit or surgical procedure, the care given to obtaining those photographs is usually inadequate. As a result, many photographs published or presented are of poor quality and suffer from poor focus, exposure, or composition. Photography should be considered an integral part of the hair restoration process, and the purpose of this discussion is to encourage hair restoration surgeons to master photographic technique in the same way they would master a new grafting technique. Fundamentals of photographic equipment and technique are reviewed, and a simple approach to determine the proper settings for any camera system in order to take perfect medical photographs is presented. In addition, recommendations are made for

> **RECOMMENDATIONS FOR HAIR RESTORATION PHOTOGRAPHY**
>
> 1. Invest in one of the systems discussed: studio, manual, or automatic. Best-quality photographs require a good-quality camera and lens and a studio setup, which can be accomplished economically in almost any office.
> 2. Obtain proper background material. Studio grey paper is ideal. Avoid dark background for dark-haired individuals.
> 3. Calibrate the system for use with manual settings as opposed to automatic settings.
> 4. For pretreatment and posttreatment photographs, use the same reproduction ratios (RRs), lighting, patient views, and background material.
> 5. Use slower film speeds, which produce excellent photographs with minimal grain. Such photographs are recommended for use in brochures and journal publications.
> 6. Follow guidelines for standard views as shown in Fig. 1-25.

the standardization of hair restoration photography. A highly technical discussion of photographic principles is avoided. Recommendations are made to simplify the process of obtaining a photography system specific for hair restoration patients (see box).

STANDARD VIEWS FOR HAIR RESTORATION PROCEDURES

Standard views for cosmetic procedures are useful for comparing results from different physicians.[1-3] They are most important, however, to ensure consistency within one surgeon's practice. Standard views of hair restoration patients are important because follow-up photographs may be taken as long as 1 to 2 years after baseline photographs. It is essential that all features of a photograph remain the same, including lighting, background material, hairstyle, lens, patient views, and reproduction ratio (RR). The RR indicates the relationship between subject size and the size of the image on film. It is determined by the distance from the film plane to the subject and by the focus setting of the lens. A photograph of a penny at an RR of 1:1 means the film image will be exactly the same size as the real penny. At an RR of 1:5, the image will be one-fifth the size of the real penny.

The patient should sit on a swivel stool facing the photographer to facilitate positioning. The patient should be situated about 2 feet in front of the background material to avoid shadows and 2 to 3 feet from the diffuser portion of the strobe units, if used. The photographer should be sitting at the patient's eye level and should focus by setting the lens at the desired RR and moving the camera forward and backward until the patient is in focus. This technique is known as *body focusing* (Slue WE: Personal communication, January 1992). Depth of field, which is the zone of clear focus in front of the camera, depends on the lens type and aperture opening and provides clear focus both in front of and behind the actual plane of focus.[4] Therefore do not focus on the closest point; otherwise clear focus will be "wasted" in front of the patient. Focus one third of the way between the near and far limits of depth of field to maximize the clarity of the photograph. In practice, for close-up photography, this point will be just behind the closest point of interest.

Our recommendations for standard views for hair restoration photography are presented in Fig. 1-25, A to K). We recommend using 1:10 and 1:6 RRs for each view. Taking two photographs at different RRs of each view increases the likelihood that an area of particular improvement will be photographed well and also provides a selection of photographs that fully protects the patient's identity.

Frontal view:	For consistent views, align the tip of the nose with the earlobes and ensure that the patient is looking straight ahead.
Lateral views:	Align the nasal tip with the earlobe so that this line is parallel to the floor. Rotate the head until the glabella is just visible.
Top view:	Tilt head down until the nasal tip appears to touch chin.
Posterior view:	Same position as frontal view but with the patient facing away from the camera. The patient should tilt his head up slightly for a better view of the vertex.
Optional views:	Some surgeons prefer 45-degree (oblique) views instead of lateral views and a slight downward tilt for the 1:6 RR frontal view. Closeup views may be taken of the hairline to demonstrate high magnification results.

CAMERA SYSTEMS FOR HAIR RESTORATION PHOTOGRAPHY

Hair restoration photography is not simply aiming a camera at a patient.[5] A hair restoration photograph should provide objective, reproducible information

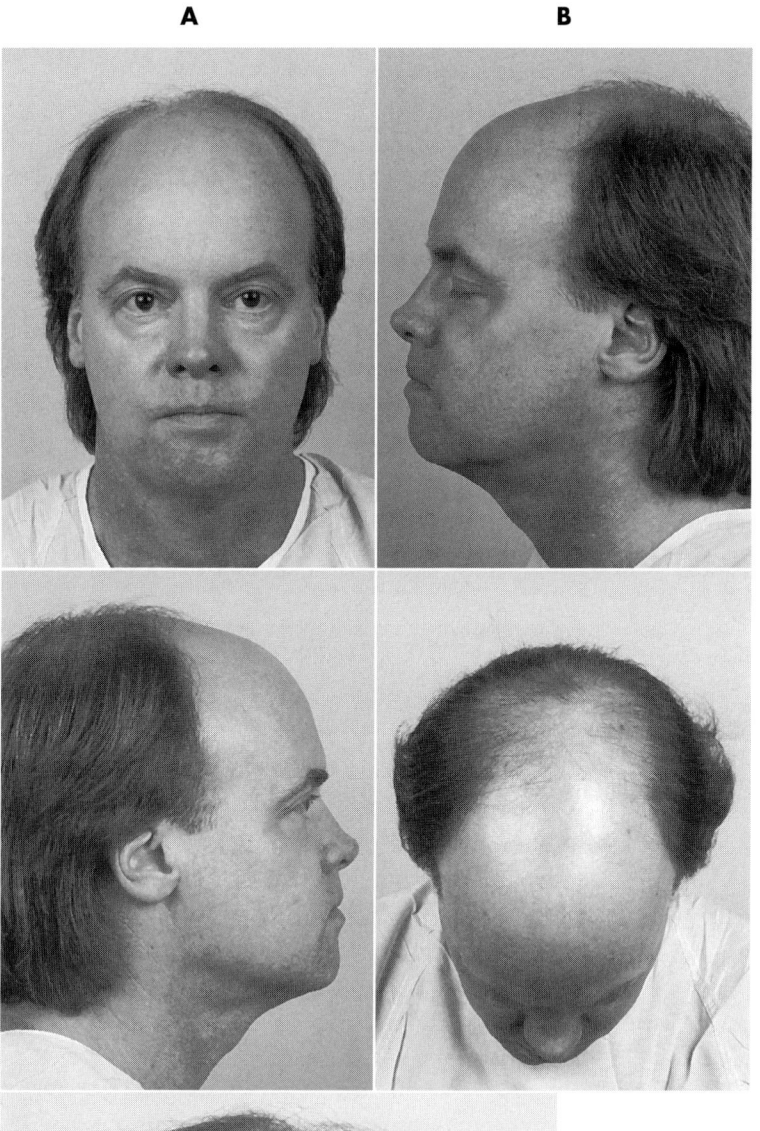

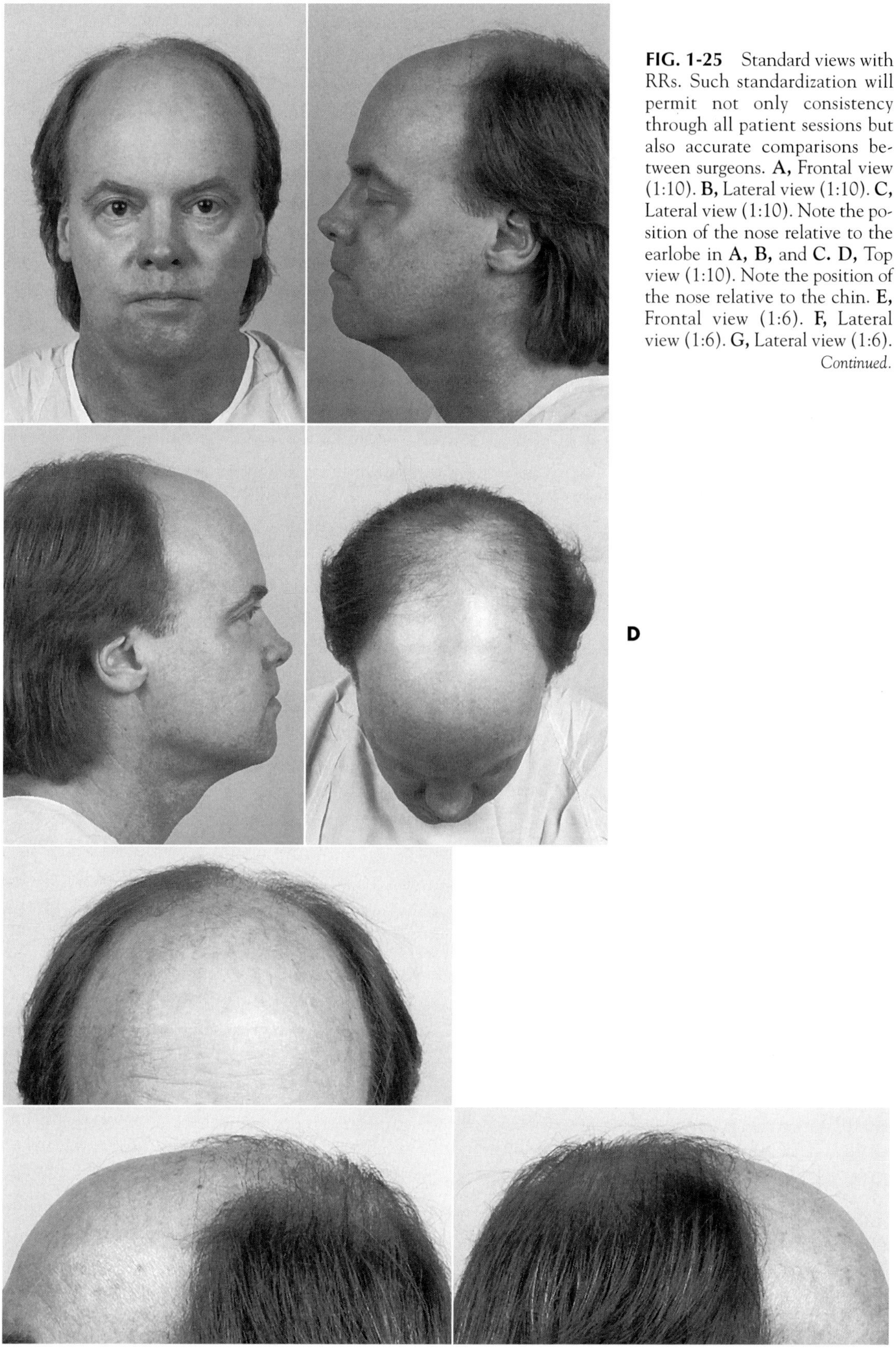

FIG. 1-25 Standard views with RRs. Such standardization will permit not only consistency through all patient sessions but also accurate comparisons between surgeons. **A,** Frontal view (1:10). **B,** Lateral view (1:10). **C,** Lateral view (1:10). Note the position of the nose relative to the earlobe in **A, B,** and **C. D,** Top view (1:10). Note the position of the nose relative to the chin. **E,** Frontal view (1:6). **F,** Lateral view (1:6). **G,** Lateral view (1:6).
Continued.

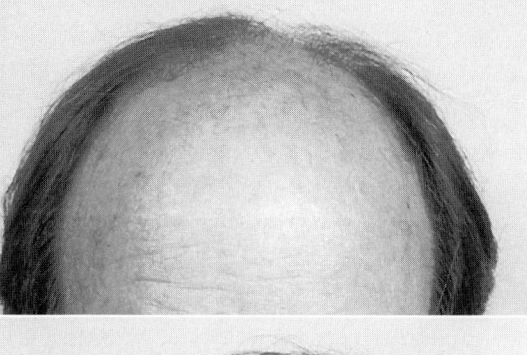

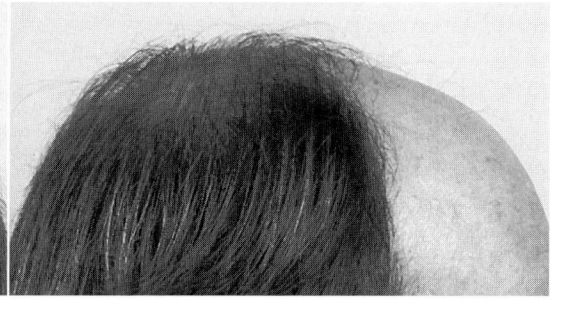

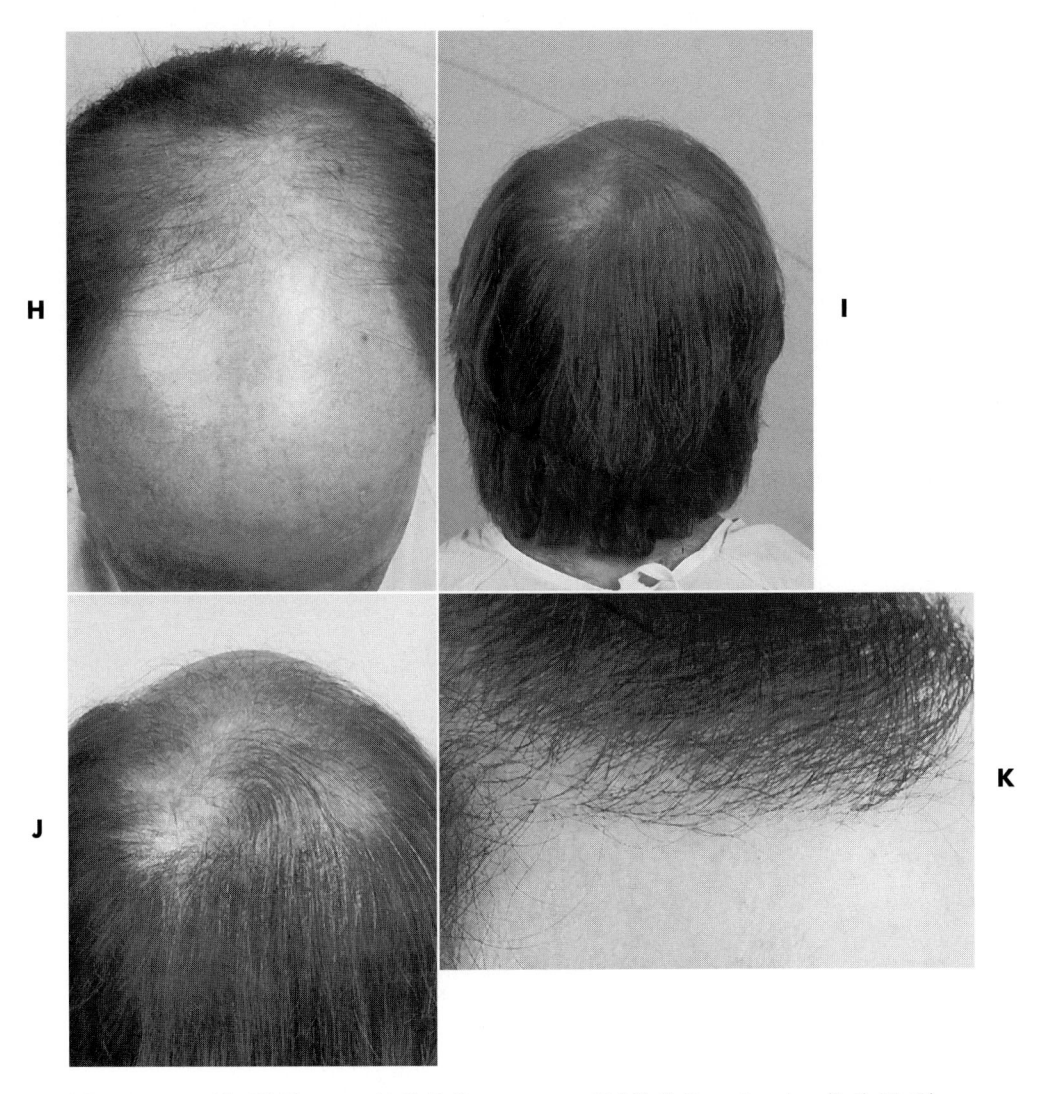

FIG. 1-25, cont'd **H,** Top view (1:6). **I,** Posterior view (1:10). **J,** Posterior view (1:6). **K,** Closeup view.

in the same way a well-designed experiment should. Hair is particularly difficult to photograph well due to the large depth of field required for the entire scalp to be in focus. Every effort should be made to avoid overemphasis or underemphasis of clinical features that might bias or mislead the viewer.[6] Overexposure may accentuate the appearance of alopecia, whereas underexposure or the use of a dark background will increase the appearance of hair density and thus must be diligently avoided. In addition, changes in hairstyle over time may alter the apparent results of surgery. Intraoperative photography of hair restoration procedures presents a special challenge because a variety of variables must be carefully timed and controlled in order to produce a high-quality result.

Studio Setup Approach

Best-quality results require a studio-type setup (Figs. 1-26 and 1-27), which includes two strobe lights with diffusers on tripods or mounted to the ceiling, a power source (Fig. 1-28), and a good-quality camera and lens (Fig. 1-29). The camera should be used with manual settings only. The benefits of this system cannot be overemphasized, and the extremely rapid, high-quality photographs that are obtained with this system should make it the standard for all hair restoration surgeons. Two strobe lights with diffusers will give a virtually shadowless effect with excellent depth of field, and identical preoperative and postoperative follow-up views can easily be obtained. We recommend a minimum light output of 400 watt-seconds for each unit and currently use two Norman LH2400B units (Norman Enterprises, Inc., Burbank, Calif.) with LiteDome 293 diffusers (Photoflex, Santa Cruz, Calif.) mounted on tripods. A power unit is required to operate the strobe lights; we use a Norman P800D unit (Norman Enterprises, Inc., Burbank, Calif.) with this system. This setup requires some dedicated space, but since tripods can be positioned against a wall when not in use and ceiling-mounted strobe lights can be retracted out of the way, the space requirements are actually minimal. This system is somewhat expensive, but the cost is well within reason for any practicing surgeon and is actually less than one might expect (Table 1-4).

Manual Camera and Flash Approach

The best alternative to a studio setup is the use of a high-quality camera body, lens, and flash that have been calibrated for use on manual settings. The type of lighting provided by the flash often will cre-

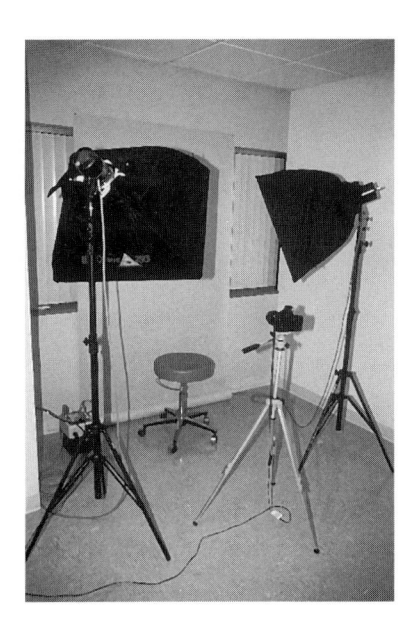

FIG. 1-26 Studio setup used to obtain all of the photographs in Fig. 1-25. All components are highly mobile and may be repositioned if the space is needed for other uses.

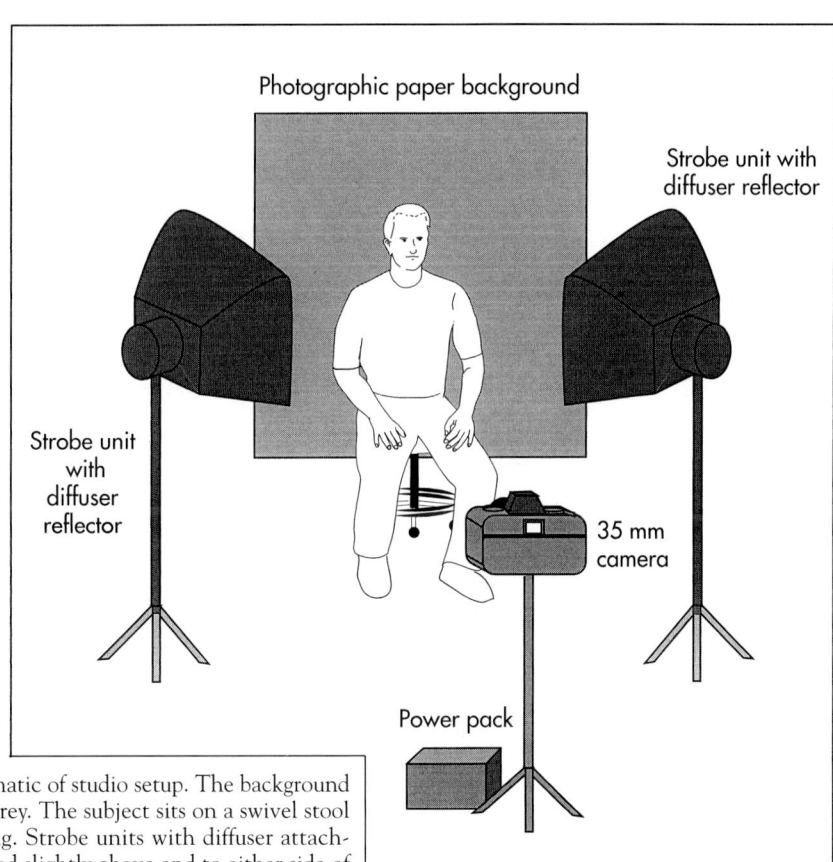

FIG. 1-27 Schematic of studio setup. The background material is studio grey. The subject sits on a swivel stool for easy positioning. Strobe units with diffuser attachments are positioned slightly above and to either side of the subject. The connecting cables are not illustrated.

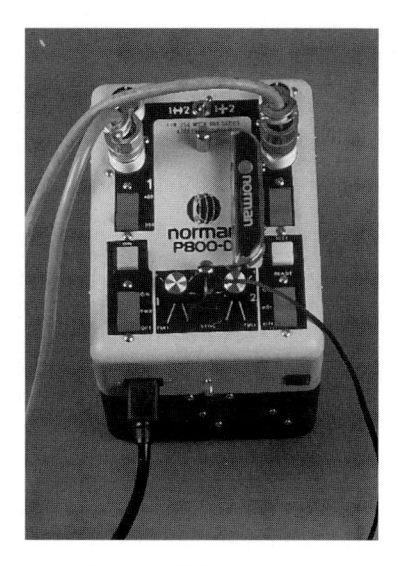

FIG. 1-28 A Norman P800-D power source is one of many versatile and effective units that can be part of a studio setup.

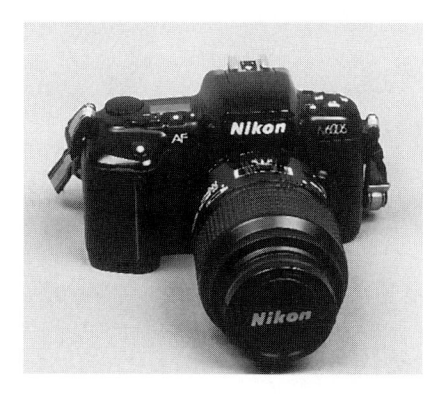

FIG. 1-29 Nikon N6006 body with Nikon 105 mm macro AF lens. Other equipment choices will also provide studio quality photographs.

TABLE 1-4 Systems for Hair Restoration Photography

SYSTEM	APPROXIMATE COST	ADVANTAGES	DISADVANTAGES
Studio Setup			
Camera	$3200	Excellent quality	Moderate expertise required
Lens		Moderately expensive	Needs dedicated space
Strobe lights (2)		Versatile	
Tripods (2)			
Power unit			
Manual Camera and Flash			
Camera	$1200	High quality	Most difficult to master
Lens		Most versatile	Need second flash to avoid shadows
Flash unit			
Automatic Camera and Flash			
Yashica Dental Eye II	$1350	Fair to good quality	Need second flash to avoid shadows
		Easiest to use	Narrow range of focus
Self-Contained System			
PDS-1 unit	$5000	Good to high quality	Not versatile
		Easy to use	Very expensive

ate unwanted shadows and will not provide quite the same depth of field as the studio setup, but if time and care are taken to master the equipment, high-quality photographs can be obtained. This approach is less expensive than the studio setup approach (Table 1-4). A second flash unit positioned behind the patient will help to eliminate shadows.

Automatic Camera and Flash or Ring Flash Approach

The lowest quality system that still provides acceptable results requires the same equipment as the manual camera and flash setup, but all settings are on automatic. An alternative would be a dedicated automatic ring flash unit such as the Yashica Dental Eye II (Kyocera America, Inc., San Diego, Calif.). With the camera making the decisions, the photographs will be well exposed but always at the expense of depth of field. Therefore in photographs taken with this system, only a narrow zone of hair is in focus. Any serious hair restoration surgeon who is planning on using slides at a meeting or in a journal should try to avoid this photographic approach. The cost of this approach depends on whether separate components are combined to create the system or a dedicated unit is used (Table 1-4).

Self-Contained System Approach

A number of manufacturers are beginning to offer self-contained units consisting of camera, lens, and high-power strobe light for use either in a fixed position or as a portable unit. An example is the PDS-1 (Photographic Documentation Systems, Inc., Los Angeles, Calif.). Although these units produce good-quality photographs, they are quite expensive (Table 1-4), can be cumbersome, and are not versatile enough for other office applications. These systems are probably best suited for a small office in which space constraints will not permit a studio setup.

EQUIPMENT
Camera Body

For hair restoration photography a 35 mm single-lens reflex (SLR) camera is ideal for cost, portability, and availability of accessories.[7-9] In this type of camera, light entering the lens is reflected to the viewfinder for composition and focusing. The photographer sees the actual image that will be reproduced on the film. We currently use a Nikon 8008S body (Nikon, Inc., Melville, N.Y.), although other models in the Nikon line, as well as similar models by other manufacturers, all perform as well.

The more expensive cameras have automatic settings, meters, and computers that help to determine the proper exposure and send commands to a lens and flash unit to assist focusing and exposure.[9] These cameras also may be operated in the manual mode, a feature useful in hair restoration photography. Many of the following features are found on modern cameras, only some of which are of use to the hair restoration physician.

EXPOSURE CONTROL

Exposure control refers to the camera options that may be used to achieve proper exposure. For hair restoration and dermatological photography, a camera with manual adjustments is desired since automatic functions do not work well at close distances.[4,9] All camera metering systems try to make all objects 18% grey. Light objects are underexposed, and dark objects are overexposed. In closeup photography, these problems are magnified. To avoid these problems, a series of test exposures at fixed camera-to-subject distances may be taken to determine proper settings for specific conditions.

FOCUSING SCREENS

The focusing screen is what is visible when one is looking through a camera's viewfinder. In addition to displaying the image, the focusing screen can provide a number of methods to permit focusing. The more expensive cameras will permit the selection of interchangeable focusing screens to best fit the subject conditions. In general, the most useful screen for dermatological photography is one with a matte surface and a central microprism, which can be used even in low light conditions and should be the choice when focusing screens cannot be changed. The least useful screen is one with a split screen since under low light conditions or high magnification half of the split screen may darken, making focusing difficult. Specialty screens with double cross hairs are most useful for very high–magnification work.

FLASH SYNCHRONIZATION

Until recently most cameras could operate with an electronic flash only at 1/60 of a second. At this speed strong artificial ambient lighting, such as that used for surgery, can adversely affect color balance. Newer camera bodies can synchronize a flash at speeds of 1/125 or 1/250 of a second, eliminating this problem. In addition, using a faster shutter speed lessens the likelihood of blurring during high magnification handheld photography. In general, the best speed for hair restoration photography is 1/125 of a second.

AUTOFOCUS

Available on many cameras today, a microprocessor determines when the film image is in sharp focus. Advances in this technology in recent years have produced systems that are remarkably fast and accurate, even in very low light conditions. Less accurate in closeup photography, this feature can be used during manual focusing as confirmation of an accurate setting. Autofocus cameras require autofocus lenses, which are more expensive and somewhat heavier than their standard counterparts.

BUILT-IN FLASH

Until recently built-in flashes were available only on snapshot cameras; now they can be found on high-quality camera bodies. Always of lower power than off-camera flash units, built-in flashes are more limiting for dermatological photography and should not be relied upon. In addition, since hair restoration photographs often include a subject's eyes, this type of flash will result in distracting "red eye" in the photograph.

Lenses

The lens is the most important and usually the most expensive component; good photographs are impossible to take through a poorly made lens. For medical photography a macro lens is necessary because these lenses are designed to be distortion free, permit focusing as close as several inches from the camera, and provide up to a life-size image on the film, with RRs usually printed on the lens barrel. Regular lenses with closeup attachments will not provide the same clarity.[4] We currently use a Nikon 105 mm macro AF lens.

Two types of macro lenses are useful in hair restoration and dermatological photography: 50 mm focal length lens (standard) and 100 mm focal length lens (short telephoto). The short telephoto 100 mm macro lenses are generally preferable for hair restoration photography since they can be used farther away from the patient and cause less distortion. To produce identical preoperative and postoperative views, a 100 mm lens is held twice as far from the subject as a 50 mm lens, which thus avoids distortion of facial features, in particular making the nose look disproportionately large. In addition, when a lens is held close to a patient, proper lighting becomes difficult and the patient may become uncomfortable. In an operating room it is clearly advantageous to be positioned farther from the surgical field when taking photographs.

Lenses called "macro-zoom" lenses are not true macro lenses, usually extend up to only one-fourth life size, and cannot be set to specific RRs. Therefore taking consistent serial follow-up photographs over time with a macro-zoom lens is very difficult. In addition, this type of lens does not provide the necessary detail required for medical photography and is usually more distorting.

Lighting

STUDIO-TYPE LIGHTING
As already discussed, this type of lighting is ideal and is far simpler and less expensive to accomplish than most people would think. The benefits include providing maximum depth of field and the ability to take many photographs in a very short time due to the almost instantaneous cycling time of the strobe light units.

POINT SOURCE FLASH UNITS
These flash units are versatile and may be camera- or bracket-mounted devices. The guide number (power) of a flash should be at least 80 (feet with ISO 100 film) in order to permit the use of a small aperture and thus maximize the depth of field in closeup photography. "Red eye" is also a potential problem with point source flash units, but this effect can be minimized with high ambient room lighting.

RING FLASH UNITS
These lens-mounted flash units are commonly used and provide a reliable source of light. They are not ideal for hair restoration photography, however, because they are usually of lower power than point source flash units and have a guide number of less than 50 (feet with 100 ISO film) that may not permit adequate depth of field.[7,9] The Dental Eye II, for instance, has a guide number of only 7.5 at ISO 100.

Film
There are an ever-increasing number of color transparency films available. The goal is to use a film that provides fine detail, good color rendition, and consistency from roll to roll. Kodachrome has been around the longest and is a simple film that requires a complex developing process. Available film speeds include ISO 25, 40, 64, and 200. Kodachrome 25 is the "gold standard" for dermatological photography due to its high resolution and its longevity.[9] Kodachrome 25 slides have lasted well over 40 years without fading or showing color change. Kodachrome tends to emphasize reds, however, which may make normal mucous membranes appear inflamed, and thus might not be desirable for intraoperative photography. We currently use Kodachrome 64 with excellent results. Clearly the most bothersome drawback is the 7- to 10-day turnaround time for film development in most areas.

Ektachrome film is newer and is a complex film with a simple development process, generally permitting same-day development. Available speeds include ISO 64, 100, 200, 400, and 800/1600. Its color rendition is considered to be more accurate than Kodachrome, although flesh tones may be underemphasized and somewhat sallow. Other film types include Agfachrome, Fujichrome, and Velvia. These films are of excellent quality, but they have not been available long enough to assess longevity.

The slower the film (or the lower the ISO), the better the color accuracy and image detail on the film. Slow films produce images that project very well, but they also require more powerful flash units for exposure. Faster films (higher ISO) will produce images with more grain and when enlarged or projected show less detail. This consideration is important to remember when designing a brochure or other patient information materials.

SPECIAL FILM TYPES
Film designated as "plus" provides higher contrast, which is useful for computer graphics and scenery, but it is not desirable for medical photography. Film designated as "professional" provides better color stability over its indicated shelf life, but it must be refrigerated until used and is more expensive. In general, special films are not necessary for hair restoration photography.

Since most photographs published in medical literature are printed in black and white and because prints made from black-and-white originals are of higher quality than those made from color originals, it is reasonable to consider using black-and-white film for photographs destined specifically for publication.

The least useful film to the medical photographer is color negative film due to the wide variations in the color quality in the finished print. In addition, there is the considerable added expense of making slide transparencies from prints if projection is desired.

PHOTOGRAPHIC BACKGROUNDS

Photographic backgrounds are essential in medical photography because they eliminate distracting background clutter and can dramatically emphasize a skin lesion.[8] The most popular colors for photographic backgrounds are black and dark blue. These dark colors are best avoided in hair restoration photography, however, because they deceptively increase the appearance of hair density and in a dark-haired subject may obscure the results of surgery, particularly in a black-and-white reproduction. Dark backgrounds can be used successfully with blond or red-headed subjects, but a medium-grey background works well for all subjects regardless of hair color. When a studio-type lighting with a deep depth of field is used, the nap of sweatshirt fleece tends to become visible. We therefore recommend using a roll of studio background paper of appropriate color.

BASELINE EXPOSURE VALUES

Regardless of the type of photographic system you select, it is necessary to expose a test roll of film to ensure that your photographs are properly exposed. The type of test required depends on the photographic system used.

If an automatic camera and flash approach is used, simply expose a roll of film using the subject views you have selected, permitting the camera to make the adjustments. In general, these photographs will be properly exposed but will lack depth of field, resulting in portions of the subject being blurred. Determine if unwanted shadows exist, and use a second flash if necessary.

For the studio setup approach described, if a combined total of 800 watt seconds of light output and ISO 64 film are used, proper exposure is generally obtained at an f-stop of 22. Closeup views of the hairline usually require an f-stop of 16. Using a test subject, start with these settings and experiment with larger and smaller apertures to determine the ideal setting for your system.

If you chose to use the manual camera and flash approach, a more detailed calibration is required. After a camera body, lens, flash unit, and film are selected, the following steps should be taken:

1. Set the camera for manual exposure
2. Set the shutter speed at the maximum synchronized speed
3. Set the flash unit on "manual"

At the manual setting the flash will deliver a maximal output each time, which will permit the use of the smallest lens aperture. On automatic settings or with through-the-lens metering, depth of field will always be sacrificed in closeup photography because flash units are not designed to be used closer than about 2 feet. Inside this zone, the camera's metering system is less able to interpret data, and the result is an overexposed or underexposed

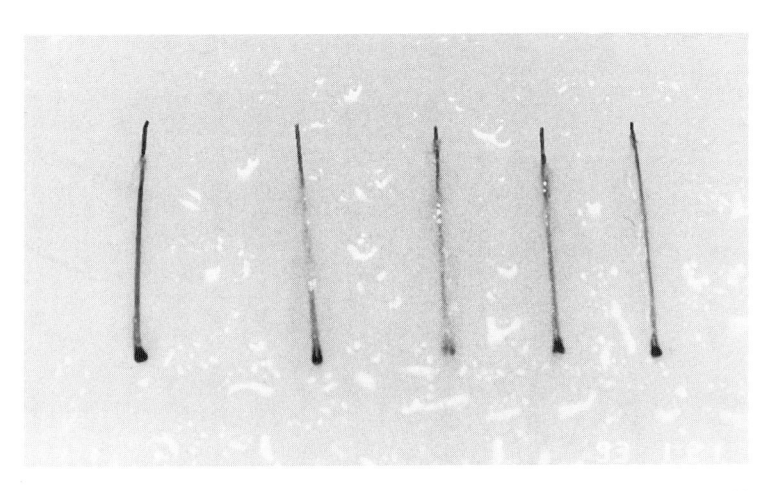

FIG. 1-30 High magnification view (2:1 RR) of single-hair grafts. See text for special lens attachment required for such a photograph.

Don'ts

Before

After

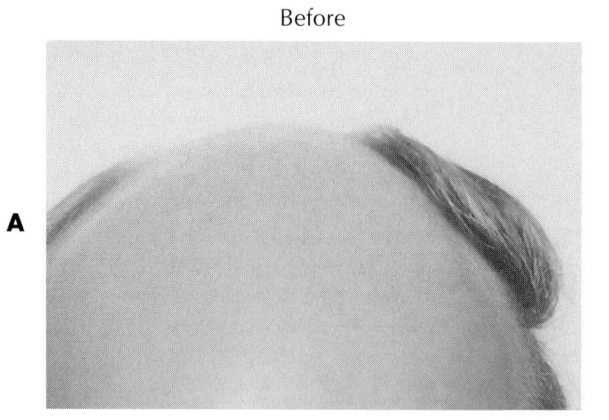

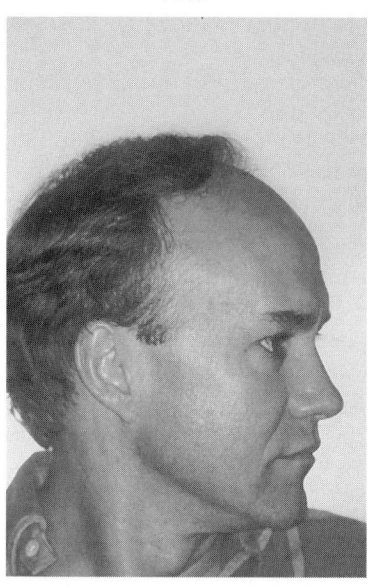

FIG. 1-31 Some of the most common photographic errors and their solutions. **A** and **B,** Do not use different views for serial photographs.

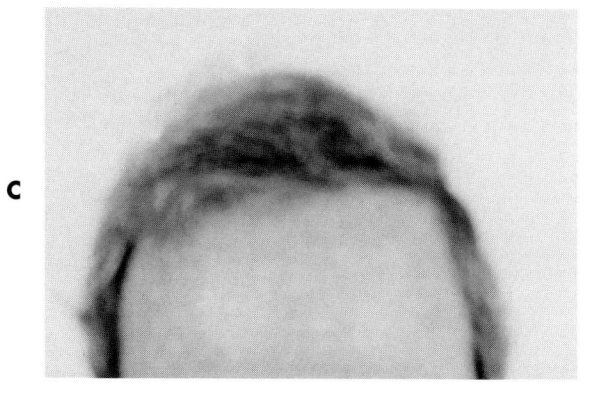

C, Do not use poor equipment and technique, which will result in overexposure, underexposure, or out-of-focus photographs.

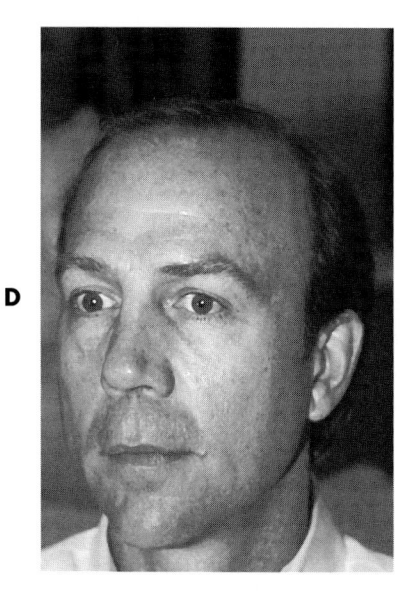

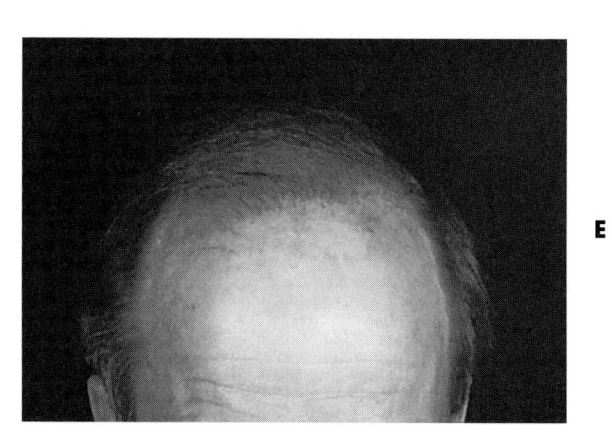

D and **E,** Do not include distracting background clutter or very dark background material.

Do's

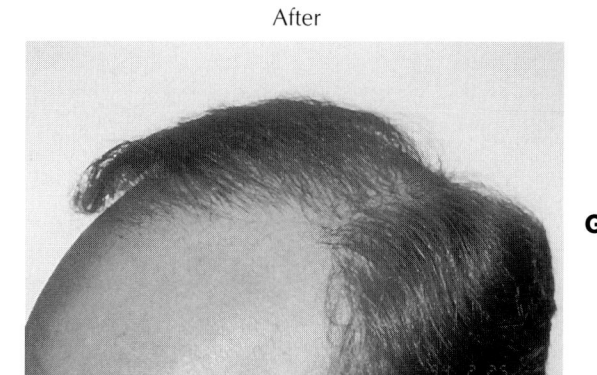

Before After

FIG. 1-31, cont'd **F** and **G,** Do match serial photographs *exactly.*

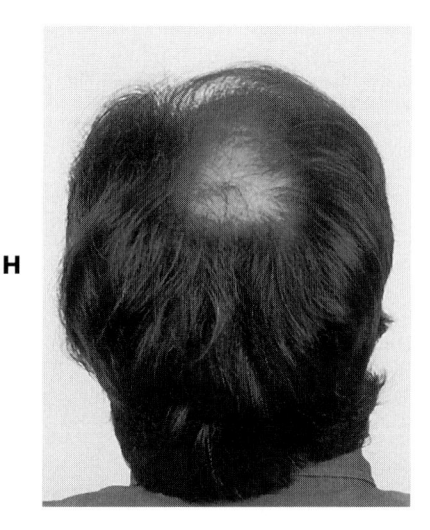

H, Do maximize depth of field and ensure proper exposure. This is accomplished with manual settings and avoiding the automatic mode.

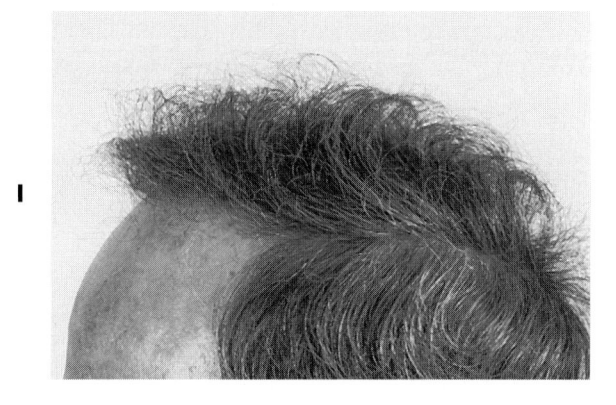

I, Do use unobtrusive background material.

Continued.

Don'ts

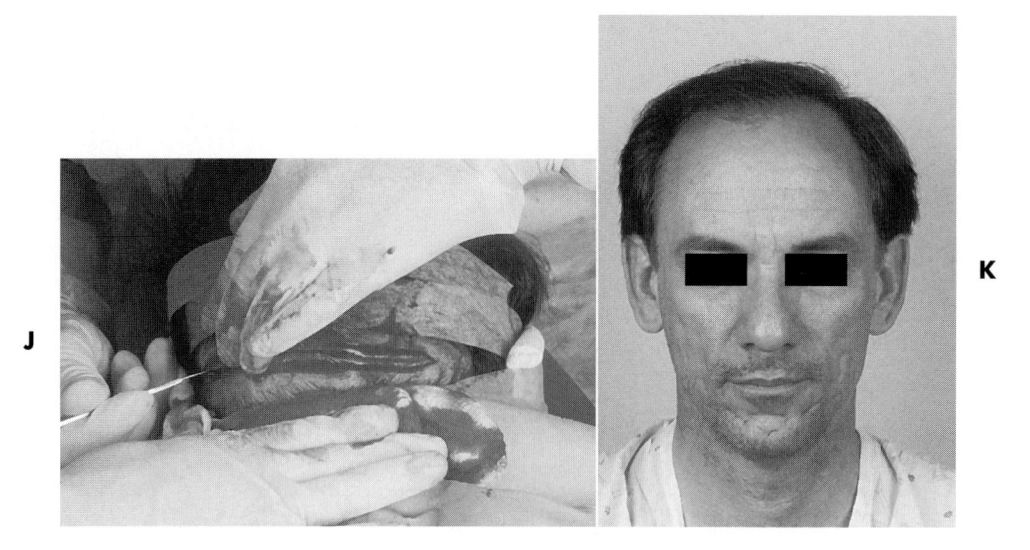

FIG. 1-31, cont'd **J,** Do not show blood or a messy surgical field in intraoperative photographs. **K,** Do not block eyes to "protect" the patient's identity.

Do's

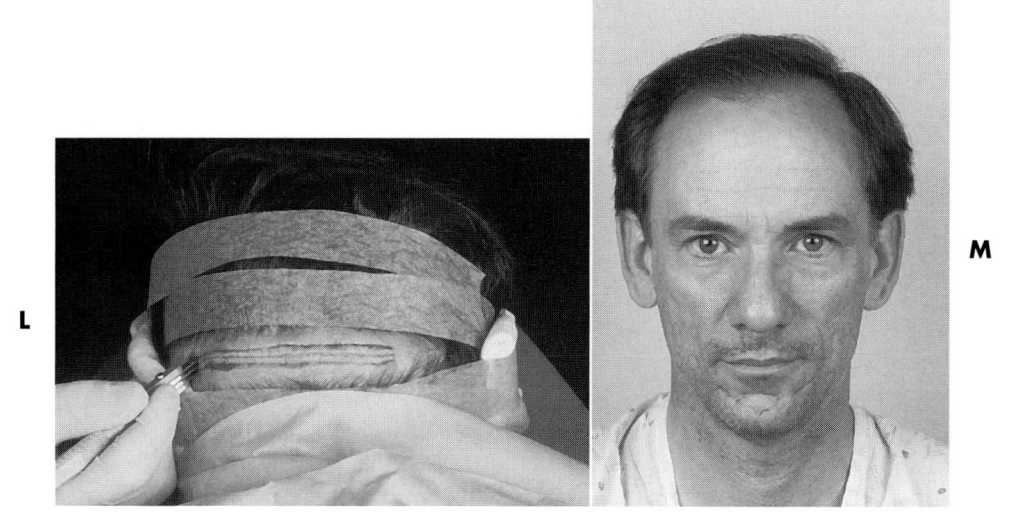

FIG. 1-31, cont'd **L,** Do take time to clean the surgical field before taking a photograph. **M,** Do obtain full patient consent for use of photographs.

photograph or an unacceptably narrow depth of field. Unfortunately, the recycling time of the flash will be longer when set on manual, and thus fresh batteries should always be on hand. As an alternative, to speed the recycling time, an adapter cord may be used to plug the flash into a wall outlet.

Choose a series of four common RRs starting with the highest magnification possible, generally 1:1 or 1:2, as well as 1:4, 1:6, and 1:10. This series will calibrate the system for the standard views as well as for the closeup views.

STEP 1. Set the lens at the highest RR.
STEP 2. Select the smallest aperture (highest f-stop).
STEP 3. Focus on the subject.
STEP 4. Expose six frames, decreasing the aperture one f-stop each time.
STEP 5. Reset the lens to the next RR.
STEP 6. Repeat steps 1 to 5 until the entire roll is exposed.
STEP 7. After development, view images on a light box and select the best image at each magnification.

The best aperture setting for each RR should be recorded and used for that combination of camera, lens, flash, and film. With all of this information listed on a card that is mounted near the camera for review, anyone should be able to take a properly exposed photograph with ease. If desired, one-half f-stop increments can be used for more precise exposure testing. Very light-skinned individuals may require one to one-half f-stop smaller aperture, whereas very dark-skinned individuals may require one to one-half f-stop larger aperture for correct exposure. Bracketing exposures on either side of the predicted exposure will ensure at least one usable photograph and will usually provide two or three.

SPECIAL SITUATIONS

Intraoperative Photography

Longer focal length lenses (approximately 100 mm) are preferable for surgical photography in order to permit the photographs to be taken from a greater distance from the surgical field and thus prevent contamination of both the patient and the photographer and avoid interfering with the surgeon. The surgical field should be as clean as possible and unnecessary instruments should be removed. As in other photographs, distracting backgrounds should be concealed with a suitable cloth.

All of the photographs of the procedure, including preoperative and postoperative views, should be taken from the same position and at the same RR. This plan requires preparation and keeping records of the view and magnification. The surgeon should be involved in the choice of the best view. Preoperative photographs are useful to document imperfections or facial asymmetry. Having preoperative photographs on file may protect against dissatisfied patients as well as lawsuits since patients tend to be more critical of their appearance postoperatively than preoperatively.

Ultra-closeup Photography

Extremely high magnification views (RRs greater than 1:1) are sometimes needed for recording individual trimmed grafts or abnormally growing hairs. Obtaining these views requires a special magnification lens that must be attached to a standard lens such as that available for the Dental Eye II. Fig. 1-30 (p. 49) represents a photograph taken with this system using the magnification lens. A device that permits a lens to be attached to the camera backwards will also permit high magnification views, but its use requires practice and patience to master.

PATIENT CONFIDENTIALITY

Historically photographic consent has not been a part of medical photography. Confidentiality was provided by applying a black strip across the subject's eyes on the photograph. This in fact remains the industry standard for all medical journals. However, the belief that concealing the patient's eyes protects the patient's identity is insulting to the patient and to the viewer.[10,11] In reality, anyone who would recognize the subject without the eyes covered can still recognize him with the eyes concealed. We are doing a disservice to our patients in a field in which privacy and confidentiality have been guiding principles for thousands of years.

Most patients readily agree to signing an unlimited consent form that permits the use of a photograph for publication in the medical or the lay literature for educational purposes. To show our patients respect, a consent form should be obtained for all patient photographs but medicolegally, patient consent must be obtained for *any* photograph that includes the face.

DO'S AND DON'TS

A variety of the most commonly seen photographic errors are illustrated in Fig. 1-31 (p. 50), along with the appropriate solutions. Remember that the most impressive surgical results will be thrown into doubt if the accompanying photographs seem misleading in any way. With only a small amount of time and effort, these errors can be avoided and your results will be clear and unassailable.

CONCLUSION

The goal of hair restoration photography is to produce consistent views over time so that results of surgical techniques can be objectively evaluated. A variety of photographic approaches can be used, and the choice of the photographic system will determine the quality of the result. A wide selection of high-quality, easy-to-use photographic equipment exists today, and any camera system can produce excellent results if a small amount of systematic testing is performed. The physician should invest in one of the systems discussed and should seriously consider using the studio-type setup because of the high quality that can be achieved at a reasonable cost. The common problems of clinical photography can therefore be eliminated with minimal effort. Protecting patient confidentiality is not difficult and must remain a priority.

REFERENCES

1. Vetter JP: Standardization for the biomedical photographic department, *J Biol Photogr* 47:3-18, 1979.
2. Davidson TM, Hoffman HT: Photographic interpretation of facial plastic and reconstructive surgery, *J Biol Photogr* 48:87-92, 1980.
3. Williams AR: Positioning and lighting for patient photography, *J Biol Photogr* 53:131-143, 1985.
4. Lefkowitz L: *The manual of close-up photography*, New York, American Photographic Book Publishing, 1979, pp 1-272.
5. Slue WE Jr and others: Snapshots versus medical photographs: understanding the difference is your key to better dermatologic office photography. *Cutis* 51:345-347, 1993.
6. Slue WE Jr: Photographic cures for dermatologic disorders, *Arch Dermatol* 125:960-962, 1989.
7. White H: Clinical photography in dermatologic office practice, *Cutis* 6:1099-1103, 1970.
8. Gibson HL: *Medical photography; clinical-ultraviolet-infrared* Rochester, N.Y., Eastman Kodak Company, 1973, pp 1-113.
9. Schosser RH, Kendrick JP: Dermatologic photography, *Dermatol Clin* 5:445-461, 1987.
10. Tarcinale MA: Medical photographer's role in protecting a patient's right to privacy, *J Biol Photogr* 48:183-185, 1980.
11. Slue WE Jr: Unmasking the Lone Ranger, *N Engl J Med* 321:550-551, 1989.

H. Medicolegal Issues in Hair Replacement

Robert Thomas Leonard, Jr.

As with all specialists in medicine, hair replacement physicians must be aware of the medicolegal aspects of their practice. Unlike patients who require the certain medical services and expertise from physicians to maintain or sustain life, our patients do not *need* hair restoration to physically survive. Despite the fact that we are not dealing with life-and-death issues, we must recognize that we are practicing at a time when members of our society are more litigious than ever before. It is important to remember that neither the physician nor the patient can accurately predict long-term hair loss. In this respect hair restoration can be regarded as a calculated risk. The physician should not be held liable for an unnatural result due to extensive progressive hair loss that ensues years after hair restoration. Therefore we as cosmetic surgeons must be diligent to practice not only exquisite medicine but also defensive medicine.

In approaching the hair restoration needs of a patient, the physician should follow the medical dictum—first do no harm. Consistent with the natural progressive nature of androgenic alopecia, the physician must always keep the patient's potential *future* hair loss in mind. Improper planning is one of the most common errors the hair restoration physician can make. Long before a hair replacement procedure is performed, the physician must practice defensively. There are several major issues to consider in order to minimize your exposure to litigation.

ADVERTISING

Advertising has become an essential aspect of the increasingly competitive practice of hair restoration. Thousands of dollars per year are invested in advertising by the physician. Often marketing experts are hired to provide services aimed at increasing the business opportunities for their physician client. The physician must carefully review both the ethical and legal ramifications of any advertising initiatives.

Some fundamental questions should be asked when preparing advertising or promotional materials. Do your promises coincide with factual reality? Does your advertising indicate that *no* scars occur with your procedures when in fact some scarring, although often minimal, results with *every* surgical procedure? Does your claim of "permanent solution to hair loss" really hold true given the progressive nature of androgenic alopecia? The use of the word "permanent" merits real caution. Although transplants have in the past been viewed as permanent, currently some individuals have pointed out that although transplants may be intact for very long durations—and often are permanent—this is not always the case. Do your hair restoration procedures actually culminate in a "full head of hair"? Are your procedures really totally "painless"? The natural state of an individual with androgenic alopecia is a thinning or balding scalp. Is it truly accurate to advertise hair restoration procedures as "natural"? Also, is it "natural" to have one's donor hair moved to the recipient site at all?

Surgical hair restoration procedures, although often multiple in nature, are marketed as being "inexpensive." When compared to nonmedical hair restoration such as the use of topical products, transplant procedures may be less expensive over a period of time. However, hair restoration surgery is certainly not inexpensive. You must personally and critically review all your promotional material for accuracy and forthrightness.

As the business aspects of a hair restoration practice become more complex, they also become extremely time consuming to the physician. Most busy hair restoration physicians hire lay consultants or medical technicians to aid in the initial consultations with prospective patients. This situation in itself can be a source of potential litigation. When physicians perform their own consultations, they know exactly what was said to the patient. Do they really know what their consultants may have told the patients? Therefore it is always wise to meet with your patients before initiating therapy or performing surgery to assess for yourself the hair loss status and the patient's expectations regarding hair restoration. You must be certain that the patient's expectations are in line with what can realistically be achieved. If not, you should postpone the procedure so that misunderstandings can be addressed. Once the patient has read a general description of a hair replacement procedure and has undergone a complete consultation with a physician and/or physician's aide, the informed consent issue should not be brought forth.

The latest ploy by the legal profession is to charge fraud and misrepresentation because it has proven difficult to win malpractice claims against hair restoration physicians. The definition of *fraud* is "dishonest practice; breach of confidence." *Misrepresentation* is legally defined as "representing falsely or imperfectly." It is imperative to know that your promotional materials are accurate, informative, and realistic.

Physician negligence is often difficult to prove in hair restoration due in part to the problem of assigning a standard of care within a given community. Currently there is such a wide discrepancy in techniques among hair transplant surgeons that the standard of care has become obscure. Likewise, if the patient grows any hair at all, it is often difficult to assess negligence on the part of the physician.[1]

The following case is an example of one of the few legal cases brought to trial in hair restoration surgery. In GK vs. JMY, the patient brought a medical malpractice suit against a dermatologist who performed hair plug transplants. In the Civil District Court for the Parish of Orleans, No. 77-17611, Division G, Judge Steven R. Plotkin dismissed the suit and the patient appealed. In the Court of Appeals, Judge Redmann held that (1) questions and answers in the dermatologist's pamphlet explaining hair transplants were not misleading and did not promise the patient anything; (2) as to the claim of lack of informed consent to cutting of the scalp, the patient had to expect some cutting; and (3) although the plaintiff was apparently one of the rare patients who experienced pain, the dermatologist's pamphlet, which stated that postoperative pain was rare, did not fail to inform him that he might experience pain. This case illustrates the issues discussed, namely an attorney's attempt to prove misrepresentation and a claim of lack of informed consent. This case was initially dismissed; the finding was then affirmed on appeal.

CONSULTATION

When you meet with patients in consultation, you must be straightforward and complete in understanding their expectations, discussing their clinical situation, explaining their diagnosis, informing them of their medical and/or surgical options, and specifically outlining their treatment plan. You must be certain to discuss every issue in terms that patients will easily comprehend and to carefully explain any medical terminology to the patients, particularly that pertaining to potential side effects of medications and adverse reactions to procedures.

Before examining a patient, you must be sure to obtain both a complete medical history and a complete history regarding his hair loss situation. Litigation can be initiated if important medical history is overlooked. Information on past adverse reactions to medications, especially to local anesthetic agents, is critical. Cardiac disease history is crucial to elicit because agents commonly administered in hair restoration surgery can adversely affect the cardiovascular system. It is important that the surgeon know prior to surgery about a history of bleeding dyscrasias and the patient's current usage of medications and vitamins that affect clotting ability. A discussion of psychiatric problems should also be addressed when a patient's history is being obtained.

A thoughtfully designed hair restoration medical questionnaire and preoperative instruction form will assist the physician in identifying potential medical difficulties that may affect the surgical and consequently the medicolegal outcomes (see Appendixes F and H). If at any time you believe that further documentation and medical evaluation may be necessary prior to initiating hair restoration surgery or treatment, you should obtain the patient's permission to speak with his primary care physician for assistance.

The estimated number of procedures to be undertaken in the immediate future (i.e., 1 to 2 years) should also be discussed with the patient. Since neither the patient nor the physician can predict the eventual extent of hair loss, the unforeseen number of procedures would not necessarily need to be estimated.

Remember that although patients may feel that for them hair restoration is a lifesaving procedure, you should never be forced to perform a procedure or initiate a treatment plan on someone who may not be a safe candidate. As with all aspects of medical practice, careful documentation of a given patient's medical conditions is the physician's best line of defense against litigation.

Although hypertrophic scarring may be a rare complication in surgical hair restoration, it is critical to inquire about a history of keloid formation. If there is any question regarding possible keloid formation, it is prudent to perform a keloid test (i.e., transplantation of a single graft and observation of its healing outcome). Of course, informed consent for this procedure must also be obtained.

A documented history of previous surgery performed or treatment undertaken on a patient is essential. If this information is not obtained, defense of possible future litigation may be difficult. A 35 mm camera for preoperative or pretreatment photographs is an important tool. With photographs, you can easily prove that possible poor results were not yours and instead were those of the previous physician. Photographic documentation of the various phases of hair restoration procedures is also helpful, particularly in noncompliant patients (see Chapter 1, Part G).

It is often difficult for a physician *not* to offer therapy to a patient in physical or psychological pain. Many patients suffering from hair loss want their hair restored to its prepubertal state: a full, thick head of hair with a straight hairline low on the forehead! This desire on the part of the patient for complete fulfillment means that one of the most important functions of the hair loss consultation is to assess the patient's expectations (see Chapter 1, Part E). Patient expectations that are not realistic and not in accordance with surgical or medical goals may precipitate a lawsuit.

In discussing the procedures and the results of those procedures with a patient, the physician must not promise in any way that the patient will achieve a complete, full head of hair. For instance, the patient must understand that the physician's skill and ability lie in placing grafts in such a way as to create the illusion of a full head of hair, but that the physician cannot actually create a full head of hair.

Physicians must guard against patients who try to coerce them to perform procedures or prescribe treatments that are not appropriate. For example, a hairline should not be transplanted too anteriorly.

The physician, not the patient, will be considered the one to know what is cosmetically correct or not. Patients often want a low, youthful hairline. Although such hairlines may look natural for several years, with the passage of time and continued hair loss, they will not be appropriate and may appear unnatural. If the patient insists on the placement of a hairline that the physician believes is not in the patient's best interest, the patient should sign an exclusionary waiver before any procedure is undertaken.

The last important component of the consultation is a discussion of the number of procedures required and the cost. It must be remembered that fraud and misrepresentation are the legal avenues that attorneys are traveling. The *initial* minimum number of visits and the cost should carefully be explained to the patient. Documentation of this discussion should be included in the patient's medical record.

Even if every precaution is taken and all of the recommended steps are followed, there is no guarantee that lawsuits will be avoided. Despite meticulous technique and acceptable results, not all patients are pleased with the results of hair restoration procedures. When dissatisfaction occurs, a lawsuit may ensue. In cases in which the patient is unhappy with the result and all of the recommended steps were followed, there should be no grounds for litigation. The patient should not be able to receive monetary remuneration simply because he is unhappy with the results. The physician's best protection, however, is accurate documentation of what was said and ultimately what was done for the patient.

INFORMED CONSENT

Experts in the field of medical malpractice litigation are well aware that specific operative consent by a patient will not prevent litigation. Lack of informed consent, however, will expedite a lawsuit. The physician should have a complete informed consent discussion with the patient. The patient should be required to sign a consent form that grants specific permission by the patient for the physician to perform the scheduled procedure or treatment. The consent form must indicate that the procedure itself was fully explained and that alternative treatments for the condition were discussed.

Surgeons should obtain permission for their assistants to perform certain parts of the procedure as needed. Consent should include permission for the administration of anesthetics and any other medication that may be required to properly treat the patient. Because complications may occur in the hands of even the most experienced and skilled physician, the most common known complications should be carefully explained to the patient and included in the consent form. These complications include excessive bleeding, infection, dysesthesia of the donor and recipient sites, reactions to medications including possible death, hypertrophic scarring, and poor hair growth. A partial list of rare complications can also be included.

Patient acknowledgment that he had all of his questions answered satisfactorily by the physician and that he understands the contents of the informed consent must be part of the form. Once again all details of the procedure should be discussed and explained so that a reasonable person could understand the operation and could therefore refuse the procedure based on the possible complications that could occur.

As hair restoration techniques continue to be refined and public interest in these procedures grows, an increasing number of physicians are including hair restoration as part of their practices. Hair transplantation can be a rewarding experience for both the patients who benefit from increased self-esteem and the physicians who provide the service. However, for the benefit of the public and the physician, it is important that the patient and the doctor acknowledge and understand every aspect of this area of medicine. In doing so, the physician can look forward to each patient with enthusiasm and confidence.

REFERENCE

1. Stough DB: Legal obligations of hair transplant surgery: covering the basics, *Cosmet Dermatol* 6:10, 1993.

2

Preoperative Stages

A. The History of Hair Restoration Surgery

David S. Orentreich

THE 1800s

As early as 1804 or 1818, Baromio had demonstrated the possibility of successful hair-bearing transplants in animals (Friederich, personal communication). However, according to Friederich, the first to have the idea of treatment of calvities by hair transplantation was Dom Unger (1822), who said "tunc calvities res rara erit" (then baldness will be a rare thing).[1]

Unger's student, Dieffenbach, published an inaugural thesis at Wurzburg in 1822.[1] In this thesis Dieffenbach described investigations in allotransplantation and autotransplantations of hair, feathers, and skin in animals. A self-autotransplantation (autograft) of hairs in prepared vulnerations (wounds) of the skin was successful.

Hair-bearing autografts for the correction of traumatic alopecia have been carried out with varying degrees of success since 1893.[2-8] Flaps and relatively large free grafts were the methods used.

THE EARLY 1900s

Autografts to the eyebrow, hand, scalp, and other areas have shown not only the hair growth desired in such grafts but also occasionally the development of unwanted hair.[9-20] The hair shaft insertion method was reported by Sasagawa[21] in 1930. In 1939, Okuda,[22,23] a Japanese dermatologist, described the use of small full-thickness autografts of hair-bearing skin for the correction of alopecia of the scalp, eyebrow, and mustache areas. This method was almost the same as N. Orentreich's technique, which was reported in 1959.[24] Okuda constructed special metal trephines (circular punches) with diameters of 2 to 4 mm and used these to bore out grafts from hair-bearing areas of the scalp. A similar instrument was used to prepare recipient sites in the area of alopecia into which the grafts were placed. He noted that better cosmetic results were achieved if slightly smaller trephines were used for the recipient holes. A total of 200 patients, most of whom had cicatricial alopecia, were successfully treated in this fashion. Okuda did not, however, specifically note its use in patients with male pattern baldness (androgenic alopecia).

In 1943, Tamura[25] reported the reconstruction of the female pubic escutcheon by grafting single hairs. Fujita[26] reported the eyebrow reconstruction in leprosy patients by punctiform hair grafting in 1953. In this technique, a free skin graft with hair is divided by scalpel or scissors into small pieces, each of which contains from two to ten hairs. The pieces are inserted separately into individual holes in the recipient area that have been prepared using a thick injection needle or a slender scalpel.

In addition, Fujita[27] reported the use of this technique to treat burn scar alopecia, eyebrow alopecia caused by x-ray therapy for hemangioma, eyebrow and eyelash defects associated with a pigmented nevus around the eyelids, absence of pubic hair in a 23-year-old woman, occipital lesion of alopecia areata, and vitiligo involving the corner of the mouth and mustache.

WORLD WAR II AND THE DECADES THAT FOLLOW

Unfortunately, because of World War II, Okuda's work was not recognized outside Japan until many years later. His original procedures were not acknowledged until recently. Thus knowledge and trial of these techniques outside Japan were long delayed.[28] However, in 1970, Friederich[29] mentioned Okuda's significant contribution and aptly designated the free punch graft method as the Okuda-Orentreich technique.

In 1950, Barsky[9] reported in the American literature a case of cicatricial alopecia of the occipital scalp that was improved by implanting small islands of hair-bearing skin and permitting the hair to grow long. He also noted that the transplantation of pubic or axillary hair-bearing skin to replace a hairy portion of the scalp or the face results in a rather bizarre effect because the donor hair is entirely different from that of the scalp or face.

The success of hair-bearing autografts (hair transplants) for the correction of androgenic alopecia and certain other alopecias was shown to depend on the phenomena of donor dominance and recipient dominance. Introduced by N. Orentreich[24] in 1959 (Fig. 2-1), the term *donor dominance* describes autografts that maintain their integrity and characteristics after transplantation to a new site; *recipient dominance* describes autografts that take on the characteristics of the recipient site. These concepts of dominance were developed as the result of studies undertaken in the mid-1950s to gain understanding of the pathogenesis and localization of various dermatological disorders, including several types of alopecia.

The research use of such autografts with appropriate and multiple controls helped to further understanding of physiological and pathological cutaneous phenomena. Many previous hair transplantation studies had either failed or produced contradictory results; moreover, confusion had resulted from transplants that had failed to "take" or had been only partially successful.

The experiment described in detail in the original publication[24] is briefly reviewed here. After administration of local anesthesia and appropriate surgical preparation of the skin, which included washing, trimming, and cleansing with alcohol, four full-thickness punch excisions below the level of the hair papilla were made (with punches of 6, 8, and 12 mm). Each graft was trimmed of excess fat. Of the punch grafts, two were excised from a site of persistent disease, and two were excised from a healthy normal skin site. The grafts were then transplanted in clockwise rotation in the following manner: (1) a normal graft was transplanted to a normal site, (2) a normal graft was transplanted to an affected site, (3) an affected graft was transplanted to a normal site, and (4) an affected graft was transplanted to an affected site. Photographs were taken both before and after the procedures and again at about monthly intervals thereafter.

Donor dominance was observed in all 52 cases of androgenic alopecia: normal graft to normal site grew hair, normal graft to bald site grew hair, affected graft to affected site remained bald, and affected graft to normal site remained bald.

At the time of publication in 1959, there were 4 years of follow-up, which showed that hair-bearing autografts had continued to grow hair of the same texture and color apparently at the same rate and with the same period of anagen as at the donor site. N. Orentreich's original article demonstrated his intent to treat androgenic alopecia and illustrates the aesthetic placement of approximately 12 grafts in the left frontal scalp area in a pattern that reconstructed the anterior hairline with allowance for an appropriate degree of temporal recession and frontal peaking.

In the prepublication follow-up period, the hairline continued to recede at its preordained pace, and grafts placed at the original hairline continued to show stable hair growth at increasing distances from the receding hairline. There are now 35 years of follow-up, and the hair is still growing. Eventually a punch size of 4 mm was chosen as optimal for transplanting the greatest number of hairs without incurring loss due to avascular necrosis of hair follicles at the center of larger, free, full-thickness grafts.

The results of N. Orentreich's experiment on autografts in androgenic alopecia corroborated the statement that "the capacity for development of baldness appears to be controlled by factors resident in localized areas of the scalp"[30]; that is, that the pathogenesis of common baldness is inherent in each individual hair follicle. This phenomenon thus would explain the common clinical finding of isolated, normally growing, terminal hairs in a sea of male pattern baldness. The study also refuted the then-popular theory of the pathogenesis of common baldness as the result of ischemia from the

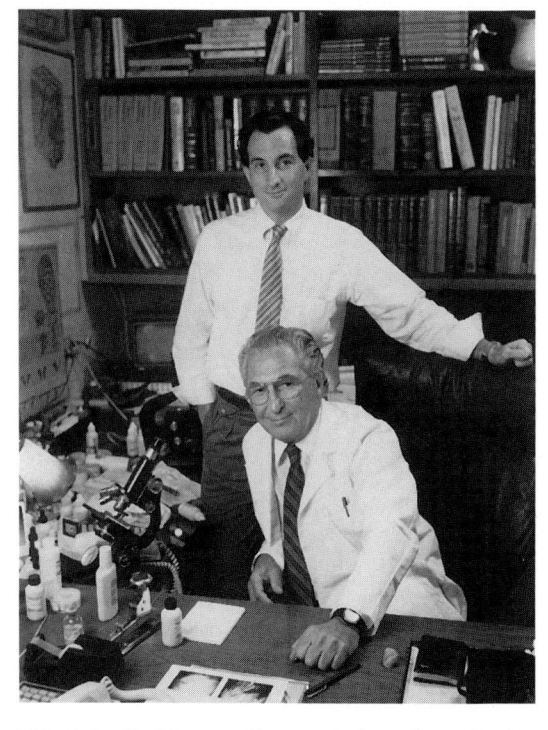

FIG. 2-1 Dr. Norman Orentreich (*seated*), credited as the "father of modern hair transplantation," shown with Dr. David Orentreich (*standing*).

chronic activity of the scalp muscles (via branches of the facial nerves), causing shearing stresses in the dermis of the scalp.[31]

IMPROVEMENTS FROM THE 1960s TO THE 1990s

Since N. Orentreich's development of punch graft hair transplantation, there have been many contributions resulting in improvements in both instrumentation and technique. Physicians with diverse surgical backgrounds entered the field of hair replacement surgery. Consequently, this field has expanded to include modalities other than punch grafting. Some innovations have endured, some have been abandoned, and others remain controversial. A noninclusive review of some of the most significant advances follows.

- Saline infiltration of the donor area[32] improved graft harvesting as did the introduction of sharper and motorized punches.[33]
- Improved methods of managing punch-harvested donor sites by using suture closure (as opposed to unassisted healing by secondary intention) reduced healing time and patient discomfort as well as improved the cosmetic appearance of the donor site scar.[34,35]
- The strip graft procedure introduced by Vallis[36] never became established; however, he may have been the first to use a double-bladed knife to obtain a strip of donor graft tissue, a popular contemporary technique for donor site harvesting.
- Free scalp flaps were reported in 1974.[37] Juri[38] introduced flaps at the 1975 International Congress of Plastic Surgeons in Paris. The flap technique was advanced by others.[39-41]
- Bald scalp reduction was first reported by Blanchard and Blanchard[42,43] and has become, with contributions by others, one of the most enduring and valuable adjuncts to grafting.[44-48]
- Kabaker and associates[40,49] have published on the use of tissue expanders for bald scalp reconstruction.
- Mini-grafting is really an old concept with a new name. In 1970, N. Orentreich[50] and Ayres[51] described the use of small circular punch grafts to refine the frontal hairline.
- Micrografts were reincarnated in the early 1980s after Marritt[52] reported on their use in eyelash transplantation and Nordström[53] reported subdividing 4 mm punch grafts into micrografts containing 2 to 4 follicles each, which were then placed into stab incisions. This work was further discussed by Marritt,[54] Bradshaw,[55] and Stough and associates,[56] who bisected or quadrisected larger punch grafts and placed them into small holes or stab wounds.
- In 1985, a method of covering the recipient area in three rather than four standardized punch graft procedures was reported.[57]
- Frechet's method of scalp extension appears to duplicate the advantages of tissue expanders without the disadvantages.[58]

• • •

Someday the limiting factor in hair restoration surgery may be overcome when hair follicle cloning will enable the surgeon to populate the bald scalp with an almost unlimited number of test tube follicles.[59]

REFERENCES

1. Dieffenbach JF: Nonnulla de Regeneratione et transplantatione. Dissertation inauguralis, 1822.
2. Dunham T: A method for obtaining a skin flap from the scalp and a permanent buried vascular pedicle for covering defects of the face, Ann Surg 17:677-679, 1893.
3. Davis JS: Scalping accidents, Bull Johns Hopkins Hosp 16:257, 1911.
4. Passot R: Cirugie esthetique pure, Paris, 1931, G. Doin et Cie.
5. Dorrance GM, Bransfield JW: Immediate covering of denuded area of skull, Am J Surg 58:236, 1942.
6. Kazanjian VH: Repair of partial losses of scalp, Plast Reconstr Surg 12:325, 1953.
7. Vallis CP, Humphreys SP: Treatment of extensive defect of scalp and skull, J Int Coll Surg 26:249-252, 1952.
8. Lamont ES: A plastic surgery transformation, West J Surg Obstet Gynecol 65:164, 1957.
9. Barsky AJ: The scalp. The eyebrow. In Barsky AT, editor: Principles and practice of plastic surgery, Baltimore, 1950, Williams & Wilkins, pp 137-140, 395.
10. Conway H, Berkeley W: Chromoblastomycosis (mycetoma form) treated by surgical excision, AMA Arch Dermatol Syphilol 66:695-702, 1952.
11. Delak Z: Successful replacement of the completely avulsed scalp, Br J Plast Surg 8:55-56, 1955.
12. Goyanes CJ: Contribucion al estudio de la blefaroplastia, Arch Oftal Hispano-Am 5:229-245, 1905.
13. Hoff F: Storungen in der Harmonie der Fettverteilung, Dtsch Med Wochschr 67:671-703, 1941.
14. Hoff F: Beobachtungen an Hauttransplantaten, Klin Wochenschr 31:56-57, 1953.
15. Matthews DN: The eyebrow. Eyelashes. In Surgery of repair, ed 2, Springfield, Ill., 1946, Charles C Thomas, pp 268-271.
16. Meister E: Scalp avulsions: attempt to restore hair growth, Br J Plast Surg 8:44-48, 1955.
17. Paletta FX: Avulsion of the entire scalp, Mo Med 53:191-192, 1956.
18. Wynn SK: Free pattern skin graft in total scalp avulsion, Plast Reconstr Surg 7:225-236, 1951.
19. Gussenhauer K: Ueber Scalpiring durch Maschinengewalt, Z Heilk 4:380-392, 1883.
20. Straith CJ, McEvitt WG: Total avulsion of scalp; review of problem with presentation of case of skin graft in which thrombin plasma fixation was used, Occup Med 1:451-462, 1946.
21. Sasagawa M: Hair transplantation, Jpn J Dermatol [Japanese] 30:493, 1930.
22. Okuda S: Klinische und experimentelle Untersuchungen

uber die Transplantation von lebenden Haaren, *Jpn J Dermatol* [Japanese] 40:537, 1939.
23. Okuda S: Clinical and experimental studies of transplantation of living hairs, *Jpn J Dermatol* [Japanese] 46:135-138, 1939.
24. Orentreich N: Autografts in alopecias and other selected dermatological conditions, *Ann NY Acad Sci* 83:463, 1959.
25. Tamura H: Pubic hair transplantation, *Jpn J Dermatol* [Japanese] 53:76, 1943.
26. Fujita K: Reconstruction of eyebrow, *La Lepro* [Japanese] 22:364, 1953.
27. Fujita K: Hair transplantation in Japan. In Kobori T, Montagna W, editors: *Biology and diseases of the hair*, Baltimore, 1976, University Park Press.
28. Kobori T, Montagna W, editors: *Biology and disease of the hair*, Baltimore, 1976, University Park Press.
29. Friederich HC: Indikation and technik der operativ-plastischen Behandlung des Haarverlustes, *Hauturzt* 21:197-202, 1970.
30. Hamilton JB: Patterned loss of hair in man: types and incidence, *Ann NY Acad Sci* 53:708-728, 1951.
31. Szasz TS, Robertson AM: The theory of the pathogenesis of ordinary human baldness, *AMA Arch Dermatol Syphilol* 61:34-48, 1950.
32. Frankel EB: Hair transplantation: additional observations, *Cutis* 15:545, 1975.
33. Tezel J: Miniature drill expedites hair transplantation, *Cutis* 5:461, 1969.
34. Carreirao S, Lessa S: New technique for closing punch graft donor sites, *Plast Reconstr Surg* 61:455-456, 1978.
35. Pierce HE: An improved method of closure of donor sites in hair transplantation, *J Dermatol Surg Oncol* 5(6):475-476, 1979.
36. Vallis CP: Surgical treatment of receding hairline, *Plast Reconstr Surg* 33:247, 1964.
37. Harri K, Obmori K, Obmori S: Hair transplantation with free scalp flaps, *Plast Reconstr Surg* 53:410, 1974.
38. Juri J: Use of parieto-occipital flaps in the surgical treatment of baldness, *Plast Reconstr Surg* 55(4):456, 1975.
39. Elliott RA: Lateral scalp flaps for instant results in male pattern baldness, *Plast Reconstr Surg* 60:699, 1977.
40. Kabaker S: Experiences with parieto-occipital flaps in hair transplantation, *Laryngoscope* 88:73, 1978.
41. Fleming RW, Mayer TG: Short vs. long flaps in the treatment of male pattern baldness, *Arch Otolaryngol* 107:403, 1981.
42. Blanchard G, Blanchard B: La reduction tonsurale (detonsuration): concept nouveau dans le traitement chirrurgical de la calvitie, *Rev Chir Esthet* 4:5, 1976.
43. Blanchard G, Blanchard B: Obliteration of alopecia by hairlifting: a new concept and technique, *J Natl Med Assoc* 69:639, 1977.
44. Stough DB, Webster RC: *Esthetics and refinements in hair transplantation*. Presented at the International Hair Transplant Symposium. Lucerne, Switzerland: February 4, 1978.
45. Sparkuhl K: *Scalp reduction: serial excision of the scalp with flap advancement*. Presented at the International Hair Transplant Symposium. Lucerne, Switzerland: February 4, 1978.
46. Unger MG, Unger WP: Management of alopecia of the scalp by a combination of excisions and transplantations, *J Dermatol Surg Oncol* 4:670, 1978.
47. Bosley L, Hope CR, Montroy RE: Male pattern reduction (MPR) for surgical reduction of male pattern baldness, *Curr Ther Res* 25:281, 1979.
48. Alt TH: Scalp reduction as an adjunct to hair transplantation: review of relevant literature and presentation of an improved technique, *J Dermatol Surg Oncol* 6:1011, 1980.
49. Kabaker S and others: Tissue expansion in the treatment of alopecia, *Arch Otolaryngol* 112:720, 1986.
50. Orentreich N: Hair transplants. In Maddin S, editor: *Current dermatologic management*, St Louis, 1970, Mosby.
51. Ayres S: Hair transplantation. In Epstein E, editor: *Skin surgery*, ed 3, Springfield, Ill., 1970, Charles C Thomas.
52. Marritt E: Transplantation of single hairs from the scalp as eyelashes, *J Dermatol Surg Oncol* 6:271-273, 1980.
53. Nordström REA: "Micrografts" for improvement of the frontal hairline after hair transplantation, *Aesthetic Plast Surg* 5:97-101, 1981.
54. Marritt E: Single hair transplantation for hairline refinement: a practical solution, *J Dermatol Surg Oncol* 10:962-966, 1984.
55. Bradshaw W: Quarter-grafts: a technique for minigrafts. In Unger WP, Nordstrom REA, editors: *Hair transplantation*, ed 2, New York, 1988, Marcel Dekker.
56. Stough DB, Nelson BR, Stough DB: Incisional slit grafting, *J Dermatol Surg Oncol* 17:53-60, 1991.
57. Orentreich DS, Orentreich N: Hair transplantation, *J Dermatol Surg Oncol* 11(3):319-324, 1985.
58. Frechet P: Scalp extension, *J Dermatol Surg Oncol* 19:616-622, 1993.
59. Yang JS, Lavker RM, Sun T-T: Upper human hair follicle contains a subpopulation of keratinocytes with superior in vitro proliferative potential, *J Invest Dermatol* 101:652-659, 1993.

B. An Approach to the Younger Patient

Jeffrey C. Weidig

PATIENT SELECTION
Judgment

Anyone who has performed hair transplantation for a considerable period of time has had the following experience: after interviewing and examining a potential patient, you feel that, from a technical point of view and from a psychological point of view, this patient is absolutely right for a hair transplant. This sense is based on one's own ability, positive interaction with the patient, quality of the patient's donor area, and degree of baldness. This sense of correctness is based on experience and can only be built up over time. Confidence in one's ability to perform a transplant in a satisfactory manner and an understanding of what it takes on the patient's part to be committed to the procedure with realistic expectations produce this feeling.

However, the physician must pay attention to the opposite feeling, that of danger and concern that things are not right with a patient. The feeling of incorrectness is based on interaction with the patient and on the patient's lack of understanding, lack of commitment to the procedure, and inability to understand what may be involved. The type and degree of baldness in relationship to the quality and quantity of the donor area also contribute to this sense. Experience has shown that regardless of the quality of the donor area, technical expertise with which a transplant is performed, and objective result, some patients will still be dissatisfied and unhappy. The transplant can become the focus for amplifying their unhappiness. Yet other patients who fall in the suboptimal candidate group but who have a very strong commitment and a great appreciation for what is involved may in fact be quite pleased and content with the result. For them, the transplant becomes a focus for furthering their own personal sense of happiness. Anyone who has been practicing hair transplantation for a long time realizes that this is essentially true.

Recognizing the Problem

Younger patients are by far the ones with whom difficulties most commonly arise. The question arises as to what is incumbent upon the physician with regard to the younger patient. How can the physician sharpen his/her sensitivity to the patient's psychological state and emotional needs? How can appropriate adjustments be made technically to bring about a satisfactory result? To illustrate, the following are two very different cases.

FIRST CASE

DW is a 42-year-old successful businessman. At the initial interview he has very thick, grey hair and an area of baldness that is rather narrow through the crown area. He has seen a number of other men who have undergone hair transplants that were performed by a certain physician, and several friends have recommended this physician to him. He is accompanied by his wife at the initial interview. She is supportive. The interview is characterized by a ready, smiling acceptance of what is involved and a clear understanding of the time interval involved and the need to make a complete commitment. DW concludes the interview by saying, "I want to be your best patient." A year later the patient is not only happy with the result but states that it has exceeded his expectations. Several months later he begins to refer patients to the physician.

SECOND CASE

RL is a 20-year-old young man who comes to the office wearing a hat. He is accompanied by his mother. The patient is uncommunicative and appears withdrawn and somewhat depressed. He does not respond directly; his mother speaks for him. The patient requests that the door be shut before he removes his hat. The examination reveals only the initial stages of male pattern baldness. There is some temporal recession and an area of thinning in the crown. His hair loss is at a stage at which it is difficult to predict with certainty the extent to which he will go bald. However, a close examination suggests that his future hair loss might be extensive indeed. There is simply no good way to know with certainty at this point. The patient has rather thin, very black hair. The scalp is quite pale in complexion. As the interview proceeds, it is evident that the patient did not come to the consultation on his own accord but was brought to the office by his mother, who was referred, via a telephone conversation, by her own physician. She is intent on doing something about her son's baldness. He is persistent in his demands that something be done for him. The interview is characterized by the patient's assertion that he is miserable and that he wants his hair back. His hair loss is the source of his problem. The patient seems ambivalent to the discussion involving the genetics of male pattern baldness. The patient is told that baldness is a developing trait and not a disease and that hair transplantation is not a cure but rather cosmetic surgery to give the appearance of a relatively normal head of hair. Furthermore, it is explained that hair transplantation must be performed over time and that a long-term commitment must be made. All of this information is to no avail. A gulf of misunderstanding remains. Since it was evident from the scalp examination that there is no need to start with a hair transplant, it is suggested that the patient return for a follow-up examination in 6 months. The dangers of doing something immediately are stressed to the patient. At the end of the interview the physician expresses concern for the patient's underlying psychological condition and suggests that perhaps he explore with a psychologist why he feels he must wear a hat continuously. This suggestion was met with hostility.

One year later the patient returns still wearing a hat. Examination reveals the presence of grafts placed at a level that is inconsistent with a natural hairline (i.e., below the rule of thirds). The patient is very anxious, angry, and desirous only of having the grafts removed.

• • •

In the above two cases, the first appears to be a success just waiting to happen. The second case appears to be a disaster waiting to happen. These two examples are extremes, of course, but one must recognize that there are very definite psychological aspects involved in patient selection and that there are also technical factors involved in patient selection. These two sets of issues definitely interact in the physician's mind. Attention must be paid to both.

PSYCHOLOGICAL APPROACH TO THE YOUNGER PATIENT

First and foremost the physician should function as a teacher and inform the patient about the process of balding. Patients should learn that the loss of hair in someone with male pattern baldness is a continuing process and that the expression of the gene for male pattern baldness varies greatly from person to person and that this trait is progressive as the patient ages. It is also true that in many individuals this process is continuous and seems to follow a straight, unbroken line of activity. In other patients this process seems to start and continue for awhile and then stop, only to start again at a later date. It must be stressed to the patient that male pattern baldness is not a disease in the truest sense of the word. It is the expression of a genetically inherited trait. The patient's perception of this genetically evolving trait may cause a feeling of unease, or if you will, "*dis*ease," but according to medically accepted terminology, it is not specifically a disease. It is remarkable and in some cases astounding how uninformed young people are with regard to developing baldness. In many instances they do look upon it as a disease, but in every event it is seen as a loss. It is on this level that the physician can empathize with the patient and discuss the patient's feelings. Listening to the patient express his concerns with regard to the continuing loss of hair is the key to discovering how realistic and how mature the patient will be in committing to a hair transplant and how satisfied he will be with the result.

In the interview the physician should find out how much research the patient has done on his own and how much inquiry he has made prior to the office visit. It is very helpful for the patient to be as informed as possible. To that end, the physician should have literature on the subject of male pattern baldness and hair transplantation available for patients, especially younger, uninformed patients. Having information available in this form is of great benefit because patients can read it on their own and any question that arises can be a point of further discussion. In addition to questioning the patient about how much research he has done, supplying the patient with literature on the topic, and exploring further questions that may arise after reading the material, it is important to find out if the patient has seen anyone with a hair transplant and what his reactions were. It is crucial to develop the idea that a hair transplant produces the appearance of a normal-looking head of hair but that evidence of surgical intervention is always visible on closer examination of the scalp. The patient should know that if the hair is separated and the scalp examined or if the hair is wet and separated, one will always be able to see evidence of the transplant itself. It is crucial for the younger patient to understand that the scalp will not be the way it used to be.

Importance of a Long-Term Relationship

With younger patients the importance of establishing a long-term relationship must be emphasized. This is a virtual given from the outset with a more mature patient who understands the nature of a continuing interaction with a physician or anyone else who provides a service. However, with younger patients it is important to explain that the nature of the commitment establishes a long-term relationship with the physician. Although a hair transplant may be performed in the immediate future, baldness continues. Further transplant plans and means of follow-up are a necessary part of both patient and physician commitment.

Supporting Roles

PARENTS

The role of a younger patient's parents can be either positive or negative, especially when the parents accompany the patient to the initial interview. Concern with their expectations is very important because how the parents react to the result of the patient's hair transplant will determine to a considerable degree how the patient will react. The most rewarding situation occurs when the younger patient is brought in by a father who has had a hair transplant. In that instance the parent is supportive and understanding and has very realistic expectations. The most dangerous situation is one in which the mother brings her son in and views his less-than-perfect condition as a reflection of herself. It is she who needs it set right more than he. It is in this case that discussing the situation with the mother is of vital importance. The younger patient's ability to interact and to deal with the issues involved independently from the wishes and pressures of the parents is a deciding factor in whether or not the patient is a candidate for a hair transplant. An honest appraisal of this situation is essential before committing a patient to surgery.

SPOUSE

It is also important to note that in young married patients a similar situation can arise. A young man may in fact be led into getting a hair transplant at the behest of his wife. In that instance, the degree of independence of his judgment and the degree of his commitment independent of his wife's wishes are important to establish. If a young married man gets a hair transplant simply to please his wife's wishes but not inherently because he deems it important for himself, there may be problems ahead. Rather than becoming a source of increased patient's happiness and self-esteem, the hair transplant may well be a source of a marital conflict.

FAMILY

Frequently, younger patients who seek hair transplants have great opposition from family members, specifically from a spouse or from the parents. Although the patient may indeed be a very good candidate for hair transplantation, a discussion of the opposition they must contend with from the family or spouse must take place. I have found it very beneficial in those instances to ask the patient to bring the family along so we can discuss in a friendly atmosphere his reasons for wanting hair transplantation and to allay their fears.

Physicians must be the advocate for the patient and look out for his best interest first. The physician must put his/her own interests and those of anyone else in the family second, regardless of their orientation toward what the patient seeks. Securing the patient's best interests at last rests on the physician's ability to recognize what indeed is in the patient's best interests and to apply those interests to the case in an unswerving manner. There are obviously many pitfalls and problems in approaching the younger patient, and often the situation can get confusing.

Periodic Reexamination

What I have found of unestimable value is waiting and reexamining patients at 4- to 6-month intervals. This approach allows several things to happen. First, it permits the physician to reexamine the patient's hair and scalp to see how rapidly the process of balding is occurring. Second, it establishes a continuing, ongoing relationship with the patient. Third, it allows further time for the patient to become more knowledgeable about hair transplantation. Fourth, it permits for more interaction with relatives, parents, or a spouse who may be involved in the decision. The patient is not rejected for hair transplantation but rather the situation is given more study. It is also a test of the maturity and commitment of the patient.

In this way over time patients who are really not good psychological candidates for hair transplants will in essence weed themselves out. This recommendation is not without its own problems. Often patients will ignore the advice to wait and they rush out and undergo an inappropriate treatment. Despite that risk, the physician should never perform a hair transplant on someone to "save the patient from himself" or feel compelled to do a hair transplant because if he/she does not do the transplant, someone else will.

Test Grafts

Another technique that I have found invaluable in treating the younger patient is performing test grafts. In an individual in whom there is a question about whether he would be a good candidate, transplanting perhaps six to twelve grafts in a location that is easily hidden and observing the growth of these grafts over time accomplishes several things.

The process establishes a long-term relationship with the patient. The patient understands what it is like to go through the surgical procedure of a hair transplant. The patient will see and observe for himself the grafts growing and begin to get a realistic idea of what is involved and thus be better equipped to make a decision about whether to continue. In some instances, test grafts prevent someone who is not a good candidate from a technical or psychological point of view from getting a hair transplant. Many times it is helpful in a positive way in that the patient now has a realistic idea of what is involved and can make a more informed decision. This technique often clears up a good deal of the confusion previously mentioned.

Age Parameters

Even with the best of intentions and with good judgment borne of experience and common sense, selecting younger patients for hair transplantation is not error free. Younger men between roughly 19 and 25 years of age who are seeking hair transplantation are in the most challenging age group. Therefore with these younger patients it is imperative that the physician bring to bear every resource at his/her disposal. Paying attention to the patient's psychological situation is important in all age groups but most essential in the younger patient.

Medical History

It must be mentioned and emphasized that the patient needs to be medically qualified for a hair transplant. Most patients are healthy and free of any chronic disease process. However, even in the younger patient, chronic underlying diseases such as diabetes or chronic liver disease must be discovered during the initial interview.

TECHNICAL APPROACH TO THE YOUNGER PATIENT

It is evident that male pattern baldness should be considered an evolving process. Once the physician is satisfied that the younger patient is a good candidate psychologically, examination of the patient's donor area for adequacy should follow. Parameters for judging younger candidates do not differ from those of older patients. However, because of the problems that frequently arise in younger patients, these parameters become even more important. Although Chapter 1, Part E deals with these factors in great detail, the following is a brief compendium of considerations especially important in the younger patient.

1. First and foremost is the color of the hair and the color of the scalp and their degree of con-

trast. People with a ruddy complexion who have gray or blonde hair are better candidates because of the lack of contrast between the scalp color and the hair color. On the other hand, the worst candidates for hair transplant have a very black hair color with a very pale or white scalp. Whereas the older patient will readily accept and understand limitations of the hair-to-skin match, the younger patient may not.

2. Density must be evaluated. By density I mean the number of hairs per unit of area. When one speaks of thickness, this term should refer to hair shaft thickness only. Although hair shaft thickness is a consideration, density is the most overriding concern.
3. Evaluation of the donor area for consistency throughout the area that will be retained is important. A careful examination will reveal whether or not the density is consistent throughout the occipital, parietal, and temporal areas. Younger patients with spotty, inconsistent density should be approached with caution or observed for six months or longer before proceeding with hair transplantation.
4. There are instances in which density is adequate but the hair shafts are so fine and so thin that coverage would be lacking.
5. The patient's hair texture is important. Wavy or curly hair is much preferred over straight hair for coverage although by no means is it an overriding concern.
6. The quantity of the donor area in relation to the potential bald area must be established at the initial consultation. It is of vital importance to determine whether the patient has a truly sufficient quantity of donor area for the potential area of baldness that may develop. Some uncertainty will always remain, and the transplant surgeon should not be afraid to state "I cannot predict your balding pattern 20 years from now."

Drawing the Hairline

It has been a well-known rule of hairline construction that one must obey the rule of thirds. That is, the hairline should never be lower than one third of the vertical dimension of the face (Fig. 2-2). The origin of this rule is from class techniques of sculpture. The dimension between the bottom of the chin and the bottom of the nose must equal the dimension between the bottom of the nose and the brow. This dimension in turn must equal the dimension between the brow and the hairline. This length is generally equivalent to the width of the palm along the metacarpal joints. Although this rule is a good general guideline, the rule must be modified when it is applied to patients with male pattern baldness and especially to younger patients. I have long considered it important to place the

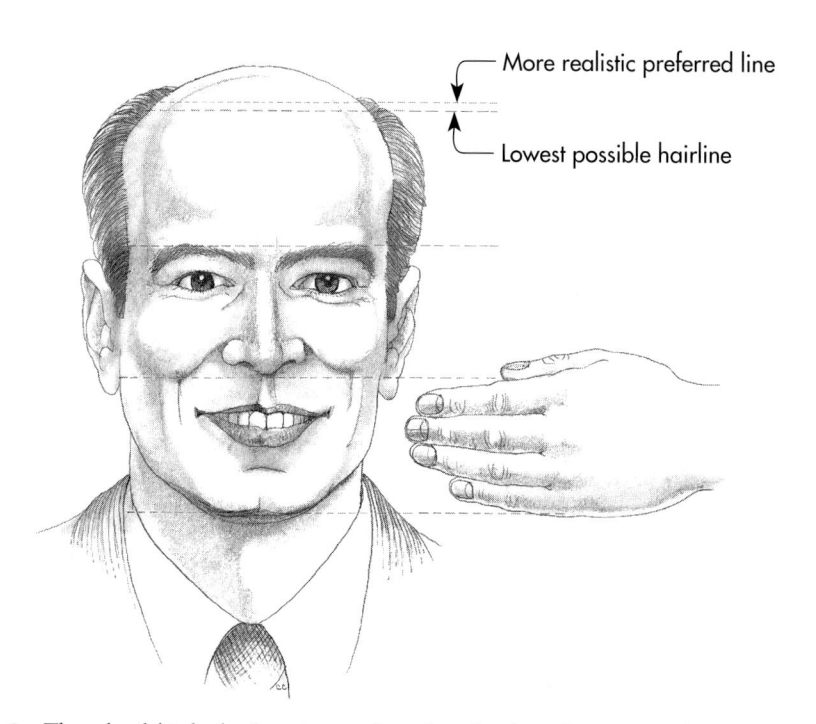

FIG. 2-2 The rule of thirds plus 2 cm is a rough guide to hairline placement in the younger patient.

hairline approximately 1 cm higher or sometimes 2 cm higher than that determined with the rule of thirds. The hairline should be drawn parallel to a line drawn between the two pupils. It is helpful in that respect to draw the hairline in while you are at eye level with the patient. In addition, it is also important to make sure that the line is drawn symmetrically without regard to asymmetrical hair loss or asymmetry of the face. Furthermore, the hairline must be drawn without concavity and must not curve in a downward direction. It is helpful when drawing the hairline to use a mirror and to look at the reverse image to correct any asymmetry that may be introduced into the drawing of the hairline because the physician is either right-eye dominant or left-eye dominant.

A higher hairline looks far better in profile and the eye is not readily drawn to it as the case if the hairline is lower. Modifying the rule of thirds to accommodate a higher hairline also results in greater preservation of the donor area. In addition, it places the grafts higher on the scalp in a flatter contour of the balding area so that coverage is better and the hairline has a more natural appearance. Another general rule in the younger patients is not to create a broken hairline. Transplantation of the bitemporal areas without creating a complete hairline should, with few exceptions, be avoided. A completed hairline and transplantation of the frontal area to a point about even with the level of the ears in profile will result in a pleasing result even if the patient rapidly goes bald and is negligent in receiving follow-up treatment.

Many times younger patients are anxious to have the hairline placed at a level that is really too low. The initial hairline that is drawn is a guideline and can be modified downward should that need eventually arise. It is necessary to intruct patients about the reasons to have the hairline high. They should be told that after the hair grows in they will see that the result will be to their liking and that the hairline can always be modified downward; however, raising a hairline is fraught with enormous difficulties. The physician may be concerned that if the hairline is too high, the area will tend to float away from the parietal area. However, connection of the transplant to the parietal area should not be a consideration at all in drawing the initial hairline. In addition, it is helpful to curve the trailing edge of the frontal transplant in a symmetrical fashion in the same manner or contour as the hairline. This design leads to a more pleasing growth pattern and aesthetically more pleasing result so that as hair loss continues, grafts are not "floating off the back." I highly recommend always grafting as symmetrically as possible and never overloading toward the part side or transplanting asymmetrically in any fashion.

CONCLUSION

Any approach to the younger patient or to the patient who has evolving baldness must in the end be conservative. First and foremost, the transplant will necessarily have to occur over a relatively long period of time in a number of sessions. The speed with which one performs the hair transplant is dictated by the rate of hair loss that the patient exhibits. Thus the relationship that one establishes with the patient will be long term and open ended. The physician must always be mindful that the patient has only so much donor area and plan accordingly. It is important to avoid any radical overuse of the donor area to any one section of baldness and to always leave some donor area for the future. The accompanying box summarizes some of the more basic and important points.

THE YOUNGER PATIENT—PSYCHOLOGICAL AND TECHNICAL CONSIDERATIONS

PSYCHOLOGICAL	TECHNICAL
• Determine patient's willingness to commit to a long-term program • Ensure that patient is well informed and understands what is involved in a hair transplant, particularly its limitations • Make sure that patient has a proper perspective on the role of hair transplantation as an enhancement of self image not as a miracle cure	• Wait until balding pattern declares itself • Create a conservative high hairline that is unbroken • Transplant at least the first third of the potentially balding area • Always transplant symmetrically and uniformly • Avoid any radical overuse of the donor area to any one section of baldness • Always leave some donor area in anticipation of future hair loss

C. Surgical Microbiology and Antibiotic Prophylaxis for Hair Restoration Surgery

John Karl Randall

Until recently, rational and scientifically based antimicrobial use for outpatient cutaneous surgery had not been well delineated.[1-3] A perusal of current textbooks with dedicated chapters on hair restoration reveals little guidance on this topic.[4-8]

The topic of antimicrobial use in hair restoration surgery can be divided into three separate but interconnected areas: (1) preoperative surgical preparation, (2) prevention of surgical wound infection, and (3) endocarditis prophylaxis.

SCALP MICROBIOLOGY

Preoperative surgical preparation begins with an understanding of the microbiology of the scalp. The scalp, like the rest of the integument, has both resident and transient flora. Transient flora lie free on the skin, usually do not multiply, and are not present in most individuals.[9-13] Interestingly, transient flora are readily removed with topical antiseptics or antimicrobial agents and surgical scrubbing, yet they are the organisms involved in most wound infections.[14-18]

Resident flora normally live harmlessly, are commensal, and are difficult to completely remove from the skin.[8,19,20] Twenty percent of resident flora live in adnexal structures such as hair follicles and pilosebaceous units, making it impossible to completely sterilize skin with surgical scrubs.[21-24] Generally speaking, resident skin flora include the organisms listed in the accompanying box. Scalp microflora are predominantly lipophilic organisms such as *Propionibacterium* organisms, *Pityrosporum* yeast, and aerobic diphtheroids.[9,19]

Many factors can affect scalp microbial ecology, including age, androgenic alopecia, scalp disorders (seborrheic dermatitis), systemic disease and medication use.[9,19] Hair restoration surgeons should be aware that a young, healthy Norwood type II patient will be colonized predominantly with lipophilic organisms, principally *Propionibacterium acnes*. An older Norwood type VI patient will have increased numbers of coagulase-negative staphylococci and decreased numbers of lipophilic organisms. If the patient described in the latter example had a condition such as diabetes, psoriasis, atopic dermatitis, seborrheic dermatitis, or HIV-related disease, then *Staphylococcus aureus* could account for 20% to 80% of the normal flora.[3,9,19,25-30]

MICROBIAL ECOLOGY OF SKIN: RESIDENT FLORA

Gram-Positive Micrococcaceae
1. Coagulase-negative staphylococci *Staphylococcus epidermidis*—90% of aerobic flora; *Staphylococcus hominis*, others
2. *Peptococcus* organisms *Peptococcus asaccharolyticus*—large numbers on forehead
3. *Micrococcus* organisms

Propionibacterium Organisms
1. *Propionibacterium acnes/Propionibacterium granulosum*—large numbers on scalp most prevalent anaerobe

Coryneform: Gram-Positive Rods/Diphtheroids
1. *Corynebacterium* organisms
2. *Brevibacterium* organisms

Acinetobacter Organisms

Pityrosporum Organisms

HOST RISK FACTORS

Knowledge of expected resident scalp flora is needed for informed use of preoperative antimicrobial cleansers and for wound prophylaxis. Preoperative preparation of the patient starts with a review of host risk factors known to increase the probability of infection. The box on p. 69 lists risk factors for the development of surgical site infections (SSIs). Cigarette use, extremes of age, remote infection, immunosuppressive therapy, diabetes, malnutrition and severe obesity are the most widely accepted.[2,16,24,31,33-39] Many other risk factors have been described, including rare genodermatoses such as hereditary hemorrhagic telangiectasia (Rendu-Osler-Weber disease).[40] The potential hair restoration patient should have as many factors controlled as possible and be informed of the probable increased risk of postoperative infection if the risk factors are not amenable to correction.

PREOPERATIVE SKIN PREPARATION

Prior to hair restoration, a patient should shampoo with chlorhexidine gluconate 4% the night prior and the morning of the surgery.[3,23,41-49] Along with proven, reduced intraoperative wound contamination, the greatest antibacterial effect is obtained with this method. No other agent has shown the same efficacy (mercurials, hydrogen peroxide, quaternary ammonium compounds, hexachlorophene, and iodophors).[3,23,41-49] Chlorhexidine gluconate is specifically labeled for use as a preoperative show-

> **NON–ANTIBIOTIC-RELATED RISK FACTORS FOR THE DEVELOPMENT OF SURGICAL SITE INFECTIONS**
>
> *Surgical Risk Factors*
> 1. Failure to use appropriate preoperative showers/surgical site scrubbing
> 2. Timing and type of hair removal (no shaving)
> 3. Poor surgical technique—dead space not closed, hematomas, devitalized tissue (compromised flap or crushed hair grafts)
> 4. Insertion of foreign bodies (implants, Silastic extenders)
> 5. Use of drains
> 6. Prolonged surgical procedures,* particularly with poor perfusion, hypoxia, and epinephrine use
>
> *Patient Factors*
> 1. Tobacco use/cigarette smoking
> 2. Immunosuppression: chemotherapy, corticosteroids, malignancy, HIV
> 3. Chronic disease: cardiac, metabolic (diabetes), pulmonary, renal, HIV
> 4. Obesity or malnutrition
> 5. Extremes of age
> 6. Occult infection: remote site—cellulitis, urinary tract
> 7. Colonization with *S. aureus* (i.e., hospital employees)
> 8. Preoperative antibiotic use (should be avoided for reasons other than those of prophylaxis; i.e., URTI, otitis media, acne)
>
> *Recent studies have discounted earlier studies that showed a relationship between wound infection rates and prolonged procedures.[31,32]

ering antiseptic/germicide.[50] The scalp and hair should be washed with 25 ml of chlorhexidine gluconate (Dyna-Hex, Exidine Skin Cleanser, Hibiclens Liquid are some brands available). The hair should be rinsed and the wash repeated.[51] The patient should then rinse thoroughly after the second application. A change in preoperative preparation that included scrubs the evening prior to surgery resulted in a decrease in SSIs from 9% to 0% in one large study of Class I procedures.[51]

Serious eye injury has occurred when chlorhexidine entered and remained in the eye during surgery.[3,49,50] Chlorhexidine binds with the stratum corneum yet is not absorbed.[52,53] The keratitis is believed to result from the detergent or solvent, not the chlorhexidine.[54,55] Numerous studies have shown chlorhexidine to be extremely safe (even when used on oral mucosa) and nonsensitizing or irritating.[56-61] Several cases of anaphylaxis associated with chlorhexidine use have been described, but these reactions are extremely rare and involve complicated situations.[3,49,50,62] Alternatives to chlorhexidine include chloroxylenol 3% (TechniCare) and liquid Dial soap.

Use of chlorhexidine for preoperative hair restoration surgery is nearly risk free. However, it should not be used in the presence of a perforated eardrum, and patients should be instructed to keep it out of the eyes while shampooing.

SSIs can be minimized by following appropriate sterile technique prior to and during surgery. A number of excellent reviews are available that examine the operating theater, surgical attire, drapes, instruments, gloves, and hand washing.[15,49,63-65]

Special mention of preoperative skin preparation as it relates to surgical scrubs and hair removal is warranted. The surgical scrub of the hair donor and recipient sites should be carried out with chlorhexidine for many of the same reasons previously mentioned in preoperative showering. A 2-minute application starting in the center of the sites and working peripherally is all that is needed.[44,66,67] Chlorhexidine will leave a prolonged residual effect and will not be removed with alcohol.[68,69] Hair removal or trimming is required with many hair restoration procedures, particularly the donor area in hair transplantation. Numerous studies have demonstrated that wound infection rates are lowest if hair is neither shaved nor trimmed.[70-73] If hair removal is required, then immediate preoperative trimming with scissors should be the method of choice.[22,41,44] The difference in postoperative wound infection rates between razor-shaved surgical sites and clipped surgical sites (0.6%) is significant.[70-73]

GUIDELINES FOR ANTIBIOTIC USE

The issue of antibiotic use to prevent SSIs as it pertains to cutaneous surgery is not well defined.[74]

Basic principles of antibiotic prophylaxis in surgical patients begins with an understanding of wound classification. Surgical wounds are classified into four types: clean (Class I), clean-contaminated

> **CLASSIFICATION OF SURGICAL SITE INFECTIONS**
>
> Class I   Clean wound (75% of all surgeries): nontraumatic wound; noninflamed; no break in technique; no entry into genitourinary, gastrointestinal, oropharyngeal, or respiratory tract.
>   Infection rate should be 1%. (Range 0->5%* in most cutaneous surgery.)
> Class II   Clean-contaminated wound: minor break in surgical technique or entry into hollow organ.
>   Infection rate 10%.*
> Class III   Contaminated wound: open, fresh, traumatic wound from relatively clean source or major break in technique, nonpurulent inflammation such as inflamed cyst and tumors with inflammation.
>   Infection rate 20%.*
> Class IV   Dirty and infected wound: devitalized tissue and necrotic tissue.
>   Infection rate 30-40%.*
>
> *References 24, 33, 35, 37, 51, 65, 71, 76.

(Class II), contaminated (Class III), and dirty and infected (Class IV)[1-3,24,75] (see box above).

Literature that specifically reviews SSI in clean cutaneous surgery and does not recommend prophylaxis far exceeds the converse, although few good placebo-controlled, double-blind studies are available for either point of view.[1-3,16,38,49,76-82] The otolaryngology and plastic surgery literature has failed to demonstrate reduced SSI rates for Class I procedures of the head and neck (multiple scalp procedures are included in these studies) with the administration of preoperative antibiotics.[16,38,78,83,84] *The Medical Letter on Drugs and Therapeutics*[85] recommends antibiotic prophylaxis in head and neck surgery only if the oral cavity is violated, and no recommendation is made for Class I (clean) cutaneous surgery.

Hair restoration literature does not address antibiotic use and SSIs, except in the form of anecdotal reports and surveys.[4-5,6-8,86-92] Unfortunately, even hair restoration surgeons who have performed thousands of procedures are as likely not to use antibiotics as the converse. The difficulty is deciding if the risk of complications from antibiotic use exceeds the estimated 0.5% wound infection rate in hair restoration.[4-8,86-92] What should be obvious when dealing with the low wound infection rates in hair restoration is that it statistically takes very large numbers of patients (in a well-controlled double-blind study) to show efficacy of preoperative antibiotic use.

A number of hair restoration surgeons have claimed decreased SSIs after instituting the standard practice of preoperative antibiotic administration, but the type of antibiotic, timing, and dose are not consistent with current acceptable use.[93]

A number of studies do support use of prophylactic antibiotics in Class I procedures.[24,32,79,94-100] If a surgeon is going to administer preoperative antibiotics in Class I procedures, then certain practices and principles need to be applied. Numerous studies have evaluated the safety of oral antibiotics in the treatment of skin infections, and generally cephalosporins had an adverse drug reaction (ADR) rate of 15% (13% gastrointestinal complaints, 2% of these diarrhea). Amoxicillin/clavulanate had an ADR rate of 29%, with 7% experiencing diarrhea. Erythromycin has been shown to cause a 35% incidence of gastrointestinal complaints.[101,102] Cutaneous reactions occur in 2.1% of those using cephalosporins, which is a much lower incidence than that with penicillin and its derivatives.[103]

Immediate allergic reactions (anaphylaxis) occur in 0.01% of those given penicillin, and 9% of these reactions will be fatal.[104] Urticarial reactions to penicillin occur in 4.5% to 10% of patients without a history of penicillin allergy.[104-108] Cephalosporin cross-reactivity in individuals with a known allergy to penicillin is probably 3% to 7%, but some sources quote 15%.[104,105,109]

The economic cost of prophylaxis includes the cost of not only the antimicrobial agent but also treatment of ADRs, treatment of associated ecological consequences, missed work for the patient, and expense to the physician.

Recommendations

Although I do not believe prophylactic antibiotics are warranted for the majority of hair restoration procedures, if a physician chooses to use antibiotics, then cephalosporins should be administered (Table 2-1). Cephalosporins are bactericidal and are the most widely used prophylactic antibiotic.[24,76,77,85] First-generation cephalosporins are probably as safe as any antibiotic. Most cephalosporins associated with bleeding abnormalities and disulfiram-like reactions contain an N-methylthiotetrazole moiety and are usually in parenteral form.[110] First-generation

TABLE 2-1 Prophylactic Antibiotic Recommendations for Prevention of Surgical Site Infections in Hair Restoration Surgery

PROCEDURE	ANTIBIOTIC*	DOSAGE SCHEDULE[†]
Uncomplicated hair transplantation	None	—
Complicated/high-risk patient hair transplantation[‡]	Cefadroxil (po)	2 g 1½ hr preop
Uncomplicated scalp reduction	None	—
Complicated/high-risk patient scalp reduction[‡,§]	Cefadroxil (po)	2 g 1½ hr preop
Uncomplicated scalp-lifting/flaps	None	—
Complicated/high-risk patient scalp-lifting/flaps[‡,||]	Cefadroxil (po)	2 g 1½ hr preop

NOTE: For prolonged procedures, an intraoperative dose of antibiotic may be warranted.
*Alternatives for penicillin-allergic patients include erythromycin (1 g po), trimethoprim-sulfamethoxazole (TMX-Sulfa) (two double-strength tablets), or clindamycin (300 mg po) 1½ hours prior to the procedure.
[†]If intravenous access is available, cefazolin (1 g IV) 30 minutes preoperatively, or another similar cephalosporin can be administered. If a center is experiencing methicillin-resistant staphylococcal infections or an alternative for penicillin-allergic patients is needed, vancomycin (15 mg/kg) 60 minutes preoperatively can be substituted. To minimize risk of hypotension and skin eruption, vancomycin must be infused over 1 hour.
[‡]See text for definition of high-risk patient (includes patients with medical problems such as diabetes, extremes of age, immunosuppression). Complicated implies a semiclean procedure or very prolonged procedure (>4 hours).
[§]In scalp reductions, the use of Silastic implantable extenders may put patients at increased risk of postoperative infections, as does the use of many prosthetic devices. The use of intraoperative balloon expansion, Miami Suture-Tension Adjustment Reel (STAR), or Sure-Closure devices have an unknown effect on SSIs.
[||]Staged procedures as well as the use of implantable tissue expanders, may increase the risk of SSIs.

oral cephalosporins should be the antimicrobials of choice. Use of any drug by the oral route also carries the added benefit of the lowest risk of allergy.

The three available first-generation oral cephalosporins (cephalexin, cephradine, cefadroxil) have excellent activity against the organisms most likely to cause SSIs in hair restoration procedures. *S. aureus* and *S. epidermidis,* both penicillinase- and nonpenicillinase-producing (but not methicillin-resistant) agents, are susceptible to first-generation cephalosporins with rare exceptions.[24,111] *Streptococcus pyogenes* (Group A β-hemolytic), Groups B, C, G, *Streptococcus viridans,* and *P. acnes* are also sensitive to first-generation cephalosporins.[107,111]

Of the available oral first-generation cephalosporins, cefadroxil has clear advantages. Cefadroxil is rapidly (1½ hours for peak serum levels) and well absorbed. The drug is the only oral first-generation cephalosporin for which food does not delay or decrease peak serum levels. Cefadroxil achieves high minimum inhibitory concentrations (28 μg/ml) after a single 1000 mg dose, and its half life is approximately twice as long (1½ hours) as cephalexin or cephradine.[112]

The dose, timing, and duration of prophylactic antibiotic use is now fairly standardized.* Optimal timing of prophylaxis is preoperatively. Most intravenous antibiotics should be given immediately prior to the incision (30 minutes) but not more than 2 hours prior to surgery. To achieve therapeutic drug levels with oral antibiotics, one and one-half to two times the standard dose should be used 1 to 2 hours prior to the procedure. The duration of prophylaxis should not be longer than 24 hours.[13,24,76,95,117] Unless a procedure is excessively prolonged, only a single preoperative dose of antibiotic is justified.* Table 2-1 lists a synopsis of recommendations for SSI prevention.

ENDOCARDITIS PROPHYLAXIS

Endocarditis prophylaxis in cutaneous surgery is another area that is poorly delineated. Endocarditis can occur despite applying current recommendations in prophylaxis. The American Heart Association does make recommendations on prevention of bacterial endocarditis (AHA 1990 guidelines), although it allows some latitude and encourages clinical judgment.[120-122] The AHA recommendations do not specifically cover cutaneous surgery, but they are based on certain axioms. The axioms include the assertion that specific cardiac conditions are associated with an increased risk of endocarditis.[120-122] Some surgical and dental procedures result in transient bacteremia (violation of mucosal surfaces) with increased risk of endocarditis.[120-122]

A number of articles specifically review bacteremia in skin surgery and endocarditis.[115,123-131] The study by Halpern and associates[115] revealed three cases out of 45—a 7% incidence of bacteremia. Of special note is that only four of all the patients underwent hair transplantation, but one of

---
*References 1-3, 16, 24, 32, 35-39, 66, 76-78, 83, 85, 94, 95, 113-117.

*References 3, 24, 38, 76, 85, 94-96, 117-119.

TABLE 2-2 Review of Literature on Endocarditis Prophylaxis and Cutaneous Surgery

AUTHOR	DRUG/DOSE/TIMING	ALTERNATIVE/SPECIAL CONSIDERATIONS
Wagner et al.[123] (1986)	Dicloxacillin (2 g po 1 hr preop and 1 g 6 hr postop)	For penicillin-allergic patient: erythromycin (1 g po 1 hr preop and 0.5 g 6 hr postop)
Sabetta et al.[129] (1987)	Dicloxacillin sodium (2 g po 1 hr preop and 500 mg 6 hr postop)	Vancomycin IV for recent prosthetic valves
Halpern et al.[115] (1988)	First-generation cephalosporin (1-2 g po 1 hr preop and 500 mg 6 hr postop)	
Terracina et al.[1] (1993)	Dicloxacillin (2 g 1 hr preop and 1 g 6 hr postop)	For penicillin-allergic patient: erythromycin (1 g 1 hr preop and 500 mg 6 hr postop)
Spelman et al.[128] (1993)	Flucloxacillin (1 g 1 hr preop for abnormal native valves) Flucloxacillin and IV or IM gentamicin (for prosthetic valves)	For penicillin-allergic patient: vancomycin (500 mg)
Hobbs[3] (1994)	Dicloxacillin (2 g 1 hr preop and 1 g 6 hr postop)	For penicillin-allergic patient: erythromycin (1 g 1 hr preop and 500 mg 6 hr postop)
Haas[2] (1994)	For contaminated skin (*S. aureus*): first-generation cephalosporin (1 g po 1 hr preop and 500 mg 6 hr postop) For contaminated skin (*S. epidermidis*): vancomycin (500 mg IV 1 hr preop and 250 mg IV 6 hr postop) For methacillin-resistant staphylococci or prosthetic valves: vancomycin (500 mg IV 1 hr preop and 250 mg IV 6 hr postop)	For penicillin-allergic patient: clindamycin (300 mg po 1 hr preop and 150 mg 6 hr postop)

three cases of bacteremia was in a hair transplant patient. *P. acnes* was the organism isolated. It must be remembered that transient bacteremias probably occur every day in individuals, and the cumulative risk of these infections is greater than the occasional surgical or medical procedure.[132] Tooth brushing, defecation, flossing, water irrigation, chewing, and sexual acts are just some of the many causes of transient bacteremias, with blood culture rates greater than 25%.[133]

The bacteria commonly responsible for surgically induced endocarditis (*S. viridans* in oral procedures and enterococci/Group D streptococci in gastrointestinal and gastrourinary procedures) should not be the causative organisms in skin surgery. Coagulase-negative staphylococci (*S. epidermidis*), which are the most common cause of early prosthetic valve endocarditis, and diphtheroids, are organisms that will be encountered in hair restoration procedures. *S. aureus* may be encountered in many patients, as previously mentioned, and is also a major pathogen in bacterial endocarditis. Table 2-2 lists currently published recommendations for endocarditis prophylaxis and cutaneous surgery.

CONDITIONS FOR WHICH ENDOCARDITIS PROPHYLAXIS IS RECOMMENDED

Prosthetic valves
Rheumatic valvular disease, most other acquired valvular dysfunction conditions
Congenital cardiac anomalies (some exceptions)
Previous episode endocarditis
Mitral valve prolapse associated with mitral regurgitation
Hypertrophic cardiomyopathy/idiopathic hypertrophic subaortic stenosis (IHSS)
Surgical systemic-pulmonary shunts

Recommendations

As with most authorities listed in Table 2-2, I agree that for high-risk patients (see box), antibiotic prophylaxis for the prevention of endocarditis is recommended. This recommendation is made as much for medicolegal considerations as it is for evidence that cutaneous surgery puts patients at risk, that prophylaxis works, and that it has a favorable cost-

TABLE 2-3 Endocarditis Prophylaxis in Hair Restoration Surgery

TYPE OF PATIENT	ANTIBIOTIC/DOSE/TIMING
Individuals with high-risk cardiac lesions (see box, p. 72)	Cefadroxil (2 g 1 hr preop and 500 mg 6 hr postop)
Individuals with cardiac pathologic conditions but not at high risk (see box, p. 72)	None

NOTE: 1. For patients with prosthetic valves less than 60 days after transplantation, use vancomycin (500 mg IV over 1 hour preoperatively and 250 mg IV 6 hours postoperatively).
2. For penicillin-allergic patients, clindamycin (300 mg po 1 hour preoperatively and 150 mg po postoperatively) or erythromycin (1 g 1 hour preoperatively and 500 mg 6 hours postoperatively) can be used.

benefit profile. It has been estimated that it costs more than 2 million dollars to prevent a single case of endocarditis in mitral valve prolapse.

The organisms mostly likely to be involved in endocarditis in hair restoration surgery should be susceptible to first-generation cephalosporins, although coagulase-negative staphylococci can occasionally be resistant to most antibiotics.[130]

Table 2-3 lists recommendations for endocarditis prophylaxis. Hair restoration surgeons should not hesitate to contact the patient's cardiologist or cardiovascular surgeon, or the local infectious disease specialist if questions arise concerning a particular patient.

PROSTHETIC JOINTS

Prosthetic joint infections occur following the same type of surgical procedures that precipitate bacterial endocarditis (oral procedures, gastrointestinal and gastrourinary procedures, and pyogenic skin processes).[108] The bacteriology is predominately staphylococci and streptococci.[108] Due to the lack of data, it is difficult to define risk, but a couple of studies seem to support the belief that transient bacteremias secondary to surgical procedures rarely are responsible for prosthetic infections.[134,135] The weight of information does not support prophylactic antibiotic administration in individuals with prosthetic joints unless infected tissues are violated.

The use of prophylactic antibiotics in individuals with arterial venous shunts or other prosthetic devices such as breast or penile implants is probably not warranted.

A brief mention should be made of the many new antimicrobials. Numerous new macrolides, fluoroquinolones, and β-lactams have been recently released. The use of these antibiotics for wound prophylaxis or endocarditis is not recommended without extensive testing and rigorous studies.

REFERENCES

1. Terracina JR, Wagner RF: Antibiotic use in dermatologic surgery. In Roenigk RK, Roenigk HH, editors: *Surgical dermatology—advances in current practice*, St Louis, 1993, Mosby.
2. Haas AF, Grekin RC: Antibiotic prophylaxis in dermatologic surgery. *J Am Acad Dermatol* (submitted for publication).
3. Hobbs ER: Surgical microbiology, antibiotic prophylaxis, and antiseptic technique. In Wheeland RG, editor: *Cutaneous surgery*, Philadelphia, 1994, WB Saunders, pp 64-75.
4. Beeson WH, McCullough EG, editor: *Aesthetic surgery of the aging face*, St Louis, 1986, Mosby.
5. Norwood OT, Shiell RC, editors: *Hair transplant surgery*, ed 2, Springfield, Ill., 1984, Charles C Thomas.
6. Stegman SJ, Tromovitch TA, Glogau RG: *Cosmetic dermatologic surgery*, ed 2, Chicago, 1990, Year Book.
7. Mitchell AJ, Krull EA: Hair disorders, *Dermatol Clin* 5(3):457-640, 1987.
8. Roenigk RK, Roenigk HH, editors: *Dermatologic surgery—principles and practice*, New York, 1989, Marcel Dekker.
9. Roth RR, James DJ: Microbiology of the skin: resident flora, ecology, infection, *J Am Acad Dermatol* 20:367-390, 1989.
10. Hobbs ER: Surgical microbiology, antibiotic prophylaxis, and antiseptic technique. In Wheeland RG, editor: *Cutaneous surgery*, Philadelphia, 1994, WB Saunders, p 65.
11. Somerville-Millar DA, Noble WL: Resident and transient bacteria of the skin, *J Cutan Pathol* 1:260-264, 1974.
12. Price PB: The bacteriology of normal skin: a new quantitative test applied to a study of the bacterial flora and the disinfectant action of mechanical cleansing, *J Infect Dis* 63:301-318, 1938.
13. Larson E: Guidelines for use of topical antimicrobial agents, *Am J Infect Control* 16:253-266, 1988.
14. Simmons BP: Guidelines for hospital environmental control, *Infect Control* 2:131-137, 1981.
15. Simmons BP: Guidelines for prevention of surgical wound infections, *Infect Control* 3:187-196, 1982.
16. Paluzzi RG: Antimicrobial prophylaxis for surgery (medical consultation), *Med Clin North Am* 77(2):427-441, 1993.
17. Evans CA and others: Bacterial flora of the human skin, *J Invest Dermatol* 15:305-324, 1950.
18. Ulrich JA: Techniques of skin sampling for microbial contaminants, *Hosp Topic* 43:121-123, 1965.
19. Leyden JJ and others: Skin microflora, *J Invest Dermatol* 88(3):65S-69S, 1987.
20. Noble WC: *Microbiology of human skin*, London, 1981, Lloyd-Luke, pp 329-357.
21. Selwyn S, Ellis H; Skin bacteria and skin disinfection reconsidered, *Br Med J* 1:136-140, 1972.
22. Mackenzie I: Preoperative skin preparation and surgical outcome, *J Hosp Infect* 11:27-32, 1988.
23. Warner C: Skin preparation in the surgical patient, *J Natl Med Assoc* 80:899-904, 1988.
24. Kaiser AB: Postoperative infections and antimicrobial prophylaxis. In Mandell GL and others, editors: *Principles and practices of infectious disease*, New York, 1990, Churchill Livingstone, pp 2245-2257.
25. White MI, Noble WC: Consequences of colonization and infection by *Staphylococcus aureus* in atopic dermatitis, *Clin Exp Dermatol* 11:34-40, 1986.
26. Aly R, Maibach HI, Shinefield HR. Microbial flora of atopic dermatitis, *Arch Dermatol* 113:780-782, 1977.
27. Leyden JJ, Marples RR, Kligman AM. *Staphylococcus aureus*

in the lesions of atopic dermatitis, *Br J Dermatol* 90:525-530, 1974.
28. Aly R, Maibach HI, Mandel A. Bacterial flora in psoriasis, *Br J Dermatol* 95:603-606, 1976.
29. Berman DS and others: *Staphylococcus aureus* colonization in intravenous drug abusers, dialysis patients, and diabetics, *J Infect Dis* 155:829-831, 1987.
30. Tuazon CV: Skin and skin infections in the patient at risk: carrier state of *Staphylococcus aureus*, *Am J Med* 76(5A):166-171, 1984.
31. Nagachinto T, Stephens M, Reitz B. Risk factors for surgical wound infection following cardiac surgery, *J Infect Dis* 156:967-973, 1987.
32. Platt R and others: Perioperative antibiotic prophylaxis for herniorrhaphy and breast surgery, *N Engl J Med* 322(3):153-160, 1990.
33. Garibald RA, Cushig D, Lerer T: Risk factors for postoperative infection, *Am J Med* 5(suppl 3B):158S-163S, 1991.
34. Simchen E and others: Risk factors for postoperative wound infection in cardiac surgery patients, *Infect Control* 4:215-220, 1983.
35. Barker GR, Brown AE: Surgical site infections in the cancer patient, *Infect Med* 2(1):20, 25-26, 1994.
36. Nichols RS: Surgical wound infection, *Am J Med* 91(suppl 3B):545, 1991.
37. Campbell LA and others: Clean surgical wound infections at an oncology center, *Infect Med* 2(4):280, 282-286, 1994.
38. Peterson LJ: Antibiotic prophylaxis against wound infections in oral and maxillofacial surgery, *J Oral Maxillofac Surg* 48(6):617-620, 1990.
39. Tabet JC, Johnson JT: Wound infection in head and neck surgery: prophylaxis, etiology and management, *J Otolaryngol* 19(3):147-200, 1990.
40. Swanson DL, Dahl MV: Embolic abscesses in hereditary hemorrhagic telangiectasia, *J Am Acad Dermatol* 24:580-583, 1991.
41. Craig CP: Preparation of the skin for surgery, *Infect Control* 7:257-258, 1986.
42. Kaol AF, Jewett VF: Agents and techniques of disinfection of the skin, *Surg Gynecol Obstet* 152:677-685, 1981.
43. Lowbury EL, Lilly HA: Use of 4 percent chlorhexidine detergent solution (Hibiscrub) and other methods of skin disinfection, *Br Med J* 1:510-515, 1973.
44. Masterson BJ: Skin preparation, *Clin Obstet Gynecol* 31:736-743, 1988.
45. Garibaldi RA and others: The impact of preoperative skin disinfection on preventing intraoperative wound contamination, *Infect Control Hosp Epidermiol* 9:109-113, 1988.
46. Van de Hoeven E, Hinton NA: An assessment of the prolonged effect of antiseptic scrubs on the bacterial flora of the hands, *Can Med Assoc J* 99:402-407, 1968.
47. Leclair JM and others: Effect of preoperative shampoos with chlorhexidine or iodophor on emergence of resident scalp flora in neurosurgery, *Infect Control* 9:8-12, 1988.
48. Kaiser AB and others: Influence of preoperative showers on staphylococcal skin colonization: a comparative trial of antiseptic skin cleaners, *Ann Thorac Surg* 45:35-38, 1988.
49. Sebben JE: Sterile technique and the prevention of wound infection in office surgery, part II, *J Dermatol Surg Oncol* 15(1):38-47, 1989.
50. Olin BR, Hebel SK, Dombek GF. *Facts and comparisons drug information*, St Louis, 1993, Facts and Comparisons, pp 637-638.
51. Olson M, O'Connor M, Schwartz ML: Surgical wound infections: a 5-year prospective study of 20,193 wounds at the Minneapolis V.A. Medical Center, *Ann Surg* 199:253-259, 1984.
52. O'Neill J and others: Percutaneous absorption of chlorhexidine in neonates, *Curr Ther Res* 31:485-489, 1982.

53. Case DE and others: Chlorhexidine: attempts to detect percutaneous absorption in man, *Chemotherapy* 3:367-376, 1976.
54. Burstein NL: Preservative alteration of corneal permeability in humans and rabbits, *Invest Ophthalmol Vis Sci* 25:1453-1457, 1984.
55. Hamill MB, Osako MS, Wilhelmus KR. Experimental evaluation of chlorhexidine gluconate for ocular antisepsis, *Antimicrob Agents Chemother* 26:793-796, 1984.
56. Bain MV: Chlorhexidine in dentistry—a review, *NZ Dent J* 76:49-54, 1980.
57. Ciancio SG: Chemotherapeutics in periodontics, *Dent Clin North Am* 24:813-826, 1980.
58. Newmann PS, Addy M: Comparison of hypertonic saline and chlorhexidine mouth rinses after the inverse bevel flap procedure, *J Peridontal* 53:315-318, 1982.
59. Rosenberg A, Alatary SD: Chlorhexidine and contaminants, *Ann Intern Med* 84:752-753, 1976.
60. Rosenberg A, Alatary SD: Safety and efficacy of the antiseptic chlorhexidine gluconate, *Surg Gynecol Obstet* 143:789-792, 1976.
61. Phillips L and others: A comparison of rabbit and human skin response to certain irritants, *Toxicol Appl Pharmacol* 21:369-382, 1972.
62. Bicknell PG: Sensorineural deafness following myringoplasty operations, *J Laryngol Otol* 85:957-961, 1971.
63. Sebben JE: Sterile technique and the prevention of wound infection in office surgery, part I, *J Dermatol Surg Oncol* 14:1364-1371, 1988.
64. Postlethwaite RW: Principles of operative surgery: antisepsis, technique, sutures, and drains. In Sabistan DC, editor: *Davis-Christopher textbook of surgery*, ed 11, Philadelphia, 1977, WB Saunders.
65. American College of Surgeons Committee on Control of Surgical Infections. *Manual on control of infections in surgical patients*, ed 2, Philadelphia, 1984, JB Lippincott.
66. Pollock AV: Surgical prophylaxis—the emerging picture, *Lancet* 1:225-230, 1988.
67. Aly R, Maibach HI: Comparative antibacterial efficacy of a 2-minute surgical scrub with chlorhexidine gluconate, povidone-iodine and chloroxylenol sponge-brushes, *Am J Infect Control* 16:173-177, 1988.
68. Laufman H: Current use of skin and wound cleansers and antiseptics, *Am J Surg* 157:359-363, 1989.
69. Dahl J, Wheeler B, Mukherjee D. Effect of chlorhexidine scrub on postoperative bacterial counts, *Am J Surg* 159:486-489, 1990.
70. Cruse PJE, Foord R: A five-year prospective study of 27,649 surgical wounds, *Arch Surg* 107:206-210, 1973.
71. Cruse PJE, Foord R: The epidemiology of wound infection: a ten year prospective study of 62,939 wounds, *Surg Clin North Am* 60:27-40, 1980.
72. Strachan C: Antibiotic prophylaxis in "clean" surgical procedures, *World J Surg* 6:273-280, 1972.
73. Seropain R, Reynolds BM: Wound infection after preoperative depilatory versus razor preparation, *Am J Surg* 121:251-254, 1971.
74. Drake LA, chairman: Guidelines of care: actinic keratosis, contact dermatitis, dermabrasion, phototherapy and photochemotherapy, *Dermatol World* (suppl) July 1993.
75. Altermeier WA and others: *American College of Surgeons manual on control of infections in surgical patients*, ed 2, Philadelphia, 1984, JB Lippincott.
76. Hurley LD, Westfall CT, Shore JW: Prophylactic use of antibiotics in oculoplastic surgery. *Int Ophthalmol Clin* 32(3):165-178, 1992.
77. Krizek TJ and others: The use of prophylactic antibacterials in plastic surgery: a 1980's update, *Plast Reconstr Surg* 76(6):953-963, 1985.

78. Sacks T: Prophylactic antibiotics in traumatic wounds, *J Hosp Infect* 11:251-258, 1988.
79. Bencini PL and others: Antibiotic prophylaxis of wound infections in skin surgery, *Arch Dermatol* 127:1357-1360, 1991.
80. Fry DE: Antibiotics in surgery, *Am J Surg* 155:11-14, 1988.
81. Chodak GW, Plaut ME: Use of systemic antibiotics for prophylaxis in surgery, *Arch Surg* 112:326-334, 1977.
82. Ma S, Chiang SS, Fung RH: Prophylactic antibiotics in surgical treatment of axillary hyperhidrosis, *Ann Plast Surg* 22:436-439, 1989.
83. Weber RS, Callender DL: Antibiotic prophylaxis in clean contaminated head and neck oncologic surgery, *Ann Otol Rhinol Laryngol* 101:16-20, 1992.
84. Johnson JT, Wagner RL: Infection following uncontaminated head and neck surgery, *Arch Otolaryngol Head Neck Surg* 113:368-369, 1987.
85. The Medical Letter on Drugs and Therapeutics: Antimicrobial Prophylaxis in Surgery. *Med Lett Drugs Ther* 35:91-94, 1993.
86. Stough DB III, Randall JK, Schauder CS. Complications in hair replacement surgery. *Facial Plast Surg Clin North Am* 2(2):219-231, 1994.
87. Quinlan P and others: *Complications of micrografting and scalp reductions.* Presented at the International Society of Hair Surgeons World Congress. Dallas, Tex.: April 30-May 2, 1993.
88. Alt TH: Hair transplantation and scalp reduction. In Coleman WP III and others, editors: *Cosmetic surgery of the skin: principles and techniques,* Philadelphia, 1991, BC Decker.
89. Unger WP: Preoperative instructions. In Unger WP, Nordstrom REA, editors: *Hair transplantation,* ed 2, New York, 1988, Marcel Dekker.
90. Tromovitch TA, Stegman SJ, Glogau RG. Sequelae and complications of hair transplantation. In Unger WP, Nordstrom REA, editors: *Hair transplantation,* ed 2, New York, 1988, Marcel Dekker.
91. Unger WP: Hair: surgical aspects. In Parish LC, Lask GP, editors: *Anesthetic dermatology,* New York, 1991, McGraw-Hill, pp 220-221.
92. Randall JK, Schauder CS: Current concepts in alopecia correction in the black patient, *Am J Cosmet Surg* 10(3):173-178, 1993.
93. Kunim CM: Problems in antibiotic usage. In Mandell GL, Douglas RG, Bennett JE, editors: *Principles and practices of infectious disease,* New York, 1990, Churchill Livingstone, pp 427-433.
94. Nichols RL: Postoperative wound infections, *Ochsner Clin Rep Serious Hosp Infect* 4(3):1-7, 1988.
95. Kaiser AB: Antimicrobial prophylaxis in surgery, *N Engl J Med* 315:1129-1138, 1986.
96. Culver DH and others: Surgical wound infection rates by wound class, operative procedure and patient risk index, *Am J Med* 91(3B):152S, 1991.
97. Ergina PL, Gold S, Meakins JL: Antibiotic prophylaxis for herniorrhaphy and breast surgery [letter], *N Engl J Med* 322(26):1884, 1990.
98. Rutkow IM, Robbins AW: Antibiotic prophylaxis for herniorrhaphy and breast surgery [letter], *N Engl J Med* 322(26):1884, 1990.
99. Byrd DR, Brown BW, Hohn DC: Antibiotic prophylaxis for herniorrhaphy and breast surgery [letter], *N Engl J Med* 322(26):1884, 1990.
100. Sebben JE: Prophylactic antibiotics in cutaneous surgery, *J Dermatol Surg Oncol* 11(9):901-906, 1985.
101. Nolen T: Skin and skin-structure infection in elderly patients, *Nurs Home Med* 1(6):25-34, 1993.
102. Heskel NS and others: Erythromycin versus cefadroxil in the treatment of skin infections, *Int J Dermatol* 31(2):131-133, 1992.
103. Bigby M and others: Drug-induced cutaneous reactions *JAMA* 256(24):3358-3363, 1986.
104. Saxon A: Immediate hypersensitivity reactions to beta-lactam antibiotics, *Ann Intern Med* 107:204-215, 1987.
105. Stern RS, Wintroub BV: Adverse drug reactions: reporting and evaluating cutaneous reactions, *Adv Dermatol* 2:3, 1987.
106. Van Arsdael PP: The risk of penicillin reactions, *Ann Intern Med* 69:1071, 1968.
107. Wang WL and others: Susceptibility of *Propionibacterium acnes* to seventeen antibiotics, *Antimicrob Agents Chemother* 11:171-173, 1977.
108. Brause BD: Infections with prostheses in bones and joints. In Mandel GL, Douglas GR, Bennett JE, editors: *Principles and practice of infectious diseases,* ed 3, New York, 1990, Churchill Livingstone, pp 919-922.
109. Olin BR, Hebel SK, Dombek GF. Facts and comparisons: drug information. St Louis, 1993, Facts and Comparisons, p 336A.
110. Smith BR, LeFrock JL: Disulfiram-like and hematologic complications of cephalosporin therapy, *Ochsner Clin Rep Serious Hosp Infect* 2:(4):1-7, 1986.
111. The choice of antibacterial drugs, *Med Let Drugs Ther* 36(925):53-60, 1994.
112. *AMA drug evaluations: cephalosporins and related compounds,* ed 5, Chicago, 1984, American Medical Association, pp 1618-1642.
113. Kaiser AB and others: Efficacy of cefazolin, cefamandole, and gentamicin as prophylactic agents in cardiac surgery, *Ann Surg* 206:791-797, 1987.
114. Hopkins CC: Antibiotic prophylaxis in clean surgery: peripheral vascular surgery, non-cardiovascular thoracic surgery, herniorrhaphy, and mastectomy, *Rev Infect Dis* 13(suppl 10):S869-S873, 1991.
115. Halpern AC and others: The incidence of bacteremia in skin surgery of the head and neck, *J Am Acad Dermatol* 19:112-116, 1988.
116. Classen DC and others: The timing of prophylactic administration of antibiotics and the risk of surgical-wound infection, *N Engl J Med* 326:281-286, 1992.
117. Scher KS, Wroczynski AF, Jones CW. Duration of antibiotic prophylaxis, *Am J Surg* 151:209-212, 1986.
118. Shapiro M, Townsend TR, Rosner B. Use of antimicrobial drugs in general hospitals: patterns of prophylaxis, *N Engl J Med* 301:351-355, 1979.
119. McCue JD: Medical and surgical use of prophylactic antibiotics, *Hosp Pract* 21:167-170, 1986.
120. Dajani AS and others: Prevention of bacterial endocarditis (recommendations by the American Heart Association), *JAMA* 264(22):2919-2922, 1990.
121. Kaye D: Prophylaxis for infective endocarditis: an update, *Ann Intern Med* 104:419-423, 1986.
122. Shulman ST and others: Prevention of bacterial endocarditis, *Am J Dis Child* 139:232-235, 1985.
123. Wagner RF: Antibiotic prophylaxis against bacterial endocarditis in patients undergoing dermatologic surgery, *Arch Dermatol* 122:799-800, 1986.
124. Larkin J: Chemoprophylaxis for infective endocarditis [letter], *Lancet* 739:932, 1992.
125. Duracek DT: Prophylaxis of endocarditis. In Mandell GL and others, editors: *Principles and practice of infectious diseases,* ed 3, New York, 1990, Churchill Livingstone.
126. Endocarditis Working Party of the British Society for Antimicrobial Chemotherapy: Antibiotic prophylaxis of infective endocarditis, *Lancet* 375:88, 1990.
127. Victorian Medical Postgraduate Foundation: *Antibiotic guidelines,* ed 7, 1992.
128. Spelman DW, Weinmann A, Spice JW: Endocarditis following skin procedures, *J Infect* 26:185-189, 1993.

129. Sabetta JB, Zitelli JA: The incidence of bacteremia during skin surgery, *Arch Dermatol* 123:213-215, 1987.
130. Carmichael JA and others: Prophylactic antibiotics for skin surgery? [letter], *Acta Derm Venereol* 72:312-314, 1992.
131. Carmichael AJ and others: Chemoprophylaxis for skin surgery [letter], *Lancet* 339:932, 1992.
132. Guntheroth WG: How important are dental procedures as a cause of infective endocarditis? *Am J Cardiol* 54:797-801, 1984.
133. Everett DE, Hirschmann JV: Transient bacteremia and endocarditis prophylaxis: a review, *Medicine* 56(1):61-77, 1977.
134. McGowan DA, Hendrey ML: Is antibiotic prophylaxis required for dental patients with joint replacements? *Br Dent J* 158:336, 1985.
135. Ainscow DAP, Denham RA: The risk of hematogenous infection in total joint replacements, *J Bone Joint Surg* 66(B):580-582, 1984.

D. Standard Terminology of Graft Sizes

Russell Graham Knudsen

Hair transplant surgeons need clear, standard terminology to accommodate the surgery's continually evolving techniques and to address the recent development of a range of graft sizes and styles. This discussion provides a historical overview of terms used in hair transplant surgery and an accurate classification of terminology that will be useful for physicians now and in the future.

HISTORICAL OVERVIEW OF TERMINOLOGY

Early Terms

Modern hair transplantation began in 1959 with Norman Orentreich's application of the punch biopsy technique to graft harvesting and transfer. These grafts came to be known as *punch grafts* or *plugs*.

Because these descriptive terms gave no indication of graft size, they were imprecise. Physicians defined size by the donor graft diameter. The donor graft, invariably cylindrical, was obtained by a circular punch. Scalp elasticity influenced the recipient hole diameter, which was usually 0.5 to 0.75 mm smaller than the donor graft's diameter.

Because the original grafts were often 5 mm in diameter, physicians considered the quantity of donor hairs an impractical means of classifying punch grafts. Graft size was associated with hair quantity and range of density. Donor diameter gave a rough approximate of hair numbers. The larger the graft, the greater the variation in individual donor scalp hair density.

The 1980s: Micrografts and Minigrafts

Classifying donor grafts by diameter proved accurate and practical until the advent of micrografting in the early 1980s. Surgeons called single- to two-hair grafts *micrografts* and inserted them into either slits cut by a scalpel blade or needle holes.

Graft sectioning into segments became popular in the mid-1980s. Depending on the method of harvesting, surgeons called these sections either *quarter grafts* or *hemigrafts* because the round grafts were cut into either quarter or halves, respectively. Some surgeons called the hemigrafts *bisected grafts* or *bi's*. These terms defined donor grafts by shape rather than size, although surgeons usually specified the donor diameter. The punch technique was the assumed harvesting method.

Leading hair transplant surgeons soon realized that sectioning made possible any number of permutations of size and shape and coined the term *minigraft* to describe any donor graft with a size between a micrograft and a traditional round graft.

The Minigraft Revolution

In addition to donor shape, recipient area shape and size became factors in minigraft definition. Surgeons could place these grafts into slits (cut by a scalpel blade) or holes (cut by the punch trephine). Minigraft definition factors still did not include the number of donor hairs, an issue later acknowledged as critical.

The 1990s

In the early 1990s, surgeons moved toward harvesting donor grafts by scalpel excision rather than by trephine punch excision. This innovation exceeded the older classification's capabilities of definition and necessitated new standards and terminology. Most surgeons now use a classification system that considers recipient site shape, size, and number of hairs per graft.

The Future

With the imminent use of lasers in hair transplantation, physicians will need to classify recipient shapes as either slits or holes to describe the surgically created linear defects, known as *trenches*, as well as the variety of possible recipient shapes. Because laser transplantation is still developing, its terminology has not yet evolved.

STANDARD GRAFT CLASSIFICATION SYSTEM

An accurate classification of grafts has some essential requirements. Because a variety of donor and recipient shapes is possible, hair transplant surgeons should define graft shape descriptively. Graft size,

TABLE 2-4 Standard Classification Terminology

CLASS	SHAPE	SIZE	EXAMPLE
Standard or traditional	Round or square	Graft size ≥2 mm	Traditional round 3 mm punch graft
Minigraft	Round, linear, or square	Must be ≤2 mm; size determined by recipient diameter (in mm) and by number of hairs	Round 1.5 mm six-hair minigraft
Micrograft	Not required	Defined by number of hairs	Two-hair micrograft
Strip graft	Strip	Defined by length × width (in mm)	30 × 2 mm strip graft

critical to accurate classification, needs to consider both the number of hairs contained and, depending on shape, the size in millimeters. Definition by hair numbers is impractical for larger grafts. For historical continuity, surgeons will still need to use common terms but more precisely.

The following terminology describes grafts by class, shape, and size. Class designators are optional. Table 2-4 summarizes the terminology and lists the three essential elements of defining or classifying grafts: class, shape, and size. Correct usage of this terminology would allow for standardization and accurate communication among hair restoration surgeons.

STANDARD GRAFTS. Standard grafts are the traditional, larger, usually round grafts, which are harvested by a trephine or by sectioning donor strips with a scalpel blade. Standard graft shapes are defined descriptively (e.g., round, square), and donor size, whether diameter or length, will be expressed in millimeters. A standard graft must have a donor diameter greater than or equal to 2 mm. An example would be a 4 mm standard round graft.

MINIGRAFTS. Minigrafts are smaller, sectioned grafts harvested either by trephine, scalpel, or laser. A minigraft must have a donor and recipient diameter of less than 2 mm. The shape will generally either be linear or round, but other shapes are possible. Surgeons will be able to apply the term *linear minigraft* to laser transplant surgery and to grafts placed in surgically created linear defects, or trenches. The shape of the recipient site and the method of harvesting are inconsequential.

With linear minigrafts, size is defined by the number of hairs contained. With round minigrafts, size is defined by the number of hairs contained, recipient hole diameter, or both.

Recipient diameter is necessary for minigraft definition because scalp elasticity affects it. Since surgeons can harvest donor grafts in several ways, they must define a minigraft's recipient diameter as less than 2 mm. Examples include a three-hair linear minigraft, a four-hair round minigraft, and a 1.5 mm round minigraft.

MICROGRAFTS. Micrografts are single- to two-hair grafts that are not defined by shape or method of insertion. An example would be a single-hair micrograft.

STRIP GRAFTS. Strip grafts are grafts harvested by scalpel or laser and are greater than 10 mm in length. Size is defined by length and width, and it is expressed in millimeters. An example would be a 30 × 2 mm strip graft.

CONCLUSION

From the first punch-excised grafts of the 1960s to laser innovations still developing, the evolution of hair transplant surgical techniques has proceeded and created the need for standard language that can describe it accurately. This standard terminology categorizes grafts by class, shape, and size. To apply the terms successfully, physicians must properly use the classes of standard graft, minigraft, and micrograft.

This terminology will facilitate simple yet more accurate classification for comparing the types of grafts that various surgeons are using. It is flexible enough to accommodate future graft forms. Its use will enhance communication among transplant surgeons.

E. The Surgical Suite

Dow B. Stough

Although differences in technique exist among all hair restoration surgeons, there is a common need for a well-equipped operating room that is comfortable for both the patient and the transplanting team. With the advent of total micrografting, the properly designed and equipped surgical suite becomes paramount (see box). The design of a surgical suite that maximizes efficiency for the transplanting team requires careful planning.

SIZE

A 10 × 11 foot room is the minimal size operating suite to perform hair transplant surgery. The ideal room size for a transplant procedure is in the range of 13 × 15 feet. Our operating suites are 15 × 16 feet and can accommodate a wide number of other procedures (Fig. 2-3). A spacious room will avoid a claustrophobic effect on the patient. Cramped rooms may be adequate to perform a procedure but ultimately will fall short on patient and staff comfort. The room design shown in Fig. 2-4 displays our current hair transplantation suite.

LIGHTING

The need for ideal lighting cannot be overemphasized. Natural light includes a balance of ultraviolet and visible color wavelengths. Full-spectrum light is the light that is optimal for sight. The spectrum balance of ultraviolet and visible light is required for lamps to be called *full spectrum*.

Older eyes require a greater quantity of light than younger eyes for the same task. An individual requires roughly 25% greater quantity of light at 50 years of age than at 25 years of age. Therefore the age of the physician and technicians and the difficulty of the task to be performed must be factored into the lighting selection for a particular space.

These concerns are paramount in hair restoration surgery. Glare is any brightness that causes discomfort or interference with vision, resulting in eye strain and fatigue. Minimal glare should be the first consideration in the selection and placement of the light source.

Proper lighting allows technicians to work effectively and decreases eye strain. Full-spectrum lamps are ideal for reduced glare in interior lighting, aiding in "see-ability." Full-spectrum lighting is more advantageous for photographic documentation since standard fluorescent lights often will cast a green hue. Standard fluorescent lamps, which produce most of their light output in the yellow-green spectral region, are high-brightness sources (such as cool white and warm white). Incandescent and high-intensity discharge lamps are high-brightness sources and require special fixture designs for glare reduction and control. Full-spectrum fluorescent lights are available from a number of manufacturers and require no special outlets (Duro-Test Corp., Newark, N.J.). With adequate fluorescent lighting, there is very little need for additional intense medical-grade illumination systems. The advantages and disadvantages of full-spectrum lights are listed in the accompanying box below.

GRAFT SECTIONING TABLE

A unique aspect of hair restoration surgery is the requirement for countertop space sufficient for technicians to trim and prepare micrografts. Many surgeons initially entering this field are unaware of these specifics. Fig. 2-5 demonstrates the correct table

---

UNIQUE ASPECTS OF THE HAIR RESTORATION SUITE

Space requirements, at least 10 × 11 ft, optimum 13 × 15 ft
Countertop space for graft preparation with ample legroom for two technicians (see Fig. 2-5)
Full-spectrum ultraviolet lighting is advisable
Minimum of nine electrical outlets

FULL-SPECTRUM LIGHTING

Advantages
Allows clearer perception of fine details of graft sectioning than standard lighting
Permits more effective performance of visually demanding tasks
Reduces glare, thereby lessening eye fatigue and strain
Reduces maintenance and replacement costs as a result of its long-life features
Provides superior conditions to standard Cool White fluorescent lights for clinical photographs

Disadvantages
Creates slightly higher initial cost
Affects room design

Data from Duro-Test Corporation, Technical Bulletin, Engineering Department.

The Surgical Suite 79

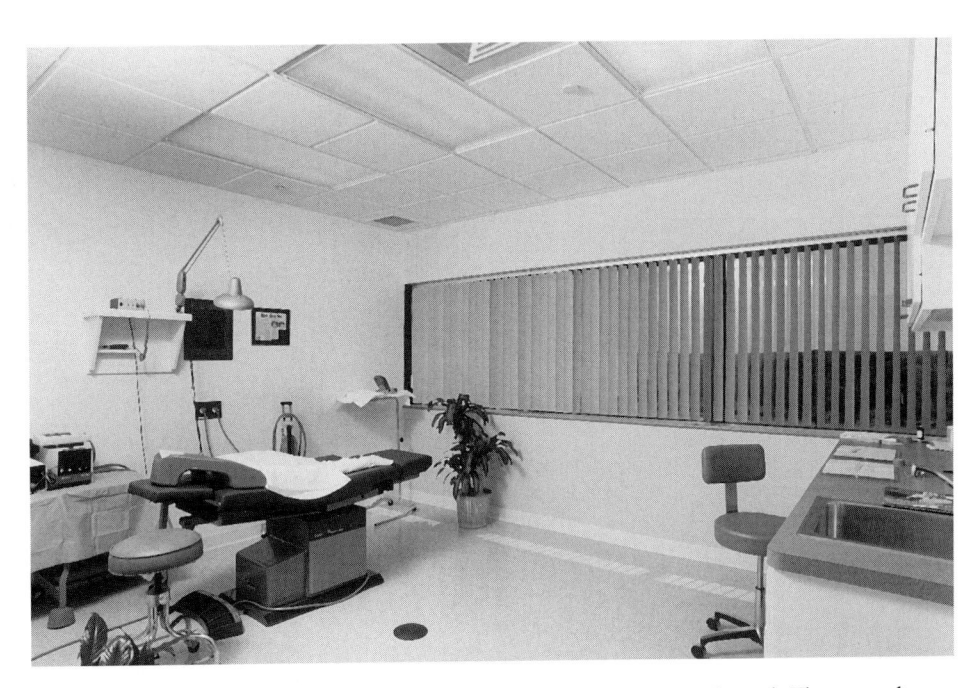

FIG. 2-3 The author's surgical suite in which hair transplants are performed. The room dimensions are 15 × 16 feet. The overhead lighting employs full-spectrum fluorescent lamps. These lights, in addition to ambient light from the windows, obviate the need for medical-grade illumination lights. The latter often produce glare and lack the effectiveness of the above system.

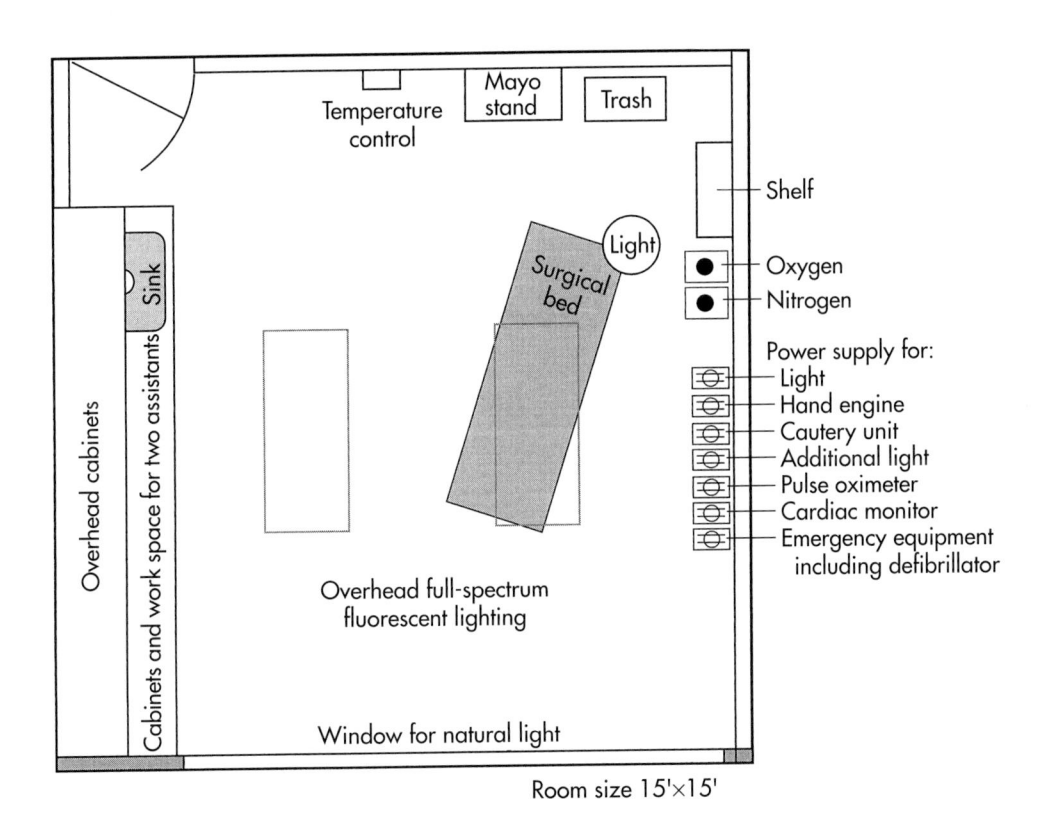

FIG. 2-4 Operating room requirements.

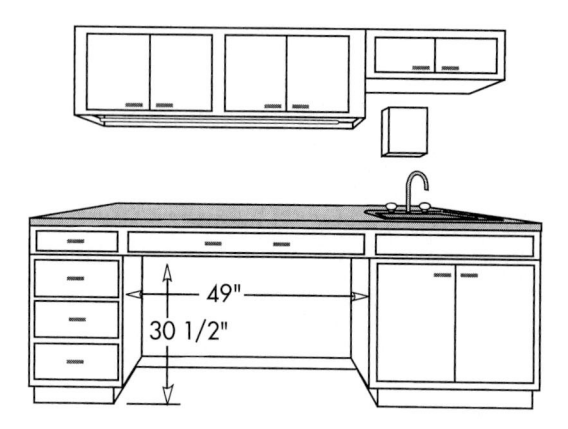

FIG. 2-5 Cabinet layout showing minimal dimensions for two assistants. It is important to have ample knee room and good undercounter lights for surgical assistants to section grafts.

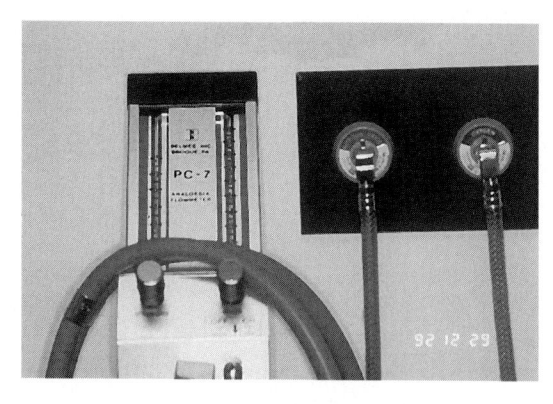

FIG. 2-6 Specialized outlets for nitrogen and oxygen allow nitrous oxide to be used as a preanesthetic agent.

height as well as leg space requirements for trimming grafts. Since the space requirements will vary depending on the type of chairs used, chair selection should be addressed in the initial surgical suite design.

ELECTRICAL OUTLETS

Determining the number of electrical outlets for a given procedure is fraught with difficulties. Techniques and technology change at such a rapid rate that initial requirements may fall short in terms of future needs. A minimum of nine electrical outlets will be needed to operate an electric surgical table and accessories with current techniques (see Fig. 2-4).

ANESTHESIA OUTLETS

I favor the use of nitrous oxide as a preanesthetic agent. Use of this anesthetic agent requires rooms that are designed with specialized outlets for nitrogen and oxygen (Fig. 2-6). Scavenger systems for nitrous oxide are also available.

3
Anesthesia

A. Local Anesthesia in Hair Transplantation

David J. Seager

IMPORTANCE OF EFFECTIVE ANESTHESIA

The importance of good pain control cannot be overemphasized. A surgeon who performs painless hair transplantation will have a competitive edge over his/her colleagues. Often patients who experience a lot of pain during their first hair transplant session will not return. The result of an unfinished case with a pluggy or thin appearance will give the public a poor impression of hair transplantation in general. One's ability to perform painless hair and scalp surgery is therefore of paramount importance.

Consideration of the Patient's Emotional State

Pain control begins at the first preoperative consultation. The process of obtaining the patient's confidence begins with the patient's initial perception of the surgeon and his/her staff. A prolonged time spent in the waiting room can increase the patient's anxiety; if there is going to be any significant delay, the patient should be sent out of the office until the appointment time. One should avoid mentioning blood, pain, or needles. Before and during surgery, sharp instruments and bloodstained swabs or gloves should be kept out of the patient's sight. There should be no distracting noises, such as bursts of laughter from the staff. Soft background music should be playing. Some patients will be more at ease watching a video of their choice immediately before and during their surgery.

Role of Premedication

Although premedication is mentioned elsewhere in this textbook, it is so fundamental to effective pain control that its importance must be reemphasized. The purpose of premedication is to reduce anxiety, raise the pain threshold, and, in the case of certain benzodiazepines, provide profound amnesia and counteract the neurological side effects of possible local anesthetic toxicity.

Nearly all of my young healthy patients receive intravenous sedation with midazolam (Versed) because of its brief duration of action and profound amnesic properties. When enough midazolam has been given to mildly impair the patient's intellect, needleless injectors, EMLA cream, 30-gauge needles, and other measures to reduce the pain of infiltration of local anesthetics are not necessary. However much these patients may wince and complain about the pain of the "needles" at the time, they all report at the end of each session that they did not feel or remember any pain at all!

In patients over the age of 60 to 65 years or those with a history of heart or respiratory disease, I avoid intravenous medication but administer intramuscularly a slightly lower dose of midazolam—1.5 to 3 mg, depending on the weight and age of the patient. For those patients reluctant to have any "injection" of a sedative, oral diazepam, 10 to 20 mg, may be administered.

LOCAL ANESTHETICS
Historical Development

Local anesthetics have been used since ancient times when the Incas chewed coca leaves and let their saliva drip into the wounds of trephination to numb pain.[1] Karl Koller was the first to use cocaine, an extract from the coca plant, in surgical practice in 1884; he initially used it as a topical agent for the eye during an operation for glaucoma.[2] The first regional nerve block using cocaine was performed in 1884 by Halstead.[2] Local anesthetics gained popularity after procaine was produced in 1904, despite the tendency of these "ester group" local anesthetics to cause local allergic reactions. Lidocaine, the first of the "amide group," was synthesized in 1943. Lidocaine is still the best known and most used local anesthetic. Local anesthetics can be classified into these two groups: the ester group and the amide group (Table 3-1). The ester anesthetics are hydrolyzed in the plasma by an enzyme called *pseudocholinesterase.* Rare individuals with abnor-

TABLE 3-1 Ester and Amide Local Anesthetics and Their Properties

GENERIC NAME	TRADE NAME	INFILTRATION DOSE (%)	ONSET OF ACTION	DURATION OF ACTION (MIN) WITHOUT EPINEPHRINE	DURATION OF ACTION (MIN) WITH EPINEPHRINE	MAXIMUM DOSE (MG IN 70 KG MAN) WITHOUT EPINEPRHINE	MAXIMUM DOSE (MG IN 70 KG MAN) WITH EPINEPHRINE
Esters							
Cocaine		Topical use only					
Procaine	Novocain	0.5-2	Fast	15-30	30-90	500	600
Tetracaine	Amethocaine (pontocaine)	0.25-1	Slow	120-240	240-480	100	—
Amides							
Lidocaine	Xylocaine	0.5-2	Fast	30-120	60-400	300	500
Bupivacaine	Marcaine	0.25-0.5	Slow (15 min)	120-240	240-480	175	225
Prilocaine	Citanest	0.5	Moderate	30-120	60-400	400	600
Etidocaine	Duranest	0.25	Slow	200	240-360	300	400

mal forms of pseudocholinesterase may experience an overdose if they are given a large dose of an ester local anesthetic. Amide anesthetics such as lidocaine are metabolized in the liver and are then excreted by the kidneys. Therefore persons with impaired liver function have reduced tolerance to amide anesthetics.

Dosage and Duration

A vasoconstrictor, usually epinephrine, is added to the local anesthetic used in hair restoration surgery. The main reason for the addition of epinephrine is to limit absorption, enabling the use of higher total dosage and prolonging the duration of action. Most local anesthetics with the exception of cocaine and prilocaine cause vasodilatation by direct relaxation of the vascular smooth muscle. Epinephrine also reduces the bleeding that would result from this increased vasodilatation. (Note that in muscle such as temporalis or occipitalis musculature epinephrine will have the reverse effect of increasing vasodilatation, thereby increasing any bleeding.)[3] Other vasoconstrictors such as phenylephrine or ornithine-8-vasopressin (not currently available in North America) have been used.

Local anesthetics such as lidocaine premixed with epinephrine in various concentrations are available; 1:200,000 is the concentration most commonly used. Studies have shown that concentrations greater than 1:200,000 are probably not necessary, and concentrations greater than 1:100,000 are associated with increased side effects.[4] The New York Heart Association believes that up to 0.2 mg of epinephrine administered subcutaneously is safe even in cardiac patients.[5] It takes 7 to 15 minutes for the vasoconstriction caused by epinephrine in these concentrations to achieve its maximum effects, which last for approximately 40 minutes. After 40 minutes further administration of epinephrine often fails to cause further vasoconstriction. Because epinephrine mixed with local anesthetics degrades with time, various acids are added to the premixed commercial local anesthetics to reduce the pH, which slows the degradation of epinephrine. This is important to bear in mind for two reasons. First, these acidic local anesthetics produce more pain on injection than neutral or alkaline local anesthetics. Sodium bicarbonate can be added in the amount of 1 ml of 8.4% sodium bicarbonate for every 10 ml of local anesthetic to reduce pain during infiltration; this mixture is less painful but seems to cause more postoperative edema. Second, acidity that remains after anesthetic effects have worn off may produce tolerance to further local anesthetic injected in the operative site. For both of these reasons, it may be better to mix plain local anesthetic with epinephrine freshly each operation day. A total of 0.1 ml of 1:1000 epinephrine mixed with 20 ml of lidocaine provides a solution of a 1:200,000 concentration of epinephrine.

DURATION OF ACTION

The two most commonly used local anesthetics in hair restoration surgery are lidocaine and bupivacaine. Lidocaine has a fast onset of action, within minutes, and with epinephrine it lasts 60 to 400 minutes.[6] The shorter duration, 60 minutes, is usually applicable to the hairline area of a young patient's head, whereas the longer duration, 400 minutes, represents the longest period the effects of lidocaine with epinephrine may last in relatively in-

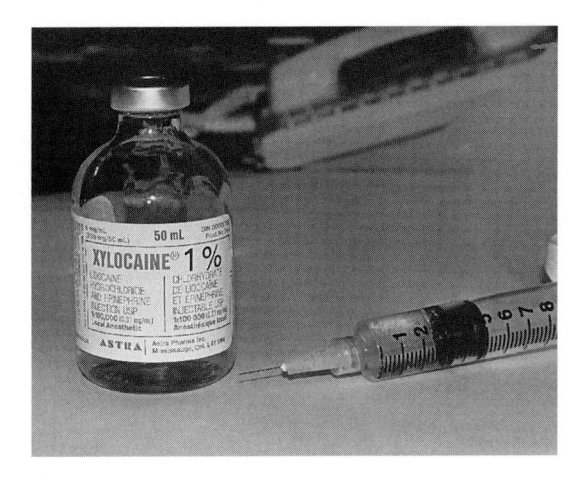

FIG. 3-1 Bottle containing 50 ml of 1% lidocaine (Xylocaine) with epinephrine (the maximum amount allowable for an average patient weighing 70 kg) with 30-gauge needle.

sensitive areas such as the donor area in an older patient. Bupivacaine's onset of action is slower; it often takes 12 to 20 minutes to work, and with epinephrine it may last 204 to 480 minutes (see Table 3-1). This duration of time applies to local infiltration; with peripheral nerve blocks these time intervals may be longer. My experience is that in younger patients the local anesthetic has a shorter duration of action. In general, it is more difficult to achieve adequate local anesthesia in younger patients than in older patients. It should be noted that it is more difficult if not impossible to locally anesthetize inflamed, infected tissues.

MAXIMUM DOSAGE

The maximum dosage of local anesthetic depends on many factors such as the vascularity of the site being infiltrated, concentration of the local anesthetic being infiltrated, age and general condition of the patient, and weight of the patient. For a person weighing 100 kg, the maximum recommended dose of lidocaine given as a 1% solution with 1:100,000 epinephrine is 70 ml or 700 mg (Fig. 3-1). If given as a 2% solution, the maximum dose is 35 ml or 700 mg. This maximum dose must be reduced (or increased) pro rata for patients with different weights (see Table 3-1). The maximum dose must also be reduced for older patients and especially for patients with any liver function impairment. The first signs of toxicity are all neurological, and benzodiazepines counteract all of these early side effects. Many physicians performing hair transplantation now believe that under adequate benzodiazepine cover, the total maximum recommended dose can be considerably increased. Various physicians say they regularly give patients double the previously recommended maximum dose. However, I believe that such high doses are inadvisable even under benzodiazepine cover, although there is no doubt that with generous intravenous or oral benzodiazepine sedation, doses higher than those previously recommended are quite safe; how high or how safe the dose has not yet been established. For hair transplantation I never have to exceed the traditional maximum dosage (as described in Table 3-1). In transplant sessions involving a large number of grafts in older patients or patients with lighter weights, I may anesthetize the donor area first and the recipient area later. With scalp reductions it is sometimes necessary to give patients high doses of local anesthetics; these patients should definitely receive higher doses of intravenous benzodiazepine if doses of local anesthetics around the maximal levels are going to be administered.

ADMINISTRATION TECHNIQUES
Topical Local Anesthetics

EMLA is the newest and most effective topical local anesthetic at this time. EMLA is a mixture of 2.5% lidocaine combined in a eutectic mixture with 2.5% prilocaine. Topical application under occlusion with plastic provides some superficial anesthesia to the skin but not enough for full-thickness surgery. It has been found to be useful in reducing the pain from needleless injectors. In my experience EMLA does not help unless it is applied in a thick coating covered with an occlusive plastic wrap for 2 hours (Fig. 3-2). (The manufacturer states that occlusive application for 1 hour is adequate, but I have not found this period to be long enough. Dr. Dow Stough and I have independently conducted as yet unpublished double-blind clinical trials that clearly demonstrate that 2 hours is necessary.) I would also stress that EMLA does not seem to make the sensation of either the piercing of skin by a needle or the injection of local anesthetic any less painful, but in double-blind trials it has definitely been found to reduce the discomfort caused by multiple injections of local anesthetics with a needleless injector. Use of occlusive plastic wrap over EMLA for 2 hours before surgery is not conducive to the smooth flow of patients through a busy hair-transplant clinic. I have found that patients either do not place it in the right locations for anesthetization of their hairlines or they do not like waiting at the office before surgery. Therefore I use it only with patients who refuse intravenous sedation or those with whom I am not comfortable administering intravenous sedation such as older patients or those with a history of heart disease. The dose of local anesthetic absorbed systemically from applying EMLA in this manner is negligible.

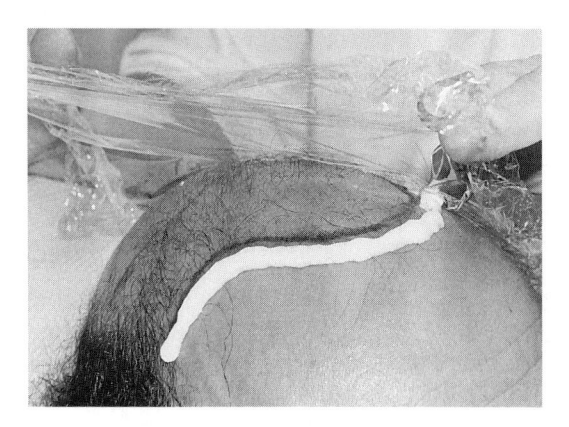

FIG. 3-2 Thick coating of EMLA cream over the hairline about to be covered by occlusive plastic.

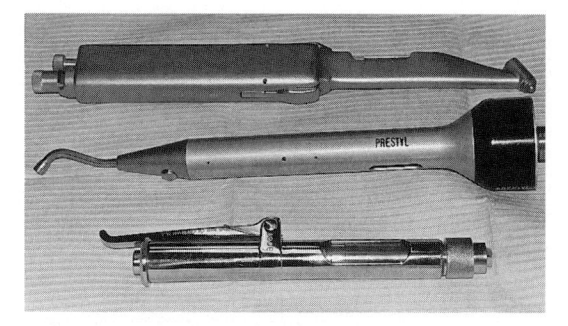

FIG. 3-3 The Syrijet (*top*) (Mizzy, Inc., Cherry Hill, N.J.) is less painful for the patient, but in my experience it is less reliable and less durable than the Dermojet. The Prestyl (*middle*) (BMA Technologies, Billere, France) is the newest and easiest to use needleless injector. It is powered by compressed air and is fired like a machine gun with foot pedal controls. The Dermojet (*bottom*) (Robbins Instruments, Inc., Chatham, N.J.) is the most reliable, commonly used needleless injector.

Other methods of applying topical local anesthetics include iontophoresis, the active transport of charged ions across membranes by an electric current. This method is still in its experimental stages.

Needleless Injectors

Several kinds of needleless injectors are available (Fig. 3-3). The most widely used and in my experience the most reliable is the Dermojet (Robbins Instruments, Inc., Chatham, N.J.) (Fig. 3-3, *bottom*). Alternative needleless injectors are the Syrijet (Mizzy, Inc., Cherry Hill, N.J.) (Fig. 3-3, *top*) and the Prestyl (BMA Technologies, Billere, France) (Fig. 3-3, *middle*). Each needleless injector holds a volume of local anesthetic mixture in a reservoir or cartridge. A lever is used to cock the mechanism, and when a trigger is pressed, the needleless injector ejects a set amount of local anesthetic mixture, usually 0.1 ml, which penetrates the skin of the patient superficially. In the case of local anesthetics with added epinephrine, a circular wheal of skin blanching is produced.

Infiltration Techniques

One method of anesthetizing skin for hair transplantation consists of using a needleless injector to make wheals every 1½ inches around the perimeter of the area to be anesthetized. The surgeon then uses a syringe filled with the local anesthetic solution attached to a 1-inch 30-gauge or larger needle. This needle is inserted to its hilt through one of these wheals in the direction of the line of the ring blockage. The plunger of the syringe is withdrawn slightly to ensure that no blood is aspirated into the syringe, indicating that the tip of the needle is not in a blood vessel. With nerve blocks one is more likely to encounter a significantly large blood vessel and the use of a 25-gauge needle is suggested because aspiration of blood as a test is more reliable with a larger bore needle. The plunger of the syringe is then pressed, injecting the anesthetic subcutaneously as the needle of the syringe is pulled backward slowly toward its insertion point in the center of the wheal created by the needleless injector (Fig. 3-4). This procedure is repeated for all adjacent wheals until local anesthetic has been infiltrated around the entire perimeter of the area to be locally anesthetized.

When the donor area is being anesthetized, it should be remembered that the nerve supply approaches from the inferior direction, and thus it is necessary to infiltrate only the lower margin of the area to be anesthetized. Similarly, if the recipient area includes hairlines and/or the vertex, most of the nerve supply to this region courses up from the face, and thus most of the local anesthetic for the ring block should be used in the hairline and less in the lateral margins of the area to be anesthetized.

Author's Technique

My own technique currently involves one of two different methods. One method is to use fairly generous intravenous sedation with midazolam and the other is to use a local anesthetic cream along with frequent use of the needleless injector. With generous intravenous sedation the patient invariably does not remember receiving the local anesthetic and one can use a longer and larger needle (such as a 1½-inch 25- to 27-gauge needle), which is more painful but faster to use. A ring block around the donor or recipient area is thus achieved, with the majority of the local anesthetic inserted into the proximal aspect of the fields to be anesthetized. Be-

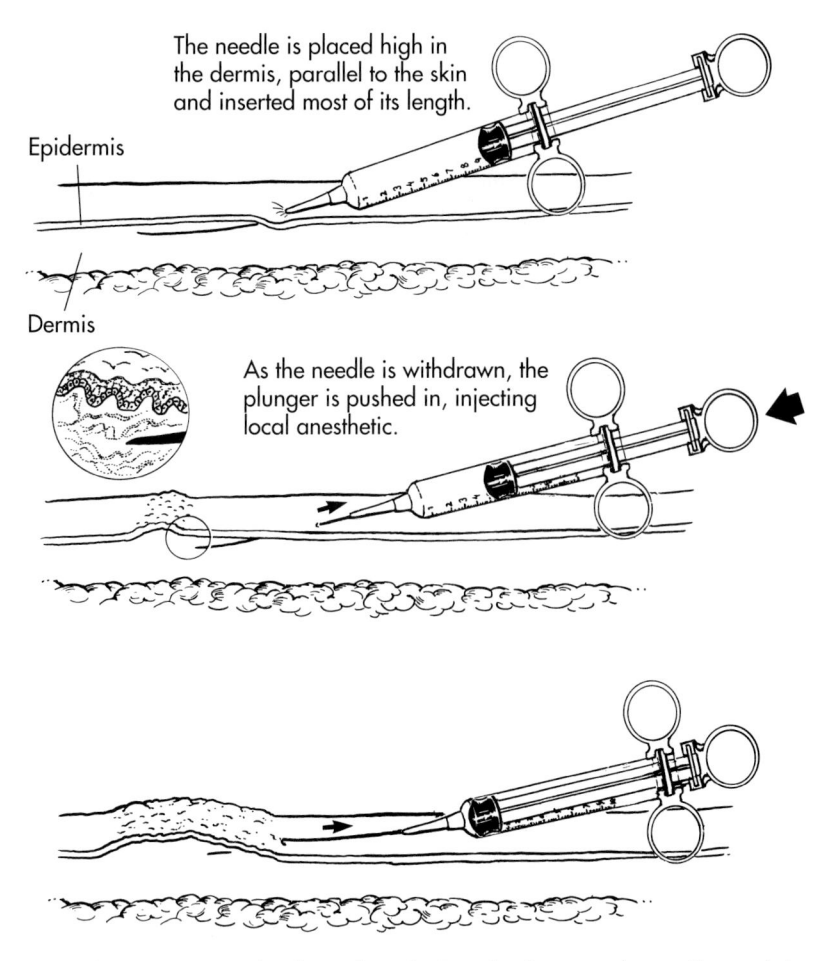

FIG. 3-4 Syringe injecting local anesthetic high in the dermis as the needle is withdrawn.

cause of the profound amnesia patients will experience, use of EMLA, a needleless injector, or a 30-gauge needle is not necessary. In my opinion this technique is the quickest, most effective, and least unpleasant method for locally anesthetizing the patient. The midazolam will counteract any early toxic neurological side effects of the local anesthetic, permitting the administration of larger doses. The disadvantage of using intravenous sedation is that close monitoring of the patient's oxygen saturation level, blood pressure, and pulse is required because intravenous benzodiazepines, especially midazolam, can depress the respiratory drive and blood pressure.

The second method is reserved for those who refuse intravenous sedation or those for whom I do not feel comfortable giving intravenous sedation, as mentioned previously. A thick coating of EMLA is applied to the area requiring infiltration of local anesthesia (see Fig. 3-2), occlusive plastic wrap (such as that used in any kitchen) is placed over it, and the patient is sent away for 1½ hours. When the patient returns, he is taken to the surgery room and the EMLA and plastic wrap are removed from the donor area, the hair is taped up, and the area is shaved and cleaned in the usual manner. A needleless injector is then used to create series of wheals immediately adjacent to each other along the inferior margin of the selected donor site and up both sides, as shown in Fig. 3-5. With the 30-gauge needle, 1% lidocaine with 1:200,000 epinephrine is injected into each of these wheals very superficially, as is done for a tuberculin test. This injection pattern will create a peau d'orange appearance of the skin. In this manner the ring block is created around the inferior and lateral borders of the donor site. A 30-gauge needle is better than a 27-gauge needle because it is easier to inject smaller doses more precisely and superficially. Injecting more slowly and using local anesthesia warmed to room temperature and buffered with sodium bicarbonate as described all help to reduce the pain of infiltration. The rest of the donor site is then infiltrated with 0.5% lidocaine with 1:200,000 epinephrine. To prepare an

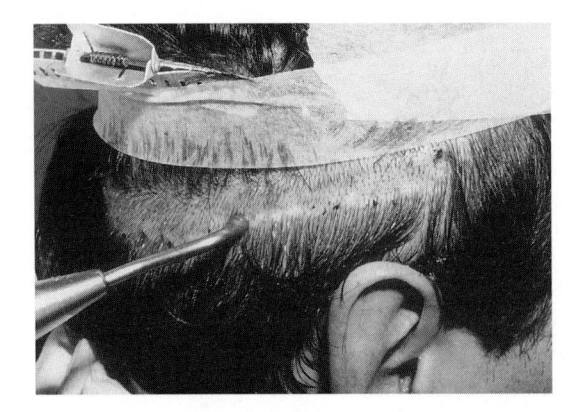

FIG. 3-5 Wheals produced by a needleless injector immediately adjacent to one another, initiating a ring block.

area 1 cm wide by 12 cm long, it generally takes approximately 5 ml of 1% lidocaine and epinephrine and approximately 7 ml of 0.5% lidocaine and epinephrine. This is the way I currently locally anesthetize a typical donor site. This method of very superficial infiltration into the dermis results in a more rapid onset of anesthesia that lasts longer than that achieved with deeper injections. Deeper subcutaneous injection is faster to give, but the effect is slower in onset with shorter duration and is less effective. I should stress that the key to successful and lasting local anesthesia is very superficial injection into the upper dermis (Fig. 3-4). However, should the local anesthesia begin to wear off before the procedure is finished (never the case in the donor area), additional local anesthetic may be infiltrated with a 30-gauge needle to create a peau d'orange effect. This reinfiltration should be timed to take place just as the patient is beginning to feel sensation in the anesthetized area, so that the discomfort of this "reanesthetizing" is easily bearable. It is remarkable how little local anesthetic is necessary to reanesthetize; often 1 to 2 ml of 2% lidocaine will reanesthetize an entire hairline. One should *not* wait until the local anesthesia has completely worn off, or the patient will complain bitterly. If necessary, additional intravenous sedation can be given, which will make the second injection better tolerated with regard to pain and total dosage of local anesthetic.

I then finish harvesting the donor grafts and suture the area closed. A pressure dressing is applied, and I then turn my attention to the recipient area. The occlusive plastic wrap is removed and the EMLA is thoroughly cleaned off (this is an important step; severe scarring erythematous reactions have occurred as a result of the needleless injector "tattooing" EMLA into the skin). The site of application of the EMLA will be apparent either by blanching of the skin or by noting the erythema created by the EMLA. With the needleless injector I then repeatedly inject this "EMLA line," typically just below the hairline, with wheals immediately adjacent to each other with 2% lidocaine with 1:200,000 epinephrine. I then inject more 2% lidocaine with epinephrine with a 30-gauge needle into each wheal very superficially into the dermis, again creating a peau d'orange effect. I use 2% lidocaine only in the hairline and 1% lidocaine for the ring block in the lateral margins of the recipient areas. I then infiltrate 0.5% lidocaine with epinephrine over the entire recipient area using a 30-gauge needle. I try to ensure that 5 ml of 2% lidocaine with epinephrine is injected into the anterior hairline in the manner described. I believe this approach is the most effective way of securing complete and lasting local anesthesia to the sensitive hairline area.

Certain details should be noted:

1. The total amount of local anesthetic used should be continuously monitored. One can assume that only approximately one third of what was used with the needleless injector actually penetrates the skin; the remainder splatters off the surface of the skin without being injected.
2. The maximum response of the vasculature from the epinephrine takes 3 to 15 minutes. When a large number of grafts are to be transplanted, I would not delay making recipient sites at all but would apply digital pressure to any bleeding incisions in the recipient area immediately. This vasoconstricting effect is fairly short-lived and will be needed more when the transplanting is actually begun; it often wears off all too soon.
3. The 30-gauge needle is particularly useful because it is easier to be more precise while injecting the local anesthetic superficially into the dermis. In this manner less local anesthetic can be used more effectively.
4. It is more difficult to achieve adequate local anesthesia in younger patients than older patients and the anesthetic wears off sooner. This observation has been an invariable finding of mine. It is well known that most medications are dose for dose more potent in older patients. In my experience younger patients, in general, also have higher anxiety levels.

Tumescent Method

Another method of administering local anesthesia is the tumescent method in which large quantities of very dilute solutions of local anesthetic solutions with epinephrine are injected into the scalp to make it balloon out. I, and most other hair transplant surgeons I have spoken to who have tried this method, find it more time consuming and difficult than traditional anesthetic techniques because the grafts tend to sink below the surface of the skin, and we find it offers no real advantage in hair transplantation. However, the tumescent method does have its proponents.

Nerve Blocks

Nerve blocks are rarely used for hair transplantation. For scalp reductions and other major hair restoration procedures I use supraorbital, supratrochlear, and occipital nerve blocks. The details of these nerve blocks are beyond the scope of this discussion.

ADVERSE REACTIONS AND THEIR TREATMENT

Toxicity

Toxicity from anesthesia can be divided into neurological and cardiac side effects. Early neurological side effects occurred frequently before the use of significant premedication with benzodiazepines. Early side effects are a chilled sensation, shivering, muscle twitching, and visual disturbances. Perioral paresthesia and numbness are said to be pathognomonic, as is a bitter taste in the mouth. Other subjective CNS symptoms involve sensations of lightheadedness and dizziness, visual and auditory disturbances, disorientation, and drowsiness. The rate of injection and rapidity with which a particular blood level is achieved will alter the toxicity of that particular blood level of the local anesthetic drug; that is, the more rapidly absorbed the local anesthetic, the lower the level at which CNS toxicity occurs. More serious signs of CNS overdose include muscle twitching and tremors involving the facial muscles and distal parts of the extremities and then generalized tonic-clonic convulsions. Ultimately these signs of CNS excitation are followed by a generalized state of CNS depression. Respiratory depression and then respiratory arrest may occur. Cardiac side effects occur much later and with a much more serious local anesthetic overdose. (To cause cardiac side effects, the blood level has to be at least double the dosage required to cause neurological side effects.) Initially a decrease in cardiac output occurs; later, profound myocardial depression followed by cardiac collapse occurs. Experimental evidence with animals and humans implies that three to seven times the dose of local anesthetic is necessary to cause cardiac collapse as compared to convulsions.[7] Bupivacaine is notorious for a more potent effect on the heart, and toxicity can cause severe cardiac arrythmias.

Drug Interactions

Monoamine oxidase inhibitors and phenothiazines are both contraindicated with local anesthetic agents, and these drugs should be discontinued 2 weeks before surgery. Amiodarone has also been reported to interact adversely with lidocaine.

Epinephrine/β-Blocker Reaction

Interaction with β-blockers has been well documented. A syndrome of severe hypertension with bradycardia has occurred when lidocaine with epinephrine has been administered to patients currently taking β-blockers. This drug interaction must be extremely rare because these drugs have frequently been given together for years, often deliberately to counter anxiety and epinephrine side effects. However, this syndrome does occur and it is dangerous. My opinion is that lidocaine and epinephrine may be given with β-blockers if the patient cannot discontinue the β-blocker but that the anesthetic must be administered with great caution and in stages, with monitoring equipment and full resuscitative facilities available. Prilocaine, with its lack of vasodilatory effect and its long duration of action, may be a good alternative in cardiac patients, although its tendency to produce methemoglobinemia should be considered in cyanotic heart or pulmonary disease.

Treatment for the epinephrine-propanolol reaction includes intravenous administration of chloropromazine in 1 mg increments with careful monitoring. No more than 5 mg is usually necessary. A hydralazine drip, 20 mg in 250 ml saline solution, also administered with monitoring, is equally effective. If bradycardia persists after control of hypertension, the patient can be given atropine.[5]

Allergic Reactions

Allergic reactions to local anesthetics are rare and are mainly associated with the ester anesthetics. These allergic reactions may be anaphylactic, delayed and urticarial, contact dermatitis, or a mixture of all three types. Because the ester and amide classes of local anesthetic are antigenically distinct, a patient may react to one group but not the other. Usually the history is somewhat vague and more typical of an anxiety or vasovagal attack or an epinephrine reaction. True allergies to the more commonly used amide anesthetics are extremely rare and are more often caused by the paraben preservatives included in commercial preparations. Preservative-free lidocaine is obtainable, but considering that patch and intradermal testing are not reliable in these cases, it is preferable to use an anesthetic from a different group or even general anesthesia in patients who seem to have had a true allergic reaction to lidocaine. If an anaphylactic reaction occurs during local anesthesia, it should be treated in the usual manner with intravenous epinephrine, intravenous hydrocortisone, and a tourniquet placed around the skull; the patient should be placed in the Trendelenburg position, given oxygen, and immediately transported via ambulance to a suitable emergency department.

Epinephrine Reactions

Epinephrine reactions are more likely to occur if the epinephrine solution is inadvertently administered intravenously, but they also occur with usual field infiltration. Epinephrine reactions are characterized by anxiety and apprehension, tachycardia, palpitations, and perspiration. These epinephrine reactions are nearly always short and self-limited. The following scenario represents a more serious epinephrine reaction: If the heart rate remains above 140 beats per minute, ventricular tachycardia, premature ventricular complexes (with a frequency of more than six per minute, or closely coupled [R on T phenomenon], multiform, or occurring together in short bursts), the administration of a 100 mg bolus of intravenous lidocaine or intravenous propanolol should be considered.

TREAMENT OF ADVERSE REACTIONS

Syncope

The first step required when an adverse reaction occurs is accurate diagnosis. Distinguishing syncope from other, more serious forms of collapse may be difficult. Syncope is common in the patients of novice, inexperienced surgeons; the patients seem to be able to sense the lack of experience and/or confidence of the surgeon and staff. Syncope is common in physically fit patients who often have high vagal tone. In my experience it is particularly more likely in a patient who has already verbalized anxiety, such as a patient who has said that he hates the smell of hospitals, cannot stand the sight of blood, has a history of syncope, or has been in the waiting room an excessively long length of time. I try to ensure that these patients take 5 to 10 mg of diazepam (Valium) by mouth before leaving home for my clinic, and when they arrive I give them atropine, 0.4 mg intramuscularly (provided they have no tachycardia or hypertension). Syncope is characterized by the patient feeling faint or having nausea and by the appearance of pallor, hypotension, and bradycardia; in fully blown cases the patient loses consciousness. Occasionally a syncopal seizure may occur with simple syncope as a result of cerebral anoxia; however, with any seizure activity one should carefully consider the possibility of local anesthetic toxicity. Usually with syncope the total dosage of local anesthetic (which should continuously be monitored during the course of the procedure) will be well below the traditional maximum amounts; thus, especially if benzodiazepines have also been given, anesthetic toxicity is extremely unlikely. Treatment consists of putting the patient into Trendelenburg position with the legs raised.

Toxicity

With local anesthetic toxicity, one usually knows that a large amount of local anesthetic has been given. Initial subjective symptoms of early toxicity may be present, such as a feeling of being chilled, a bitter taste in the mouth, paresthesia, circumoral and lingual numbness, difficulty hearing, visual disturbance, and drowsiness and confusion. (Drowsiness from benzodiazepines may mask these symptoms.) The next objective signs of toxicity are shivering, muscle twitching, tremors, and loss of consciousness, followed by convulsions.

Treatment of a local anesthetic overdose consists of immediate administration of intravenous benzodiazepine—perhaps midazolam, 5 mg, lorazepam, 3 mg, or diazepam, 15 mg—whichever one the surgeon is most familiar with. This medication should be given by slow intravenous injection over 1 to 5 minutes depending on the urgency. I always leave an intravenous "butterfly needle" in place and keep it flushed with saline solution to keep it patent precisely in case of this sort of eventuality; once a patient has become hypotensive or is convulsing, inserting an intravenous line can be next to impossible.

Administration of oxygen and hyperventilation is the next step. An open airway must be secured and the patient, if conscious, should be asked to hyperventilate. If the patient is unconscious and/or the airway is obstructed, the patient should be intubated and hyperventilated with an Ambu-bag or its equivalent. This is necessary because higher levels of arterial carbon dioxide increase blood flow to the brain, bringing higher amounts of local anesthetic there sooner. In addition, diffusion of carbon dioxide into the nerve cells of the brain lowers their intracellular pH, which results in increased local anesthetic CNS toxicity.[7] In cats, increasing the $PaCO_2$ from an average of 32.5 mm Hg to 73 mm Hg decreased the convulsive threshold of prilocaine, lidocaine, and bupivacaine by 50%.[6] While these first two steps are being effected, one's staff should call for an ambulance. The patient should by now be placed in the Trendelenburg position. Should cardiovascular collapse take place, cardiopulmonary resuscitation must be performed. The staff of any office using intravenous sedation or large amounts of local anesthesia should be trained in basic and advanced cardiac life support and necessary equipment must be on hand.

REFERENCES

1. Greenbaum SS, Greenbaum CH: Local anesthesia. In Parish LC, Lask GP, editors: *Aesthetic dermatology*, New York, 1991, McGraw-Hill, p 19.
2. Fink R: Leaves and needles: the introduction of surgical local anesthesia, *Anesthesiology* 63:77-83, 1985.
3. Monheit GD: Anesthesia. In Unger WP, Nordstrom REA, editors: *Hair transplantation*, ed 2, New York, 1988, Marcel Dekker, p 135.
4. Dinehart SM: Topical, local and regional anesthesia. In Wheeland RG, editor: *Cutaneous surgery*, Philadelphia, 1994, WB Saunders, p 102.
5. Winton GB: Anesthesia for dermatologic surgery, *J Dermatol Surg Oncol* 14:1, 1988.
6. Stromberg BV: Regional anesthesia in head and neck surgery, *Clin Plast Surg* 12(1):123-136, 1985.
7. Englesson S: The influence of acid-base changes on central nervous system toxicity of local anesthetic agents. I. An experimental study in cats, *Acta Anaesthesiol Scand* 18:79, 1974.

B. Nerve Block Anesthesia of the Scalp

Robert S. Haber, Sajjad Khan, and Dow B. Stough

The fear of pain is one of the chief concerns of potential hair transplant patients. Minimizing the discomfort of the anesthetic process is an important aspect of the refinement of the surgical approach. Standard scalp anesthesia in the past has consisted of establishing a ring block with lidocaine and epinephrine, chosen for rapid onset and hemostasis, followed by bupivacaine for more prolonged anesthesia.[1,2] In our experience the most painful area of the ring block occurs along the frontal hairline. Nerve blocks are useful in this regard because they can substitute a single injection for a larger number of injections and anesthetize a large area with a small amount of anesthetic.[1-4] Nerve blocks can also be used in conjunction with tumescent anesthesia. The performance of nerve blocks is rarely taught in residency programs, and for this reason many physicians are uncomfortable with the procedure, believing that it requires a high degree of skill and training. Although a detailed knowledge of regional anatomy is required, this procedure is readily learned.

A nerve block involves the infiltration of a small volume of anesthetic around the trunk of a nerve that has a specific and defined anatomical distribution to provide anesthesia to that entire region.[3,5] Its advantages include the production of a large area of anesthesia with a minimum of discomfort to the patient, as well as a reduction of the total volume of anesthetic required.

ANATOMY

Although scalp anatomy was addressed in Chapter 1, Part D, this section reviews scalp sensory innervation as related to nerve blockade. Sensory innervation of the forehead and frontal scalp is supplied by branches of the frontal nerve, itself a branch of

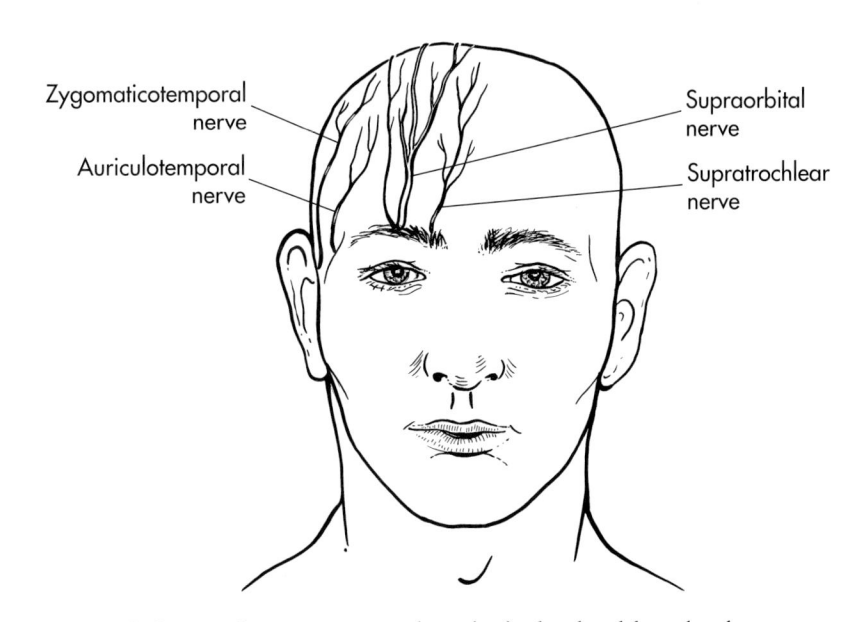

FIG. 3-6 Sensory nerve supply to the forehead and frontal scalp.

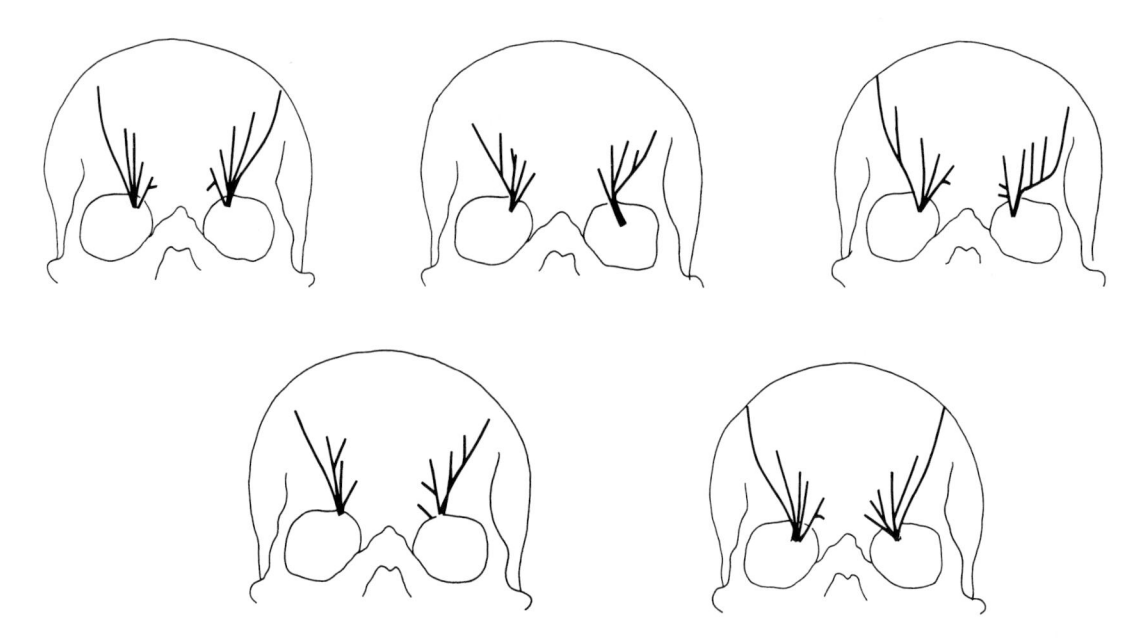

FIG. 3-7 Variations in the pattern of division of frontal nerve outside the orbit. (From Fatah MF: *Br J Plast Surg* 44:351-358, 1991.)

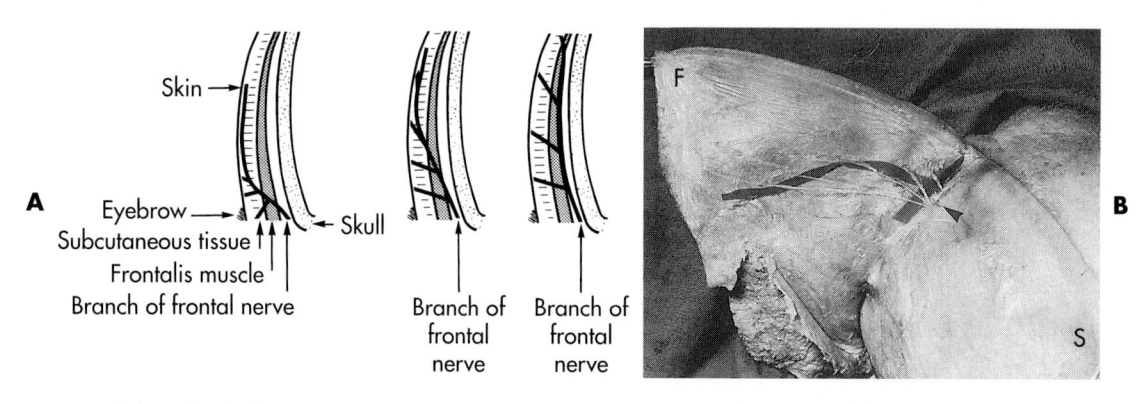

FIG. 3-8 A, Diagrammatic representation of sagittal views of the different branches of the frontal nerve in the forehead demonstrating how each subsequent nerve changes plane from submuscular to subcutaneous, starting from medial *(left)* to lateral *(right)*. **B,** Anatomical dissection demonstrating the points made in **A.** S is on the skull. F is on the inner aspect of the reflected forehead skin on the left side. The *black arrow* is pointing at the left supraorbital rim. The points at which each subsequent branch changes plane and penetrates the muscle are highlighted by a strip of dark background. (From Fatah MF: *Br J Plast Surg* 44:351-358, 1991.)

the ophthalmic division of the trigeminal nerve. Traditionally these branches are known as the supraorbital and supratrochlear nerves and are believed to follow the general course diagrammed in Fig. 3-6.[1-9] The supraorbital nerve is believed to emerge in the midpupillary line through a foramen located along the supraorbital ridge, whereas the supratrochlear nerve is believed to emerge as a separate trunk closer to the medial aspect of the supraorbital ridge. According to this model the medial aspect of the forehead is innervated by the supratrochlear nerve, whereas the more lateral aspect is innervated by the supraorbital nerve (Fig. 3-6).

Notably, however, a series of detailed anatomical dissections by Fatah[10] casts doubt on this prevailing view. A widely variable and asymmetrical pattern of nerves was identified, and in only one of 20 sides dissected were the traditional supraorbital and supratrochlear divisions seen (Fig. 3-7). The most notable consistency found was that the most me-

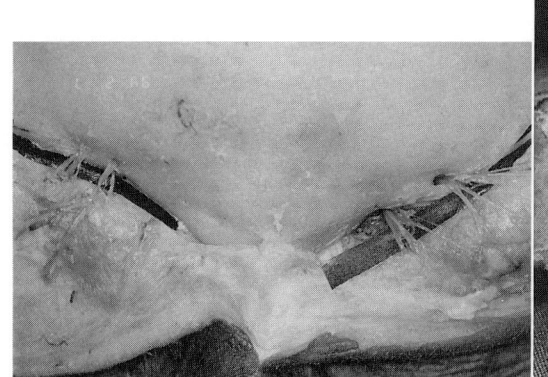

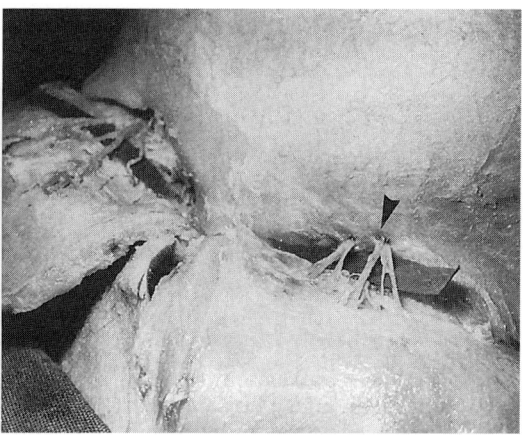

FIG. 3-9 **A,** Cadaver dissection demonstrating the emergence and course of the supraorbital and supratrochlear branches of the frontal nerve innervating the forehead and frontal scalp. **B,** Cadaver dissection with the forehead skin reflected down and split vertically in the midline. The *black arrow* points at the left supraorbital groove that is converted into two fibrous canals through which the two main branches of the frontal nerve are emerging. On the right side the periosteum is dissected to show the bony groove. (From Fatah MF: *Br J Plast Surg* 44:351-358, 1991.)

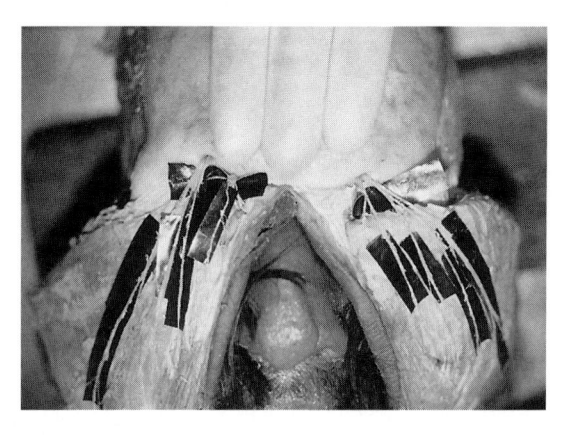

FIG. 3-10 Three-finger rule. Note the position of the fingers and the emergence of the major nerve branches just lateral to the outer fingers.

dial branch always becomes superficial within a short distance from the orbit, whereas the most lateral branch always remains in a very deep plane below the frontalis muscle until reaching or passing the hairline (Fig. 3-8). In addition, true bony foramen were rarely seen and varied considerably in their location. Therefore, although it is convenient to discuss nerve blocks using traditional anatomy, it should be kept in mind that the classical anatomical branching pattern as seen in Fig. 3-1 may only rarely be encountered.

A large series of cadaver dissections performed by one of the authors (SHK) further corroborates this modified anatomical model. Fig. 3-9 is a photograph of one of these dissections, demonstrating the emergence and course of the nerves. The nerves sometimes emerged from two foramen but more often emerged from one foramen and one notch; often no foramen were found at all. One major consistent feature was noted, however. When three fingers were placed vertically over the lower forehead and centered over the glabella, both major nerve branches were noted to emerge just lateral to the outer fingers (Fig. 3-10). We refer to this finding as the "three-finger rule," and it can be used to help to guide the administration of the nerve block.

TECHNIQUE

Most surgeons recommend approaching this dual nerve block via an injection of anesthetic above the eyebrow.[1,5,7] Suboptimal anesthesia may be achieved with this approach because of the wide separation of the two nerves above the orbital rim and the variability in depth of the two nerves as previously discussed. In addition, although some surgeons recommend concentrations of lidocaine up to 2% for greater effect,[5] we have found that a lower concentration of 0.5% provides excellent results and further minimizes toxicity.

Our approach involves the palpation of the supraorbital notch (Fig. 3-11, A) and inserting a ½-inch 30-gauge needle just *under* the eyebrow until it rests on the bone above the notch (Fig. 3-11, B). We do not attempt to enter the notch or elicit paresthesias. After aspiration, 2 ml of 0.5% lidocaine is infiltrated into the periosteum at this spot. The needle is then partially withdrawn and redi-

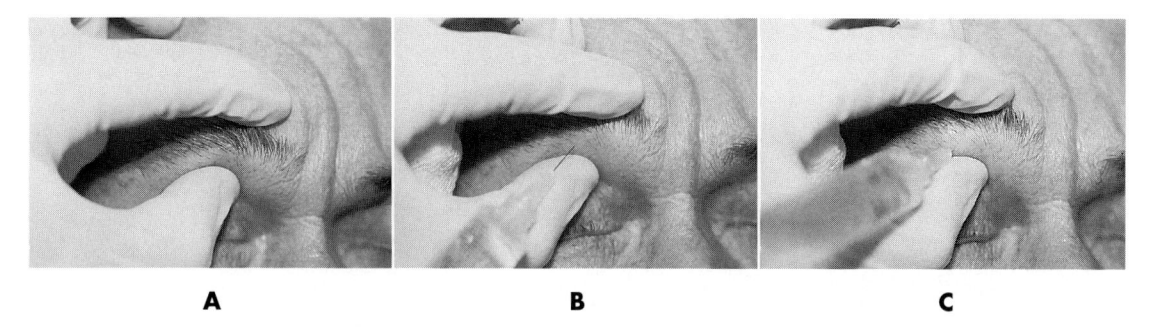

FIG. 3-11 **A,** Technique for locating the supraorbital notch. **B,** Proper position and direction of needle during infiltration of anesthetic for nerve block. **C,** Needle redirected medially to block supratrochlear nerve.

rected 0.5 cm medially, without exiting the skin, and an additional 0.5 ml of anesthetic is again injected into the periosteum (Fig. 3-11, C). In a small percentage of patients no supraorbital notch is palpable on one or both sides. When this occurs, the three-finger rule can be used or the infiltration can be carefully directed at the supraorbital ridge at the midpupillary line. The patient will often note a sensation of "heaviness" of the upper eyelid because of anesthesia of a branch of the supraorbital nerve that innervates the upper eyelids; this is a sign of a successful nerve block.

This procedure is followed on the contralateral side as well, and both sides are then massaged briefly to help to distribute the anesthetic. We believe that with the needle in contact with the periosteum, the anesthetic is forced along this tissue plane and effectively envelopes the nerves as they emerge from their foramen. Maintaining contact of the needle on bone is therefore an important aspect of the technique.

COMPLICATIONS

Potential drawbacks to nerve blocks include the risk of nerve damage because of close approximation of the needle to the nerve.[11] Careful technique and knowledge of anatomy can help to lessen this risk. In addition, because larger vessels are generally in close proximity to nerve trunks, inadvertent intravascular injection can occur.[5,6] Aspiration of the syringe while advancing and before each injection serves to lessen these risks.

Paresthesias, such as burning or tingling sensations, should be considered a complication because it indicates direct contact of the nerve trunk by the needle.[11] For this reason deliberately eliciting this response is not recommended. When paresthesia is noted with resolution of anesthesia, the patient can be reassured that normal sensation generally returns over days, weeks, or months. In rare cases paresthesia can be permanent.[11]

A very rare complication of a nerve block is infection. When reported, infection has generally been the result of injection through an infected area or injections at multiple sites with use of the same needle.[11] Other rare complications, such as CNS or systemic cardiovascular toxicity, are extremely unlikely if basic local anesthetic precautions are taken.

RESULTS

We perform nerve block anesthesia of the scalp every day and have used this procedure on more than 400 patients; a complete block is achieved in more than 95% of our patients. Although many studies report delays from 3 to 20 minutes before nerve block anesthesia takes effect,[1,5,8] we have found that complete anesthesia generally takes place within 30 seconds of the injection. In approximately 5% of the most fortunate patients, this block provides complete anesthesia to the entire scalp, extending beyond the vertex. More often, though, the lateral aspects of the frontal hairline, as well as the vertex scalp, are not affected by the block. The remainder of the scalp is anesthetized in the usual manner for both prolonged pain control and hemostasis.

In theory, it should be possible to use nerve blocks to anesthetize other areas of the scalp.[7] The zygomaticotemporal nerve, auriculotemporal nerve, great auricular nerve, and greater and lesser occipital nerves also innervate portions of the scalp (Figs. 3-6 and 3-12), but in practice these nerves are more difficult to successfully block because of greater inconsistency in their course and the absence of very reliable landmarks. In addition, there is a great degree of overlapping innervation among these nerves, making a partial block essentially useless.

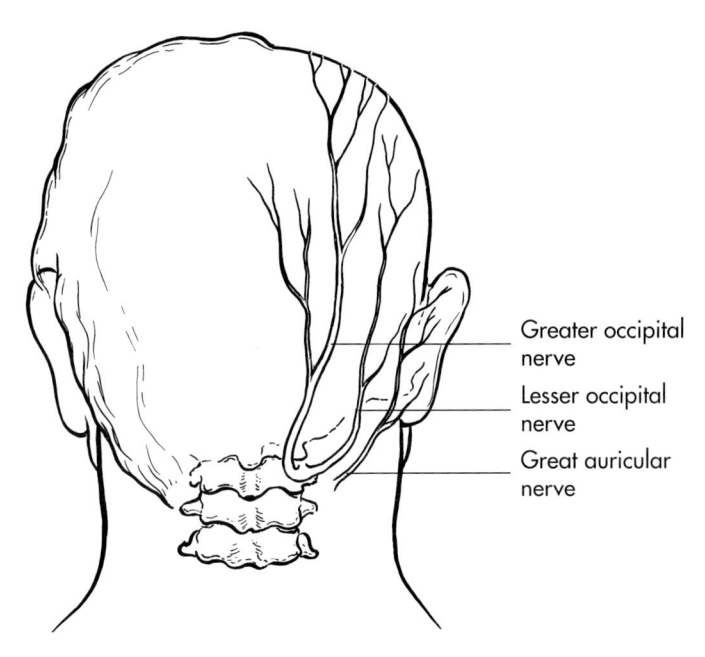

FIG. 3-12 Nerve supply to the posterior scalp.

For these reasons it is generally impractical to rely on nerve blocks for regions other than the frontal scalp.

CONCLUSION

Nerve blocks are tolerated extremely well in all but the most pain-intolerant patients, and these patients may be pretreated with nitrous oxide with great success. Patients previously treated with standard ring block and subsequently treated with the supraorbital and supratrochlear blocks have reported that the discomfort of the anesthetic process was significantly diminished. We highly recommend this procedure because it is easy to learn, is highly effective, and offers a high margin of safety.

REFERENCES

1. Grekin RC, Auletta MJ: Local anesthesia in dermatologic surgery, *J Am Acad Dermatol* 19:599-614, 1988.
2. Stromberg BV: Regional anesthesia in head and neck surgery, *Clin Plast Surg* 12:123-136, 1985.
3. Winton GB: Anesthesia for dermatologic surgery, *J Dermatol Surg Oncol* 14:41-54, 1988.
4. Greenbaum SS, Greenbaum CH: Local anesthesia. In Parish LC, Lask GP, editors: *Aesthetic dermatology*, New York, 1991, McGraw-Hill.
5. Dinehart SM: Topical, local, and regional anesthesia. In Wheeland RG, ed: *Cutaneous surgery*, Philadelphia, 1994, WB Saunders.
6. Laskin DM: Diagnosis and treatment of complications associated with local anesthesia, *Int Dent J* 34:232-237, 1984.
7. Meyer TG, Fleming RW: Anatomy and physiology of the scalp and hair. In *Aesthetic and reconstructive surgery of the scalp*, St Louis, 1992, Mosby.
8. Randle HW, Salassa JR, Roenigk RK: Know your anatomy, *J Dermatol Surg Oncol* 18:231-235, 1992.
9. Salasche SJ, Bernstein G, Senkasik M: Forehead and temple. In *Surgical anatomy of the skin*, Norwalk, Conn., 1988, Appleton &Lange.
10. Fatah MF: Innervation and functional reconstruction of the forehead, *Br J Plast Surg* 44:351-358, 1991.
11. Giovannitti JA, Milam SB: Anesthesia and pain control. In Waite DE, editor: *Textbook of practical oral and maxillofacial surgery*, ed 3, Philadelphia, 1987, Lea & Febiger.

C. Tumescent Anesthesia for Surgery of the Scalp

William P. Coleman III

Providing anesthesia for scalp surgery presents unique challenges. Athough the scalp is relatively insensitive to pain compared with other areas of the body, extensive surgical procedures have the potential to be uncomfortable and may result in considerable swelling and cause headaches. Furthermore, the scalp is richly endowed with blood vessels, and bleeding during or after scalp surgery is annoying for both the surgeon and the patient.

Excluding local excisions and small flaps, many surgical procedures performed on the scalp are quite extensive. Dermabrasion, scalp reduction, hair-bearing flaps, occipital advancement techniques, and hair transplantation require that large areas be anesthetized. The ideal local anesthetic is painless to administer, effective, hemostatic, and convenient to use. Although not perfect, tumescent anesthesia has many of these advantages.[1-4]

Classically, hair transplantation and other scalp surgeries have been performed with field blocks created by transcutaneous injections of lidocaine usually mixed with epinephrine. In recent years sodium bicarbonate has been added to these solutions in the hope of decreasing the pain on injection. Although injections are less painful when sodium bicarbonate is used, there is wide suspicion that this additive increases swelling and bleeding.[5]

One of the main difficulties encountered when stock solutions of lidocaine (1% to 4% with 1:100,000 epinephrine) are used is that the maximum recommended dose is 7 mg/kg.[6] This dose works out to a total of 500 to 650 mg for the average-sized male patient. Consequently, only 50 to 65 ml of 1% lidocaine can be safely used. In more sensitive patients who require 2% lidocaine, this total maximum volume is only 25 to 32 ml. The use of more concentrated solutions reduces the safe volume even further. To exceed these recommended dosages may be to risk neurotoxicity or cardiotoxicity.

The tumescent anesthetic technique involves the injection of large volumes of very dilute lidocaine and epinephrine. This anesthetic approach was first developed for patients undergoing liposuction.[1] It has been shown that tumescent anesthesia significantly reduces the total milligrams of lidocaine required.[2] This approach also maximizes the vasoconstrictive benefits of epinephrine, thus decreasing bleeding. These same advantages have been demonstrated when the tumescent technique is used for extensive scalp surgery.[3] The tumescent approach to anesthesia has gained increasing popularity during the past several years.

When the tumescent anesthetic technique is compared with the standard field block anesthetic technique for scalp surgery, several advantages of the tumescent technique become clear:

1. There is significantly less bleeding.
2. Fewer total milligrams of lidocaine are required.
3. The process of injecting the anesthetic is much less painful for the patient.
4. There is a reduced need for systemic sedation.

ANESTHETIC SOLUTION

Although tumescent anesthesia refers to a variety of low-concentration lidocaine and epinephrine solutions, the most popular mixture for scalp surgery can be prepared in the following manner: Into a 250 ml bag of normal saline solution from which 13.5 ml has been removed, add 12.5 ml of plain 2% lidocaine and 1 ml (one vial) of 1:1000 epinephrine for a final concentration of 0.1% lidocaine with 1:250,000 epinephrine.

TECHNIQUE

As with all new methods, it is important for the neophyte to precisely duplicate the approach presented here. Any variation in this method may produce inferior results. Once one is certain that he/she has mastered this technique, future experimentation will lead to other variations.

Recipient Area

The recipient area should be anesthetized first. A small wheal is raised bilaterally within the temporal hairline using 1% lidocaine with epinephrine (stock solution). After 1 or 2 minutes, an 18-gauge spinal needle is advanced through one of these wheals and 10 to 20 ml of tumescent anesthetic fluid is injected without moving the needle further. Once the area is sufficiently swollen, the needle may be advanced slowly to the edge of the tumesced tissue and approximately 10 ml of additional fluid injected. Each time the needle is moved, the surgeon should draw back on the plunger to ensure that the needle is not in an intravascular location. This process of gradually advancing the needle through previously tumesced tissue should cause the patient no discomfort. It is normal, however, for the patient to report a feeling of tightness or swelling. The patient may remark that it feels as if there is a rubber band around the head. The entire recipient area is tumesced in this manner until the ridge of swelling extends 2 cm beyond any areas that will be operated on (Fig. 3-13).

Donor Area

A small wheal is then raised in the center of the proposed site for graft harvesting. If extensive havesting is planned, wheals should be raised at close enough intervals for the spinal needle to reach all of the necessary areas. The injection is performed slowly, depending on the patient's tolerance for the unusual sensation of stretching skin. Once again the zone of tumescence should extend 2 cm beyond the proposed surgical site.

Other Areas

Tumescing the vertex of the scalp as a recipient area can often be accomplished through one central wheal. The spinal needle can then be rotated in a 360-degree pattern from the central injection site. When the vertex is infiltrated for scalp reduction, the same technique is used (Fig. 3-14). The surgeon must be sure to extend the tumesced ridge beyond the area planned for undermining. For dermabra-

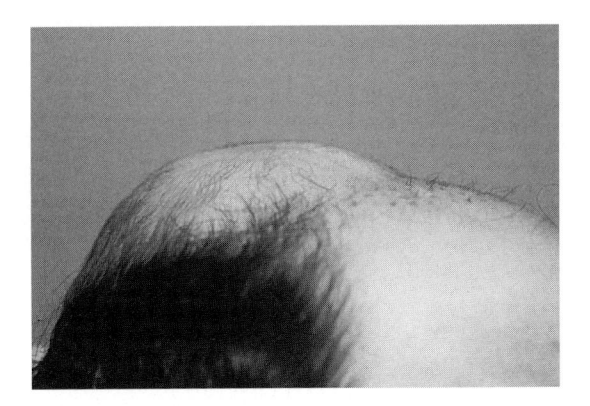

FIG. 3-13 Tumescent recipient site before surgery. A consistent blanching signified excellent vasoconstriction. (Used with permission from William P. Coleman III, M.D.)

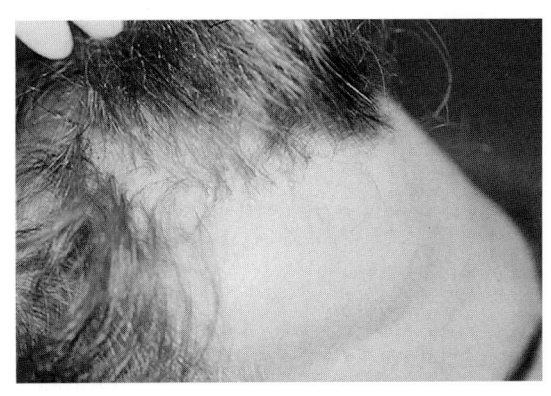

FIG. 3-14 Scalp vertex tumesced before reduction surgery. Note from the side view that the site is significantly swollen to allow complete infiltration of lidocaine and epinephrine throughout the operative area. (Used with permission from William P. Coleman III, M.D.)

sion or massive scalp-lifting, the same techniques are used, but larger amounts of the tumescent anesthetic fluid must be injected to anesthetize the large areas of scalp that will be operated on.

RESULTS

Surgeons who have performed scalp surgery with use of traditional field block anesthesia will immediately be impressed with the significant decrease in bleeding afforded by the tumescent anesthetic technique. Bleeding has always been an annoying facet of surgery on the scalp. Blood obscures the surgical field and makes the procedure less precise. Tumescent anesthesia minimizes bleeding so completely that only a few 4 × 4 gauze pads may be needed for an entire hair transplantation procedure.

Patients who have had scalp surgery performed previously with field block anesthesia often report that the injection phase is less painful with the tumescent approach. The tumescent technique is less painful because only one or two small areas need to be injected to obtain a wheal through which the remainder of the anesthetic can be infiltrated, thus minimizing needle sticks through unanesthetized skin. Once a sufficient amount of tumescent anesthetic has been infiltrated, anesthesia should be consistent throughout the entire operative site.

POTENTIAL PROBLEMS

Some surgeons worry that the increased turgor of a scalp anesthetized with the tumescent technique makes implantation of very small grafts more difficult. This effect can be minimized by infiltrating the recipient area first; a minimum of 45 minutes can then elapse before grafts are inserted, thus allowing much of the swelling to dissipate.

Adding sodium bicarbonate to the tumescent solution (or, in fact, to any local anesthetic solution) may increase swelling.[5] This can be a problem not only during surgery but also postoperatively. There is no need to use sodium bicarbonate in the tumescent solution because the dilution effect of the saline solution raises the pH to a nearly physiological level, thus neutralizing the acidity of the lidocaine solution.

When some surgeons begin to use the tumescent technique, they report that the expected vasoconstriction is not achieved. In this case, the error is often in preparing the tumescent fluid with premixed solutions of lidocaine and epinephrine rather than adding the epinephrine separately from an individual ampule. Use of fresh epinephrine from a 1 ml ampule provides far better vasoconstriction than the premixed stock solutions that contain preservatives.

Sodium chloride solutions are available in small bottles for injection. These solutions often contain preservatives such as benzyl alcohol. There is no need to add this additional variable to the procedure. Intravenous bags containing 0.9% sodium chloride without preservatives are widely available. It is also much more convenient to mix large volumes of the tumescent mixture in a single 250 ml bag than in small 30 ml bottles.

As with the field block technique, there may be "hot spots" that are not completely anesthetized. This is especially true in patients with scar tissue from previous surgeries. These areas can be further anesthetized with small amounts of 1% lidocaine. Because the skin is already fairly numb, these additional transcutaneous injections are usually painless.

On rare occasions a patient will be quite sensitive to the tumescent effect. These persons simply do not like the feeling of massive swelling. This is a natural psychological response because swelling of the head is intrinsically associated in our psyche with injury. These persons may prefer increased bleeding and more pain on injection to the swollen feeling of a tumesced scalp.

Some surgeons who perform hair transplantation have privately voiced concerns about the use of tumescent anesthesia in the recipient area because of the potential for increased forehead swelling postoperatively. After using this technique for 3 years, I have found that forehead swelling is extremely rare after the recipient area is tumesced. In fact I suspect that such swelling occurs less often with tumescent anesthesia than when field blocks are used. To minimize the potential for swelling, however, it is wise to limit the edges of the tumesced zone to 2 cm beyond the surgical site. There is no need to advance this ridge down onto the forehead where no surgery will be performed. Furthermore, supraorbital nerve blocks are unnecessary with tumescent anesthesia. These nerve blocks may contribute to forehead swelling and are also quite painful. Edema after hair transplant surgery can also be reduced by applying ice packs the day of surgery and by administering short-action intramuscular corticosteroids.

CONCLUSION

Tumescent anesthesia appears to be superior to field block anesthesia for all forms of scalp surgery. The tumescent anesthetic approach provides better vasoconstriction, more consistent anesthesia, and more patient comfort on injection than traditional anesthetic approaches.

REFERENCES

1. Klein JA: The tumescent technique for liposuction surgery, *Am J Cosmet Surg* 4:263-267, 1987.
2. Coleman WP III: L'anesthesie locale de la lipo-suction, *J Med Esthet* 16:241-243, 1989.
3. Coleman WP III, Klein JA: Use of the tumescent technique for scalp surgery, dermabrasion, and soft tissue reconstruction, *J Dermatol Surg Oncol* 18:130-135, 1992.
4. Klein JA: Tumescent technique for regional anesthesia permits lidocaine doses of 35 mg/kg for liposuction: peak plasma lidocaine levels are diminished and delayed 12 hours, *J Dermatol Surg Oncol* 16:248-263, 1990.
5. Straub P: The cause of poor growth? *Hair Transplant Forum* 3(5):17-18, 1993.
6. Benowitz NL, Meister W: Clinical pharmacokinetics of lidocaine, *Clin Pharmacokinet* 3:177-201, 1978.

D. Buffered Lidocaine and Postoperative Edema

Paul M. Straub

To prolong the shelf life of lidocaine, it is dispensed as a solution with a pH of 3.3 to 5.5. Sodium citrate and/or hydrochloric acid is added for pH adjustment. This acidic lidocaine solution is painful on injection. Buffering the solution with 1 ml of 8.4% sodium bicarbonate to each 10 ml of lidocaine (1% or 2%) brings the pH closer to 7 (Fig. 3-15). This solution is less painful on injection; however, I noted an apparent increase of postoperative edema with the addition of sodium bicarbonate.

A study was therefore carried out in which one group of patients was anesthetized with sodium bicarbonate–buffered lidocaine and another group was anesthetized with nonbuffered lidocaine. The patients were asked to report any significant swelling. Postoperative edema with nonbuffered lidocaine was noted in 10 of 305 cases (3.25%), and postoperative edema with buffered lidocaine occurred in 42 of 328 cases (12.8%).

Norwood[1] then suggested adding 0.75 ml triamcinolone acetonide suspension to each 10 ml lidocaine to diminish the frequency of postoperative edema. Postoperative edema following the administration of sodium bicarbonate–buffered lidocaine plus triamcinolone acetonide was seen in seven of 85 cases (8.23%).

CONCLUSION

The addition of sodium bicarbonate to lidocaine diminishes the pain of injection but increases the

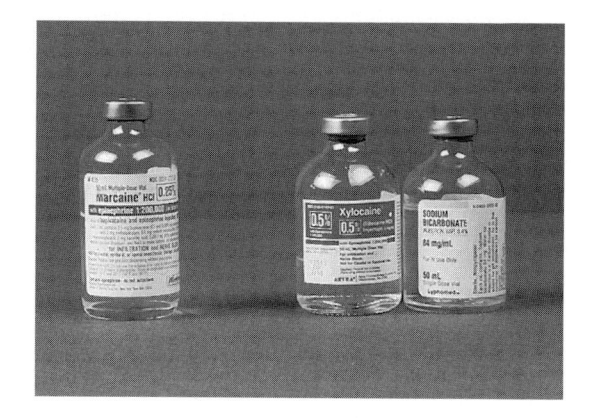

FIG. 3-15 The addition of sodium bicarbonate (*far right*) to lidocaine (*middle*) will decrease pain on injection. Bupivacaine (Marcaine) will remain painful on injection despite buffering with sodium bicarbonate.

probability of postoperative edema. The mechanism is thought to be the addition of Na$^+$ ions.

REFERENCE

1. Norwood OT: Say goodbye to postoperative edema, *Hair Transplant Forum* 1(1):13, 1994.

E. The Use of Monitored Anesthesia Care as an Adjunct to Local Anesthesia for Scalp Surgery

Dwight A. Scarborough and Emil Bisaccia

Hair transplant surgical techniques have become increasingly sophisticated during the past few decades. Commensurate with this evolution, recently developed anesthetic agents and an established anesthesia technique called *monitored anesthesia care* (MAC) have been used to enhance patient comfort and safety.

Providing office anesthesia of any type is a serious responsibility for the physician. The comfort, safety, and well-being of patients is of foremost concern when anesthesia options are being considered. MAC is being increasingly used in the United States for surgical procedures of the scalp because some patients are reluctant to undergo local or regional anesthesia without supplemental medication because they are concerned about pain and awareness during surgery. MAC refers to instances in which an anesthesiologist or certified registered nurse anesthetist (CRNA) is called on to provide specific anesthesia services to a particular patient who is undergoing a planned procedure that requires local anesthesia. In such a case the anesthesiologist or CRNA provides specific services to the patient, is in control of the patient's nonsurgical care including the responsibility of monitoring of his vital signs, and administers anesthetics as appropriate.

Intravenous conscious sedation, when used in MAC as an adjunct to local anesthesia, can enhance the surgical experience for both the patient and the surgeon. This method of anesthesia induces a brief period of deep sedation, permitting painless infiltration of local anesthetic into the operative field. Subsequent mild sedation in conjunction with periodic reinforcement of local block provides optimal anesthesia for hair transplantation in appropriately selected patients.

OFFICE SURGERY PREREQUISITES FOR MAC

Although outpatient surgery in an office setting is appropriate for patients undergoing hair transplantation, the site where MAC is administered should meet the appropriate standards of a hospital setting. However, compliance with those standards does not guarantee that problems will not occur. A well laid out plan must exist to deal with all office emergencies. Crisis planning should be performed at the onset, with written algorithms covering each prospective problem. The facility's floor plan and design must allow for the administration of lifesaving care, and hospital transport mechanisms should be prearranged.[1-4] The overriding concern of the facility staff must be for the patient's well-being, and this obligation transcends all others while providing for the patient's comfort and convenience. Key members of the surgical team should be certified in advanced cardiac life support.

The members of the office operating staff are principally responsible for the patient's well-being, but the final responsibility resides with the surgeon. Therefore the surgeon who administers anesthesia must be thoroughly familiar with the anesthetic agents that are used and he/she must be prepared to deal with any complications or untoward events that might arise from their use. A list of drugs used in office surgery is found in the box on p. 98. The surgeon must also understand physiological monitoring and possess demonstrable competence in airway management because the CRNA, although a highly skilled professional, is under the direction of the physician.

PREOPERATIVE CONSIDERATIONS FOR MAC

Candidates for office surgery with use of MAC are selected on the basis of the classification system of the American Society of Anesthesiologists. Healthy patients undergoing routine procedures (class I) and those with mild to moderate systemic disease (class II) are generally suitable candidates for office surgery, whereas patients with severe systemic disease (class III) are not. Using the services of a CRNA or equivalent contributes to the success of the surgical team. For MAC sedation, the intravenous anesthetic should be administered only by persons experienced in providing anesthesia. Patients should be continually monitored and facilities for maintenance of a patent airway, artificial ventilation, and oxygen enrichment and circulatory resuscitation must be immediately available.

During the initial stages of the procedure, the monitoring and management of the anesthesia may consume a large portion of the surgeon's energy. This task becomes less demanding as the procedure

DRUGS COMMONLY USED IN OFFICE SURGERY	
Acetazolamide (Diamox)	Isoproterenol (Isuprel)
Albuterol (Proventil)	Ketamine (Ketalar)
Alfentanil hydrochloride (Alfenta)	Labetalol (Trandate)
Aminophylline	Lidocaine (Xylocaine) (for infiltration)
Atenolol (Tenormin)	Lidocaine (Xylocaine) (for treatment of arrhythmias)
Atropine	Mannitol
Benzquinamide (Emete-Con)	Metaproterenol (Alupent)
Bretylium (Bretylol)	Metoclopramide (Reglan)
Calcium chloride	Midazolam (Versed)
Calcium gluconate	Nalbuphine hydrochloride (Nubain)
Chlorpromazine (Thorazine)	Naloxone (Narcan)
Dexamethasone (Decadron)	Nitroglycerin (Nitrostat)
Dextrose	Phenylephrine hydrochloride (Neo-Synephrine)
Diazepam (Valium)	Prochlorperazine (Compazine) (injectable, suppository, and "spansule")
Digoxin (Lanoxin)	Propofol (Diprivan)
Diphenhydramine (Benadryl)	Propranolol (Inderal)
Dopamine (Intropin)	Secobarbitol (Seconal)
Epinephrine (Adrenalin)	Sodium bicarbonate
Furosemide (Lasix)	Sufentanil citrate (Sufenta)
Glycopyrrolate (Robinul)	Terbutaline
Hydralazine (Apresoline)	Trimethobenzamide (Tigan)
Hydrocortisone	Verapamil (Isoptin)
Hydrocortisone sodium succinate (Solu-Cortef)	

gets underway because after local anesthetic infiltration, patients are only lightly sedated. Patients undergo a preliminary medical evaluation before their procedure, and a final decision about the appropriateness of MAC sedation for the elective procedure is made at that time, particularly with regard to patients who are overly anxious, who have a history of anesthetic difficulties, or who have significant medical problems.

The preoperative history and physical examination include an evaluation and medical clearance from the patient's family physician or internist (see Appendix E). This evaluation may include a chest x-ray film, ECG, urinalysis, complete blood cell count with differential, platelets, chemistry profile, thyroxine, prothrombin time, partial thromboplastin time, fibrinogen, hepatitis B surface antigen, and human immunodeficiency virus screen, preferably obtained within 2 weeks of the elective procedure.

A preoperative visit takes place in which informed consent to the procedure and an agreement not to drive on the day of surgery is obtained.[5] Photographs are taken and financial arrangements are made.

Preoperative medications are prescribed, including transdermal scopolamine, which is to be applied 24 hours before surgery, and diazepam, 10 mg, taken the night before and the morning of surgery. In addition, depending on the procedure to be performed, administration of an oral cephalosporin antibiotic may be initiated 24 hours before the procedure.

PERIOPERATIVE MONITORING

All patients who receive anything more than a small quantity of lidocaine should be monitored during the procedure. It is standard to use a transcutaneous pulse oximeter, an automated noninvasive sphygmomanometer, and a real-time electrocardiograph throughout the procedure. The pulse oximeter provides the most important information and should be considered an indispensable part of each patient's care. The pulse oximeter is a noninvasive device that measures the oxygen saturation of hemoglobin in the cutaneous circulation through a transducer placed on the fingertip. This information is reported as a percentage and is generally referred to as the "SaO_2" or "O_2sat." Newer machines also supply a perfusion waveform that allows monitoring of trends in skin blood flow. Maintenance of an adequate SaO_2 is a physiological imperative that depends on but supersedes in importance the maintenance of blood pressure. The SaO_2 reflects the complex concerted interactions of the cardiovascular and respiratory systems. Maintenance of adequate blood pressure is but one part of a larger scheme in which oxygen, the cornerstone of cellu-

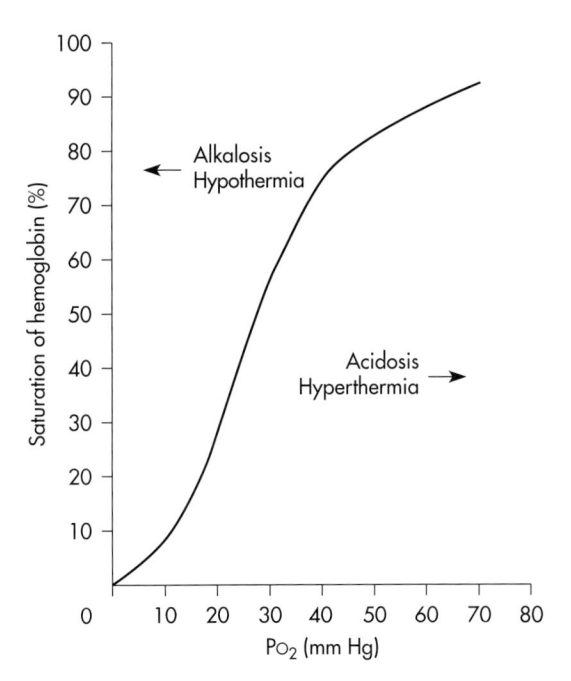

FIG. 3-16 The hemoglobin-oxygen dissociation curve is such that small changes in SaO_2 reflect a significant change in PO_2.

QUALITIES OF THE IDEAL ANESTHETIC AGENT

Rapid onset
Controllable duration
Levels of anesthetic depth are easily identified, achieved, measured, and changed
Technically easy to administer
No unwanted effects on vital organs
No toxic metabolites
Predictable, controllable elimination independent of hepatorenal function
Pharmacokinetics independent of altered physiology
High degree of specificity
High margin of safety
Useful in all age groups

---

lar metabolism, is delivered to cells. Pressure and flow are superfluous if oxygen is not provided.

Review of the hemoglobin-oxygen dissociation curve (Fig. 3-16) graphically illustrates the physiological importance of the maintenance of an adequate SaO_2. The curve is logarithmic and not linear, and therefore small changes in hemoglobin saturation can reflect immense changes in oxygen delivery. Although the shape of this curve is influenced by metabolic factors and the overall oxygen-carrying capacity is dependent on the total hemoglobin concentration in the blood, physiological reserve is lost at an SaO_2 of approximately 90%. This warning occurs before clinical signs of physiological aberration and cellular compromise.

Transcutaneous monitoring of SaO_2 assumes that adequate saturation in the skin circulation parallels adequate oxygen delivery to the myocardium. This is generally a safe assumption, but because myocardial oxygen delivery depends on adequate flow in the coronary arteries during diastole, situations may exist in which this relationship is not true. For this reason, actual cardiac performance must be monitored as well. In the absence of noninvasive monitoring of cardiac output, sphygmomanometry and electrocardiography provide adequate information on cardiac performance in the outpatient setting.

In contrast to early changes in the SaO_2, disturbances in blood pressure, heart rate, and rhythm generally follow some physiological compromise. Possible underlying causes must be carefully considered. Hypovolemia resulting from blood loss or loss of peripheral vascular resistance will lead to hypotension and concomitant tachycardia, whereas vagally mediated processes (vasovagal reflex and oculocardiac reflex) are usually manifested as hypotension and bradycardia. However, any patient who has hypotension without tachycardia should be suspected of experiencing myocardial ischemia (unless he is taking β-blockers). Depression of the ST segment, T-wave inversions, ectopy, and heart block must be watched for and demand prompt attention. Conversely, hypertension may indicate pain, anxiety, urinary retention, drug (epinephrine) effect, or fluid overload.

It is the responsibility of the entire surgical team to monitor the patient's condition. The physiological data being monitored must be periodically and systematically recorded for them to be useful and applied in a meaningful way. This responsibility must rest with a designated individual, either the CRNA or the anesthesiologist. Their training and expertise provide a wide margin of safety for the patient. Trends more than numbers are often diagnostic if recognized and interpreted, and monitoring devices alone are no substitute for careful scrutiny by trained personnel.

PHARMACOLOGICAL ASPECTS OF PROPOFOL AND MIDAZOLAM

Propofol is a versatile intravenous anesthetic agent that closely approximates would-be ideal characteristics[6] (see box above). The pharmacological properties of propofol are derived from its unique alkyl phenol chemical structure (Fig. 3-17).

The original formulation of propofol incorporated polyoxyethylated castor oil (Cremophor EL) as a solubilizing agent. However, a high incidence of pain on injection and an association with anaphylactoid reactions were noted, leading to its reformulation in 1984.[7-9] The chemical structure 2,6-diisopropylphenol is almost insoluble in water and is thus formulated as an oil-in-water emulsion. This emulsion consists of soybean oil, glycerol, and purified egg-yolk lecithin, not egg-white protein and therefore is not contraindicated in patients allergic to eggs. Propofol has no known active metabolites but is extensively metabolized in the liver to glucuronide and sulfate conjugates, which are excreted primarily in the urine. Less than 0.3% is excreted as the parent drug.[10]

No statistically significant alteration in pharmacokinetic parameters was found in patients with mild to moderate kidney insufficiency or cirrhosis, which suggests that propofol can be used in both groups of patients.[11] Finally, studies have reported that the in vitro inhibition of cortisol secretion by propofol has not been found to be clinically significant; in addition, there are no significant changes in plasma levels of histamine after propofol administration.[12,13]

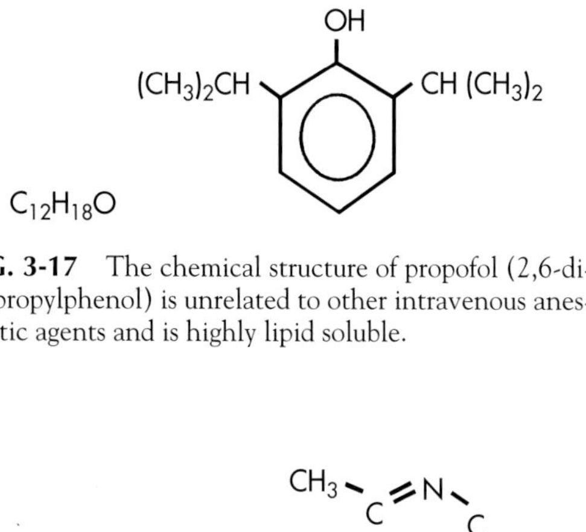

Midazolam is a relatively new benzodiazepine also suited for outpatient use. The chemical structure of midazolam varies from that of classic benzodiazepines by the presence of a fused imidazole ring (Fig. 3-18). This ring, which is rapidly metabolized, is responsible for the short-acting nature of midazolam. In addition to its short-acting characteristics, its chemical properties include minimal local irritation when administered intravenously or intramuscularly and high solubility in water and acidic media; it is also highly lipophilic at physiological pH. Indications include outpatient use for intravenous sedation, premedication, or induction and maintenance of general anesthesia. Its pharmacodynamics are characterized by a potency one and one-half to two times greater than that of diazepam. It has an anxiolytic, hypnotic, and antegrade amnesic effect. It also has anticonvulsant muscle-relaxant properties and is reversible with flumazenil.[14]

The cardiovascular, respiratory, and CNS effects of midazolam are outlined in the accompanying box. The cardiovascular effects are characterized by a slight decrease in the left ventricular stroke volume. There is a decrease in systemic vascular resistance and in systolic and diastolic blood pressure. This corresponds with a slight increase in reflex peripheral vasoconstriction and heart rate increase, and there is an increase in the coronary artery blood flow. The CNS effects result in a decreased ventilatory response to carbon dioxide and a decrease in minute ventilation. There is little effect on respiratory mechanics. However, there has been a rare but potentially serious respiratory depression associated with the use of midazolam, prompting a Food and Drug Administration (FDA) warning

FIG. 3-17 The chemical structure of propofol (2,6-diisopropylphenol) is unrelated to other intravenous anesthetic agents and is highly lipid soluble.

FIG. 3-18 Chemical structure of midazolam compared with diazepam.

> **SUMMARY OF EFFECTS OF MIDAZOLAM ON THE CARDIOVASCULAR, RESPIRATORY, AND CENTRAL NERVOUS SYSTEMS**
>
> *Cardiovascular System*
> Slight decrease in left ventricular stroke volume
> Decrease in systemic vascular resistance
> Slight decrease in systolic and diastolic blood pressure
> Slight increase in reflex peripheral vasoconstriction and heart rate
> Increase in coronary artery blood flow
>
> *Respiratory System*
> Ventilatory response to carbon dioxide is increased
> Decrease in minute ventilation
> Little effect on respiratory mechanics
> Rare but potentially serious respiratory depression (dose-related and function of injection speed)
>
> *Central Nervous System*
> Protective against cerebral hypoxia by decrease in cerebral blood flow and in cerebral metabolic rate for oxygen
> Anticonvulsant properties

> **ADVERSE EFFECTS OF MIDAZOLAM**
>
> Ataxia and motor uncoordination
> Impairment of mental and psychomotor function
> Confusion, dysarthria
> Retrograde amnesia, paradoxical effects
> Nausea and vomiting (rare)
> Local venous complications (rare)
> Respiratory depression

concerning potential respiratory arrest and subsequent morbidity. It is of note that this described apnea is dose- and age-related and is also a function of the injection speed.[15] The respiratory depressant effects of midazolam are not reversed by naloxone but they are reversed by flumazenil.[14] Midazolam has protective effects against cerebral hypoxia by reducing cerebral blood flow and reducing the cerebral metabolic rate for oxygen. Awareness persists, however, and therefore no true state of general anesthesia can be produced by this agent alone. Adverse effects are summarized in the accompanying box. Nausea and vomiting are rare, as are local venous complications. It is important to note that the potential of midazolam to produce respiratory depression may be augmented by barbiturates and narcotics.

INTRAVENOUS SEDATION

The patient is placed in the supine position on the surgical table after the donor and recipient areas of the scalp have been marked, prepared, and scrubbed for sterility. Most patients are somewhat tranquil and anxiety-free but responsive by the time of surgery because of their preoperative medications. If this is not the case, small quantities of midazolam (Versed) are sometimes administered intravenously as necessary immediately before surgery. Midazolam can be given in an average initial dose of 0.03 to 0.05 mg/kg administered intravenously over a 2-minute interval. The patient response varies according to the preoperative medication effects, age of the patient, and inherent medication tolerance level of the patient. The action of these medications is reinforced and enhanced by reassurance from the surgeon, and they also engender a desirable degree of amnesia for the patient. Extreme caution must be observed when administering midazolam to older patients or patients taking narcotic analgesics because even small doses can result in profound apnea.

At this stage some patients are ready for the administration of local anesthetic. However, if the patient is particularly anxious or if the desire for complete comfort has been expressed, a brief period of deep sedation is required for painless administration of the local anesthetic. This deep sedation is achieved through the administration of small quantities of propofol. For initiation of MAC sedation, either an infusion or a slow injection method is used while cardiorespiratory function is closely monitored. With the infusion method, sedation is initiated by infusing propofol at 100 to 150 µg/kg/hr for approximately 3 to 5 minutes and titrating to the desired level of sedation while closely monitoring respiratory function. This is the method of choice for older patients. For other patients the slow injection method is used, whereby approximately 0.5 mg/kg propofol is administered over 3 to 5 minutes and titrated to clinical response. This will produce a window of adequate anesthesia as measured by loss of the eyelash reflex. Immediately before induction, the patient is instructed to take a few deep breaths. Supplemental oxygen is administered via nasal cannula throughout the procedure. Pain at the injection site, which occurs relatively frequently with propofol, can be reduced significantly by intravenous administration into relatively large veins in the forearm or the antecubital fossa.

The proper end point of propofol administration is most appropriately gauged through skilled observation of the patient. As the proper threshold is reached, characteristic slackening of the jaw occurs along with a distinctive relaxation of the face in conjunction with the absence of the eyelash reflex. Frequently the patient will begin to snore softly at this point, indicating the need for gentle elevation of the mandible, extension of the neck, or forward thrust of the jaw. In the majority of cases no change in SaO_2 will occur. In the unusual case in which a change occurs, proceeding with the injection of the local anesthetic will produce enough stimulus to correct this situation, especially if one is working in particularly sensitive areas of the scalp. If this fails, ventilation can be supported and an adequate SaO_2 level can be maintained with a mask-valve-bag unit (Ambu-bag) and oral airway until the sedative effect has abated, which usually takes no more than 1 or 2 minutes. If sedation is administered judiciously and as described, ventilation support will rarely if ever be necessary.

ADMINISTRATION OF LOCAL ANESTHESIA

In Chapter 3, Part A, Seager outlines the guidelines for administration of local anesthesia in hair restoration surgery. The reader is referred to this section for an extensive discussion of local anesthesia. The brief discussion that follows outlines our own approach to local anesthesia when combined with MAC sedation.

The surgeon begins the administration of local anesthetic as soon as the desired level of sedation is reached. Lidocaine, a synthetic amide derivative, is our current agent of choice for local anesthesia because of its low allergenicity, short onset of action, and relatively long duration of effect. Buffering commercially available preparations to a physiological pH has been shown to significantly reduce the pain on injection.[16] The addition of sodium bicarbonate is considered to diminish hemostasis, although some reports do not substantiate this belief.[17] The initial injections of 1% buffered lidocaine with 1:100,000 epinephrine are used in 3 ml increments with a 30-gauge 1-inch needle to establish regional sensory nerve blocks of the scalp in the standard fashion. This approach follows generalized infiltration of the operative site with a greatly reduced degree of stimulation.[18] A 27-gauge 1½-inch needle is used to deliver 0.5% buffered lidocaine with 1:200,000 epinephrine to the recipient scalp sites; an adequate volume is used to attain moderate tumescence. The patient's head is then turned to one side and the same local anesthetic mixture is administered to the donor scalp to produce the desired turgor. A total volume of 20 to 30 ml of the 0.5% lidocaine solution is used for the entire operation depending on the extent of the procedure.

INTRAOPERATIVE MAINTENANCE OF ANESTHESIA

Once the procedure has begun, most patients require minimal additional sedation if unnecessary stimulation is avoided. The local block can be reinforced in sensitive areas if there are any signs that the local anesthetic effect is wearing off. These signs include restlessness, tachycardia, hypertension, grimacing, flinching, withdrawing, and motion of the extremities. Such signs may occur if more than 90 minutes have lapsed since the initial injection; however, most of our procedures typically are completed before 90 minutes have elapsed. Occasional gentle verbal reassurances may in some way enhance the outcome, but the temptation to substitute "vocal" anesthesia instead of local anesthesia as a bridge to closure should be avoided. The surgeon should instead stop operating and reinfiltrate the surgical site at the first sign of discomfort regardless of whether he/she is nearly finished and not rely on the amnesic effect of the intravenous anesthetic agents.

Should the patient become agitated or restless during the procedure, the underlying cause should be sought before further sedation is arbitrarily administered. Frequently, nose itching, urinary retention, low back strain, or loss of the lidocaine effect will be the cause of the agitation or restlessness. The other possibilities that must be considered include hypoventilation, hypoxemia, airway obstruction, lidocaine toxicity, dystonia, and intraocular hypertension.

It is often desirable that the patient have greater consciousness for subsequent intervals during the procedure, enabling the patient to be placed in the upright position for the transplantation procedure.

PATIENT RELEASE CRITERIA

Alert, oriented, and responds coherently to questioning
Hemodynamically stable when standing and sitting
Neurologically intact and ambulates with minimal assistance
Has voided after the procedure
Oral intake has been maintained
Released to a responsible third party

MAC sedation with propofol is titrated by dosage and rate to maintain the desired clinical effect. A variable rate infusion technique is preferable to an intermittent bolus method. With the variable rate infusion method, patients will generally require maintenance rates of 25 to 75 µg/kg/min (1.5 to 4.5 mg/kg/hr) during the first 10 to 15 minutes of sedation maintenance. Infusion rates should subsequently be decreased over time to 25 to 50 µg/kg/min and be adjusted to clinical responses. When titration to clinical effect is being performed, approximately 2 minutes should be allowed for onset of peak drug effect.[19] If the intermittent bolus method is used, incremental bolus doses of 10 or 20 mg can be administered when changes in consciousness are accompanied by a response to surgical stimulation. With the intermittent bolus method of sedation maintenance the potential exists for respiratory depression, transient increases in sedation depth, and prolonged recovery. In older patients, rapid single or repeated bolus administration should not be used, and for such patients the adult dose should be reduced by at least 20%.

POSTOPERATIVE RECOVERY

Recovery from MAC sedation with propofol is characterized by rapid emergence with minimal confusion. Early recovery, as measured by time to eye opening, response to command, and orientation, occurs on an average of 3 to 7 minutes on discontinuation of infusion. Even so, because of the continuity of local anesthesia, little sedation is generally given toward the end of most procedures, and the patient is thus already "awake." Washing the operative sites, dressing the wounds, and, if needed, applying the postoperative wrap stimulates the patient and further signals the completion of the procedure. At this point most patients can be assisted in walking to the recovery area.

Each patient remains in the recovery room under observation for a minimum of 30 minutes and is not released until he fully meets the criteria for release (see box, p. 102).

Patients are monitored with pulse oximetry until they are alert and free from significant residual sedation. Patients are given hot tea or hot chocolate to drink to assist in rewarming from the cool surgical suite air and surgical site washing. The administration of intravenous fluids is completed and the patient is assisted to the bathroom to void. The patient can then be released in stable condition to a responsible adult; it should be confirmed that the written postoperative instructions are readily at hand, the physician's phone numbers for emergencies have been given, and a postoperative appointment has been made.

CONCLUSION

Midazolam used alone or in combination with propofol appears to be the near-ideal MAC sedative agent for outpatient ambulatory scalp procedures. Midazolam is not recommended for office use outside the suitable setting or by untrained individuals. Used as described, midazolam and propofol produce varying degrees of rapid sedation, which allows for the painless administration of local anesthesia followed by rapid recovery to a clear-headed, street-ready state. Transient apnea and hypotension are possible adverse reactions that can be minimized and are manageable. In addition, the signs of local anesthetic toxicities, although rare in commonly used dose ranges, must be understood, recognized, and treated. We have found that MAC sedation with midazolam and/or propofol in conjunction with local anesthetics is a highly satisfactory anesthesia technique from the standpoint of the surgeon, anesthetist, and patient.

REFERENCES

1. AAAHC guidelines, Skokie, Ill., AAAHC.
2. Courtiss EH, Kanter MA: The prevention and management of medical problems during office surgery, *Plast Reconstr Surg* 85:1227-1236, 1990.
3. Elliott RA, Hoehn JG: The office surgical suite—the physical plant and equipment, *Clin Plast Surg* 10:225-246, 1983.
4. Gilbert DA, Adamsom JE: Procedure manuals in office surgery, *Clin Plast Surg* 10:269-272, 1983.
5. Scarborough DA, Bisaccia EB: The preoperative evaluation visit for cosmetic surgery, *Cosmet Dermatol* 6(2):10-12, 1993.
6. Saidman and Stanley, American Society of Anesthesiologist Refresher Course 123 A/B, 1985.
7. Sebel PS, Lowdon JD: Propofol: a new intravenous anesthetic, *Anesthesiology* 71:260, 1989.
8. Clarke RSJ and others: Adverse reactions to intravenous anesthetics, *Br J Anaesth* 47:575, 1975.
9. Dye D, Watkins J: Suspected anaphylactic reaction to Cremophor EL, *Br Med J* 280:1353, 1980.
10. White PF: Pharmacology of propofol, *Anesth Clin North Am* 297-318, 1988.
11. Kanto J, Gepts E: Pharmacokinetic implications for the clinical use of propofol, *Clin Pharmacokinet* 17(5):308, 1989.
12. Sebel PS and others: Propofol infusion for sedation in intensive care, *Anesthesia* 42:929, 1987.
13. Doenicke A and others: Effects of propofol on histamine release, immunoglobulin levels and activation of complement in healthy volunteers, *Postgrad Med J* 61(suppl):15, 1985.
14. Flumazenil package insert brochure, Nutley, N.J., March 1993, Roche Laboratories.
15. Reeves JG and others: Midazolam: pharmacology and uses, *Anesthesiology* 62:310-324, 1985.
16. McKay W, Morris R, Mushlin P: Sodium bicarbonate alternates pain on skin infiltration with lidocaine with or without epinephrine, *Anesth Analg* 66:572, 1987.
17. Ragland P, Coleman W, Guilotte R: Does sodium bicarbonate buffered lidocaine increase ecchymoses in cosmetic surgery? *Am J Cosmet Surg* 10(4):255-257, 1993.
18. Scarborough DA, Bisaccia E: Anesthesia for the dermatologic surgeon, *Int J Dermatol* 28(10):629-637, 1989.
19. Propofol package insert brochure, Wilmington, Del., March 1992, Stuart Pharmaceuticals.

F. Nitrous Oxide in Hair Restoration Surgery

Neil S. Sadick and Dow B. Stough

Most hair restoration surgery is performed with the use of regional anesthesia. We favor a combination of nitrous oxide (N₂O), regional nerve blocks, and supplemental local anesthetics. Nitrous oxide, a colorless gas with a slightly sweet odor, is an excellent agent for the induction phase of local anesthesia. An excellent review of nitrous oxide in 400 hair transplant procedures was presented by Sadick.[1] For a complete review of this subject, readers are referred to other sources.[2,3]

Although the use of nitrous oxide with local anesthetics is highly effective, these agents are less likely to achieve the same degree of sedation and level of anesthesia as a combination of intravenous agents such as midazolam (Versed), fentanyl, and meperidine (Demerol).

The use of intravenous agents with monitored anesthesia care is outlined by Scarborough and Bisaccia in Chapter 3, Part E.

DELIVERY SYSTEMS

The greatest risk in the use of nitrous oxide is the potential for the delivery of a hypoxic mixture (<21% oxygen). This situation is simply avoided with use of proper equipment[1] (Fig. 3-19). Three basic features that ensure safety in this setting include a fail-safe system, a flowmeter arrangement, and proportioning systems.

To ensure that nitrous oxide and oxygen are delivered from separate tank devices, the tanks are connected to the delivery system by flowmeters designed to prevent hypoxic mixtures. The system should also have a fail-safe device that sets off an alarm and automatically turns off the nitrous oxide tank should the oxygen tank pressure be lost.

A nasal inhaler that provides a snug fit over the nose for both the delivery and scavenging of nitrous oxide vapors is used (Fig. 3-20). For additional safety, the patient's oxygen saturation (SaO₂) should be monitored with pulse oximetry (Fig. 3-21).

TECHNIQUES OF NITROUS OXIDE ADMINISTRATION

It is important to explain to patients that nitrous oxide will produce euphoria and mild acral tingling. The nasal inhaler should have a snug fit. Initial flows should consist of 3 L/min of oxygen. Once established, the flows are adjusted to provide 35% nitrous oxide and 65% oxygen.

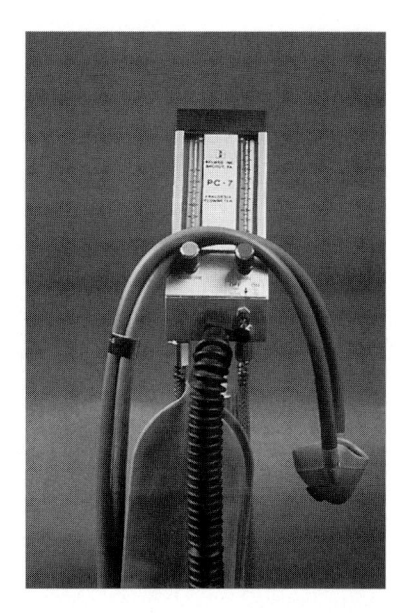

FIG. 3-19 Nitrous oxide unit (Belmed, Inc., Brogue, Pa.).

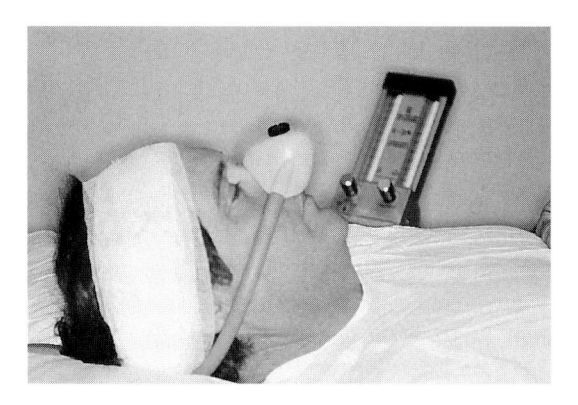

FIG. 3-20 A nasal inhaler provides a snug fit for both the delivery and scavenging of nitrous oxide vapors.

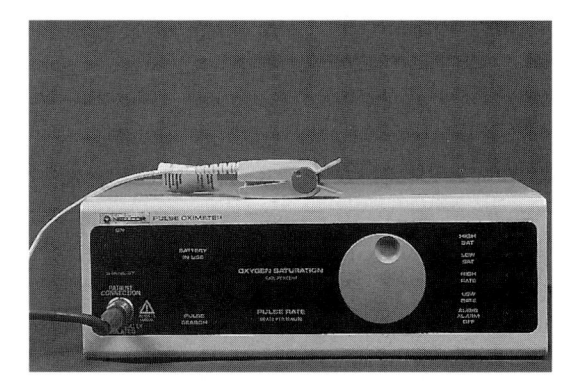

FIG. 3-21 Pulse oximeter (model N-100C; Nellcor, Inc., Hayward, Calif.).

Approximately 3 minutes is required for full effect, allowing subsequent injection of local anesthetic. If sedation is inadequate, flows may be safely adjusted to provide 50% nitrous oxide and 50% oxygen. This ratio usually provides sufficient sedation for local anesthetic infiltration in hair transplantation surgery. Concentrations of nitrous oxide as high as 66% have been used without toxic effect.[3] Clearing of mentation usually occurs 10 to 20 minutes after cessation of nitrous oxide administration.

SIDE EFFECTS*

Nitrous oxide is the most commonly used inhalation agent and is considered to have the highest margin of safety of all drugs currently in use for conscious sedation. It has a minimal depressive effect on the respiratory or cardiovascular systems.[4] However, because of its poor solubility, nitrous oxide exits the bloodstream rapidly and enters the alveoli with cessation of administration. This rapid diffusion of nitrous oxide into the alveoli dilutes alveolar oxygen, so-called diffusion hypoxia, which may last from 1 to 2 minutes. This effect can be minimized by administering 100% oxygen for 3 to 5 minutes after discontinuing the nitrous oxide administration. Nausea and vomiting may occur postoperatively in up to 15% of patients. According to our own data, the incidence of nausea is less than 10% in patients undergoing hair restoration surgical procedures.[1]

---

*This section is taken in part from Sadick NS: Use of nitrous oxide in hair transplantation surgery, J Dermatol Surg Oncol 20(3):186-190, 1994.

CONCLUSION

Nitrous oxide is an excellent agent for the preanesthetic induction phase of hair transplantation surgery (see box). It is of great help in reducing pain from local anesthetic infiltration and has an extremely low complication profile, most commonly producing transient, minor mood alterations. It produces significant augmentation of pain threshold for local anesthetic infiltration, causes short-term dissociative effects, and produces no hypersensitivity reactions in contradistinction to other previously described preanesthetic agents.

Nitrous oxide should be added to the armamentarium of preanesthetic agents used during hair transplantation surgery. This modality has been tested in thousands of patients undergoing hair transplantation and has proved to be a useful and safe preanesthetic agent.[5]

REFERENCES

1. Sadick NS: Use of nitrous oxide in hair transplantation surgery, J Dermatol Surg Oncol 20(3):186-190, 1994.
2. Eger EL II: Cardiovascular effects of nitrous oxide. In Eisele J, Jown N, editors: Nitrous oxide/N_2O, New York, 1985, Elsevier.
3. Griffin G, Campbell U, Jones R: Nitrous oxide-oxygen sedation for minor surgery, JAMA 245:2411-2413, 1981.
4. Gilman AG and others: General anesthetics. In Price HL, Dripps RD, editors: The pharmacological basis of therapeutics, New York, 1985, Macmillan.
5. Miller FL, Marshall BE: The inhaled anesthetics. In Longnecker DE, Murphy FL, editors: Introduction to anesthesia, ed 8, Philadelphia, 1992, WB Saunders.

G. Pain Control and Management of the Postoperative Period

David J. Seager

POSTOPERATIVE PAIN

Usual Course

Pain after hair transplantation or scalp reduction is variable both in intensity and duration, between different patients, and even in the same patient between different sessions.

The most common description of pain after hair transplantation by patients in my practice is fairly consistent. Approximately 1 hour after the transplant session has finished, which is usually about 2 hours after the infiltration of local anesthetic into the recipient area, the patient reports a burning or stinging sensation over the recipient area. Patients with low pain thresholds call it pain, but most patients refer to it as mild discomfort. This sensation lasts for approximately 1 to 2 hours. During this

---

NITROUS OXIDE

Advantages
Analgesia
Rapid uptake and elimination
Little cardiac or respiratory depression

Disadvantages
Sympathetic stimulation
Expansion of closed air spaces
Interferes with B_{12} metabolism
Limits FIO_2

Modified from Miller FM, Marshall BF: The inhaled anesthetics. In Longnecker DE, Murphy FL, editors: Introduction to anesthesia, ed 8, Philadelphia, 1992, WB Saunders.

time the local anesthetic in the donor area seems to remain effective, and patients do not complain of pain in the donor area yet. However, 1 to 2 hours later, when the recipient area begins to feel better, the donor area begins to hurt. The pain now felt in the donor area is usually of moderate intensity and remains moderate for 3 to 12 hours, at which time it lessens in intensity and usually becomes quite mild for approximately another 24 hours. One to two days after surgery, this pain usually regresses into a "tenderness to touch" only, which lasts 1 week to 10 days. These intensities and durations can be variable; a fair number of patients (perhaps 25%) say "there was no pain at all," but a few patients (perhaps 1% to 3%) report excruciatingly severe pain in the donor area starting 1 or 2 hours after surgery; on occasion, the pain is severe enough to cause vomiting and diaphoresis. This pain stops immediately after reinfiltration with local anesthetic, first lidocaine with epinephrine for its almost immediate effect and shortly thereafter bupivacaine (Marcaine) with epinephrine for its long duration of action. This is the only instance in which I use bupivacaine in hair transplantation surgery; bupivacaine is longer lasting than lidocaine but more toxic.

Treatment

Treatment of postoperative pain varies tremendously from physician to physician. Shiell rarely if ever prescribes anything stronger than plain acetaminophen (Shiell R: Personal communication, 1992). He says that preparations containing codeine are rarely necessary and do more harm by upsetting stomachs than good by relieving pain. On the other hand, Unger[1] gives patients acetaminophen with 30 mg codeine and usually gives packets of six Percocet (oxycodone and acetaminophen) and six meperidine (Demerol) tablets in case they are needed.

My own routine is to provide every patient who undergoes hair transplantation with a prescription for 20 tablets of Tylenol No. 3 (acetaminophen, 325 mg, and codeine, 30 mg). Extremely rarely, when patients have described severe pain in the donor area before leaving the clinic, I have injected the donor area incision with lidocaine and bupivacaine with dramatic relief of pain. Thankfully, postoperative pain rarely warrants this step, and thus most patients are offered one or two Tylenol No. 3 tablets before leaving the clinic. Approximately 60% of my patients accept them. Some say that they only require plain Tylenol, and a few say they do not require any analgesics. Patients who have particularly severe pain on leaving the clinic, those with a history of severe postoperative pain, or those with a tolerance to codeine are given a prescription for 12 tablets of Percocet with instructions to take one to two every 4 hours as required.

NEURALGIA
Usual Course

Another type of pain sometimes experienced is neuralgia, which usually if not always is felt only in the donor area. Neuralgia generally takes a few days to develop and occurs after a nerve has been either severed or otherwise damaged (e.g., injury by cautery, suture material wrapped around a small branch of a nerve). Neuralgia varies from being fairly mild and lasting only a few days to being extremely severe and lasting for weeks, then lingering for months with milder intensity. Neuralgia is characterized by continuous and/or shooting pains ("like electric shocks") and tingling and hypersensitivity distal to the nerve injury. Patients say that water from the shower falling on the area, combing their hair, or even the blowing of wind causes pain in the hypersensitive area. I perform an average of approximately 20 hair transplant procedures per week in my practice, and about one patient per month complains bitterly about neuralgia, which usually lasts a couple of weeks. However, if every patient is carefully questioned about his postoperative pain, milder forms of neuralgia are found to occur much more commonly but are usually insufficiently severe for the patient to mention. Dr. Pierre Porteaux of France has commented that neuralgia may be more common with the scalpel technique than with the traditional hand engine technique.[2] Stough has had one extremely severe case of neuralgia after transplantation combined with scalp reduction. The neuralgia was described as severe, excruciating, shooting pains across the occiput. The symptoms persisted for 4 months. During this time, local anesthetics led to complete, albeit temporary, relief. The patient was treated with nonsteroidal antiinflammatory agents with limited benefit. Complete resolution occurred after 6 months (Stough DB: Personal communication, April 1994). One patient of mine had severe neuralgia for 6 months that responded partially to amitriptyline (Elavil); hyperesthesia distal to the nerve injury was the principal symptom. Eventually the pain completely resolved.

Neuralgia is definitely a patient-specific phenomenon. When the main neurovascular bundle of the greater occipital nerve is severed completely and then cauterized, many patients feel no pain whatsoever afterward, whereas others report neuralgia after almost any significant incision into skin anywhere on their bodies.

Treatment

Neuralgia can be very difficult to treat. I try to convince patients that after they use all of their original prescription of Tylenol No. 3, they should try to make do with plain Tylenol only because the codeine in the Tylenol No. 3 can become very addictive. When the prescription is renewed once, it is more difficult to say no the third time, and it is easy to fall into the trap of creating an addict.

Other medications are commonly used for treating neuralgia. First-line medications after simple analgesics are tricyclic antidepressants such as amitriptyline followed by anticonvulsants such as carbamazepine (Tegretol) or phenytoin (Dilantin), and lastly by membrane stabilizers such as mexiletine (Mexitil). After all these agents have been tried (and in my extensive experience while pain control physician at a large general hospital, none of these more complex drugs are very effective) and have failed, local anesthetics and long-lasting cortisone agents (such as methylprednisolone acetate [Depo-Medrol], triamcinolone diacetate [Aristocort], or triamcinolone acetonide [Kenalog]) can be injected into the affected nerve. These treatments usually provide only temporary relief. In my experience of treating occipital neuralgia (the usual type of neuralgia encountered in patients who have undergone hair transplantation), firm reassurance regarding the subjective and self-limiting nature of the condition and temporizing is my usual approach. In most cases this suffices.

POSTOPERATIVE EDEMA

Usual Course

After hair transplantation to the front one third of the scalp there is usually some edema of the forehead and periorbital areas. This edema usually does not appear the day after surgery but begins the second day after surgery. It varies tremendously in its extent and duration, but nearly everyone who has even a fairly minimal number of grafts inserted into the front of the scalp will have at least enough edema to eliminate the wrinkles in the forehead. At the other extreme end of the spectrum are those who, after a fairly minor session of hair transplantation, experience massive, disfiguring facial edema that closes one or both eyes. As stated, this process begins on the second postoperative day, usually reaches a peak on the fourth postoperative day, and has usually resolved completely by the sixth or seventh postoperative day. In about 1 in 50 patients, especially after the first transplant session, one or two "black eyes" will develop. This edema starts at the hairline and then drifts inferiorly, affecting next the forehead and the bridge of the nose, then the eyelids, and by the fifth or sixth day it usually resolves through the cheeks. Unfortunately, there is no way of predicting which patients will experience edema or the degree of edema and therefore there is no way to determine exactly who will need prophylactic corticosteroids. Some of my patients have had almost no significant edema after the first and second sessions, yet with a smaller third session, huge periorbital edema developed. In my experience, once edema has begun, ice packs and sleeping while sitting in an upright position have little effect. Because of the lag time it takes for corticosteroids to work, the late institution of cortisone has hardly any effect on shortening the natural course that the edema would have taken to resolve without it.

Prevention

Most experienced hair transplant surgeons routinely administer some type of corticosteroid preparation to most patients without contraindications who are undergoing hair transplant surgery. Perioperative and postoperative steroids have been found to reduce the incidence and degree of postoperative edema (and to a lesser extent, discomfort) after head and neck surgery.[3,4] These steroids are usually given immediately before or after the surgery. The three most common methods of administering steroids are as follows:

1. *Celestone Soluspan (a commercially available preparation of a mixture of betamethasone sodium phosphate and betamethasone acetate), 1 to 2 ml administered intravenously or intramuscularly, often with a sedative at the start of a procedure.* This regimen provides effective blood levels of betamethasone for 5 to 7 days. The downside of this method of administration in my opinion is that once given, it cannot be stopped. Should a serious side effect develop, such as cortisone psychosis, or worse still, a bleeding ulcer, one cannot prevent further worsening effects of the cortisone from continuing. However, this method is an extremely convenient way of administering a corticosteroid, and is probably slightly easier on the gastrointestinal tract than oral preparations, although cortisone by any route can cause a silent ulcer to bleed.

2. *Oral cortisone preparations.* The most common method of using oral cortisone preparations is to prescribe prednisone (physicians usually prescribe doses between 15 to 60 mg) in a single daily dose to be taken as early as possible in the morning with food. This dose is repeated daily for 3 to 5 days, often on a sliding scale. The advantage of the oral route is that

at the first hint of any side effect the prednisone can be stopped. Because of the short half-life of prednisone, side effects and complications usually then cease immediately.

3. *Cortisone preparations added to the local anesthetic to be used to infiltrate into the recipient area.* Norwood[5] advocates adding triamcinolone acetonide to the lidocaine to achieve a concentration of 1 mg/ml of lidocaine solution. This preparation is used in addition to injected and oral steroids. Whether the reduction in postoperative swelling that results from this method is caused by the local effect of the triamcinolone acetonide being injected directly into the dermis or by the systemic effect of the (usually) extra 50 mg of triamcinolone acetonide thus administered is unknown. I suspect that the reduction of postoperative swelling is simply a function of the total dose of steroid received by whichever route. The more cortisone that is administered, the lesser the swelling but with a greater potential for serious side effects. Arnold has reported the occurrence of a folliculitis-like reaction that occurred at injection sites after the addition of triamcinolone acetonide to lidocaine (Arnold J: Personal communication, Jan. 1994).

There are more complex and esoteric protocols for administering cortisone. For instance, some advocate administering 100 mg of hydrocortisone intravenously 1 hour before surgery in addition to oral prednisone because this combination will be effective in preventing damage to the microcirculation as surgery takes place; these drugs are given in addition to large doses of prednisone afterward.

The previously described three methods are frequently used and, with large enough doses, work well. However, even with the use of cortisone doses at the upper limits mentioned, there is often some minor swelling and rarely considerable swelling.

My policy is to discuss with the patient the possible need for the reduction or elimination of probable edema by the use of cortisone and the potential side effects and complications of steroids. Each patient who elects to take cortisone is given a packet that contains four tablets of 50 mg prednisone with instructions to take one whole tablet with his next meal, three fourths of a tablet the next morning with food, one half of a tablet the next morning with food, and a one quarter of a tablet the next morning with food.

CRUSTING

The day after surgery, crusts will form over every graft. These crusts vary in color; they are usually straw-colored but may possibly be white or blood-stained dark red or brown. The duration of time they remain on the scalp depends on the size of the graft. Micrograft crusts usually remain adherent for 5 to 7 days and minigraft crusts usually remain 10 to 14 days, whereas 4 mm graft crusts are usually firmly adherent for at least 2 to 3 weeks. If shortly after surgery these grafts are coated with some moisturizing agent such as an antibiotic ointment or Vaseline or vitamin E oil, they will look a lot messier, but the crusts will come off slightly sooner. These moisturizing agents both decrease the amount of crusting (especially if applied within hours of the end of the procedure) and make the crusts softer and less adherent to the grafts, allowing them to be removed earlier and more easily.

ADVICE TO PATIENTS WHO WEAR HAIRPIECES

Patients who habitually wear a hairpiece before hair transplantation are usually extremely reluctant to abandon wearing the hairpiece. Traditional advice has been that, provided the base of the hairpiece is made of open mesh rather than solid plastic, it may be worn a few days after surgery (provided, of course, no tape is placed over the grafts; clips to existing fringe hair are generally recommended to attach hairpieces after hair transplantation). However, I have spoken to a hair transplant surgeon who performed hair transplantation on a set of identical twins who were identically bald and gave each man the same number of grafts in the same pattern. One wore a hairpiece daily after surgery and the other did not. The twin who wore the hairpiece had noticeably poorer growth than the other (Bedard P: Personal communication, 1992). It was after hearing about this anecdotal evidence that after my own hair transplant, I abandoned the use of the hairpiece I had previously worn daily. I therefore feel dutybound to advise patients in general that they may have better hair growth if they minimize the use of the hairpiece after surgery. Since Dr. Bedard communicated this observation to me, I have more closely inspected the hair growth of many of my patients who continued to wear hairpieces soon after hair transplantation, and it is my opinion that these patients as a whole experience a slightly higher incidence of poor growth than the rest of my patients who have not worn hairpieces. Nonetheless, conventional teaching is that mesh hairpieces do not affect growth.

HAIR GROWTH

Most of the transplanted hair in the grafts will fall out from 1 to 6 weeks after surgery. Much of the transplanted hair that comes out is attached to the crusts; most of the rest looks as if it is continuing to grow, but it eventually falls out also. Usually only a very small proportion of hairs (especially micrografts in the hairline) will continue to grow continuously from the day of transplantation without shedding. The rest of the transplanted hair in the scalp will begin to regrow anywhere from 7 weeks with minigrafts (especially anteriorly) to 10 to 14 weeks for larger grafts (especially further back from the hairline). With some patients I observed that 20 weeks passed before any hair at all grew after any of the transplant sessions, and yet ultimately they experienced good growth. Some hair transplant surgeons have said that in their experience an occasional graft has not grown until 1 year after hair transplantation (Shiell R: Personal communication, 1993). Not all hairs in the same graft begin to grow at the same time, and a five-hair graft that has only three hairs growing from it 12 weeks after transplantation may well have all five growing by 20 weeks after transplantation. I have observed that hair transplanted at third and fourth sessions may take slightly longer to begin growing than hair transplanted at the first or second sessions, probably because of slightly impaired vascularity. It has also been my observation that these subsequent sessions of slit incisional grafting may actually accelerate the onset and rate of hair growth from previous sessions. This accelerated growth is probably because of the increased blood flow resulting from the inflammation caused by the most recent hair transplant.

MINOXIDIL USE

Many hair transplant surgeons, including myself, believe that hair growth after hair transplantation starts sooner and is more rapid with the topical use of minoxidil. It is also believed that a greater proportion of hairs will not initially shed with minoxidil use. I know of no evidence that hair growth will be any better eventually with or without the use of minoxidil. Because of the expense and some of the fears regarding the potential side effects of minoxidil, I do not offer it routinely to all patients. However, I prescribe it postoperatively to certain selected patients in cases in which I believe I may have crowded the grafts excessively closely together or when I am otherwise concerned about the impaired vascularity of the recipient area. Those patients who are in a hurry for their hair to grow (e.g., grooms-to-be who wish to look good in their wedding photographs) or anyone who requests it because they have heard about it elsewhere will receive a prescription for 2% minoxidil solution (after a discussion about potential side effects) to be applied twice daily until new growth occurs. Some physicians recommend its use the first day after transplantation. However, at this point the scalp is inflamed, and therefore systemic absorption is greatly increased. When I routinely prescribed minoxidil starting the day after surgery, several patients reported palpitations. I now advise patients to wait 1 week before they cautiously begin to use it.

BANDAGING

Bandaging is another subject about which different experienced and successful hair transplant surgeons hold rigid and opposing opinions. For approximately the first two decades of hair transplantation, virtually all hair transplant patients were fully bandaged postoperatively in turbanlike dressings, and even today following most hair transplants the patient's head is bandaged. Either Vaseline gauze covered with antibiotic ointment or sofra-tulle is applied directly to the recipient area (although some surgeons prefer a dry nonstick dressing such as a Telfa pad). These dressings are then adhered to the patient's head by bandaging them into place with a slightly elastic gauze bandage, such as Kling. Many surgeons generally apply some tension around the donor area when applying the bandage so that the bandage acts as a pressure dressing, lessening the risk of hematoma formation. There are a variety of different bandaging techniques (Figs. 3-22 and 3-23) (see Chapter 8, Part B). Those that are wrapped un-

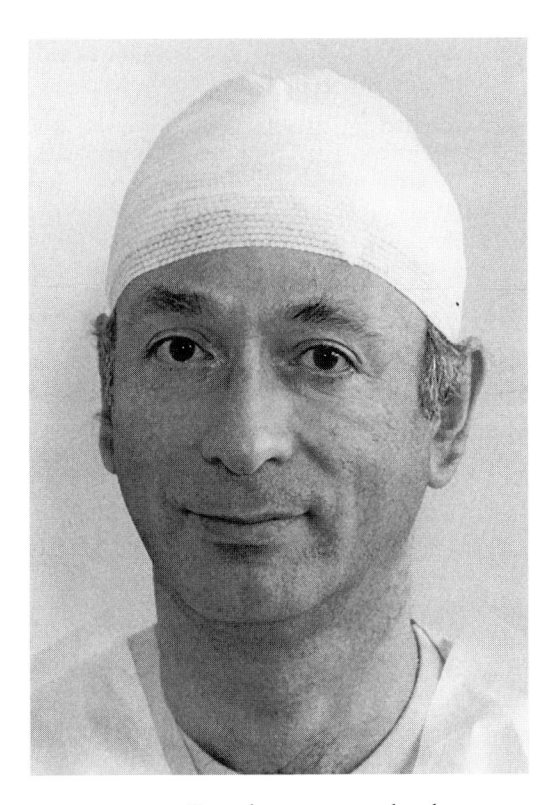

FIG. 3-22 Typical postoperative bandaging.

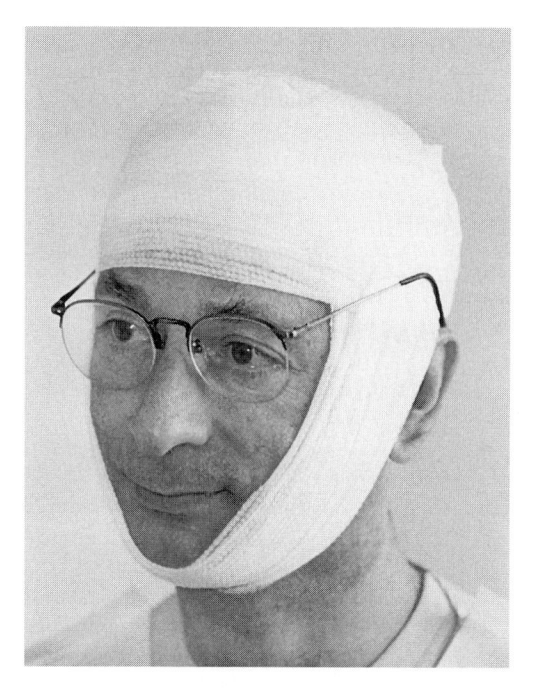

FIG. 3-23 Bandaging continued under patient's chin is more secure but less tolerated by patients.

der the chin are the most secure but are slightly less accepted by the patients. In fact, being sent home with a turban-type bandage is generally not very well accepted by a lot of patients. A growing number of hair transplant surgeons are sending patients home from surgery without any bandaging at all.

The advantages of bandaging are the following:

1. Any spotting of blood, which is quite common, is concealed. This spotting of blood is worrisome to patients and makes them look all the more unsightly.
2. A great deal of evidence indicates that certain types of bandaging encourage earlier epithelialization and more rapid healing.
3. Should the patient bump his head or let it roll on a pillow, a graft is less likely to be lost.
4. These bandages can be applied immediately after surgery and the patient can be released from the office without delay.
5. A pressure dressing around the donor area helps to lessen the risk of hematoma formation.

Usually the patient is asked to return to the office the next day for the removal of the bandage, at which time the nursing staff washes the patient's hair and cleans off any spotting of blood that may have stained the scalp. The patient is then sent home looking relatively clean.

On the other hand, if the patient is kept in the office for 1 or 2 hours after the completion of surgery, any beading or spotting of blood is meticulously cleansed from around the grafts as it occurs, and pressure is applied to any bleeding points, in most cases the patient's scalp eventually stays clean and spotless. The patient is then sent home and does not need to return the next day or have the psychologically traumatic task of removing a dressing at home. I find that patients prefer to go home wearing a baseball cap rather than a conspicuous turbanlike dressing. The extra work and inconvenience of having the patient wait at the office afterward is more than made up for by not having to tend to him the next day. If the patient sleeps sitting upright, as he should to help prevent swelling, a graft is almost never lost. I have not found any practical difference in the rate of healing or epithelialization by sending patients home without a dressing on the recipient area. However, I apply a dry dressing over the donor area by means of a moderately tight pressure dressing that looks like a headband. I believe this helps to prevent hematoma formation and allows one to be somewhat less meticulous in achieving hemostasis in the donor region (i.e., less cautery and/or use of hemostats). The patient is instructed to remove the pressure dressing 24 hours later. I find that this method of bandaging is more acceptable to patients. However, several patients refuse to wear even the pressure dressing around the donor area, and these patients have the pressure dressing removed before leaving the office. Chapter 8, Part B discusses in detail the specific steps in bandaging.

GENERAL POSTOPERATIVE ADVICE

My advice to patients after hair transplantation is presented in my postoperative handout instruction pamphlet (see Appendix H). Again, much of this advice regarding when to first wash the hair or touch the grafts or perform various types of exercise is determined by each surgeon partly by tradition and partly empirically. My aftercare instructions have been modified from those of several other hair transplant surgeons including Dr. Richard Schiell. I have found they work well in practice and have faced no complications as a result of these instructions.

REFERENCES

1. Unger WP: Postoperative course. In Unger WP, Nordstrom REA, editors: *Hair transplantation*, ed 2, New York, 1988, Marcel Dekker.
2. Porteaux P: Written communication to Dr. Dow Stough, Paris, March 23, 1994.
3. Griffies WS and others: Steroids in rhinoplasty, *Laryngoscope* 99(11):1161-1164, 1989.
4. Hoffman DF: Steroids and rhinoplasty–a double-blind study, *Arch Otolaryngol Head Neck Surg* 117:990-993, 1991.
5. Norwood O: Say goodbye to postoperative swelling, *Hair Transplant Forum* 2(6):13, 1992.

4
Instrumentation

A. Instrumentation for Hair Transplantation and Scalp Reduction

James M. Swinehart

An expert skier could probably ski straight down the fall line in a steep mogul field in Aspen or Vail with leather boots and wooden skis. A top figure skater could certainly execute elaborate aerial maneuvers with dull skates. These athletes, however, would not dream of entering a competitive event without the finest available equipment. In similar fashion, the hair replacement surgeon should complement his/her skills with state-of-the-art instrumentation.

Hair replacement surgery is in a state of rapid change. The exciting new hair and scalp surgical methods practiced today, including extensive micrografting, single-hair cloning and implantation, scalp-lifting, scalp extension, scalp expansion, and repair work, have spawned a new generation of "tools" to assist the specialist. These items are described here as the surgeon would use them during a procedure.

INSTRUMENTATION FOR HAIR TRANSPLANTATION

Preparation and Anesthesia

PREPARATION TRAY
A separate tray (Fig. 4-1) containing instruments necessary for preparing the donor site for graft removal should include the following:

- Surgical marking pen
- Stainless steel comb
- Hair clips
- Tape or Hypafix
- Alcohol or povidone-iodine (Betadine) for cleansing

NOTE: The author has no proprietary interest in any of the instruments mentioned in this discussion.

- Stainless steel ruler
- Fine, long, curved scissors (such as Metzenbaum) and/or electric trimmer (set to trim hair approximately 2 to 3 mm long so that angle of hair growth can still be ascertained)
- Densitometer, to determine density per square millimeter or density per square centimeter of hair follicles under magnification, or otoscope with a 4 mm speculum
- Proper photographic equipment as described in Chapter 1, Part G

LOCAL ANESTHESIA
Even in sedated patients, the injection of local anesthetic may sting considerably in the donor and recipient areas. The four-step approach of ice/saline solution/lidocaine (Xylocaine)/tumescent solution can provide for a nearly bloodless procedure. Ice can be in the form of cryogel "pillows" for smaller areas (e.g., supraorbital block sites) or "blue ice" packs for the donor area. The ice decreases the sting of the needle; normal saline solution containing 0.9% benzyl alcohol provides partial anesthesia without stinging. Administration of the local anesthetic (a 50/50 mixture of 1% lidocaine with epinephrine and 0.5% bupivacaine [Marcaine]) then follows. The tumescent solution (0.1% lidocaine

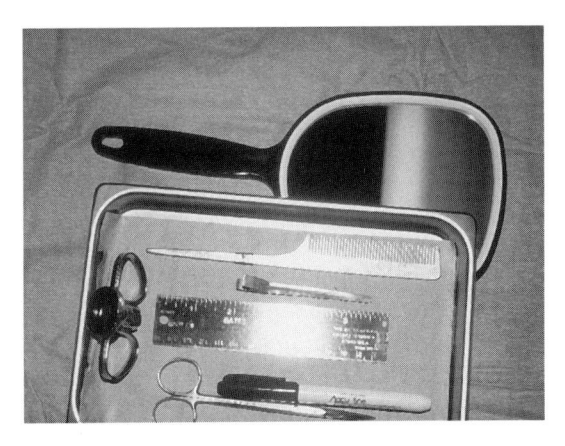

FIG. 4-1 Hair transplantation preparation tray.

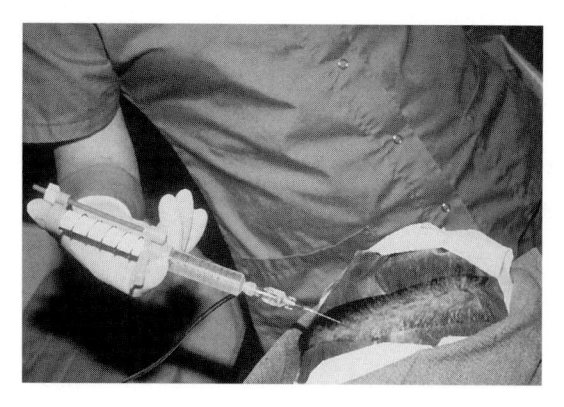

FIG. 4-2 Infiltration of donor area with dilute tumescent solution using McGhan tissue expander fill kit.

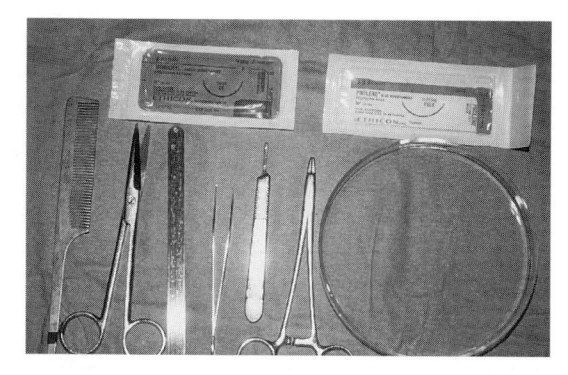

FIG. 4-3 Hair transplantation donor strip removal tray, including suture and iced saline solution dish to receive donor strip.

with 1:1,000,000 epinephrine) can be skillfully administered via a McGhan tissue expander fill kit (spring-loaded automatic fill syringe) connected to a 500 ml intravenous bag of solutions (Fig. 4-2). The induction of tumescent anesthesia is addressed by Coleman in Chapter 3, Part C.

Donor Site

DONOR GRAFT HARVESTING
Multibladed knives, producing one, two, or three hair-bearing strips 1.5 to 4 mm wide are in widespread use. Alternatively, an elongated ellipse can be removed en bloc with a single No. 10 Personna blade on a scalpel handle assisted by Adson forceps (Fig. 4-3).

CLOSURE MATERIALS
Subcutaneous placement of newer sutures such as 0 Monocryl or PDS aids in skin closure and greatly decreases the spreading of the donor scar with time. Monocryl possesses the advantages of high tensile strength, ease of manipulation, and more rapid dissolution as compared with PDS. The surgeon should choose a large needle with a relatively long cutting edge (Ethicon Y-958 with Taper CT needle).

Cutaneous sutures such as 2-0 Prolene on a cutting FSLX needle (Ethicon 8689) are less painful than staples postoperativly, but surgical staples can be placed more rapidly. Surgical staples are available in a great variety of sizes and dispensers. The U.S. Surgical 25W stapler has proved useful for donor site closure.

Graft Preparation

A comfortable, well-lit graft dissection area is indispensable (Fig. 4-4). Lighting should come from two directions if possible and should be far enough away to avoid heat production. The dissection table contains a sterile surgical drape overlying a bed of flat, self-contained ice packs. Grafts, as they are pre-

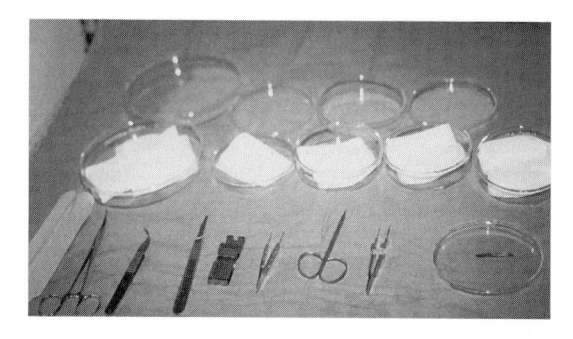

FIG. 4-4 Hair transplant dissection area, including dishes of chilled saline solution placed on ice packs underneath a sterile drape.

pared, are graded and sorted by size (or other variables), into petri dishes containing chilled saline solution.

Long ellipses are first sectioned into 2 to 1.5 mm "loaves" with gas-sterilized single-edged razor blades, using tongue blades above and below the strips as stabilizers. These "loaves" as well as strips from multibladed knives are then sectioned using a Foerster forceps and a No. 10 Personna blade. These blades can be rapidly removed via a Miltex blade remover. Iris or gradle scissors are often used for the removal of micrografts containing one to two hairs (Fig. 4-5).

Magnification is essential to accurate graft dissection. Inexpensive magnifocusers (approximately 2.5×) are usually sufficient, although a 10× stereoscope may be used for the finest dissections.

Recipient Site

PREPARATION
Should the surgeon elect to remove bald skin from the recipient site (e.g., in very bald individuals or in patients requiring plug repair), a number of small

Instrumentation for Hair Transplantation and Scalp Reduction   **113**

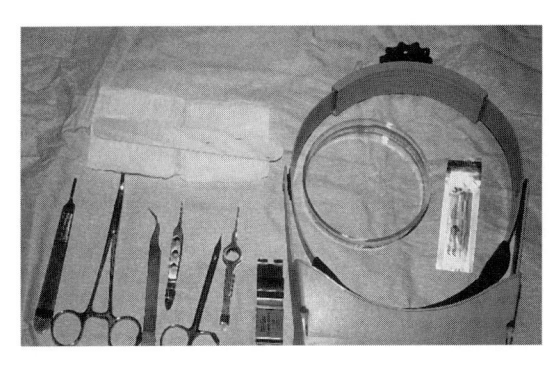

FIG. 4-5 Closeup view of hair transplant dissection materials including magnifocusers and a variety of forceps and scissors.

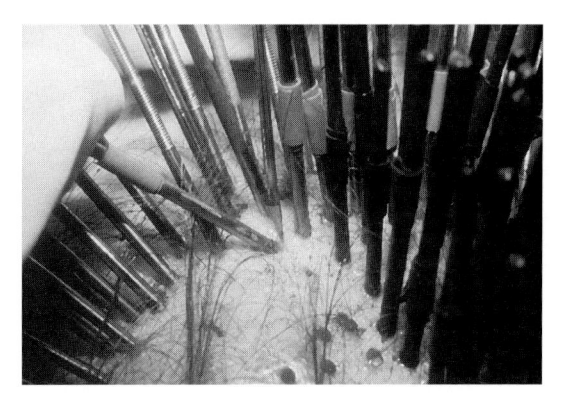

FIG. 4-7 Insertion of two-hair microdilator following the creation of a small needle hole anteriorly. In the central crown, 1 mm holes have been removed to accommodate three- to four-hair micrografts.

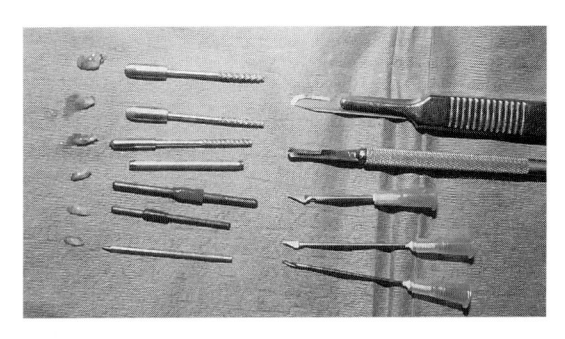

Fig. 4-6 Closeup view showing matching devices for slit creation, dilators, and graft sizes ranging from minigrafts to single-hair micrografts.

punches, graduated in increments of 0.25 mm starting at 1 mm, are available. These small punches may be attached to variety of variable speed hand engines whose handles can be protected by a sterile plastic sleeve (Fig. 4-6).

Alternatively, microslits, which receive microslit grafts, can be prepared with a variety of surgical devices. The finest recipient sites are prepared with 18- or 20-gauge needles; slightly larger sites are created with No. 18 or No. 16 NoKor needles on a 3 ml empty syringe. A Sharptome blade or small Beaver blade can be used either to create microslits or to enlarge "microholes" into ellipses. No. 64 Beaver blades or No. 15 scalpel blades create larger slits, which are suitable for minigrafts (see Fig. 4-6).

Finally, ultrapulsed carbon dioxide lasers can be used to create microslits as well.

Once the slits are created, dilating rods may be inserted temporarily prior to graft insertion. Although the use of these microdilators increase operative time and instrumentation, they can provide hemostasis, aid in accurate graft spacing, facilitate graft insertion, prevent missed recipient sites, and avoid "piggy backing" of grafts. Dilators are manufactured by several suppliers in a number of sizes and shapes. Alternatively, microdilators can be custom crafted from stainless steel or high-quality brass wire available in hardware or welding supply shops. Other possible dilators include blunted needles, sterilized wooden toothpicks, and small cotton swabs for punch graft recipient sites (Fig. 4-7).

GRAFT INSERTION

Micrografts are removed from a tray (or the sterile, gloved, nondominant index finger) and inserted into the recipient site with a jeweler's forceps. In the dominant hand the surgeon holds a fine, curved, diamond-jawed jeweler's forceps, which is used for grasping the fat pad beneath the hair follicle. The nondominant hand holds a straight, stainless steel jeweler's forceps that is used first to stabilize the skin (since the dilators are removed by an assistant using a curved hemostat) and then to "tease" the graft to the desired depth in the recipient hole (Fig. 4-8). Optical magnifiers and good lighting are of obvious importance for single-hair micrografting. A spring-loaded plunger implantation device that contains a single hair follicle in a partially open, hollow surgical needle has been developed by Choi in Korea (see Chapter 4, Part D).

The Future

The long, tedious, manual process of transplanting one graft at a time could be facilitated by the invention of a number of devices. An "auto-tissue dissector" would take a single block of hair-bearing tissue and, with proper programming, automatically laser-dissect it into the desired number and size of micrografts. Recipient slits could be perfectly crafted by a "smart" laser incisor programmed to miss existing hair follicles and to space the desired number and size of microslits exactly. An automatic

114 Instrumentation

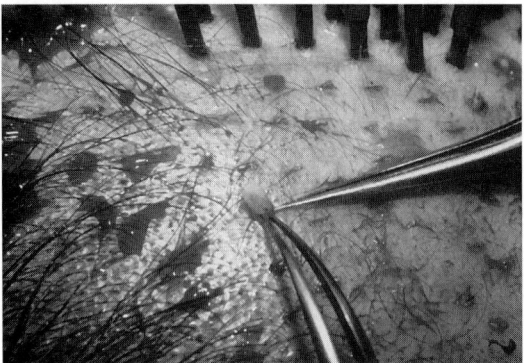

FIG. 4-8 Implantation of a single-hair graft along the hairline using curved and straight jeweler's forceps. Note that the graft is grasped on the fat pad beneath the hair follicle.

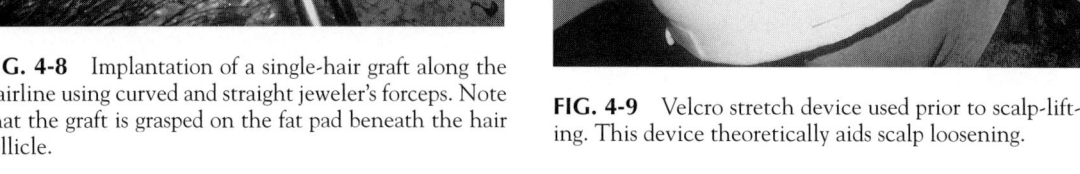

FIG. 4-9 Velcro stretch device used prior to scalp-lifting. This device theoretically aids scalp loosening.

implantation device could insert perfect grafts into these slits, closely approximating the appearance of normal human scalp hair. Finally, hair follicle cloning may someday be accomplished by automatic dissection and incubation devices in tissue culture.

INSTRUMENTATION FOR SCALP REDUCTION AND SCALP-LIFTING
Preparation for Surgery

The loosening effect of scalp massage, although often performed manually by the patient, can be facilitated considerably by a Velcro scalp stretch device worn for 30 to 60 minutes a day by the patient and retightened every 2 to 3 minutes during this time (Fig. 4-9).

Prior occipital artery ligation greatly decreases the risk of necrosis and bleeding during extensive scalp-lifting. A Weitlaner retractor, inserted into the vertical slit over each occipital artery, affords optimal exposure for this preparatory procedure (Fig. 4-10).

A handheld Doppler device is essential for accurate assessment of the location and course of both temporal and occipital arteries (Fig. 4-11). In addition, a high-quality fiberoptic headlamp is a must for distant undermining of large flaps, especially in vascular portions of the scalp.

Anesthesia and Hemostasis

Scalp reduction is often performed with the patient under local anesthesia with oral or intramuscular sedation. In contrast, intravenous sedation may be chosen during the longer, more extensive scalp-lifting procedures. For such procedures there should be complete patient monitoring with intravenous line, pulse oximeter, and cardiac and blood pressure

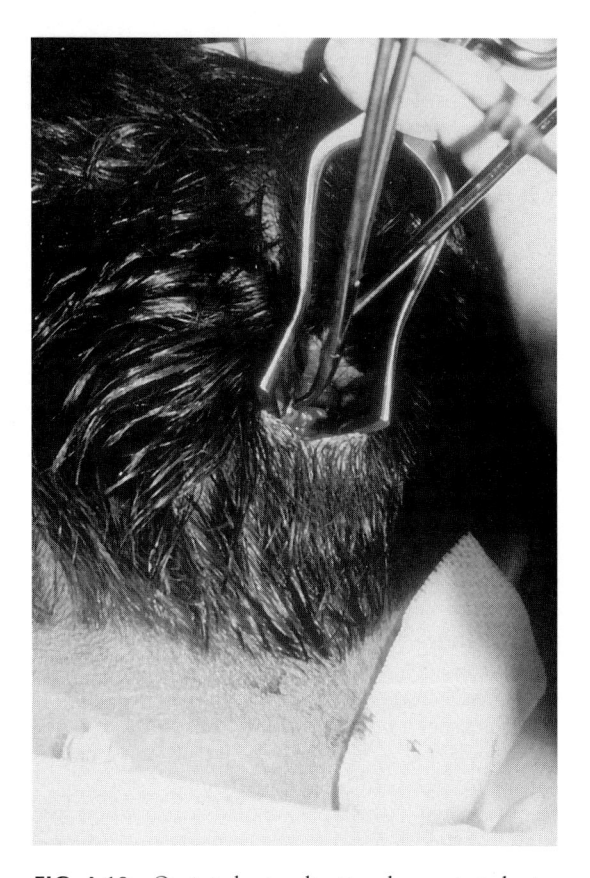

FIG. 4-10 Occipital artery ligation demonstrated using Weitlaner retractor and grounded electrosurgical device with hemostat to grasp occipital vessels.

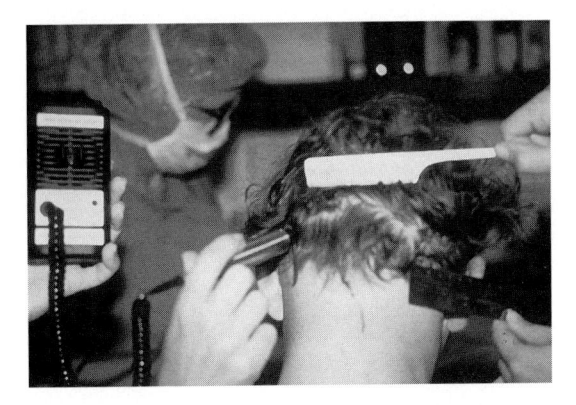

FIG. 4-11 Determining the exact location of the occipital artery with a handheld Doppler device.

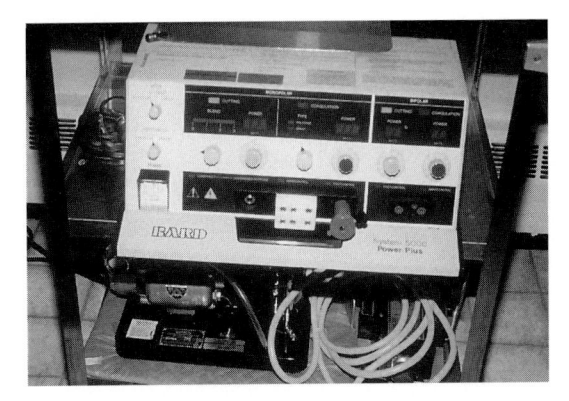

FIG. 4-13 Bard 5000 electrosurgical unit with suction device underneath.

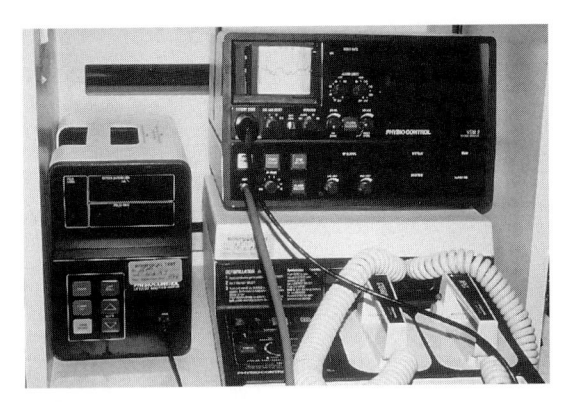

FIG. 4-12 Cardiac monitor, blood pressure monitor, pulse oximeter, and defibrillator are ready for each procedure.

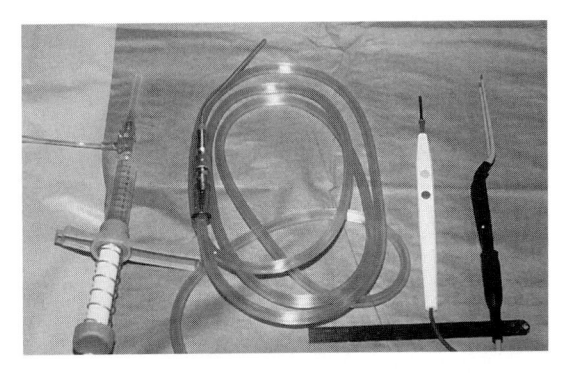

FIG. 4-14 *Left to right:* McGhan tissue expander fill kit, French suction, pen-tip cautery unit for cutting through occipitalis muscle, and custom-designed monopolar finger-switch bayonet forceps.

monitors (Fig. 4-12). In addition, the nurse anesthetist may use intravenous pump infusion devices for propofol or similar drugs.

Once a ring block has been performed prior to scalp-lifting, the McGhan tissue expander fill kit can be used to infiltrate the vascular area inferior to the nuchal ridge with tumescent solution. A good suction device, attached to either a suction retractor or a hollow suction electrocoagulation device, is a must. The surgeon must be prepared to control significant bleeding during scalp surgery. A powerful electrocoagulation machine, such as a Bard 5000 or Valleylab generator, capable of supplying cutting current, coagulation current, or a blend thereof is certainly preferable (Fig. 4-13). A "hot scalpel" affords hemostasis but may induce scarring if used near the cutaneous surface.

I use a custom-designed monopolar fingerswitch bayonet forceps electrocoagulation device for scalp-lifting. The teeth at the end aid in gripping distant vessels; current is initiated by pressure on the center of the device, bringing the contact tips together and sending current through the teeth without the need for a footswitch. Bipolar current is generally too weak for larger scalp operations (Fig. 4-14).

The newer argon beam coagulators offer great promise for extensive scalp-lifting. With these devices, first a pressurized beam of argon gas clears the operative field; the electric current then travels down the "beam" of gas to provide rapid hemostasis (Fig. 4-15).

Surgical Instruments

Incisions are generally created with a No. 10 surgical blade (such as a Personna blade) but could of course be effected with a carbon dioxide laser set at a fine cutting mode. Once the initial incisions have been made, the galea can be undermined with scissors or another blunt instrument. Blunt and sharp dissection beyond the nuchal ridge, however, is best

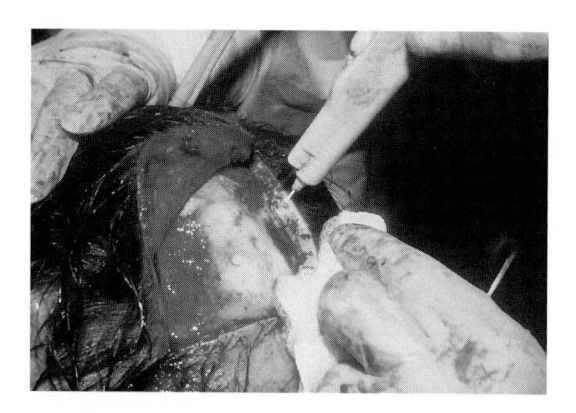

FIG. 4-15 Use of argon beam coagulator during a scalp-lifting procedure.

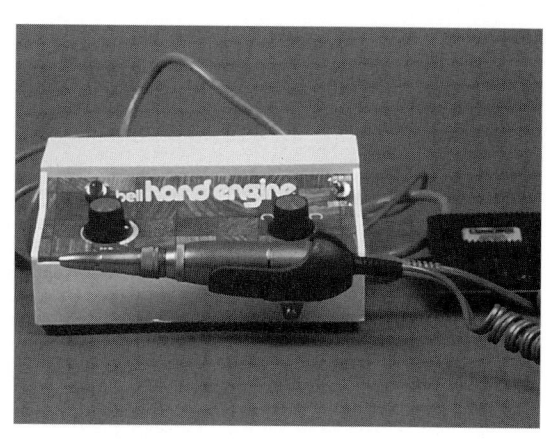

FIG. 4-18 Bell hand engine. This device is useful for creating small recipient sites. Its use for donor harvesting has been replaced with strip harvesting techniques. (Courtesy Dr. Dow Stough.)

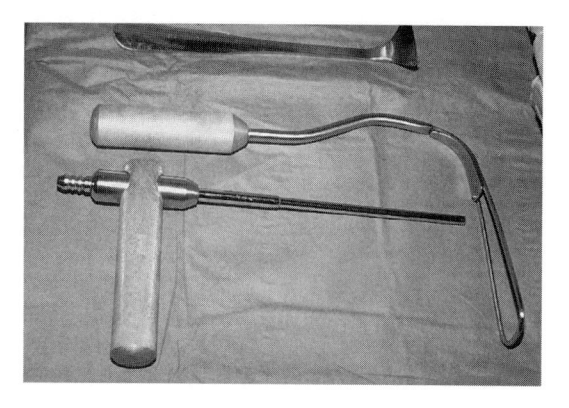

FIG. 4-16 *Top to bottom:* Special device used for implantation and removal of Frechet extender, skeleton retractor, suction retractor.

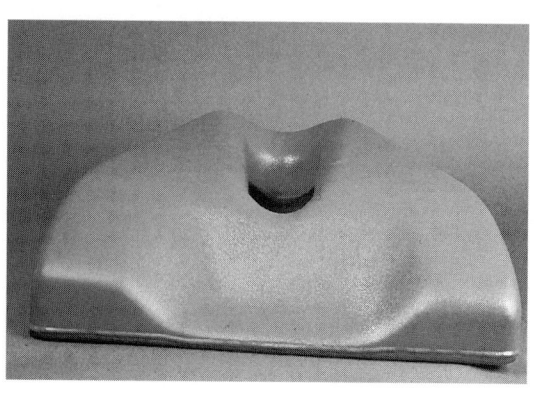

FIG. 4-19 Prōn Pillō (Robbins Instruments, Inc., Chatham, N.J.). (Courtesy Dr. Dow Stough.)

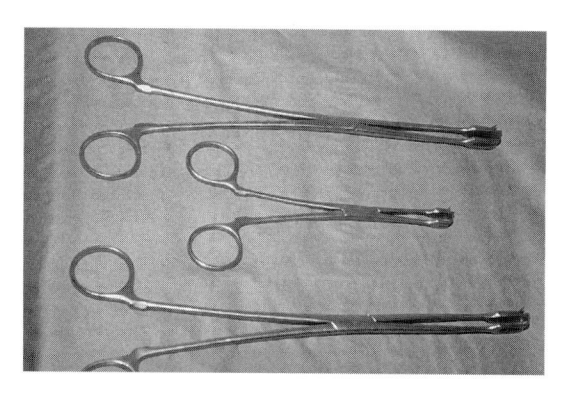

FIG. 4-17 Three different D'Assumpcao retractors used during scalp-lift advancement.

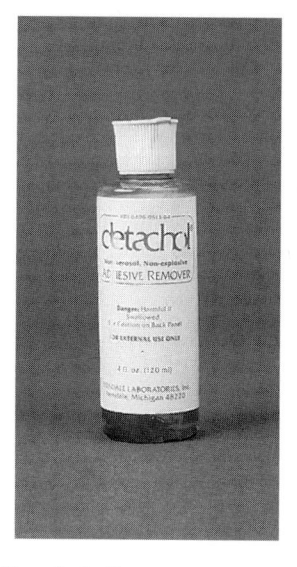

FIG. 4-20 Detachol adhesive remover (Ferndale Laboratories, Ferndale, Mich.), which is helpful in achieving painless removal of adhesive bandage tape. (Courtesy Dr. Dow Stough.)

performed by supercut scissors; long, narrow face-lift scissors can be used in the postauricular region. Heavy-gauge Mayo scissors are excellent for excising excess bald scalp. Cutting current, often guided between hemostats, provides hemostasis while the occipitalis muscle is transected.

A custom-designed skeleton retractor aids in flap retraction while simultaneously providing visualization during the electrocoagulation of bleeding vessels. The surgeon can improve visualization of the surgical field by using a suction retractor held in the nondominant hand while dissection is carried out with the scissors (Fig. 4-16). Flap advancement is exactingly accomplished with a D'Assumpcao retractor (also used in face-lift surgery) (Fig. 4-17). With this device, the overlap can be precisely measured at each part of the flap. Closure is achieved with suturing and/or stapling devices as described earlier.

The reader can contact the manufacturers listed in Appendix B for further information on product usage, safety, and design and should observe these devices in an actual operation performed by an experienced surgeon before trying these instruments. It is hoped that the reader will be stimulated to add to existing knowledge by developing further advances in instrumentation technology for hair transplantation and scalp-lifting (Fig. 4-18 to 4-22).

B. The Multibladed Knife for Donor Harvesting

Emil Bisaccia and Dwight A. Scarborough

The art of hair transplantation has continued to develop, allowing correction with an enhanced outcome. In light of the fact that the patient's hair continues to thin because of the relentless advancement of hair loss, the conservation of the donor site hair ultimately dictates the limits achievable by hair transplantation.[1] Recently introduced graft harvesting instrumentation has redefined the standard approach to hair transplantation planning and has led to more latitude in terms of the harvesting of donor grafts and the use of the donor hair. This discussion presents a brief history of the multibladed knife and the various harvesting approaches with the options they afford.

HISTORY

In 1968, Vallis[2,3] was the first to report strip harvesting of donor hair with the use of a double-bladed knife. He described the results of a strip method of harvesting and graft transplantation in 15 patients who underwent surgery for a receding hairline during a 2-year period. This incisional strip of donor hair was placed into a thin slit along the frontal hairline. In 1976, Coiffman[4] described a double-bladed knife in the Central American literature and then in the U.S. literature.[5] Coiffman introduced a parallel scalpel to harvest tissue and a four-sided blade that he used to cut recipient sites to receive square grafts.

We introduced the triple-bladed knife for donor harvesting in 1990[6] and reported additional applications in 1991 and 1994.[7-9] These applications included the harvesting of donor plugs of varied sizes for minigrafting and micrografting. We currently use the Tiemann multibladed instrument (Hauppage, N.Y.) and have abandoned the use of the

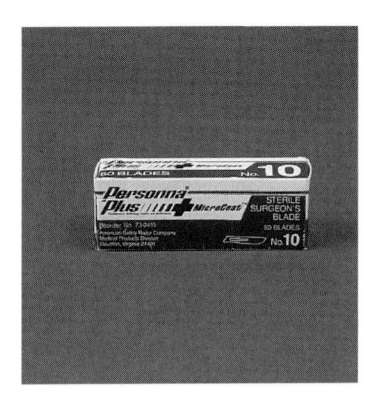

FIG. 4-21 Personna Plus blades. These blades are favored by many hair restoration surgeons because of their superior cutting ability. (Courtesy Dr. Dow Stough.)

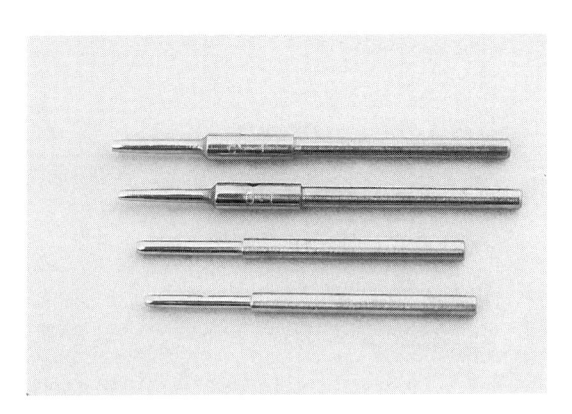

FIG. 4-22 Hair transplantation trephines. *Top*, 1 mm and 1.25 mm punches (Benn Instruments Pty. Ltd., Australia). *Bottom*, 1 mm and 1.25 mm punches (George Tiemann & Co., Hauppage, N.Y.). Motor-driven trephines are superior to handheld punches for large sessions of total micrografting.

hand engine for punch harvesting. The Tiemann handle allows the surgeon to convert the instrument into a two-, three-, or four-bladed knife (Fig. 4-23). It also allows for different-sized spacers, which can vary the size of the cut of the donor grafts from 1 to 5 mm in width in 0.25 mm increments. The Universal blade handle is a three- or four-bladed scalpel handle that allows the blades to be either staggered or set in a straight configuration. We favor the blades staggered for harvesting and straight for sectioning of the donor tissue. Depending on the procedure plan, we generally use 1 to 4 mm spacer sizes. With respect to scalpel blades, our choice of blades is the Personna blade.

Variations of the multibladed knife have also been introduced. In 1992, Brandy modified the triple-bladed knife (Robbins Instruments, Inc., Chatham, N.J.) by introducing an angulation to the blades (Fig. 4-24). The angulation of the blades was intended to minimize cutting off hair follicles while obtaining donor tissue. Brandy[10] nicely detailed the use of the multibladed knife and the strip-minigrafting technique. Stough[11] and Straub[12] also each introduced a triple-bladed knife. Straub worked with the Brandy instrument and concluded that a 30-degree angulation of the blade was the best angle to minimize transecting of a hair follicle during harvesting. The Brandy multibladed knife is available with a 30-degree canted angle or with a 20-degree canted angle. Stough designed the Van Sickle triple-bladed knife (Van Sickle, Bedford, Tex.)(Fig. 4-25) and favors this knife because he believes the blades do not move when pressure is exerted on them. They remain stable during the incision, and the staggered blades result in a more even plane with less transection. The Van Sickle knife also has variable-sized spacers and is made of cast aluminum as opposed to the stainless steel blades offered by Robbins Instruments, Inc., and George Tiemann & Co.

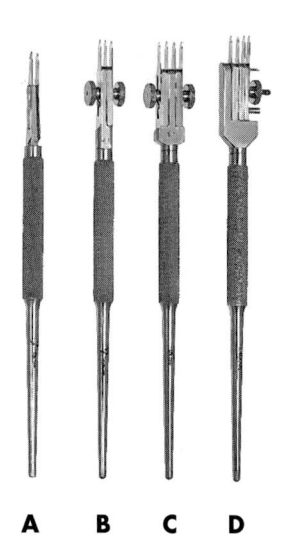

FIG. 4-23 Multibladed knife handle with two, three, and four blades. **A,** Double-bladed scalpel handle allows the surgeon to obtain a single strip. It is available in sizes 2 to 5 mm in 0.25 mm increments and is great for cutting plugs out of the strip. The blades are preset and not staggered. **B,** Triple-bladed scalpel handle is designed to harvest two strips with one cut. It is available in sizes 2 mm to 5 mm in 0.25 mm increments. The handle allows the surgeon to stagger the blades in either direction or to set them straight. One spacer is preset and permanently attached to the handle. However, different-sized spacers are available to create different-sized strip widths. **C,** Four-bladed scalpel handle is similar to the triple-bladed scalpel handle, except it allows the surgeon to obtain three strips with only one cut. **D,** Universal multibladed handle allows the surgeon to make the handle a two-, three-, or four-bladed handle and vary the space size as needed. Unlike the other handles, there is no preset spacer attached. It is available in sizes from 1 to 5 mm in 0.25 mm increments. (Courtesy George Tiemann & Co., Hauppage, N.Y.)

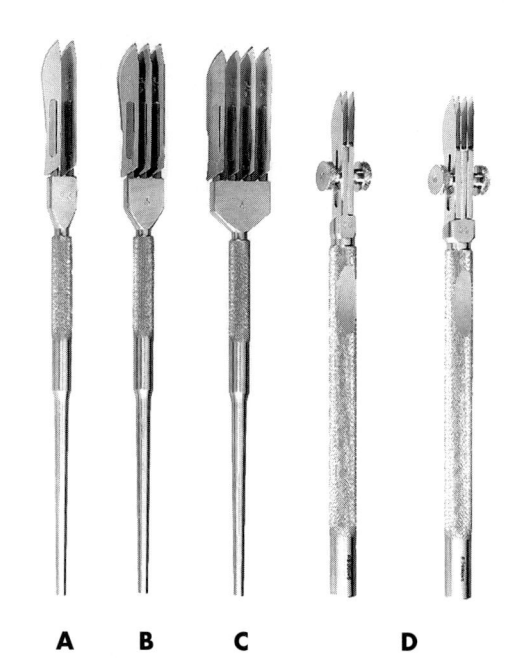

FIG. 4-24 Multibladed knife. **A,** Brandy double-bladed scalpel handle cuts one strip. It is available in 3 mm, 4 mm, and 5 mm widths with a straight or staggered blade configuration. **B,** Brandy triple-bladed scalpel handle cuts two strips. It is available in 3 mm and 4 mm widths with a straight or staggered blade configuration. **C,** Brandy quadruple-bladed scalpel handle cuts three strips. **D,** It is available in 3 mm and 4 mm widths with a straight or staggered beveled blade configuration. (Courtesy Robbins Instruments, Inc., Chatham, N.J.)

The appearance of these various multibladed knives details the 1990s as the decade in which the knife came into its own. There are a number of distinct advantages of the multibladed surgical instrument, which appear to ensure a place for this instrument in the diverse armamentarium of the hair transplant surgeon.

USE FOR HARVESTING DONOR TISSUE

Harvesting with the multibladed knife begins with achieving adequate initial anesthesia in the donor area. We use a variation of the tumescent technique at the donor site.[7,13] This technique enhances the skin turgor, thereby facilitating the incision and removal of donor tissue (Fig. 4-26). In addition, it expands the subcutaneous plane, which essentially creates an additional buffer area, distancing the base of the hair follicle from the underlying occipital arteries and their arborizing arterial branches. In addition, the dilute solution of lidocaine and epinephrine helps in achieving hemostasis with incision.

The correct depth of the incision made with the multibladed instrument is to just below the hair bulb, approximately 6 to 8 mm. A depth guard is available, which can be attached directly to the instrument and may help to prevent an inordinately deep incision. To initiate the incision, the multibladed instrument is inserted in the donor area at an angle parallel to the angle of hair growth. The actual cutting is performed with a slow, sawlike linear motion until the appropriate length is reached (Fig. 4-27). The removal of this incised strip requires direct visualization with careful attention to the location of hair bulb (Fig. 4-28). The edge of the incision is cut first with a scalpel placed along hair root growth to separate the tissue from its lateral attachment. Following this, a Metzenbaum scissors is used to advance the separation by releasing the donor tissue from its base attachment.

Once removal of the strip is complete, the donor tissue is transferred to a petri dish well moistened with saline solution (Fig. 4-29). The donor site is inspected for hemostasis. Once hemostasis is obtained, the site is partially closed with a skin stapler, leaving one end of the incision open until all grafts are placed. This partial closure allows for obtaining additional grafts, which may be needed to complete the procedure.

The harvested strips are then cut with a single- or double-bladed instrument into a variety of geometric forms, including strips, plugs, slits, mini-

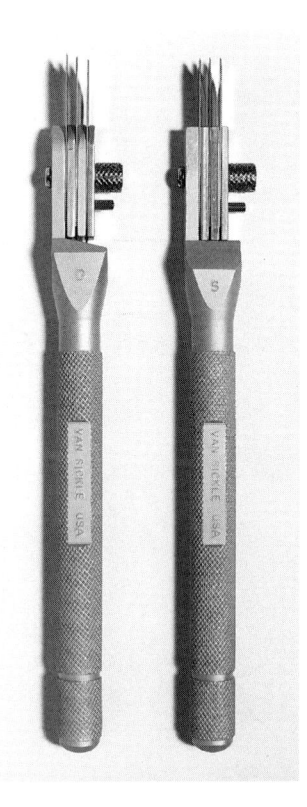

FIG. 4-25 Multibladed knife with interchangeable spacer size. Both straight and staggered blade configurations are available. (Courtesy Van Sickle, Bedford, Tex.)

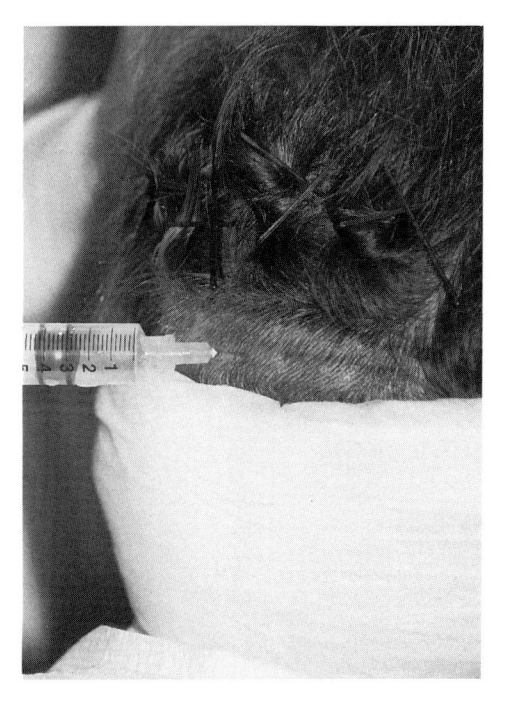

FIG. 4-26 Hair has been trimmed to accommodate the excision of multistrip donor hair. Tumescent anesthesia is now being performed. (From Unger WP: *Hair transplantation*, ed 3, New York, 1995, Marcel Dekker.)

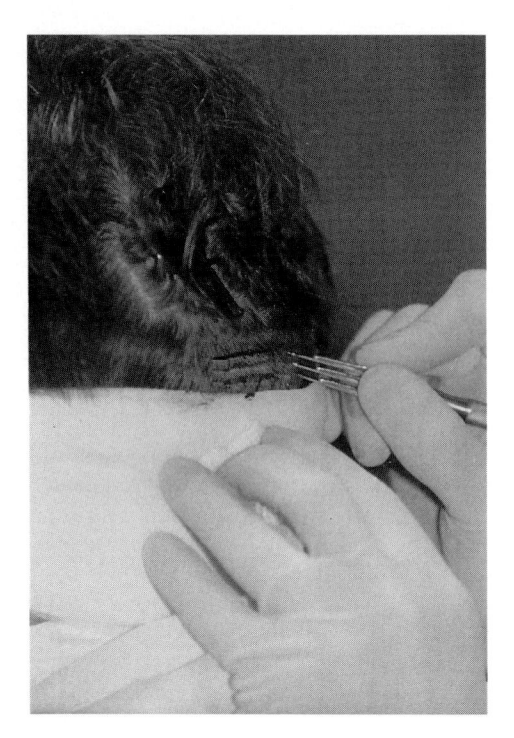

FIG. 4-27 Actual donor site cutting is performed in a slow motion until the appropriate length is reached. (From Unger WP: *Hair transplantation*, ed 3, New York, 1995, Marcel Dekker.)

grafts, and micrografts of appropriate size.[8] Several cutting surfaces have been successfully used. We favor a 4 × 4 inch gauze pad that is well moistened with saline solution and is opened across a sterile metal surgical tray; wooden and rubber or plastic surfaces have also been used. The trimming of the donor strips, depending on their size, may require the use of a lighted magnifying loupe. The sectioning of the harvested strips involves the continuation of transverse cuts over the length of the harvested strips; any variations in size and shape required by the planned procedure can be obtained by simply changing the width of the cross-cuts (Figs. 4-30 and 4-31).

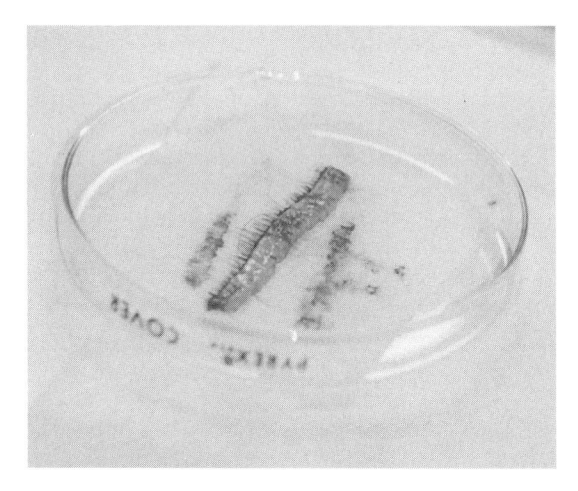

FIG. 4-29 Donor tissue is transferred to a petri dish well moistened with saline solution. (From Unger WP: *Hair transplantation*, ed 3, New York, 1995, Marcel Dekker.)

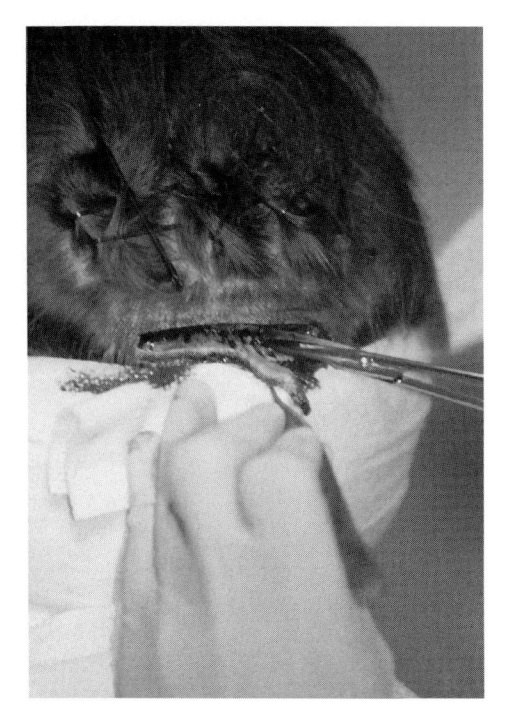

FIG. 4-28 Removal of the incised strip requires direct visualization with careful attention to the location of the hair bulb. (From Unger WP: *Hair transplantation*, ed 3, New York, 1995, Marcel Dekker.)

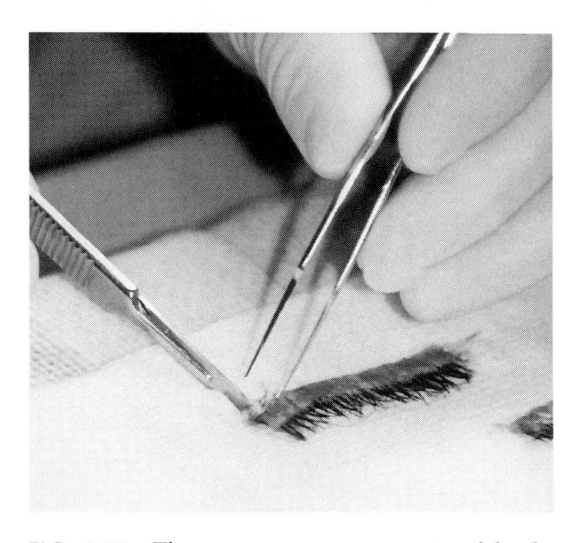

FIG. 4-30 The transverse cuts are continued for the length of the strips, and variations in size and shape can be obtained by simply changing the width of the cross-cuts. (From Unger WP: *Hair transplantation*, ed 3, New York, 1995, Marcel Dekker.)

To maintain effective sectioning, a generous supply of scalpel blades is required. There are various blades (No. 15, 10, or 11 Personna, Beaver, or standard) available for use depending on the surgeon's preference, and the blades must be changed frequently at the slightest sign of dullness.

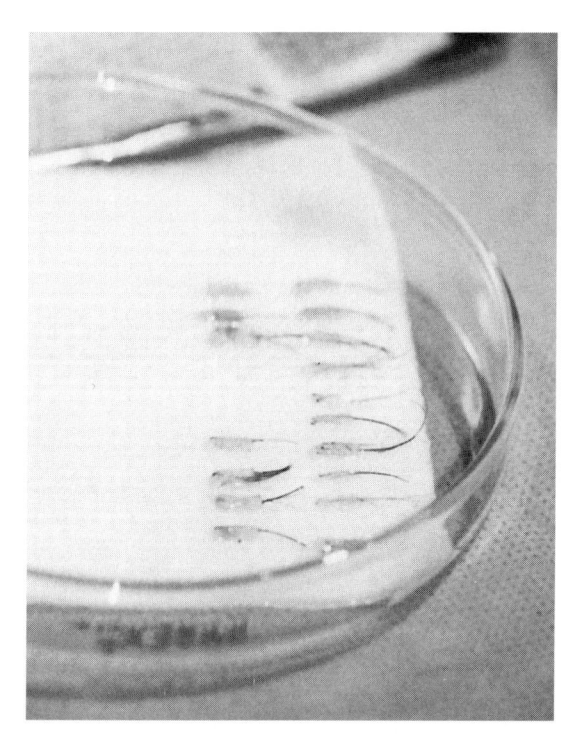

FIG. 4-31 Single-, two-, and three-hair micrografts produced after sectioning. (From Unger WP: *Hair transplantation*, ed 3, New York, 1995, Marcel Dekker.)

After all the strips have been harvested and donor sites have been transplanted, the remainder of the donor site incision is closed. While the staples are in place, they are well hidden by existing hair; the staples are removed about 10 days following surgery. The scar created by this procedure can be removed with the next procedure, ultimately resulting in one linear scar posteriorly after multiple harvesting procedures. The technique of linear scar harvesting is illustrated in Chapter 5, Part A.

CONCLUSION

Incisional harvesting not only allows the donor site to be closed transversely but also facilitates the harvesting of grafts of various sizes and shapes for a particular procedure or a series of procedures. The advantages of this approach appear to be many, including shortened procedure time, fewer hair follicles destroyed in harvesting the strips, enhanced donor site use with the elimination of "dead space" between procedures, variation in graft sizes available during a single procedure, avoidance of dull punches, elimination of the aerosol spray of blood that can occur with the use of the power punch, less time trimming or removing cut hairs, and the customizing of grafts for a better "fit" and overall result.[12]

The disadvantage of the multibladed knife is that it requires a level of developed skill that is not automatically present in a surgeon skilled with only the round punch. This is especially true with regard to the angulation of the blade for graft harvesting, production of consistent graft size, and development of a standardized systematic method to cutting the strips.[12]

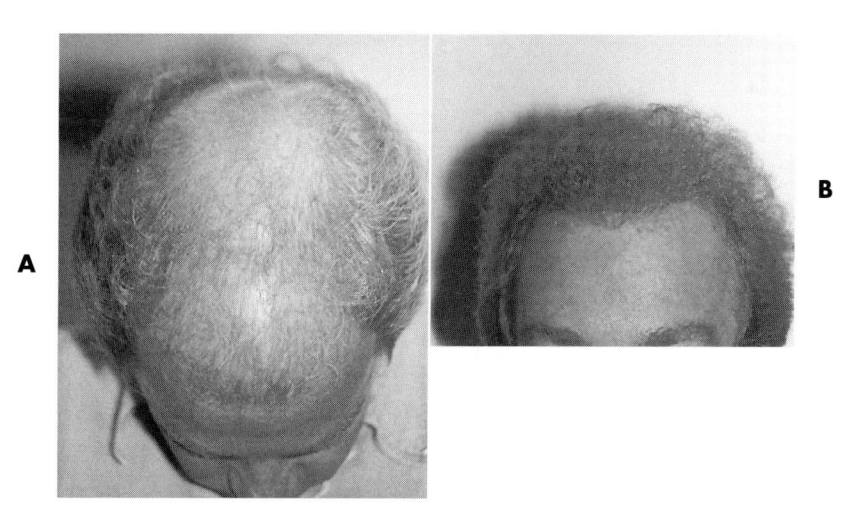

FIG. 4-32 A, Preoperative view. **B,** Postoperative view following donor site harvest with the multibladed knife and hair transplantation.

ADVANTAGES OF THE MULTIBLADED KNIFE FOR DONOR HARVESTING
1. Shortened procedure time
2. Facilitation of the harvest of grafts of varied sizes and shapes
3. Harvest of very clean strips with minimal follicular transection
4. Enhanced donor site use
5. Avoidance of dull punches
6. Elimination of aerosol spray of blood produced during rotary punch harvesting
7. Precise customizing of graft size
8. Less time trimming or removing cut hairs

The demand for better results in hair transplantation has driven the further refinement in technique. The creative use of combinations of geometric-shaped grafts harvested with the multibladed knife allows for natural hairline feathering, a gradient of increasing density, minimal visible scarring, and ultimately an aesthetically pleasing hair restoration customized to each patient[8-10] (Fig. 4-32). The multibladed knife has supported the contemporary refinements in restorative surgery of the scalp (see box).

REFERENCES

1. Norwood O: Single row donor site harvesting, *J Dermatol Surg Oncol* 16:5, 1990.
2. Vallis CP: Surgical treatment of the receding hairline, *Plast Reconstr Surg* 33:247, 1968.
3. Vallis CP: Surgical treatment of the receding hairline, *Plast Reconstr Surg* 44:271-278, 1969.
4. Coiffman F: Injertos cuadrados de cuero cabelludo. Presented at the First Iberoamerican Congress of Plastic Surgery, Quito, Ecuador, 1976.
5. Coiffman F: Use of square scalp grafts for male pattern baldness, *Plast Reconstr Surg* 60:228-232, 1977.
6. Bisaccia E, Scarborough D: A technique for square plug hair transplantation, *Am J Cosmet Surg* 7(4):219-222, 1990.
7. Scarborough D, Bisaccia E: Square-graft hair transplantation: an aesthetic surgical correction for baldness, *Cosmet Dermatol* 4:10-13, 1991.
8. Bisaccia E, Scarborough D: Hair transplant by incisional strip harvesting, *J Dermatol Surg Oncol* 20:443-448, 1994.
9. Bisaccia E, Scarborough D: Geometric-square hair transplant. In Unger WP, editor: *Hair Transplantation*, ed 3, New York, 1995, Marcel Dekker, pp 485-497.
10. Brandy D: A new instrument for the expedient production of minigrafts, *J Dermatol Surg Oncol* 18:478-472, 1992.
11. Stough DB: Hair transplantation by the feathering zone technique: new tools of the nineties, *Am J Cosmet Surg* 10:243-248, 1993.
12. Straub P: Graft harvesting: a third generation, *Hair Transplant Forum* 2(4):2-4, 1990.
13. Coleman W, Klein J: Use of tumescence technique for scalp surgery, dermabrasion and soft tissue reconstruction, *J Dermatol Surg Oncol* 18:130-135, 1992.

C. NoKor Microslit Grafting Technique

Michael A. Meshkin

HISTORY

The first attempt to accomplish refinement of a hairline with small grafts was reported by Nordstrom[1] in 1981. He described a technique in which the surgeon initially made multiple incisions with a No. 15 Bard-Parker blade immediately anterior to the hairline and subsequently placed grafts of three to six hairs into these slits. In 1984, Marritt[2] popularized the use of even smaller single- and two-hair grafts. A few years later, he introduced the concept of using dilators, which he proposed would widen the recipient sites, create hemostasis, and help to organize the procedures.[3] Marritt recommended making an incision with a 20- or 18-gauge hypodermic needle, briefly inserting a dilator, removing the dilator, and finally placing the micrograft. Since the publication of these initial articles, several other techniques,[4,5] including the use of 1.5 mm punches[6] and No. 11 blades,[7] have been reported. In 1991, I developed the NoKor microslit grafting technique, which is simple and time efficient and obviates the need for dilators. A review of the NoKor technique was published by Brandy and Meshkin[8] in 1994.

Special needles, called NoKor needles, are used with this grafting technique (Fig. 4-33). These needles are available from Becton-Dickinson and Co. (Rutherford, N.J.) and come in two sizes: 16 and 18 gauge. There is a small lancet-shaped blade at the distal tip of these cutting instruments. Early experience with these needles demonstrated that they possessed several distinct advantages over hypodermic needles. When NoKor needles were inserted into the rubber stoppers of medication bottles, they were superior to hypodermic needles in the following ways:

1. They required less force to penetrate the rubber stoppers.

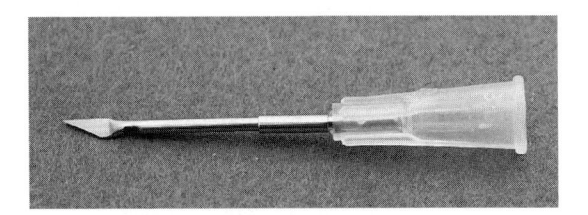

FIG. 4-33 The NoKor needle is available in both 16- and 18-gauge sizes. Note the lancet-shaped blade at the distal tip of this instrument.

2. They did not get clogged by any residual remnants of rubber.
3. They did not "core out" the stoppers.
4. They did not leave puncture holes in the surface of the rubber stoppers.

In view of these exceptional features, I hypothesized that the NoKor needle would make an ideal tool for microslit grafting.

TECHNIQUE

The 16- and 18-gauge NoKor needles may be used with or without a handle. There are two types of handles available: the Meshkin NoKor handle (Robbins Instruments, Inc., Chattam, N.J.) and the Van Sickle NoKor needle handle (Van Sickle, Bedford, Tex.) (Fig. 4-34). Personal preference will dictate the surgeon's choice. It is crucial to position the NoKor needle at 90 degrees relative to the plane of the scalp. After the needle has penetrated the scalp, a deep, 45-degree back-cut is made (Fig. 4-35). This incision opens up a pocket, which greatly enhances the surgeon's ability to place the micrografts very close together (1 to 2 mm), thereby minimizing dead space and popping problems (Fig. 4-36). Not all surgeons advocate a back-cut. Routinely, we use 18-gauge needles to place single-hair grafts in the first one or two rows of the hairline and 16-gauge needles to place grafts of two or three hairs immediately behind the hairline (Fig. 4-36). A single needle can be used in a sequential nonstop fashion to prepare up to 500 microslit stabs. However, dullness may occur after making as few as 75 stab incisions, necessitating a change in needles.

The grafts are placed into the microslits using jeweler's forceps. It should be emphasized that the placement of grafts into these small slits requires a high degree of skill. For those with little experience in micrografting, it is advisable initially to perform the technique with a 16-gauge NoKor needle, which has a larger tip and allows easier placement of the grafts than the 18-gauge NoKor needle. With experience, the advantages of the 18-gauge needle become obvious. Namely, the smaller slits created with the 16-gauge needle allow for denser placement of grafts.

ADVANTAGES

1. NoKor needles, in contrast to hypodermic needles, do not "core out" an area of bald skin (see Fig. 4-36). Consequently, since the recipient skin receives less trauma, there is less likelihood of noticeable scarring and posttransplant epidermoid cyst formation (see Chapter 10, Part F). Theoretically, a better cosmetic result can be achieved (Fig. 4-37 and 4-38).

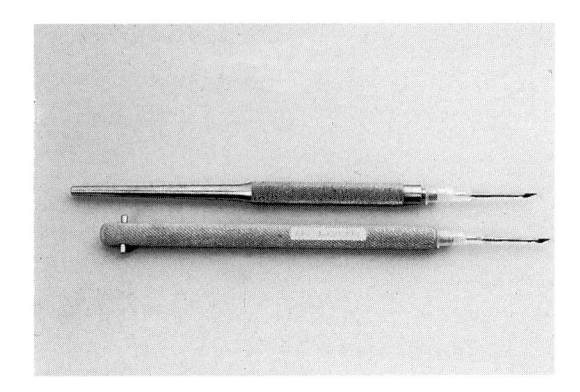

FIG. 4-34 The NoKor handle can improve control. There are two types of handles available: the Meshkin NoKor handle (Robbins Instruments, Inc., Chatham, N.J.) (*top*) and the Van Sickle needle handle (Van Sickle, Bedford, Tex.) (*bottom*).

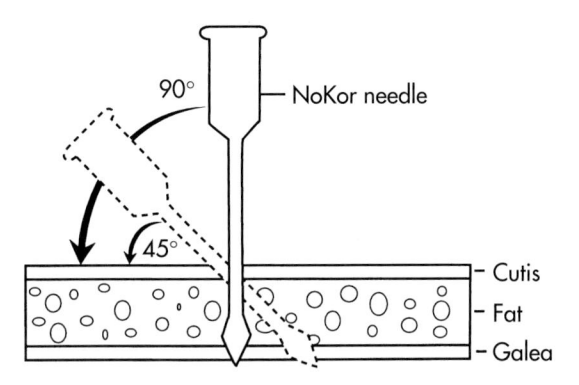

FIG. 4-35 NoKor penetration method. Note 45-degree back-cut following the penetration. (Courtesy Dr. Dominic Brandy.)

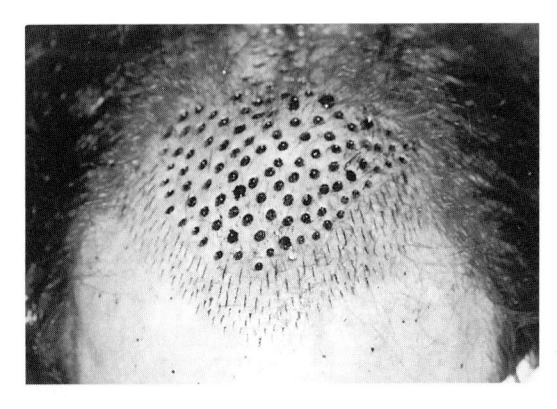

FIG. 4-36 Closeup view of slits made with 16- and 18-gauge NoKor needles. Note the lack of dead space and the reduced trauma.

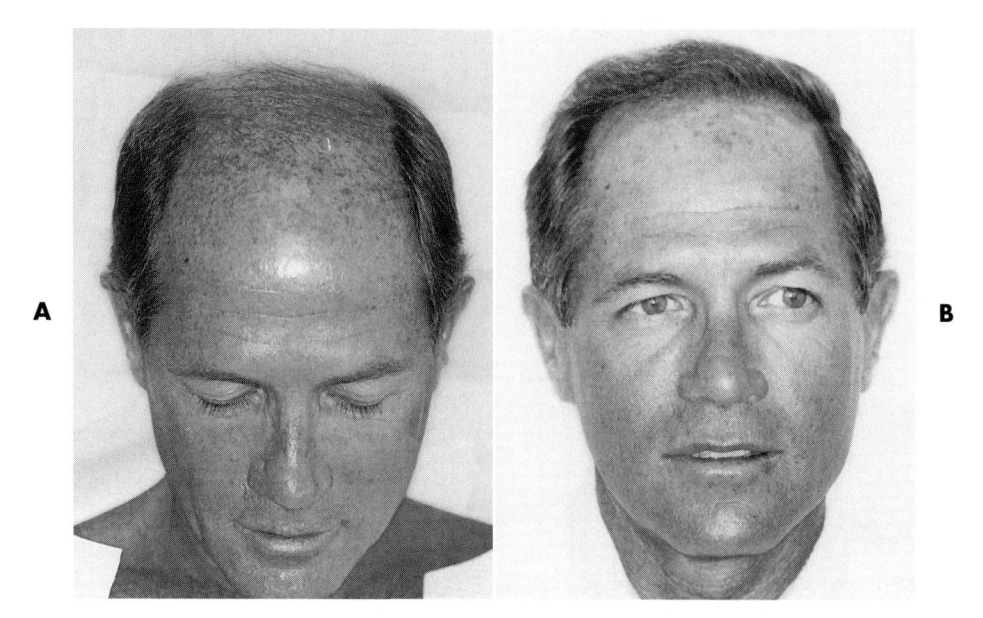

FIG. 4-37 **A,** Preoperative view of patient with frontal baldness. **B,** Postoperative view after completion of the hairline using microslit grafting. Single-hair micrografts were placed in the anterior hairline region, whereas minigrafts were placed posterior to the hairline.

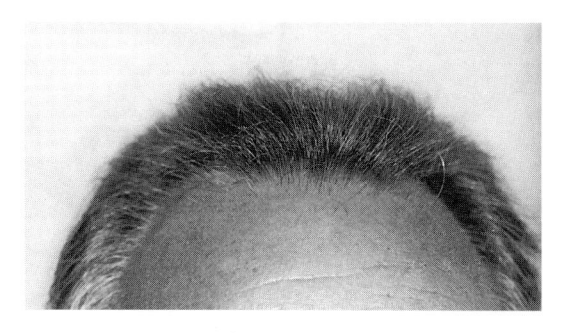

FIG. 4-38 Closeup view of hairline following two sessions of microslits and minigrafts. Note the lack of scarring around the microslit grafts.

2. The micrografts stay embedded in the NoKor needle slits more securely than they do in the puncture holes created by hypodermic needles regardless of whether or not dilators are used. Dilator techniques allow the micrografts to almost "swim" in the recipient sites. The NoKor needle slits, on the other hand, seem to grasp the micrografts and hold them in place.
3. Micrografts are more easily placed into NoKor needle microslits than they are into graft sites prepared by hypodermic needles with or without dilators. This is true even when the incisions are made 1 to 2 mm apart.
4. With the NoKor microslit grafting technique, surgeons can easily visualize the recipient field and control the placement of micrografts (see Fig. 4-36). In contrast, the presence of hundreds of dilators in the scalp at one time greatly interferes with the surgeon's ability to insert and visualize micrografts in and around the dilators.
5. The NoKor microslit grafting technique is more time efficient compared with the dilator technique. The NoKor method involves making a slit and inserting a micrograft. Conversely, the method of punching a hole with a hypodermic needle, inserting a dilator, taking the dilator out, then finally placing the micrograft, is time consuming.
6. The NoKor needle requires less force to penetrate the skin than a hypodermic needle because of its lancet-shaped tip.
7. A cleaner surgical field is maintained with the NoKor method than with the dilators, which are left in place for some time (see Fig. 4-36).
8. The NoKor needles are disposable and discarded after each use. Most dilators must be cleaned and resterilized after each use.
9. NoKor needles are less expensive than dilators.

DISADVANTAGES

1. Obtaining hemostasis may be a problem in a small number of slit sites. In these instances, bleeding can be controlled by applying direct pressure to the site or by placing dilators in the bleeding sites for a few seconds.

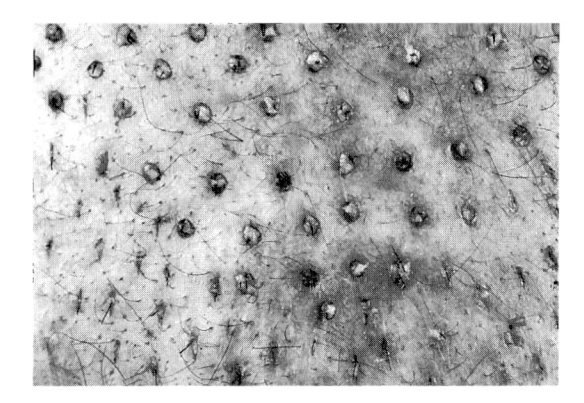

FIG. 4-39 Single-hair micrografts placed into holes (*top*) vs. single-hair micrografts placed in NoKor needle slits (*bottom*).

2. Graft popping may occur. To eliminate problems with graft retention, slit sites must be properly prepared by creating a pocket for the graft by back-cutting with the NoKor needle (see Fig. 4-35). A second way to eliminate graft popping is to ensure that the graft size is correctly matched with the size of the slit.

RESULTS

When the microslit grafting technique is properly performed, the NoKor needle creates a recipient site that is tailored to hold a single- or two-hair micrograft. The majority of micrografts will grow, and no disturbing scars are produced. This technique has been well received by surgeons and successfully used in clinical practice in well over 1000 cases. Whether single-hair micrografts perform better in growth and cosmesis in slits vs. 1 mm holes is unknown (Fig. 4-39).

CONCLUSION

Each microslit should contain no more than three hairs in order to avoid an unnatural tuftlike effect. Ideally grafts of only one or two hairs should be used. The angle of the graft placement is crucial. Slight irregularity of the placement of micrografts mimics the normal irregularity of the hairline.[9]

NoKor needles can provide invaluable benefits in the field of micrografting for surgeons who use dilators as well as for those who do not. The NoKor microslit grafting technique may be effectively used in patients who have scarring alopecia and female pattern baldness.

Similarly, patients who require eyebrow or eyelash transplants, post-scalp reduction scar coverage, and all forms of single-hair graft transplantation are ideal candidates for this procedure. This method also can be used for hairline refinement in patients who have had scalp flaps, punch grafts, or scarring following a forehead lift. In addition, because of the simplicity and efficiency of this technique, NoKor microslit grafting can be especially valuable for surgeons who perform large graft sessions with 200 to 1000 grafts per session.

REFERENCES

1. Nordstrom RE: "Micrografts" for improvement of the frontal hairline after hair transplantation, *Aesthetic Plast Surg* 5:97, 1981.
2. Marritt E: Single-hair transplantation for hairline refinement: a practical solution, *J Derm Surg Oncol* 10:962-963, 1984.
3. Marritt E: Micrograft dilators: in pursuit of the undetectable hairline, *J Derm Surg Oncol* 14:268-275, 1988.
4. Nelson BR and others: Hair transplantation in advanced male pattern alopecia, *J Derm Surg Oncol* 17:567-573, 1991.
5. Norwood O, Sheil RC: Micrografts and minigrafts. In *Hair transplant surgery,* ed 2, Springfield, Ill., 1984, Charles C Thomas.
6. Frechet P: Micro and mini hair grafting using the standard hair implantation procedure, *J Derm Surg Oncol* 15:533-536, 1989.
7. Uebel CO: Micrografts and minigrafts: a new approach for baldness surgery, *Ann Plast Surg* 27:476-487, 1991.
8. Brandy DA, Meshkin M: Utilization of NoKor needles for slit-micrografting, *J Derm Surg Oncol* 20:336-339, 1994.
9. Stough DB: The feathering zone technique: new tools for the nineties, *Am J Cosmet Surg* 9(3):242-248, 1992.

D. Single-Hair and Bundled-Hair Transplantation Using the Choi Hair Transplanter

Yung-Chul Choi and Jung-Chul Kim

Scalp hairs consist of three groupings: a single hair, a bundle with two hairs, and a bundle with three hairs.[1] Only rarely will groups of four hairs emerge from a single follicle. We refer to each grouping as a *bundled hair* when two or three hairs have a common trichilemma or common orifice but separate trichilemma. Transplantation of single-hair and bundled-hair grafts can give a more natural appearance for male alopecia treatment and hairline refinement. However, single-hair transplantation is required for the eyebrows, eyelashes, beards, and pubic regions because only single hairs predominate in those areas.[2] For those areas, after the donor site is harvested, all two- and three-bundled hair groups should be divided into single hairs.

The occipital hair-bearing area to be harvested is outlined with an indelible pen, and the surrounding area is shaved. The hairs in the donor area are cut to 2 cm lengths. After the donor area is anesthetized, an elliptical incision is made. The strip is excised from the undersurface, and the wound is closed using pulley sutures.[3] The excised strip is placed on a block of birchwood and sectioned into smaller segments using a No. 20 scalpel blade, with careful positioning of the blade between the visible hair follicles. With the same blade, each segment is then cut again into single- or bundled-hair grafts. Fig. 4-40 shows isolated single hairs and two-hair bundles. Birchwood is so hard that it allows sectioning without creating wood fragments, which could induce foreign body reactions. Hair grafts are inserted onto the needle of the hair transplanter using jeweler's forceps. The hair grafts are placed into recipient sites using the disposable Choi hair transplanter (Fig. 4-41).

There are three types of disposable Choi hair transplanters for implanting single- or bundled-hair grafts: Type L (18-gauge needle) for implanting bundle-hair grafts, type M (20-gauge needle) for fine single-hair grafts, and type S (22-gauge needle) for fine single-hair grafts (Fig. 4-42). Types L and M are used for male pattern baldness treatment and hairline refinement, and type M is used for eyebrows, beards, and pubic hair reconstruction. Type S is used only for the reconstruction of eyelashes.

Fig. 4-43 demonstrates how the Choi hair transplanter works. First, a single- or bundled-hair graft is placed onto the needle of the hair transplanter. Next, the needle is inserted into the skin and the plunger is pushed. The needle is automatically withdrawn, leaving the hair graft neatly tucked under the skin because the ring around the needle holds the hair shaft in place while the needle is withdrawn.

In a 3-hour session, 1000 single- and bundled-hair grafts can be transplanted. A surgeon and three specially trained nurses are required to perform the procedure.

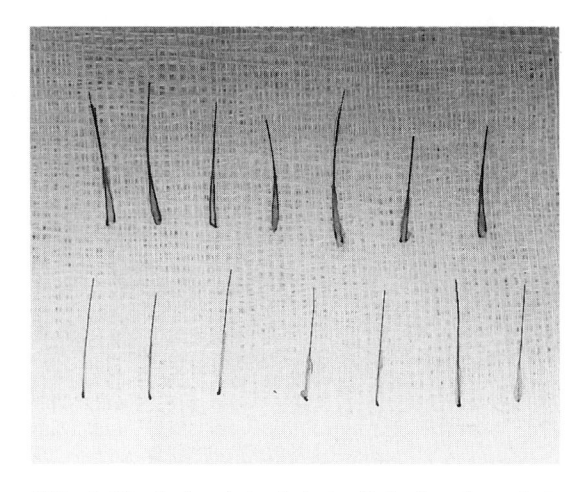

FIG. 4-40 Isolated single hairs (*below*) and two-hair bundles (*above*).

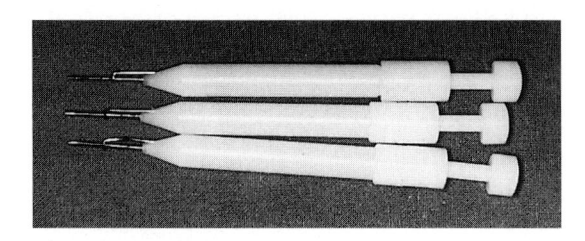

FIG. 4-41 Choi hair transplanter.

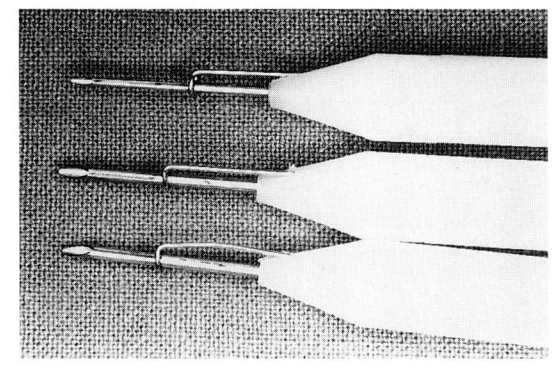

FIG. 4-42 Choi hair transplanters: type L (*bottom*), type M (*middle*), type S (*top*).

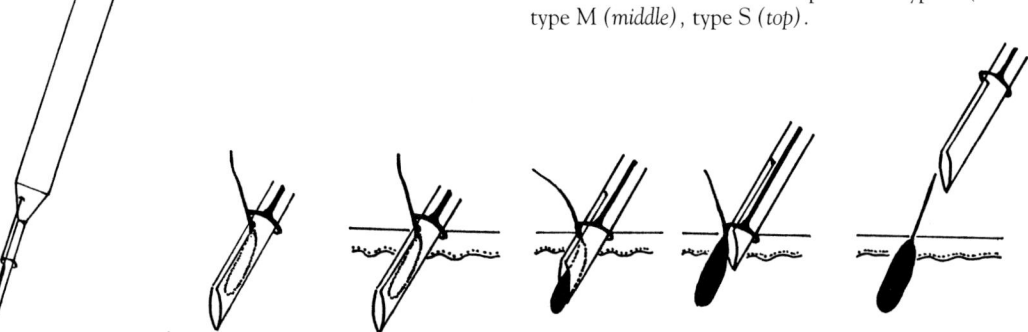

FIG. 4-43 Diagram showing how the Choi hair transplanter works.

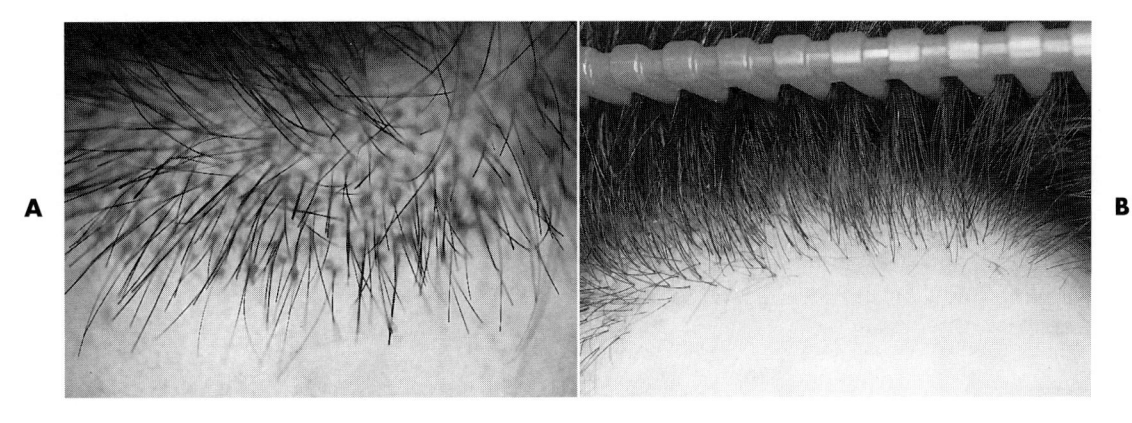

FIG. 4-44 Hairline refinement. **A,** Immediate postoperative view. **B,** One-year postoperative view.

The advantages of this method are (1) no scarring and tufting, (2) no cobblestoning, (3) minimal bleeding, and (4) natural hair direction (Fig. 4-44). Thus this technique can provide an aesthetic pattern of hair growth in hairline refinement, treatment of male pattern baldness, and reconstruction of eyebrows, eyelashes, beards, and pubic region.

REFERENCES

1. Ackerman AB and others: *Neoplasms with follicular differentiation*, Philadelphia, 1993, Lea & Febiger.
2. Choi Y-C, Kim J-C: Single hair transplantation using Choi hair transplanter, *J Dermatol Surg Oncol* 18:945-948, 1992.
3. Hitzig GS: Pulley suture, utilization in scalp reconstruction surgery, *J Dermatol Surg Oncol* 18:220-222, 1992.

Editor's Note

The technique using the Choi hair transplanter is much more effective with Asian (large-caliber) hair than fine-textured hair.

E. Retraction-Sectioning

Joseph Greco

A hair transplant surgeon can be highly skilled, meticulous, and conscientious, but the quality of the results will be directly proportional to the quality of grafts that his/her team is capable of producing.

Two of the most important stages in hair transplantation are harvesting and sectioning because follicular damage is greatest during these phases. Artistic design in graft placement is meaningless without quality grafts.

One of the primary reasons that strip harvesting with multibladed knives and elliptical harvesting

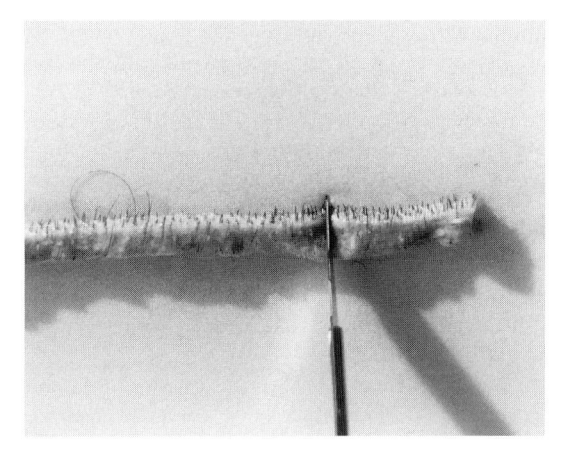

NOTE: The author has no proprietary interest in any of the instrumentation mentioned in this discussion.

FIG. 4-45 Tissue distortion occurs when scalpel pressure is applied to the donor strip without retraction of the tissue.

with a scalpel have replaced the punch method is that the incidence of tissue distortion and follicular transection is decreased during harvesting. Another advantage is reduced operative time during harvesting, thus allowing more grafts to be transplanted during a session.

Although reduced operative time and decreased tissue distortion and follicular transection have been achieved in donor site harvesting, the issues of follicular transection and tissue distortion must still be addressed in terms of graft sectioning. Although unproved, graft distortion and follicular transection seem to result from progressive scalpel pressure and the use of a firm, hard, cutting surface such as tongue blades (Fig. 4-45).

The cycle of scalpel pressure, which causes tissue distortion and thus causes follicular transection, must be eliminated to consistently achieve quality grafts.

Tension and elasticity are physical properties of fibers within the skin.[1] *Tension* accounts for the fact that the skin resists stretching by weak forces, whereas *elasticity* refers to the skin's ability to resume its original shape after external force has been applied to cause deformation.[1]

Applying tension to the skin and other tissue is a basic technique taught in surgery and is used every day. When tension is applied to tissue strips, the skin's physical properties are being used to allow more visibility of individual hair shafts for finer dissection. Thus retraction-sectioning is derived from this basic technique learned in surgery: traction-countertraction.

TECHNIQUE

With retraction-sectioning the strip or ellipse is placed on a 1 × 5 × 8 inch sterile, disposable, foam cutting block. Anchoring the tissue in the middle with a 27-gauge needle, the surgeon gently applies contralateral tension with fine tissue forceps, always grasping either the epidermal or subdermal layer. The elasticity of the tissue strip allows better visualization of individual hair shafts when tension is applied, thus reducing tissue distortion and decreasing follicular transection. With better visualization of the tissue, a precise cut is then made between the hair shafts with a scalpel, razor blade, electric knife, or other instrument. The box below lists the advantages and disadvantages of retraction-sectioning.

It is difficult to know if tissue distortion and follicular transection can ever be completely eliminated because of the human factor, but retraction-sectioning either manually or with the electric knife brings us closer toward that goal. In the final analysis, regardless of technique or instrumentation, the quality of grafts produced is directly proportional to the clinicians' skills.

THE MICRO-PEN (ELECTRIC KNIFE)

Over the past 30 years, hair transplantation has evolved from the traditional, large 4.5 mm punch grafts of the 1960s to the minigrafts of the 1970s to the single- to three-hair micrografts of today. During that time we have advanced from 50 grafts per session to 1000 or more grafts per session. Unfortunately, instrumentation has not kept pace with the techniques; in fact, some assistants are asked to section hundreds of grafts using 1960s vintage instrumentation.

The Electric Knife (Robbins Instruments, Inc., Chatham, N.J.) is the first generation of power instruments designed to section micrografts and minigrafts.[2] The components of the Electric Knife are the Bell hand engine, the Micro-Pen, the Greco blade adaptor, and the Greco cutting block (Fig. 4-46).

Many hair transplant surgeons already own a hand engine since it serves as the control box for the power handpiece used to harvest circular punch grafts. The Micro-Pen was originally designed as a micropigmentation instrument, but it converts to a reciprocating scalpel when attached to the Greco blade adapter. A No. 11 Personna Plus blade is suggested for sectioning because of its superior sharpness. The cutting block is a 1 × 5 × 8 inch double-packaged, gamma-sterilized, disposable foam cutting surface. The foam cutting block is necessary to reduce vibration when using the Electric Knife,

---

RETRACTION-SECTIONING

Advantages
1. Better visualization of individual hair shafts
2. Less tissue distortion because of gentle contralateral tension on the strip
3. Less follicular transection because of better visualization and less distortion
4. A precise cut while sectioning
5. Choice of working manually with any sectioning instrument or electrically with the Micro-Pen
6. Use of foam cutting block, which is sterile and disposable, cannot damage the tissue and will not dull blades

Disadvantages
1. Difficult with circular punch grafts
2. Need for a foam cutting block or a softer surface to anchor the strips with a fine-gauge needle

---

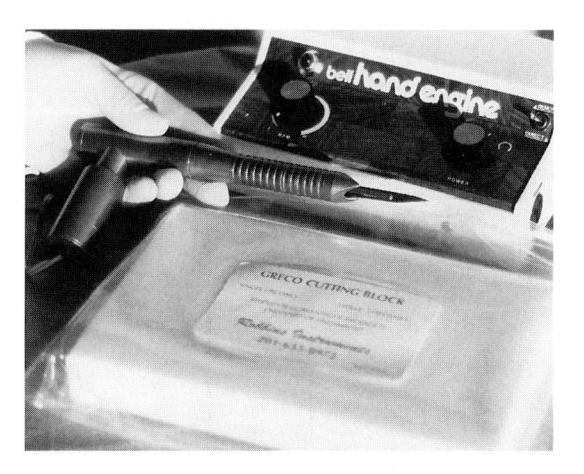

FIG. 4-46 Components of the Electric Knife: (1) Bell hand engine, (2) Micro-Pen, (3) Greco blade adapter, and (4) Greco cutting block. (Courtesy Dr. J. Greco.)

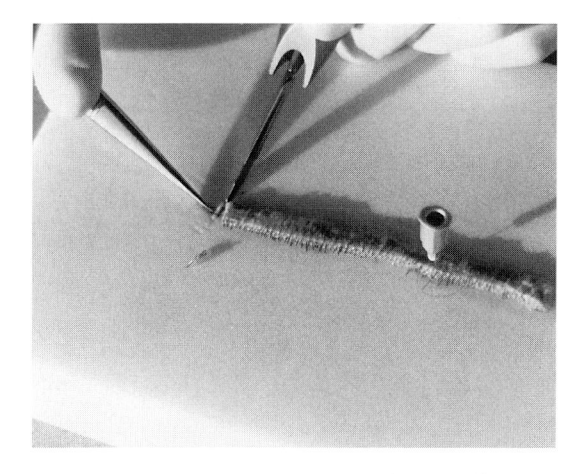

FIG. 4-47 Retraction-sectioning technique of a 2 mm × 5 cm donor strip into single- to three-hair micrografts using the Electric Knife. Note that any instrument including a scalpel, razor blade, or multibladed knife can be used to section strips using this technique.

but it is also used in manual dissection of grafts and cannot dull the blades.

When used with the retraction-sectioning technique, the Electric Knife is designed to cut without scalpel pressure and eliminates repetitious back-and-forth hand movements (Fig. 4-47). The surgeon must get the feel of "gliding" the knife over the tissue strip, thereby allowing the reciprocations of the knife to cut the tissue.

I have found it easy to train assistants to use the knife who do not have extensive prior experience sectioning. Some clinicians, highly skilled in transplant sectioning, may find it frustrating "getting the feel" of cutting with a power instrument or may just feel more comfortable manually sectioning.

Our first proclivity with something new is to be hesitant until we determine if it fits our overall scheme. Just as instrumentation changes, so must clinicians' attitudes change toward new technology. We are in the computer age of hair transplantation and must reprogram ourselves to use the most advanced instrumentation available.

REFERENCES

1. Schwartz SI and others: *Principles of surgery*, ed 2, New York, 1979, McGraw-Hill.
2. Greco J: Retraction-sectioning of micrografts and the Micro-Pen (Electric Knife), Am J Cosmet Surg 2:11-13, 1994.

5
The Donor Site

A. The Donor Area

Dow B. Stough and Robert S. Haber

HARVESTING PATTERNS

Traditional Donor Harvesting

Traditionally, transplant surgeons have begun donor harvesting by making a midline horizontal incision. The incision line was usually located midway between the ears (Fig. 5-1). In sessions two, three, and four, the incision was made above or below the initial harvesting site. If more hair was needed for later procedures (i.e., sessions 5, 6, and 7), this donor hair could be harvested from the area above the ears in the parietal zone (Fig. 5-1). However, harvesting in the parietal area often produces a very small amount of donor tissue and may require bilateral harvesting sites for a single session.

Refined Donor Harvesting

A more efficient method of harvesting uses the hair of the parietal area from the onset. We refer to this technique as *refined donor harvesting*. Instead of beginning with central incisions, lateral incisions are made, starting in the parietal area and extending toward the midline of the back of the occiput. With the traditional method, hair from the parietal zone is not used until the later sessions. The refined method involves the harvesting of this area in the earlier sessions. Fig. 5-2 demonstrates the concept of refined donor harvesting. This method has no disadvantages and has the benefit of avoiding small harvesting zones in sessions 4, 5, and 6.

Linear Scar Harvesting

Many surgeons harvest the previous linear scar when obtaining donor hair. This technique leaves the patient with a single scar, which is beneficial (Fig. 5-3). After strip removal, technicians must separate useless scar tissue from viable donor hair. This drawback can result in a longer preparation time for micrografts. Linear scar harvesting does not completely obviate the need of harvesting in the parietal areas. Thus, even with scar harvesting, surgeons must eventually harvest in three areas, that is, the right parietal, left parietal, and occipital areas.

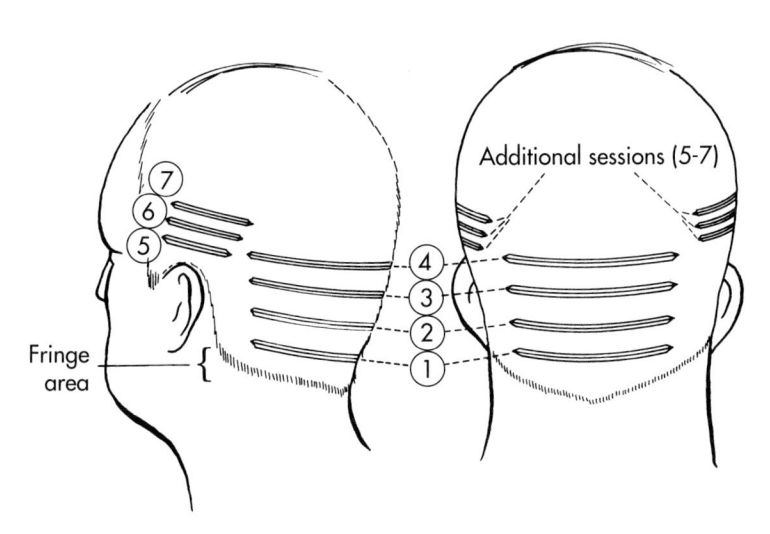

FIG. 5-1 Traditional harvesting pattern. Strip grafts obtained during sessions 5, 6, and 7 are frequently half the length of those obtained during the first four sessions, necessitating bilateral harvest.

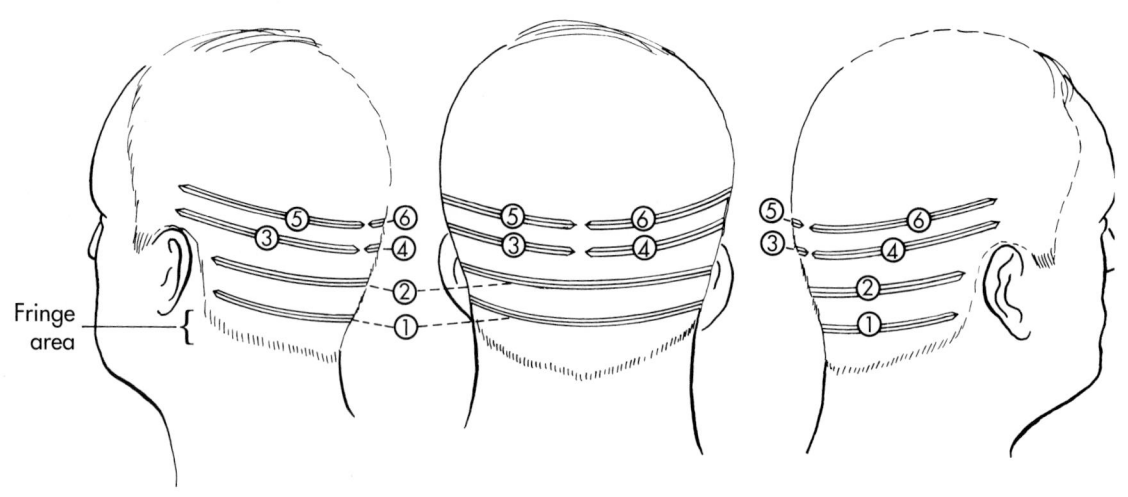

FIG. 5-2 Refined donor harvesting. All strips are of equal length.

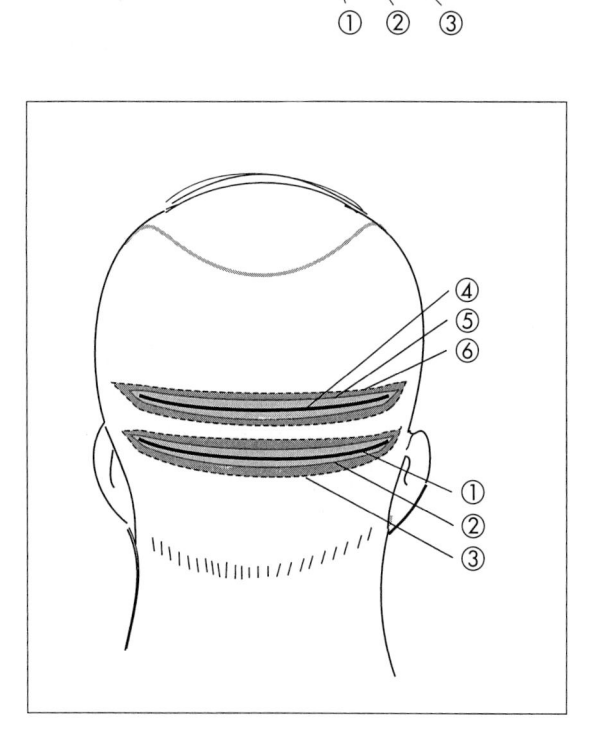

FIG. 5-3 Linear scar harvesting.

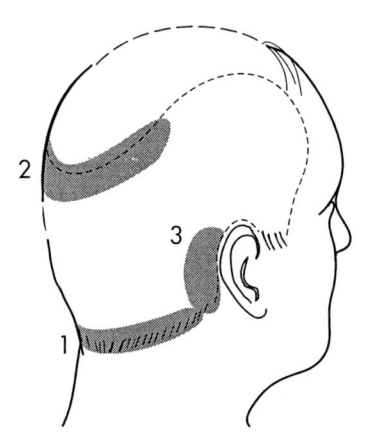

FIG. 5-4 Potential problem areas of the donor region. Areas to avoid harvesting are *1*, the lower occipital zone; *2*, the upper occipital zone; and *3*, the retroauricular zone.

PROBLEM AREAS OF THE DONOR REGION

Lower Occipital Zone

Lower occipital zone harvesting should be performed cautiously since this area is prone to extensive thinning secondary to male pattern hair loss (Fig. 5-4). We have seen numerous cases in which hair harvested from the lower occipital zone initially did well after transplantation, but with the passing of years, graft loss ensued.

Retroauricular Zone

The hair-bearing zones adjacent to the retroauricular folds can produce cosmetically observable scarring. Therefore incisions should not extend to the fringe of the scalp. Incision should begin at least 1 cm into the scalp (see Fig. 5-4). These areas are prone to hair loss from the process of androgenic alopecia. These areas can occasionally display curly whisker hair, a sign of ongoing alopecia.

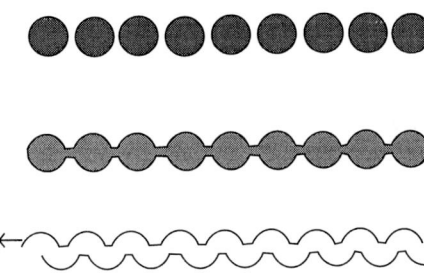

1. Single row of grafts

2. Bridges separating each graft are transected

3. Top and bottom of wound are offset

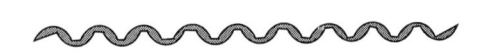

4. Wound is closed and sutured using a running lock

FIG. 5-5 Linear hand engine harvesting and steps in the Pierce closure method.

Upper Occipital Zone

The upper occipital zone can appear as a source of dense viable donor hair, only to experience thinning years after harvesting. The scars from inadvertent harvesting in this area can become quite noticeable (see Fig. 5-4).

Parietal Zone

This area can be harvested for transplantation. However, in rare instances patients will have a marked decrease in subcutaneous tissue in the parietal zone as compared with the occipital zones. This observation stresses the importance of scrutinizing blade depth during harvesting. The surgeon should always maintain a depth of incision 1 mm below the terminus of the hair follicles.

HARVESTING METHODS

Linear Hand Engine Harvesting—The Pierce Closure

Linear hand engine harvesting is a time-proven, effective technique for harvesting donor hair. The scars from this method are generally acceptable. After removing the small islands of tissue between each graft site, the surgeon closes the wound with sutures. In comparison with strip harvesting using knives, marginal loss of hair is more extensive with the hand engine technique. This loss is a result of the scalloped borders, which must either be trimmed to produce a straight incision or sewn together in a "ragged" manner (Fig. 5-5). Because of better tissue apposition, wound healing is more rapid with the knife method of harvesting, and micrograft preparation is simpler and quicker.

Shotgun Hand Engine Harvesting

Shotgun hand engine harvesting is a technique developed prior to linear hand engine harvesting (Fig. 5-6). This technique has the advantage of not re-

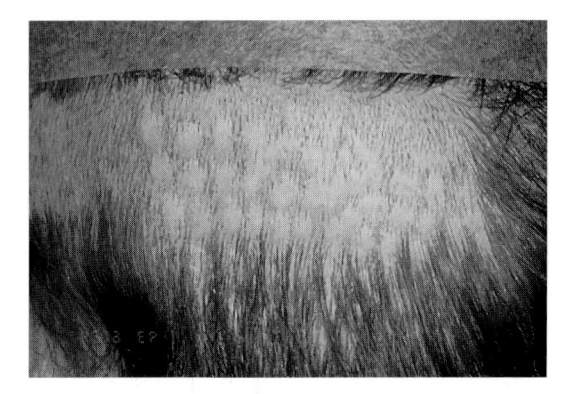

FIG. 5-6 Shotgun hand engine harvesting is now an obsolete method.

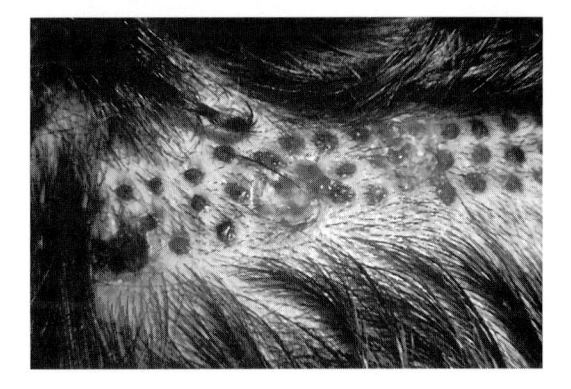

FIG. 5-7 Segmental donor area necrosis is an uncommon complication of shotgun harvesting. (Courtesy Dr. Marcelo Gandelman.)

quiring suture closure. However, its disadvantages are numerous. The technique is extremely inefficient for maximizing use of donor area. With the shotgun hand engine harvesting method, a surgeon could "tap out" the donor area after only four sessions. The healing process often created a cobblestoning effect with numerous white scars (Fig. 5-6).

TABLE 5-1 Comparison of Donor Harvesting Techniques

	HEALING	COSMESIS	SPEED OF PROCEDURE	SPEED OF CLOSURE	EFFICIENCY OF PRESERVING DONOR AREA*	MICROGRAFT PREPARATION TIME	COMPLICATIONS	DISCOMFORT AFTER PROCEDURE	SPECIALIZED SURGICAL EQUIPMENT
Single-knife elliptical harvesting	Rapid	Excellent	Rapid	Rapid	Excellent	Rapid	Few	Mild to moderate	None
Strip harvesting with multibladed knife†	Rapid	Excellent	Rapid	Rapid	Good to excellent	Rapid	Few	Mild to moderate	Multibladed knife
Linear hand engine harvesting	Good	Good to excellent	Moderate	Slow	Good	Moderate to fast	Few	Mild to moderate	Hand engine, constant supply of sharp punches
Shotgun hand engine harvesting	Slow	Poor	Slow	No closure required	Poor	Slow	Moderate	Mild to moderate	Hand engine or hand punch

*Efficiency refers to optimal usage of existing donor hair with minimal marginal loss.
†Most expeditious method of micrograft preparation.

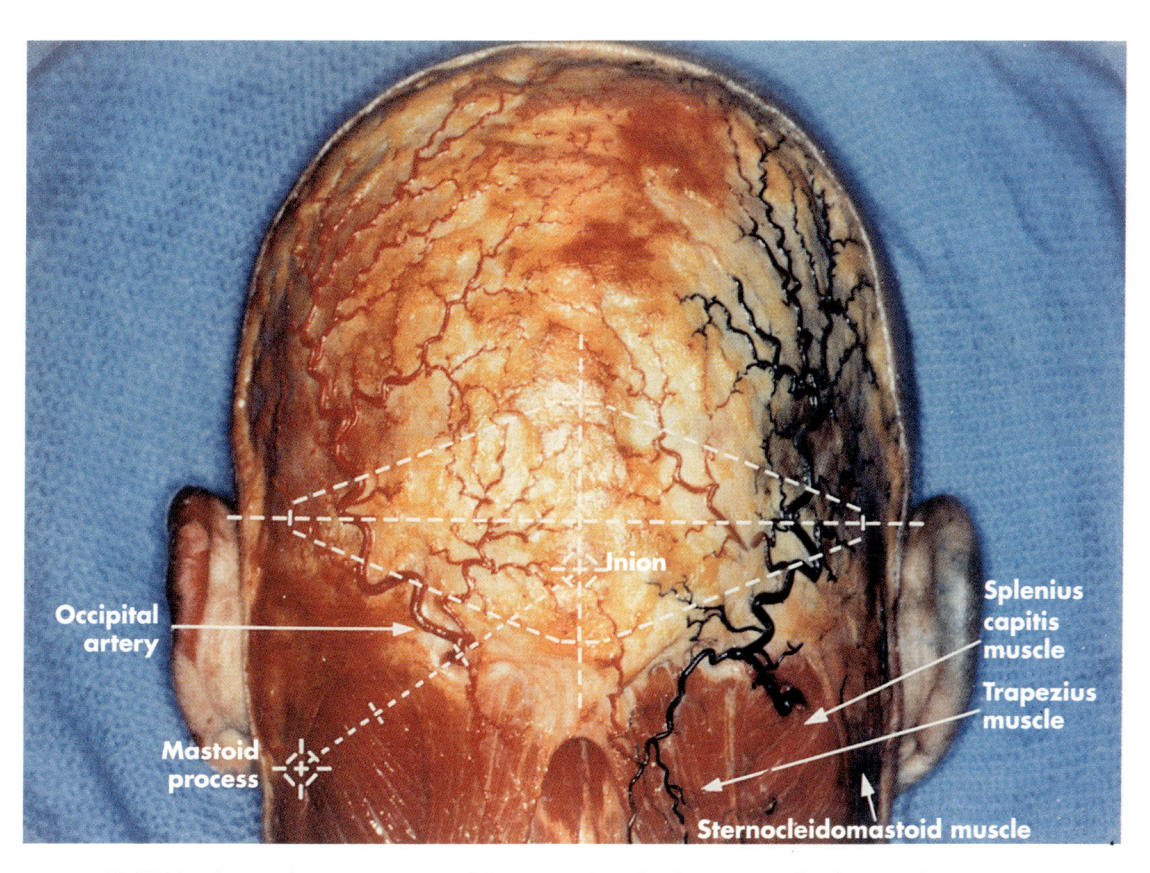

PLATE I Occipital artery anatomy. Often ignored in the description of scalp arterial anatomy is the occipital artery. Ascending and transverse branches and robust anastomoses across the midline make the occipital area a useful donor free flap site.

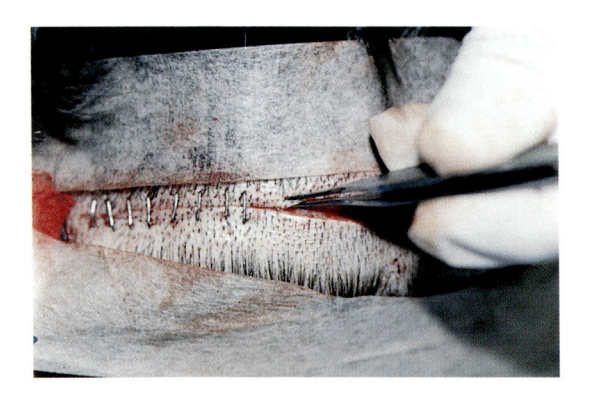

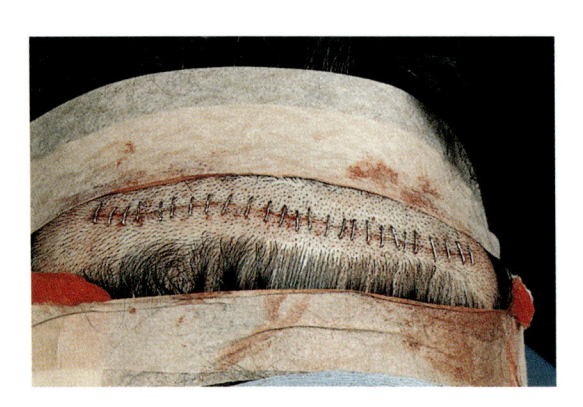

PLATE X Direct wound edge approximation is accomplished with staples.

PLATE XI Completed closure with staples.

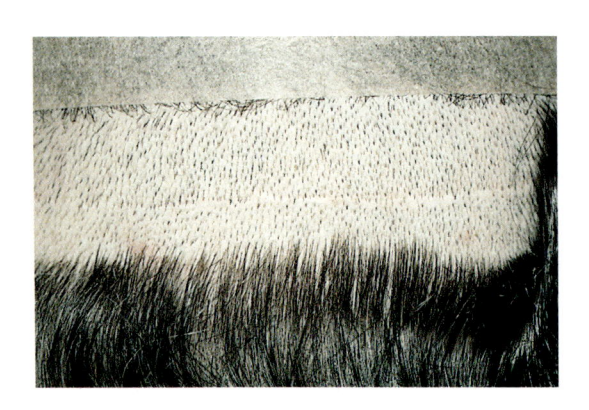

PLATE XII Donor scar after the use of a triple-bladed knife and staple closure.

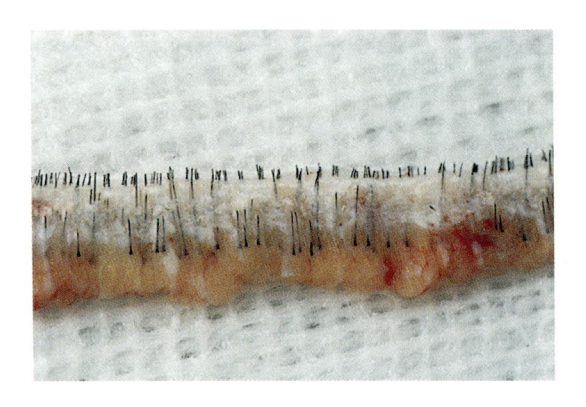

PLATE XIII Closeup view of a single 2 mm–wide strip harvested with a triple-bladed knife. The appearance of the follicles indicates that the level of incision was 1 mm too deep.

Segmental donor area necrosis is a rare complication of this harvesting method (Fig. 5-7). This technique should be discouraged in view of newer, more effective harvesting methods.

Strip Harvesting

The donor area is one of the most critical but least discussed aspects of hair restoration surgery. Regardless of the technique used, the ultimate result of hair restoration surgery will depend on the hair density and quality of the donor area. Without quantitative studies, harvesting techniques with strips as opposed to punches allow for a more efficient harvesting with better cosmesis.[1] Thus strip harvesting has replaced older punch harvesting methods.

Elliptical Harvesting

The elliptical incision method advocated by Limmer and Uebel in Chapter 5, Part C and Chapter 6, Part D accomplishes basically the same goal as that of the multibladed knife technique. The theoretical advantage of a multibladed knife lies in the ease of micrograft preparation.

• • •

Regardless of the technique, the use of a knife as opposed to traditional hand engine punch graft harvesting appears to be the direction of graft harvesting in future hair transplantation (Table 5-1). Instrumentation changes rapidly, and more refined harvesting instruments are being developed.

DONOR SITE CONSIDERATIONS
Incisions

From the epidermis to the base of a hair follicle, the tissue usually extends to a depth of 4 to 6 mm (Fig. 5-8). The dermal papilla, which lies just below the base of the hair follicle, is an important structure for the regrowth of transplanted hair. Therefore tissue that is more than 1 mm below the hair follicle does not appear to be essential to producing a viable transplant (Fig. 5-9). It is helpful to be aware of the approximate blade depth at all times. Many hair transplant surgeons trim the excess fat from the grafts prior to transplantation. This extra step can be significantly reduced if adequate forethought is given to the initial depth of the incision. An incision that is more than 7 mm deep is not required and only causes unnecessary injury to major arteries and veins and removal of superfluous amounts of subcutaneous tissue (see Fig. 5-9). Color Plates II to XIII depict the strip removal process. The multibladed knives are held at an angle parallel to the hair shafts. This angle is critical to avoid hair shaft transection. The angle varies from person to person but usually is in the range of 100 to 120 degrees. After the initial stab incision, a single pass is made in one smooth, deliberate motion. Sawing movements are specifically avoided. The blade is held at a constant depth. With practice, excellent strips can be routinely obtained. The majority of the strips we harvest are 11 to 15 cm in length. Naturally this length will vary with desired graft count. However, we generally plan for most strips to be within this range. Following the initial pass with a multibladed knife, the ends of the strips are tapered with a single No. 10 blade to create an elliptical shape. Therefore we have produced a long elliptical incision. The tapered ends generally do not exceed a length of more than 1 cm.

Donor Strip Release

Good visualization with a dry field is critical when harvesting donor strips. Foremost is the concern over avoiding the transection of hair follicles. Scis-

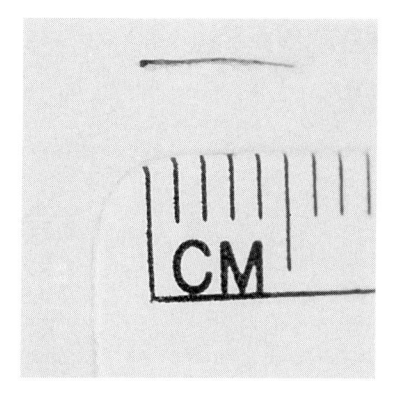

FIG. 5-8 From the epidermis to the base of a hair follicle, the tissue usually extends to a depth of 4 to 6 mm.

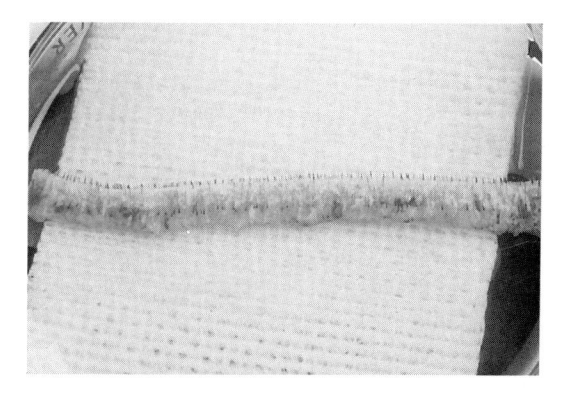

FIG. 5-9 Since the follicles are anatomically positioned in the upper subcutaneous tissue, the depth of incision should not extend to the galea. The strip above demonstrates the maximum necessary depth of blade incision.

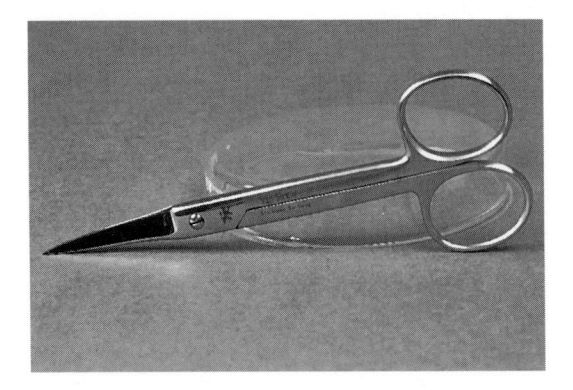

FIG. 5-10 Heavy-gauge, straight 5⅛-inch scissors with a serrated lower blade.

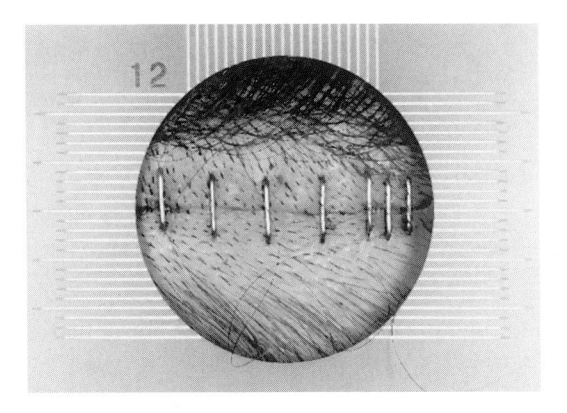

FIG. 5-11 Twenty-four–hour postoperative view demonstrating partial epithelialization. The advantages of using staples rather than sutures are numerous.

sors will allow for a rapid, even release of the donor strips from the subcutaneous bed. The use of standard tenotomy scissors, Iris scissors, or Metzenbaum scissors usually produces suboptimal donor strips because these types of scissors do not have an extremely sharp cutting edge that can be directed along a precise plane. A heavier gauge scissors with a refined, super-sharp cutting edge is the best choice. Several types of scissors made by a wide variety of manufacturers are suitable for this purpose. Small, super-sharp, delicate scissors, although effective, dull quickly and require frequent sharpening. Heavy-gauge scissors with serrated edges hold up to repeated usage and are the scissors of choice for this procedure (Fig. 5-10).

Infiltration for Donor Area Turgor

The injection of normal saline solution into the donor site has been advocated for more than a decade. This maneuver produces increased turgor in the donor area before the grafts are harvested. The additional turgor facilitates the ease with which the strips are obtained, allows a cleaner incision to be made, and to a small degree elevates the hair follicles above the underlying blood vessels. The follicles also assume a more perpendicular orientation. This slight shifting and straightening of the hair follicle after saline solution infiltration may result in the need for a decreased angle of incision. Hair direction is more easily gauged when saline solution infiltration is performed, and the depth of the incision is more easily controlled. Moreover, the injected normal saline solution can be made more effective by the addition of 0.1 ml of 1:1000 epinephrine to each 15 ml syringe of normal saline solution. The epinephrine increases the hemostatic effect of the injected solution. In this way the loss of blood from donor harvesting can be reduced to an absolute minimum.

Despite these advantages, excellent donor strips can be obtained consistently without the injection of saline solution. The use of saline solution appears more beneficial in some patients than others. The disadvantages of this technique include increased edema secondary to the additional saline solution. This edema later resolves and can result in a marked loosening of the closure and a resultant loss of hemostasis. However, we have found that this problem occurs in a very small number of patients. A second theoretical disadvantage may be "follicular shock" secondary to saline solution injection, resulting in delayed or diminished growth after transplantation. This has not been proved to occur.[2]

Bleeding

When the incision is made at the correct depth, no major vessels (i.e., occipital arteries) are encountered (see Plate VIII). We have not experienced any significant problems with excess vascularity impeding strip removal. Small bleeders are coagulated with bipolar forceps; large bleeders are ligated with 3-0 Vicryl absorbable suture. Suture ligation is required in less than 10% of cases.

DONOR SITE CLOSURE

In the past, donor site closure has been achieved by various methods.[3] To evaluate the best method of closure, we undertook a very small five-patient study in which half of a donor incision was sutured and the other half was stapled. The average incision was 12 cm long. Wound healing was accelerated in four of the five patients in the stapled area vs. wound healing in the sutured area. All five patients preferred staples. All of these patients had previously had transplants in which donor site closure was achieved with sutures. Staples may be uniquely suited for scalp surgery. A possible explanation may be the lack of damage to the underlying adnexal structures with the use of staples. In a small

TABLE 5-2 Donor Site Side Effects and Complications

SIDE EFFECTS/COMPLICATIONS	FREQUENCY	TREATMENT
Pruritus	Common	Topical antibiotics and/or steroid ointments
Hyperesthesia/anesthesia	Common	Resolution with time
Persistent suture reaction/folliculitis	Uncommon	Substitute staples
		Spontaneous resolution
Seborrheic dermatitis reaction	Uncommon	Topical steroids
Bleeding	Uncommon	Pressure
		Additional suture (rarely)
Neuralgia	Rare	Nonsteroidal antiinflammatory agents
Scar widening	Moderately common	Reexcision (of limited value)
Hypertrophic scarring	Uncommon	Intralesional steroids
Keloid formation	Rare	Intralesional steroids
		Carbon-dioxide laser surgery
Wound dehiscence	Uncommon	Oral antibiotics
		Delayed closure
Telogen effluvium	Rare	None

number of patients, sutures cause a persistent reaction, with mild erythema and a slight cobblestone texture to the suture line. A similar reaction has not been observed when staples are used. Although both methods are highly effective, staples offer the additional benefit of rapid wound healing, very quick closure, and lack of reactivity. Fig. 5-11 demonstrates epithelialization just 24 hours after closure. The principal disadvantage of staples lies in their additional cost. We remove staples in approximately 7 to 9 days in contrast to suture removal at 12 to 15 days. The use of staples in the donor area has been extolled for years by Dr. Ed Griffin (Personal communication, Jan. 1990).

DONOR SITE COMPLICATIONS

Table 5-2 lists side effects and complications of the donor area. A brief discussion of the more important complications follows.

Folliculitis

Some individuals develop a folliculitis-like eruption that is limited to the donor area and lasts for up to 6 months after the procedure. This problem is encountered less frequently when staples rather than sutures are used for donor site closure.

TREATMENT. Resolution takes place slowly over a 6-month period. Topical steroids can be of some benefit. Only rarely are antibiotics necessary. With time these reactions generally subside.

Wound Dehiscence

Occasionally a donor area will dehisce after sutures or staples are removed. If this opening is due to infection, it is best managed with antibiotics and closure by secondary intention. However, for clean dehiscence, staples can achieve excellent apposition of the wound with rapid healing. Simple reassurance to the patient is often required in these instances.

Widening of Scars

The cosmesis of the donor area is seldom a problem. Rarely, patients with dark hair color and white skin can develop scars that are obtrusive. When observed, this problem can be minimized by harvesting strips of smaller width (i.e., 4 mm or less in width). Despite these measures, some patients seem prone to develop wide scars. This problem is not unique to any donor removal technique and is probably encountered by all transplant surgeons. Scar widening is addressed in more detail in Chapter 10.

Seborrheic Dermatitis Reaction

After transplantation some patients develop an intense seborrheic dermatitis reaction, which may be limited to the donor or recipient area or may be spread over the entire scalp. Patients usually begin to notice this reaction about 2 weeks after the procedure. This reaction is self-limited and usually will resolve in 6 to 12 weeks. This complication is most common in patients who have some degree of seborrheic dermatitis prior to transplantation, but often the condition is so mild before the procedure that it may go unnoticed until afterward. The majority of patients who experience a seborrheic dermatitis reaction fail to shampoo their hair daily postoperatively and are often afraid of vigorous scrubbing to remove any scales.

TREATMENT. Steroid lotions such as Temovate and DermaSmooth FS Oil can be massaged into the scalp before bedtime and shampooed out in the morning. These products can effectively treat most seborrheic dermatitis reactions. For severe cases, referral to a dermatologist is recommended.

Keloid Formation

Rarely, keloids can form in the donor area. Their occurrence is more common in blacks. Individuals with a previous history of keloids are at highest risk.[4,5] More commonly, hypertrophic scarring is experienced. Both conditions can be treated with intralesional steroids in the dosage range of 10 to 40 mg/ml.

Ingrown Hairs in Suture Line Margins

There appears to be a predisposition among certain patients to develop hairs within the suture line. These ingrown hairs can be treated with gentle extraction. The incidence of this problem can be minimized by using staples for donor site closure.

Neuralgia

I have had two patients who complained of severe sharp intermittent shooting pains that began approximately 1 week after hair transplant surgery. Both patients had experienced no similar problems with scalp reduction procedures. The patients stated these shooting pains were transitory, lasting less than a second but were severe in nature. A diagnosis of possible postoperative neuralgia secondary to transection of occipital nerves was made. In one patient, local infiltration of lidocaine afforded complete albeit temporary relief. These patients were treated with nonsteroidal antiinflammatory agents, which provided minor pain relief. The condition resolved within 6 months in both patients. Arnold reports observing a similar case, which also resolved with time (Arnold J: Personal communication, April 1994). Seager addresses this subject in greater detail in Chapter 3, Part G.

Pruritus

Any surgical incision will provoke a normal healing response and should be an anticipated annoyance of transplant surgery. The use of topical antibiotic and/or steroid ointment will accelerate healing and decrease pruritus to a small degree.

CONCLUSION

The proper management of the donor area is a critical aspect of hair transplantation surgery. An evaluation of donor density, present and future, must be made prior to embarking on hair restoration surgery. This evaluation will aid the hair transplant surgeon in candidate selection. The refined donor harvesting presented in this discussion is a more efficient method than the traditional techniques of donor harvesting. When refined donor harvesting is combined with the use of multibladed knives, the hair transplant surgeon can approach the donor area in a much more efficient manner than previously possible.

REFERENCES

1. Brandy DA: A new instrument for the expedient production of minigrafts, *J Dermatol Surg Oncol* 18:487-492, 1992.
2. Rassman WR, Pomerantz MA: The art and science of minigrafting, *Int J Aesthetic Restorative Surg* 1(1):27-36, 1993.
3. Devine JW, Howard PS, Nordstrom RE: *Treatment of male pattern baldness: update*, Chicago, 1986, Year Book, pp 273-308.
4. Unger WP, Nordstrom REA: Hair transplantation in blacks. In *Hair transplantation*, ed 2, New York, 1988, Marcel Dekker, pp 300-301.
5. Brown MD, Johnson TM, Swanson NA: Extensive keloid formation following hair transplantation, *J Dermatol Surg Oncol* 16(9):867-869, 1990.

B. Accurate Estimation of Graft Requirements When Using Multibladed Knives

Robert S. Haber and Dow B. Stough

A transplant session begins with a determination by the surgeon of the number of grafts of each size to be placed. This estimation will be influenced by a variety of factors, including the pattern and extent of alopecia and the experience and skill of the surgical team. Harvesting with a multibladed knife will generate a strip of donor skin that must be sectioned into the appropriate-sized grafts. To ensure that the correct number of grafts is obtained, the surgeon must accurately determine the amount of donor scalp to be excised.

MEASUREMENT TECHNIQUES

In the past with round graft harvesting, one simply harvested the number of plugs to be transplanted. Formulas based strictly on surface area measurements were available to help to harvest efficiently.[1] With the advent of micrograft techniques and the development of strip harvesting, this process has become far more complex. Most experienced hair surgeons determine the appropriate length of donor tissue to harvest for a session of particular size by "feel," a skill honed by experience. For surgeons unfamiliar with the use of multibladed knives, a more objective technique is required to arrive at this estimate.

Calculations based on surface area alone are inaccurate. Due to the elastic property of the skin, 1 cm^2 drawn on the intact skin surface is no longer 1 cm^2 once excised because of contraction. The area of this skin fragment may decrease by as much as 15%.[2] In addition, during the hair graft preparation process, some excess skin is trimmed away to prepare micrografts, minigrafts, and single-hair grafts.

A 1.25 mm diameter graft has a surface area of 1.23 mm[2]. A 10 cm tapered strip obtained with a triple-bladed knife using 2 mm spacers has a surface area of 360 mm[2] (80 × 4 mm for a straight portion, plus 10 × 4 mm for tapered portions). If there were no skin shrinkage, one could theoretically obtain 292 grafts from this strip (360 mm ÷ 1.23 mm). Assuming 15% skin shrinkage, this number drops to 248. In practice, however, these numbers are not realistic because of factors difficult to quantitate such as the presence of damaged shafts in the strip, changes in density from one portion of the strip to another, and the amount of trimming necessary.

DETERMINING HAIR DENSITY

Hair density varies considerably depending on the age of the patient, location on the scalp, and individual variation. Published reports of adult hair density are inconsistent, with histological estimates varying from 150 hairs/cm[2] to 485 hairs/cm[2] [3-5] and clinical estimates varying from 80 hairs/cm[2] to 320 hairs/cm[2].[1] It is not clear why such discrepancy exists among evaluation techniques. Most researchers agree that hair at the occiput is considerably more dense than hair in the postauricular or temporoparietal areas.[1,6]

The pioneering work in hair density as related to hair transplant surgery can be attributed to Rassman and Pomerantz.[7] These surgeons have long emphasized the need for accurate determinations of hair density prior to beginning a transplant. A variety of techniques may be used to determine hair density. For standardization purposes, hair density is the number of hairs present within a 4 mm wide circle. A ruler with a 4 mm hole placed over the donor site provides an appropriate size field to count but provides no magnification and is therefore tedious and potentially inaccurate (Fig. 5-12, *bottom*). A device known as the Hair Densitometer (Robbins Instruments, Inc., Chatham, N.J.) developed by Rassman and Pomerantz illuminates a 4 mm circle and provides 10× magnification[7] (Fig. 5-12, *middle*). The Hair Densitometer provides adequate magnification but suffers from distortion resulting from poor optics. In addition, it is difficult to properly clean and virtually impossible to sterilize, and its objective lens and housing tend to become cloudy with repeated surface cleaning.

A handheld otoscope with a 4 mm ear speculum provides illumination and 2× magnification[8] (Fig. 5-12, *top*). Since contamination with patient's blood may occur during measurements if injections have already been administered, this equipment has the additional advantage of a disposable tip. Unfortunately, 2× magnification requires close scrutiny to discern all hairs in a hair bundle, leading to potential inaccuracies.

The most accurate and convenient approach involves the use of a new device known as the Trichoscope (Welch Allyn, Skaneateles Falls, N.Y.), which is a modified epiluminescent skin surface microscope with a sterilizable patient contact plate (Fig. 5-13). This device provides 10× magnifica-

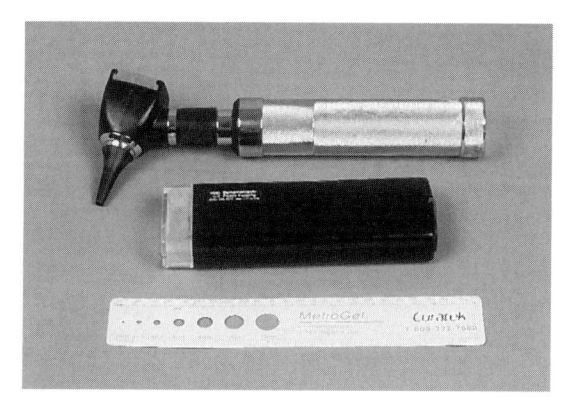

FIG. 5-12 The use of a ruler with 4 mm circle could result in a potentially inaccurate hair count (*bottom*). The Hair Densitometer produces reliable results but is not well constructed and cannot be sterilized (*middle*). The otoscope is readily available, but its relatively low magnification makes it somewhat difficult to use (*top*).

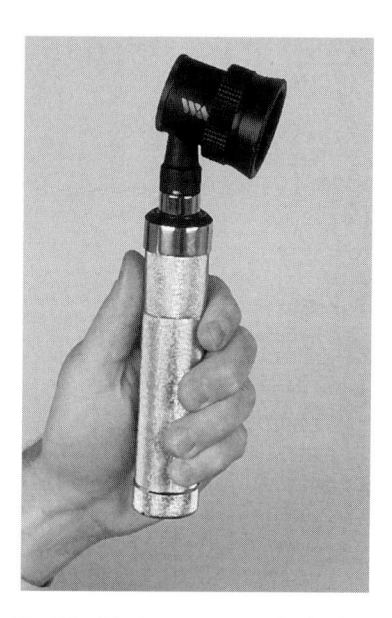

FIG. 5-13 The Trichoscope provides high magnification and strong illumination and is the most reliable device for hair density determination.

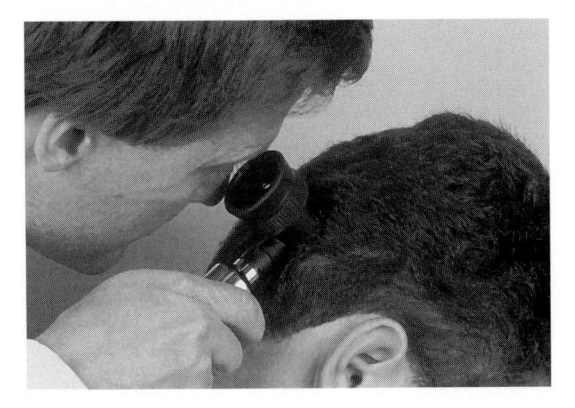

FIG. 5-14 The technique used to obtain a hair density reading through the Trichoscope.

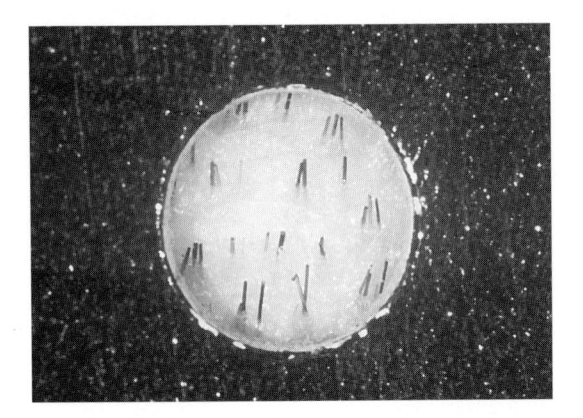

FIG. 5-15 View through the Trichoscope demonstrating the 4 mm wide field with excellent clarity of all hair shafts. The count of the view shown here is roughly 30 terminal hairs.

TABLE 5-3 Harvest Length Requirements for Three Graft Sizes Based on Graft Quantity Desired*

NO. OF GRAFTS DESIRED	DONOR STRIP LENGTH (CM)		
	SINGLE-HAIR GRAFTS	1 MM GRAFTS	1.25 MM GRAFTS
50	1.25	2	3
75	2	3	4.5
100	2.5	4	6
125	3	5	7.5
150	3.75	6	9
175	4.5	7	10.5
200	5	8	12

*Figures are based on the use of a triple-bladed knife and 2 mm spacers on a patient with average hair density.

tion and strong illumination of a 4 mm wide field and may be focused for individual needs, making the task of density determination simple and reliable (Fig. 5-14). Fig. 5-15 represents the view through the Trichoscope, illustrating its high clarity and resolution.

It should be noted that infiltration of the donor site with anesthetic or saline solution will decrease the density reading because of expansion of the hair-bearing scalp. The surgeon must therefore make this measurement at a consistent point in the evaluation process to ensure reliability. Each of these estimation techniques measures hair density in a 4 mm circle, which encompasses an area of 12.5 mm^2. Hair counts in this area usually range from 10 to 28 and correspond to counts of 80 to 224 hairs/cm^2, respectively.

Of interest is the observation under magnification that the majority of hair in the donor area emerges not as single hairs but in groups of two, three, and four hairs. Casual inspection with the naked eye will often overlook this fact; therefore, if magnification is not used, a patient's hair density rating might be underestimated.

Hair density determinations were made on a large series of patients, and meticulous data were collected regarding the number of grafts of each size that could be sectioned from unit-size strips of skin. The average hair density of patients undergoing hair transplantation was found to be 18 to 22 hairs/12.5 mm^2 (4 mm circle). Based on these data, we determined that for patients with average hair density, a 1 cm segment of a donor strip will yield 32 single-hair grafts. Likewise, a 1 cm segment could produce 24 1 mm grafts or 16 1.25 mm grafts. We refer to a 1 cm segment taken from a standard double 2 mm wide donor strip. These figures account for the tapered ends of these strips. These numbers were used to generate Table 5-3.

DETERMINING DONOR STRIP LENGTH

We measure hair density at four points along the trimmed donor site. The patient is assigned a density count based on the average of these readings. Patients are then categorized according to Table 5-4 into excellent, above average, average, below average, and poor ratings.

Required strip length is then calculated based on the desired number of grafts of each size, according to Table 5-3. All figures assume the use of a triple-bladed knife with 2 mm spacers. Strip length is increased or decreased for patients with below- or above-average density, respectively, according to the adjustment factors listed in Table 5-4. The tables are useful as a starting point, but if graft counts not in Table 5-3 are desired, a more exact estimation method can be used, which is described in the accompanying box. Slight adjustments would be required for different-sized spacers. Since we rarely

TABLE 5-4 Hair Count Determinations Correlated with Standard Density Measurements, Density Rating Category, and Adjustment Factor

DENSITY (NO. OF HAIRS/4 MM CIRCLE)	STANDARD DENSITY (NO. OF HAIRS/CM^2)	RATING	ADJUSTMENT FACTOR (%)
>26	>208	Excellent	−15
23-26	184-208	Above average	−10
18-22	144-176	Average	—
14-17	112-136	Below average	+10
<14	<112	Poor	+15

EXACT METHOD OF ESTIMATING GRAFT NUMBER*

1. Determine the graft number desired for each size graft.
   Example: 80 single-hair grafts, 100 grafts of 1 mm size, and 120 grafts of 1.25 mm size
2. Calculate strip length required for average patient hair density (see text for discussion).
   Based on: 40 single-hair grafts/cm of double strip
   25 1 mm grafts/cm of double strip
   17 1.25 mm grafts/cm of double strip
   Example: 80 single-hair grafts ÷ 40 single-hair grafts/cm = 2 cm
   100 1 mm grafts ÷ 25 1 mm grafts/cm = 4 cm
   120 1.25 mm grafts ÷ 17 1.25 mm grafts/cm = 7 cm
   TOTAL = 13 cm
3. Determine patient's hair density.
4. Adjust strip length determined in Step 2 based on patient's hair density.
   Example:

Density	Adjust by	
28 (excellent)	−15%: 13 − 15%	= 11 cm
25 (above average)	−10%: 13 − 10%	= 11.7 cm
19 (average)	no change	13 cm
16 (below average)	+10%: 13 + 10%	= 14.3 cm
12 (poor)	+15%: 13 + 15%	= 15 cm

5. Round to closest reasonable size and harvest.

*All figures are based on the use of a triple-bladed knife with 2 mm spacers.

CRITICAL ASPECTS IN DETERMINING HAIR DENSITY

Purpose	Determination of hair density allows for a precise, consistent method of estimating graft count before embarking on a hair transplant procedure. The average hair density of patients undergoing hair transplantation was found to be 18 to 22 hairs/4 mm circle.
Hair bundles	The majority of hairs on the scalp emerge not as single hairs but in groups of two, three, and four hairs. This observation is important when producing single-hair grafts.
Trichoscope	Produced by Welch Allyn, this instrument is a modified epiluminescent skin microscope designed to facilitate scalp hair density counts. The Trichoscope "reads" a 4 mm circular field.
Technique	Although not difficult to master, the use of the Trichoscope does involve a learning curve. The most critical aspect is the ability to visualize and count all hairs in a given hair bundle.
Tables	The tables and other box presented in this discussion can be used to accurately estimate graft requirements. The surgeon must employ a triple-bladed knife with 2 mm spacers. The tables are based on the results of tests on hundreds of hair transplant patients.

use grafts larger than 1.25 mm, we have not included other sizes in Table 5-3.

CONCLUSION

As hair transplantation techniques become more refined, more potential patients will be willing to undergo the procedure and will expect high-quality results. Accurate determination of hair density for donor site harvesting is essential if surgical results are to be predictable. We recommend these guidelines for the beginning surgeon. As experience is gained by both the surgeon and the technicians, less reliance on these figures will be needed, and it may be necessary to modify the yield counts to adjust for differences in technique. Eventually, most busy surgeons and often the best technicians can accurately predict the harvest requirements at a glance. The critical aspects of hair density determination are listed in the box at the bottom of p. 141.

REFERENCES

1. Alt T: The donor site. In Unger WP, Nordström REA, editors: *Hair transplantation*, ed 2, New York, 1988, Marcel Dekker, pp 209.
2. Tromovitch TA, Stegman SJ, Glogau RG: *Flaps and grafts in dermatologic surgery*, Chicago, 1989, Year Book.
3. Ebling FJG: The biology of hair, *Dermatol Clin* 5:467-481, 1987.
4. Headington JT, Novak E: Clinical and histologic studies of male pattern baldness treated with topical minoxidil, *Curr Ther Res* 36:1098-1106, 1984.
5. Abell E: Embryology and anatomy of the hair follicle. In Olsen EA, editor: *Disorders of hair growth: diagnosis and treatment*. New York, 1994, McGraw-Hill.
6. Meyer TG, Fleming RW: Punch graft hair transplantation. In *Aesthetic and reconstructive surgery of the scalp*, St Louis, 1992, Mosby, pp 75-91.
7. Rassman WR, Pomerantz MA: The art and science of minigrafting, *Int J Aesthetic Restor Surg* 1:27-36, 1993.
8. Norwood OT, Shiell RC: *Hair transplant surgery*, ed 2, Springfield, Ill., 1984, Charles C Thomas.

C. Elliptical Donor Harvesting

B.L. Limmer

Donor site preservation should be the goal of all follicular harvest methods. Donor site depletion is the only absolute limiting factor in hair transplantation. For these reasons donor harvesting methods should have as their goal the avoidance of any follicular wastage caused by transection during the harvesting process. The most efficient method of harvesting to date is the simple elliptical excision using the single-bladed knife technique and careful, microscopically assisted dissection of the ellipse of donor tissue. This technique results in full preservation of more than 95% of the follicles present within donor tissue.

HISTORY

Since Okuda and Orentreich's descriptions,[1,2] most hair transplantation techniques have been performed by punch harvesting of plug tissue. A number of alternatively designed methods have been described that use plug harvesting methods more efficiently. Excellent reviews of these plug harvest methods are provided by Norwood[3,4] and critical analysis of plug harvest technique by Alt.[5] The reader is encouraged to review these references since they constitute the history of plug harvest methods by which most hair transplantation has been done. Cohen[6] and Swinehart and Griffin[7] excise the residual tissue between plug sites to use for minigrafts and micrografts. Various closure methods for such donor-harvested areas have also been used to hasten healing, reduce scarring, and preserve donor scalp for future harvest.

Vallis[8] first described the use of double-bladed knife excision of donor scalp for strip graft hair transplantation purposes. Coiffmann[9] and Bisaccia and Scarborough[10] later used double-bladed knife techniques to harvest strips for ease of dissection into square grafts. Brandy[11] has pointed out that such multibladed harvesting methods offer the surgeon and assistants premeasured strips and speed the rate of graft creation. Simple surgical elliptical excision of donor scalp has been used by Uebel[12] and Limmer.[13] This technique uses a single-bladed knife to harvest a preset number of follicles based on the size of the ellipse and the density of follicles contained therein. Donor sites harvested by single-bladed and multibladed knife methods are closed by single- or double-layer suture technique or staple closure methods depending on the choice of the surgeon. It may be argued that excisional methods offer the advantage of harvesting all follicles within the donor site, and since the number of follicles exposed to potential transection wastage at the surgical margins is reduced, the harvested follicles are preserved more efficiently than with the plug harvest methods. Alt[5] has pointed out that if careful technique is followed, experienced hair transplant surgeons can generate plug grafts with minimal marginal wastage. Hair transplant surgeons who wish to use plugs as their donor harvesting method must diligently adhere to the principles pointed out by Alt. Single-bladed knife harvest reduces the risk of follicular transection by virtue of the ratio of surgical margin length to number of harvested follicles. The single-bladed knife technique also offers the surgeon better direct visualization of the excision process than either punch or multibladed knife techniques.

MATHEMATICAL RELATIONS

The mathematical relationship of harvest techniques and marginal exposure of follicles to potential wastage is demonstrated in Fig. 5-16. Compared with harvest by simple elliptical excision method, quadruple-bladed knife harvest using blades set 3 mm apart requires 2.45 times greater surgical margins and 4 mm plug harvest requires 4.95 times greater surgical margins to harvest the same surface area and thereby the same number of follicles. Experienced surgeons using any donor harvest technique become efficient in minimizing marginal loss of follicles, but the mathematical relationships clearly support simple elliptical excision as the most efficient donor technique in reducing marginal follicular wastage during the donor harvest process. An elliptical donor area of 100 × 15 mm bears an average of 1500 hairs with a range of 1200 to 2400 depending on the density of donor site follicles. The number of hairs contained in the donor area can be predetermined by Hair Densitometer measurements as described by Rassman and Pomerantz[14] or by 4 mm diameter otoscopic cone technique as described by Stough (Dow Stough: Personal communication, June 20, 1994). Such density measurements may be converted to numbers of grafts, graft sizes, and number of hairs per graft within the specified donor site to be harvested prior to procedure if the surgeon desires (see Chapter 5, Part B). Based on the principle of maximal preservation of donor site follicles for current and future transplantation, I favor the technique of simple elliptical donor harvest and careful dissection of the donor ellipse into micrografts and minigrafts by stereoscopically assisted methods. Meticulous attention to detail during such donor removal and graft preparation maximizes follicular preservation for grafting the recipient area.

ELLIPTICAL DONOR STEREOSCOPICALLY ASSISTED TECHNIQUE

The donor area is prepared by clipping the donor site hair to 2 to 4 mm in length. Injection of a local anesthetic and preparation of the sterile surgical field are carried out in standard fashion. An elliptical excision of approximately 100 × 15 mm is performed (Fig. 5-17). The donor wound is repaired by double-layer suture closure. Other surgeons have found single-layer suture or staple closure to be adequate. A wound dressing is applied to the donor site prior to beginning the grafting of the recipient area. The donor tissue is placed in chilled isotonic saline solution after removal from the donor site and divided in halves. One half is placed in refrigeration at 4°C while the other half is dissected into micrografts. Dissection is carried out with the assistance of stereoscopic 10× magnification (Fig. 5-18). Under such magnification the donor tissue is first reduced to thin segments to facilitate final reduction into small grafts. Care is exercised throughout the process of dissection to preserve all follicles from the epidermis to the follicular bulbs. Micrografts thus created (Fig. 5-19) are transplanted into recipient sites previously marked. Using a 16-, 18-, or 20-gauge needle, the

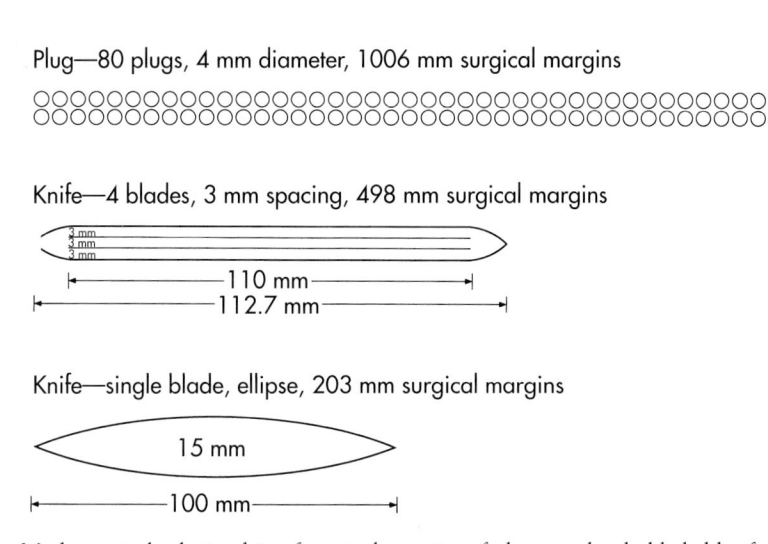

Plug—80 plugs, 4 mm diameter, 1006 mm surgical margins

Knife—4 blades, 3 mm spacing, 498 mm surgical margins

3 mm
3 mm
3 mm

|←——————110 mm——————→|
|←——————112.7 mm——————→|

Knife—single blade, ellipse, 203 mm surgical margins

15 mm

|←——————100 mm——————→|

FIG. 5-16 Mathematical relationship of surgical margins of plug, quadruple-bladed knife strips, and simple ellipse. Each technique removes 1002 ± 3 mm² donor surface area and thereby identical numbers of follicles, assuming no loss of follicles at surgical margins.

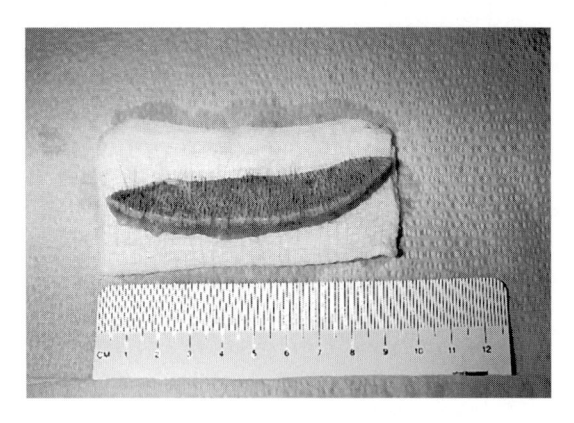

FIG. 5-17 Donor tissue harvested by elliptical excision technique. Note careful preservation of follicles at margins.

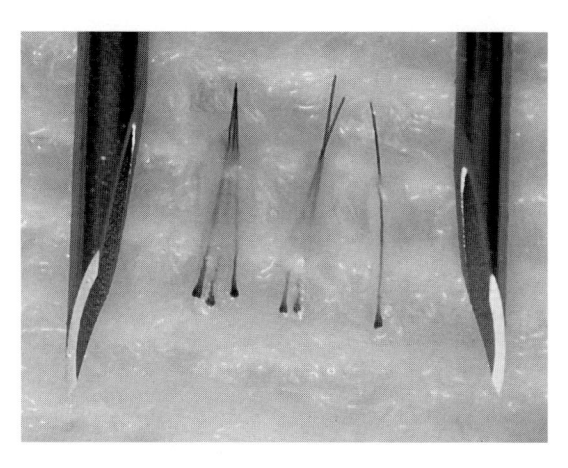

FIG. 5-19 Micrografts containing one to three hairs shown between 16- and 18-gauge needles for size comparison.

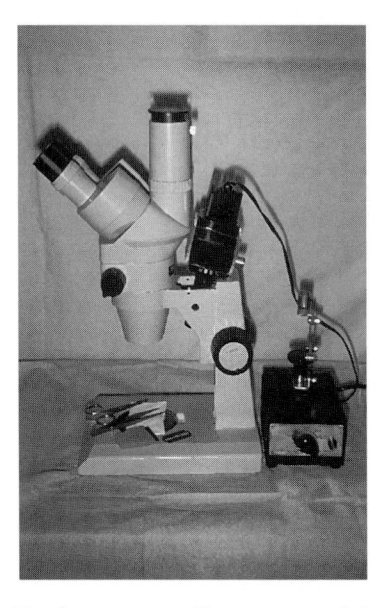

FIG. 5-18 Stereoscope, illuminator, and dissection instruments.

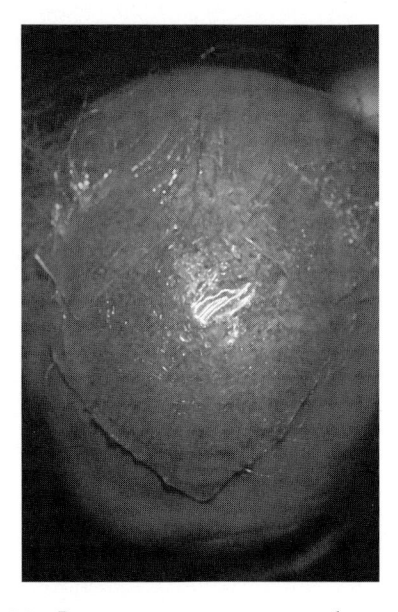

FIG. 5-20 Postoperative recipient area dressing application using antibiotic ointment under hydrocolloid dressing (Spenco 2nd Skin Dressing Kit; Spenco Medical Corp., Waco, Tex.).

surgeon creates tunnels by piercing the scalp to the level of the subcutaneous tissue. On withdrawal of the needle, a graft is immediately inserted into the recipient tunnel with fine-tip jeweler's forceps. The graft is held in place with the index finger as the next adjacent tunnel is made. This process is continued until all grafts created are implanted. Other surgeons have found NoKor needle slits, small blade-created slits, or tunnels produced by small-diameter punches to be preferred methods of recipient site creation.

On completion of grafting, the recipient area is cleaned with saline solution, antibiotic ointment is applied, and the site is covered with hydrocolloid dressing (Fig. 5-20). A disposable paper surgeon's cap constitutes the final layer of dressing. Postoperative care includes daily shampooing of the scalp, reapplication of antibiotic ointment to the donor site, and reapplication of antibiotic ointment and hydrocolloid dressing to the recipient site for 3 days. After 3 days, the hydrocolloid dressing is discontinued, but antibiotic ointment application

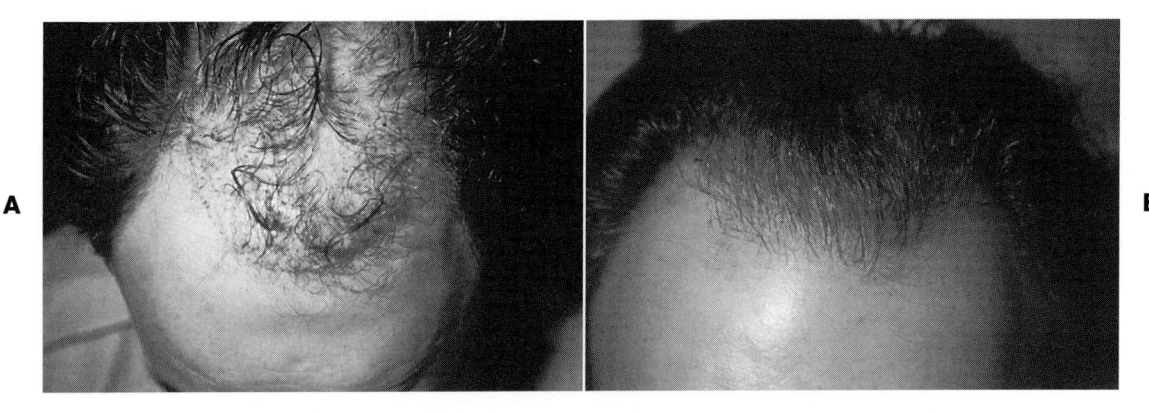

FIG. 5-21 A, Top view of scalp immediately after placement of approximately 300 micrografts. **B,** Six-month postoperative view.

continues through the seventh postoperative day. After 7 days, the grafted recipient sites may be shampooed and treated as normal scalp.

THE STEREOSCOPE

Although small grafts can be produced without magnification by skilled technicians, most hair transplant teams use some type of magnification device during the donor harvest and dissection into small grafts. I believe that the stereoscope is of great assistance during the process of dissection of donor tissue. Magnification allows for extremely precise cutting of small grafts, thereby avoiding the loss of follicles. Less than 2% loss by transection during the dissection process is routinely achieved. The stereoscope provides a very clear visual field with adjustable magnification of choice for varying tasks. Higher magnification is especially helpful when working with follicles devoid of pigmentation. Sterility is maintained by autoclavable cutting stages large enough to access the entire donor tissue until the tissue can be dissected into smaller, more workable units. The stereoscope assists the technician in accomplishing maximal precision and speed of dissection. A skilled technician can produce 200 to 300 small grafts per hour.

MICROGRAFTS AND MINIGRAFTS

Many advantages are inherent in the use of small-graft techniques. In my practice the average graft contains 2.3 hairs with a range of one to five hairs. Such methodology obviously necessitates the implantation of large numbers of grafts if sizable areas of alopecia are to be treated.

The most obvious advantage of small-graft procedures is the elimination of tufting, a characteristic of all large grafts. Preservation of preexisting hair in the recipient zones helps to disguise the ongoing transplantation process. Because of the natural appearance created by small-graft transplantation, the procedure does not commit the patient to any scheduled series of procedures, allowing flexibility of future sessions based on density and distribution desired and personal financial considerations. The cosmetic quality of previously implanted large grafts may sometimes be improved by interspersing small grafts among the large ones. Patients who are not candidates for large-graft procedures because of limited donor hair may be candidates for small-graft procedures if they are willing to accept either a thin dispersal of grafts or the creation only of a frontal tuft to frame the face.

Rapidity of healing and lack of significant scarring characterize both donor and recipient areas. Healing is typically complete in the recipient areas within 7 days. Careful shampooing is permitted from the first postoperative day and normal shampooing and grooming is allowed after 7 days. No bulky postoperative dressings are worn.

The survival of hair in small grafts is characteristically very high. My studies[15] indicate that an 89% to 95% survival of follicles as manifested by terminal hair growth is expected when such grafts are stored in chilled saline solution and transplanted to recipient sites within 8 hours of removal from the donor site. Storage of grafts for 24 and 48 hours in chilled saline solution at 4°C before recipient site implantation results in survival and growth of terminal hair in 79% and 54%, respectively (see Chapter 5, Part D).

Small-graft procedures are time and labor intensive. Exacting attention to detail is required in donor removal, graft dissection, and implantation. Additional equipment and personnel training are necessary. A well-trained team should be able to complete 500 to 1000 small grafts in a 5- to 7-hour procedure.

146 The Donor Site

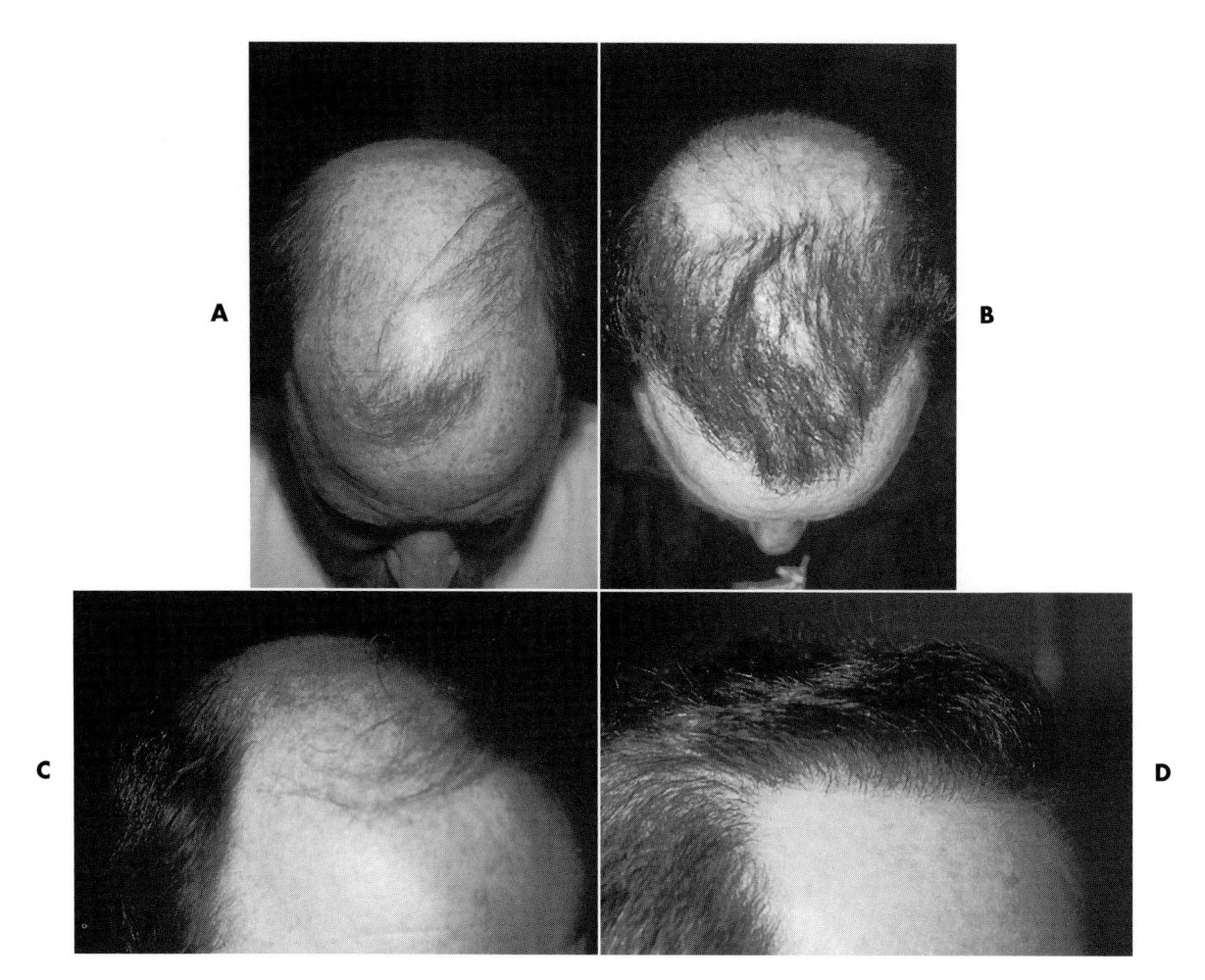

FIG. 5-22 **A,** Top view of scalp prior to grafting. **B,** Top view of scalp after two sessions of micrografting. **C,** Right lateral view of frontal scalp prior to grafting. **D,** Right lateral view of frontal scalp after two sessions of micrografting.

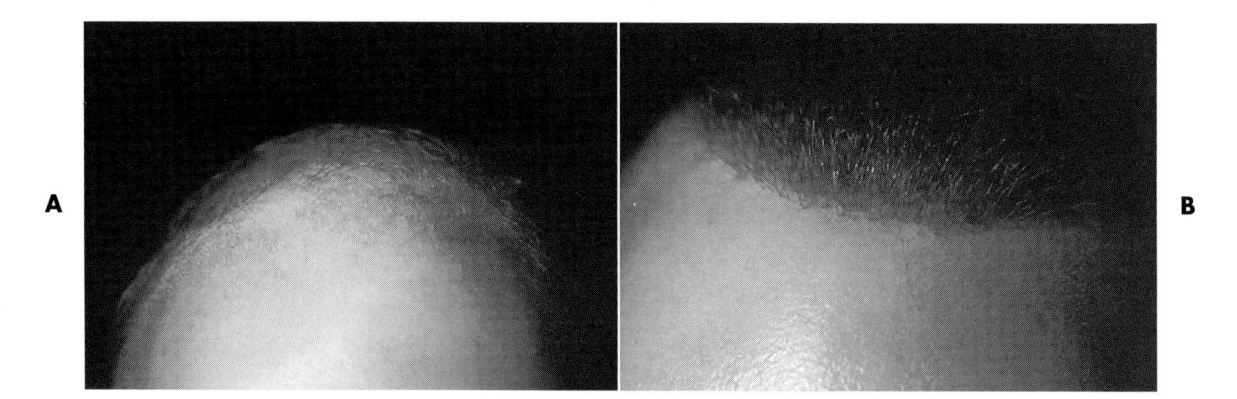

FIG. 5-23 **A,** Frontal scalp prior to grafting. **B,** Frontal scalp after four sessions of micrografting.

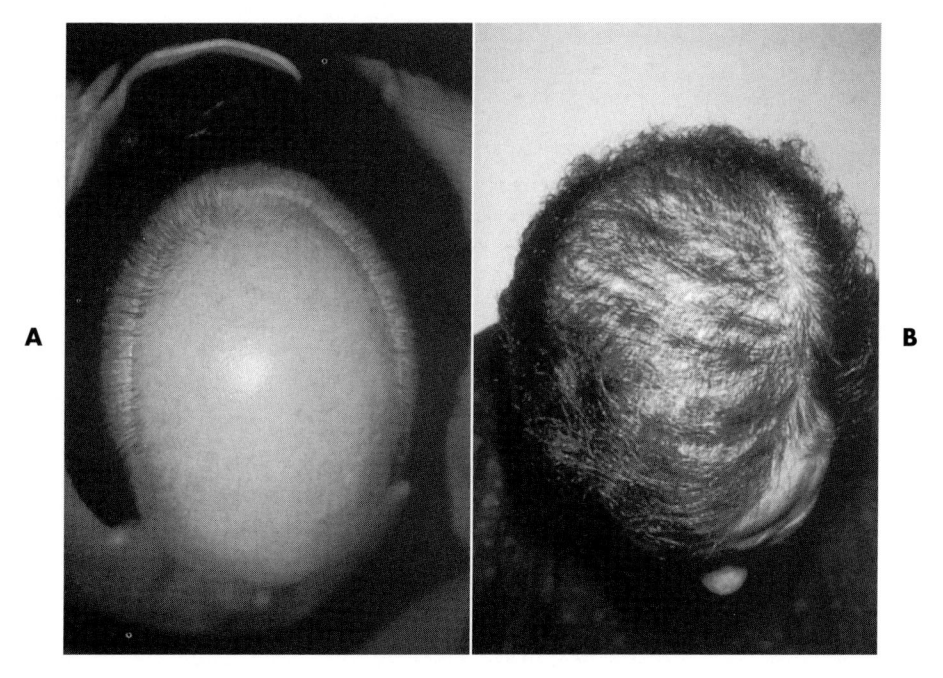

FIG. 5-24 A, Top view of scalp of patient with Norwood type VI androgenic alopecia prior to grafting. **B,** Top view of scalp after 12 sessions of micrografting.

DENSITY VS. NATURALNESS DEBATE

It may be argued that small-graft procedures do not accomplish the density of large-graft and flap techniques. Although admitting that this often may be true, I believe that any appearance of lesser density is more than compensated for by the gentleness of the procedure on the patient and the natural elegance of the final results achieved with small grafts. Representative results using this method are shown in Figs. 5-21 to 5-24.

REFERENCES

1. Okuda S: The study of clinical experiments of hair transplantation, *Jpn J Dermatol Urol* 46:135, 1939.
2. Orentreich N: Autografts in alopecias and other selected dermatologic conditions, *Ann NY Acad Sci* 83:463, 1959.
3. Norwood OT: Single-row donor-site harvesting, *J Dermatol Surg Oncol* 16:453-455, 1990.
4. Norwood OT: The donor site: a renewed interest, *Hair Transplant Forum* 1(4):1-5, 1991.
5. Alt TH: Evaluation of donor harvesting techniques in hair transplantation, *J Dermatol Surg Oncol* 10:799-806, 1984.
6. Cohen IS: Donor island harvesting for micro- and minigrafting, *J Dermatol Surg Oncol* 15:384-385, 1989.
7. Swinehart JM, Griffin EI: Slit grafting: the use of serrated island grafts in male and female alopecia, *J Dermatol Surg Oncol* 17:243-253, 1991.
8. Vallis CP: Surgical treatment of the receding hairline, *Plast Reconstr Surg* 40:138, 1967.
9. Coiffmann R: Square grafting. In Unger WP, Nordstrom REA, editors: *Hair transplantation,* ed 2, New York, 1988, Marcel Dekker, pp 423-434.
10. Bisaccia E, Scarborough D: *Am J Cosmet Surg* 7:219-222, 1991.
11. Brandy DA: A new instrument for the expedient production of minigrafts, *J Dermatol Surg Oncol* 18:487-492, 1992.
12. Uebel CO: Micrografts and minigrafts: a new approach for baldness surgery, *Ann Plast Surg* 27:476-487, 1991.
13. Limmer BL: Elliptical donor stereoscopically assisted micrografting as an approach to further refinement in hair transplantation. *J Dermatol Surg Oncol* (in press).
14. Rassman WR, Pomerantz MA: The art and science of minigrafting, *Int J Aesthetic Restor Surg* 1:27-36, 1993.
15. Limmer BL: Presentation at First Meeting of International Society of Hair Restoration Surgeons, Dallas, 1993.

D. Micrograft Survival

B.L. Limmer

Extensive micrografting techniques in hair transplantation require a significant period of time to prepare grafts from donor tissue and to implant them in recipient sites. The following study was undertaken to determine the survival of micrografts implanted at varying time intervals after removal from the donor site.

HISTORY

Hair transplantation has been accomplished by grafting techniques originally described by Okuda[1] and subsequently by Orentreich.[2] Few studies of hair survival within grafts have been undertaken. Counting terminal hair growth in 4 mm punch grafts, Adamson, Horton, and Mladick[3] reported 8 to 15 hairs per graft, Muhlbauer[4] 11 to 14 hairs per graft, and Norwood[5] 8 to 10 hairs per graft. After carefully controlled, magnified counts of donor hair in grafts and subsequent hair survival after implantation, Nordstrom[6] found an average of 22.6 hairs per 4 mm donor plug (range, 13 to 30 hairs) and a survival average of 20 hairs for a survival rate of approximately 90%. Alt[7] has discussed in detail technical factors related to follicular survival in the punch graft technique. No previous studies addressing the survival rate of single- and two-hair micrografts have been reported.

OBJECTIVE

The objective of this study was to determine the survival of micrografts implanted into the recipient scalp at intervals of 2, 4, 6, 8, 24, and 48 hours after removal from the donor site.

METHODS

Two male volunteers with androgenic alopecia were selected for the study. A template based on scalp tattoos provided the anatomical location of grafts in specific, well-defined rectangular areas (Fig. 5-25). With the replacement of the template on the tattoo marks, the areas of micrograft implantation were easily determined for later counting of termi-

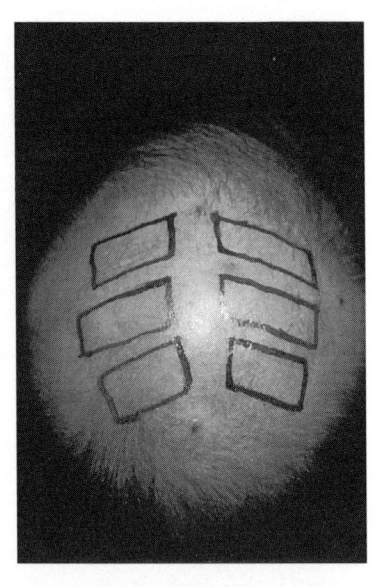

FIG. 5-25 Tattoo and micrograft implantation sites as marked through template prior to implantation.

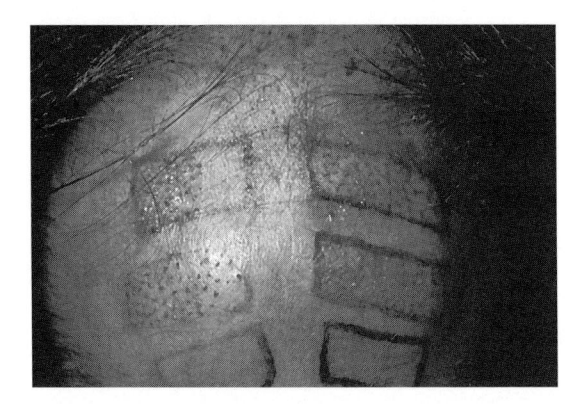

FIG. 5-26 Micrografts in 2-, 4-, 6-, and 8-hour implantation sites before implantation of 24- and 48-hour sites.

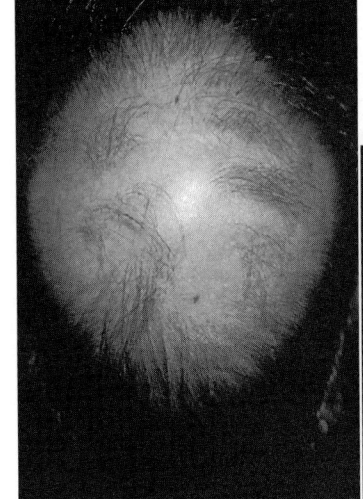

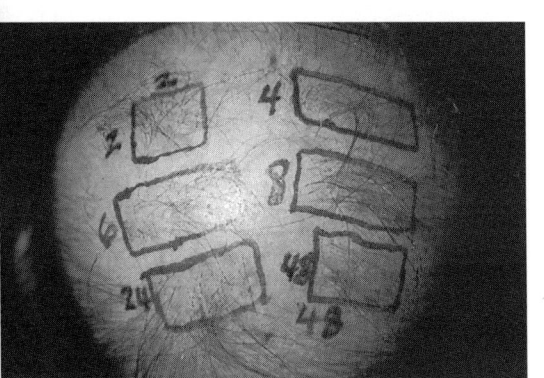

FIG. 5-27 A, Growth of hair in implantation sites 5½ months after placement. **B,** Sites marked for counting of hair shafts 5½ months after implantation of micrografts.

nal hair-shaft production. Donor hair was removed from the occipital scalp by the elliptical excision technique and placed in chilled isotonic saline solution at 4°C. Micrografts containing one or two hairs were produced by careful dissection of donor tissue under 10× stereoscopic magnification. These micrografts were transplanted into specified recipient sites at 2, 4, 6, 8, 24, and 48 hours after removal (Fig. 5-26). Approximately 5½ months later, the follicular survival was determined by counting terminal hair growth in these recipient sites (Fig. 5-27).

RESULTS

Terminal hair growth from micrograft implantation is summarized in Table 5-5. Terminal hair production in the experimental sites, as expressed as a percentage of follicular survival, was for donor grafts transplanted after 2 hours, 95%; 4 hours, 90%; 6 hours, 86%; 8 hours, 88%; 24 hours, 79%; and 48 hours, 54%.

DISCUSSION

Hair transplantation as originally described by Okuda and Orentreich involves the use of hair-bearing grafts removed from the occiput. Techniques using grafts from 1 to 5 mm in diameter have been described. The use of progressively smaller graft sizes has been described by many researchers[8-19] in recent years. Small-graft transplantation along the frontal hairline creates a more subtle and natural-appearing presentation. This method of placing micrografts along the frontal hairline in an irregular pattern creates what has been referred to as a "feathering zone" or a "no hairline hairline." The transplantation of micrografts, particularly in extensive cases in which hundreds of such micrografts are placed, is a time-consuming procedure. For this reason, it is imperative that graft survival be adequate at the time intervals required for such procedures.

TABLE 5-5 Hair Survival in Micrografts (Two Cases)

NO. OF HOURS BETWEEN HARVEST AND TRANSPLANTATION	NO. OF TRANSPLANTED HAIRS	NO. OF HAIRS SURVIVING AT 5½ MONTHS POST-TRANSPLANTATION (%)
2	257	244 (95%)
4	200	180 (90%)
6	200	173 (86%)
8	227	219 (88%)
24	200	158 (79%)
48	200	109 (54%)

CONCLUSION

Although the study population was limited, these cases support what many hair transplantation surgeons already know: follicular micrografts indeed can be expected to survive and to produce terminal hair growth in a high percentage of follicles implanted. However, survival decreases with the length of time between removal from the donor site and implantation in the recipient sites. Storage of the donor tissue in chilled saline solution between the time of donor site removal and recipient site implantation seems to contribute to these high survival rates.

REFERENCES

1. Okuda S: The study of clinical experiments of hair transplantation, *Jpn J Dermatol Urol* 46:135, 1939.
2. Orentreich N: Autografts in alopecias and other selected dermatologic conditions, *Ann NY Acad Sci* 83-463, 1959.
3. Adamson JE, Horton CE, Mladick RA: The surgical treatment of male pattern baldness, *J Am Med Wom Assoc* 24:897, 1969.
4. Muhlbauer WD: Haartransplantation bei posttraumatischer Alopezie, *Munch Med Wochenschr* 112:1655, 1970.
5. Norwood OT: *Hair transplant surgery*, Springfield, Ill., 1973, Charles C Thomas.
6. Nordstrom REA: Evaluating the efficacy of the punch hair grafting technique, *J Dermatol Surg Oncol* 15:404-408, 1989.
7. Alt TH: Evaluation of donor harvesting techniques in hair transplantation, *J Dermatol Surg Oncol* 10:799-806, 1984.
8. Pouteaux P: The use of small punches in hair transplant surgery, *J Dermatol Surg Oncol* 6:1020-1021, 1980.
9. Nordstrom REA: Micrografts for improvement of the frontal hairline after hair transplantation, *Aesthetic Plast Surg* 5:97, 1981.
10. Marritt E: Single-hair transplantation for hair transplantation for hairline refinement: a practical solution, *J Dermatol Surg Oncol* 10:962-966,1984.
11. Shiell R, Norwood OT: Micrografts and minigrafts. In Norwood OT, Schiell RC, editors: *Hair transplant surgery*, ed 2, Springfield, Ill., 1984, Charles C Thomas.
12. Bradshaw W: Quarter grafts: a technique for minigrafts. In Unger WP, Nordstrom REA, editors: *Hair transplantation*, ed 2, New York, 1988, Marcel Dekker.
13. Brandy DA: Conventional grafting combined with minigrafting: a new approach, *J Dermatol Surg Oncol* 13:60-63, 1987.
14. Lucas MWG: The use of minigrafts in hair transplantation surgery, *J Dermatol Surg Oncol* 14:1389-1392, 1988.
15. Stough DB IV, Nelson BR, Stough DB III: Incisional slit grafting, *J Dermatol Surg Oncol* 17:53-60, 1991.
16. Uebel CO: Micrografts and minigrafts: a new approach for baldness surgery, *Ann Plast Surg* 27:476-487, 1991.
17. Rassman WR, Pomerantz MA: The art and science of minigrafting, *Int J Aesthetic Restor Surg* 1:27-36, 1993.
18. Inaba Y, Inaba M, Mikami M: Single hair-bearing graft transplantation: Inaba aesthetic surgery, *J Jpn Soc Aesthetic Surg* 27:187-193, 1990.
19. Stough DB: Single-hair grafting for advanced male pattern alopecia, *Cosmet Dermatol* 6:11-15, 1993.

6

Technique—Small-Graft Hair Transplantation

A. The Art and Science of Small-Graft Hair Transplantation

William R. Rassman

Hair transplant grafts greater than 2 mm are intrinsically "pluggy." Grafts less than 1.5 mm or those with hair counts between one and four hairs each in substantial quantities produce relatively undetectable results and the appearance of a normal distribution of natural hair. A mathematical model is presented to analyze this phenomenon. Transplantation with small grafts (minigrafts and micrografts), once mastered technically, is generally a forgiving procedure, but it requires substantially more hours of work and involves considerably more procedural details than transplantation with traditional 3 to 4 mm grafts. Development of a "master plan" in hair transplantation requires merging the artistic and scientific elements of the donor hair and balancing these factors with the patient's expectations and budget. The end results are strongly influenced by hair and skin color, hair texture, hair density, hair bulk, microscopic hair growth patterns, and anticipated final stage of hair loss. The random placement of grafts in substantial numbers will avoid the appearance of inadequate density and minimize cobblestoning and donutting. Ultimately, a uniform distribution of small grafts in very large quantities, when the spaces between the grafts themselves more closely approximate the spaces between growing hair groups, results in a natural appearance. Therefore this approach may be the ideal solution to hair restoration for most physicians.

The exclusive use of very small grafts has moved from the experimental stage to the forefront of hair transplantation surgery. Dense packing of these small grafts (≤1.5 mm) in combination with single- or two-hair grafts in the hairline offers the appearance of comparable density and undetectability while making efficient use of donor hair. The use of small grafts in large quantities offers many advantages normally unavailable with traditional large hair transplantation grafts in small quantities.

QUANTIFIABLE ASPECTS OF HAIR TRANSPLANTATION

Many components of a hair transplant procedure, such as hair density, are quantifiable.[1-8] Thus if each component of the "building blocks" of hair transplantation is identified and assessed, the end results of the process should be predictable. The hair restoration physician must attempt to match the predictable end result with the patient's expectations.

To address the appearance of density in the final result with the exclusive use of very small grafts, it is critical to analyze the issue of density both scientifically and logically. If the number of hair follicles present in the microscopic field of vision is counted, a measurement of hair density (as the number of hairs per square millimeter) is easily obtained[5] (Fig. 6-1). The configuration of growing hair groups (in groups of two, three, four, or five), bulk of the individual hair shafts for that person, and amount of telogen effluvium must be analyzed. Assessment of the amounts of telogen effluvium allows anticipation of the rapidity of hair loss or the loss of hair associated with the transplantation process (see Fig. 6-1).

Nonmathematical Elements Contributing to the Appearance of Hair Density

There are three important qualitative hair attributes that dictate the appearance of the final result of a hair transplantation procedure.

CONTRAST BETWEEN HAIR AND SKIN COLOR. The contrast between hair and skin color is probably the most important qualitative element in determining the appearance of hairiness. With hair that closely matches skin color the appearance of balding is less dramatic than with hair that has a color in high contrast with that of the underlying skin. Therefore better results are easier to achieve in persons with low-contrast hair-to-skin color.[3,6]

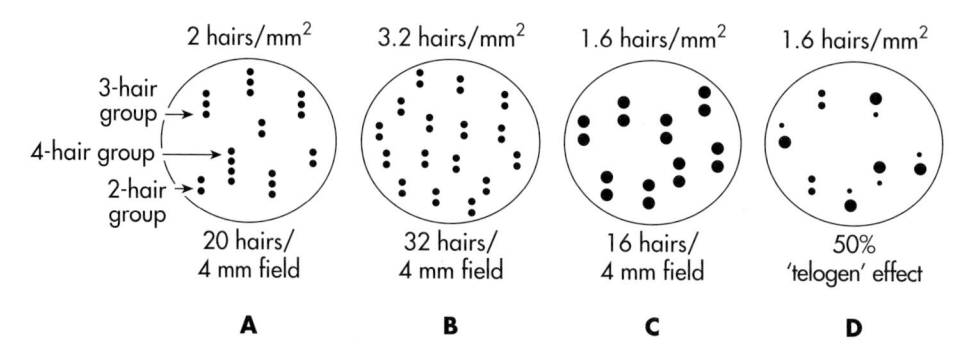

FIG. 6-1 Simulated view through a Hair Densitometer. **A,** Growing hair groups of two, three, and four hairs per group and an average hair density. **B,** A more usual growing pattern of two hairs per growing hair group but with a high density. **C,** Coarse hair and a low density count. **D,** Coarse hair with significant telogen present. Note the contrast in hair bulk of the different hair follicles.

HAIR BULK. The bulk of each hair follicle clearly adds to the appearance of hair.[3,6,9] Coarse hair may have many times more bulk than fine hair, and as a result coarse hair will carry more visual weight in creating a hairy appearance. But with greater hair bulk, as in persons of Japanese or Korean ancestry, the transplant surgeon needs to adjust the transplant technique to accommodate the increased bulk to avoid plugginess.

CHARACTER AND STRENGTH OF HAIR. The character and strength of each hair follicle can have a significant impact on altering the reality imposed by density. The curlier the hair (i.e., as in persons of African descent), the fuller the hair appears.[3,6] Wavy hair offers increased coverage, whereas straight hair, commonly found in persons from Asia, Japan, Korea, South America, India, the Middle East, and Mexico, allows the eye to follow the hair shaft to the scalp, thereby accentuating the contrast between the scalp and the color of the hair shaft. Straight hair "points" to the scalp, and in persons with thinning hair, the condition becomes evident earlier than in those with wavy or curly hair.

Mathematical Elements Contributing to the Appearance of Hair Density

Because every person is born with a particular hair population, the numbers of hairs per square millimeter can be ascertained scientifically.[6,10,11] Hair populations vary from a low of 1.2 hairs/mm^2 to a high of 4 hairs/mm^2. On the basis of my direct assessment of the hair of thousands of patients, the most common hair population measures approximately 2 hairs/mm^2 and translates into an average hair population of 100,000 hairs in an 80-square-inch area of hair-bearing scalp.

Transplant surgeons use the wreath of permanent donor hair, which grows around the back and sides of the head. This wreath represents approximately 25% of the hair-bearing area or 25% of the original hair population (20 square inches). It is a generally accepted principle that the hair transplant surgeon can reduce the wreath of permanent hair by a factor of 50% without having a significant impact on the visual appearance or "fullness" of this area. Thus in an average person, the available, movable hair population is limited to 12,500 hairs (half of the 25,000 hairs found in the wreath of permanent hair or 10 square inches of removable donor scalp). The amount of hair that can be redistributed changes if the density of the donor hair is greater or lesser than average. Subsequently, the amount of hair bulk and curliness will also influence the amount of hair that can be redistributed.

The determination of the number of grafts that can be extracted from the donor area is based on the direct mathematical calculation of the targeted number of hairs per graft and the area of donor skin removed. In an average person born with 100,000 hairs, the donor area can supply approximately 3125 four-hair grafts (12,500/4), 2083 six-hair grafts (12,500/6), 1041 12-hair grafts (12,500/12), or 521 24-hair grafts (12,500/24). These estimates are purely theoretical, however, because the density of the donor wreath decreases with each successive transplant procedure as the skin stretches to accommodate for the removed hair-bearing skin. These theoretical numbers should be adjusted for the unique attributes associated with each patient's hair characteristics. The nontransplantable donor hair may be an absolute number in most persons, making the number of transplantable hairs disproportionally higher in high-density persons.[1-6,10,12-15]

The donor area may easily tolerate the removal, on average, of 10 square inches of scalp (1 inch wide by 10 inches long) in any one procedure. Furthermore, the amount of donor hair available in any person consequently increases disproportionally as the donor density increases.

In hair transplantation the frontal hairline requires the highest density hair to make the process appear natural. Therefore the first transplant session, which yields the highest donor hair density, should focus on the frontal hairline where the highest density is needed. The center of the crown represents an area that requires as much detail and consideration as the frontal hairline because of the change of hair direction and the "vortex" effect created by this swirl. Many hair transplant surgeons perform scalp reductions before beginning the transplant process, which theoretically can dramatically reduce the density of the donor area and hence the fullness of the hairline. The perceived value of this approach to the patient in the final end result may be significantly less than what would have been obtained had the process been performed in reverse because the donor grafts will have a lower density after scalp reductions.

HAIR GROWTH PATTERNS

Hairs grow in groups, most frequently in pairs, sometimes in groups of three, and more rarely in groups of four or five. These patterns are often mixed (weighted to pairs in most persons). Understanding this architecture is critical if the incorporation of the patient's growing hair groups are to be exploited in the design of the restoration.

WHAT IS PLUGGINESS?

The spaces between the hairs within the growing hair groups (determined microscopically) are substantially less than the spaces between the grafts. The lower the density, the greater the spaces between the growing hair groups; from a transplant perspective this means that the spaces between the hair groups are large enough to accommodate a growing two-, three-, or four-hair graft placed between existing grafts. The use of larger small grafts (four to six hairs) may be critical in moving adequate quantities of hair in persons with low-density hair (except those with coarse hair). High-density hair tends to produce a more pluggy appearance unless the number of hairs in each graft are reduced significantly. Plugginess,[5] which primarily is a matter of granularity, results from the contrast between the bald skin surrounding the transplanted grafts and the appearance of hair density in the grafts; this causes problems heretofore not reported in persons with hair of high density.

HEALING AND SCAR CONTRACTION

Assuming that all of the techniques of the use of very small grafts are performed properly so that hair survival and growth progress as expected, healing in the recipient site can alter the end result in distinct ways:

1. Cobblestoning occurs when the skin graft surface is elevated or depressed below the surrounding skin edge.[3,5,6] In traditional hair transplants, in which cobblestoning has been a common problem, a large number of patients experience skin distortions in the recipient area of the scalp. This complication is less likely to occur with smaller grafts.
2. In the round punch hole, scar contraction is circular; as a result the mechanical effect of contraction reduces the diameter of the healing graft "ever so slightly" and has the effect of increasing the density of the hairs within the graft. Fortunately this visual effect can be exploited to the advantage of the patient if used as part of the "master plan" and the design of the transplant array.
3. Scar contraction in slits is very common[16,17] and causes the hairs to either line up one behind the other or exit from a common hole somewhere in the slit scar.
4. Depigmentation, which is a common finding in hair grafts, reflects the large surface area found in the skin that accompanies the hair in the grafts. With follicular transplants, which use the hair in their natural groupings (clusters of two, three, or four hairs that normally grow close together), the amount of skin can be significantly reduced, thus minimizing the effects of the skin transplant on pigmentation changes and scar contraction that are visible.

Some scarring is to be expected in the donor site. After multiple harvesting procedures, scar tissue may become extensive. I use the following procedures to address this problem:

1. Repeating the surgery at exactly the same site with successive procedures often removes the old scar at the time of harvesting. Since the scarred area is minimized, greater yields can be obtained from progressive procedures, which produces a cosmetic end result that is much more acceptable to the patient.
2. Packing the grafts as close as possible in each procedure minimizes the number of surgeries required. The density of the packing reflects the mechanical limits of the instruments used for creating the recipient wounds, not the blood supply of the scalp as previously thought.

From a practical point of view, a person with a Norwood type VII pattern of hair loss has lost 75%

of the hair population in the front, top, and crown. Traditional hair transplantation procedures attempt to restore hair by moving half of the donor hair (12.5% of the original hair population) to replace the 75% of the lost hair (illogical at best). If dense clustering attempts to produce a 1.2 to 1 surface area ratio between the recipient and donor areas under the conditions shown in Fig. 6-2 (i.e., larger traditional transplants), there cannot be enough donor hair to cover the bald area under any reasonable argument. The same logic applies to scalp reductions, hair flaps, and all other forms of surgical hair restoration. The ratios of bald skin and movable donor hair (with use of any available method of hair restoration) are critically dependent on the geometry of the process modified by the aesthetic skills of the surgeon and the attributes of the patient's hair. Therefore physicians must establish realistic goals with each patient and communicate them in a manner consistent with "informed consent" principles.

MEGATRANSPLANT SESSIONS

In the discussions by Lucas, Stough, Uebel, Griffin (Chapter 6, Parts B, C, D, and E) and Limmer (Chapter 5, Parts C and D), the underlying element is the extensive use of small grafts, that is, "megatransplant sessions" (>500 grafts per session). Although each surgeon presents a different technique, the nuances described in this discussion apply to all cases regardless of the variations in technique.

Megatransplant sessions (involving >500 grafts per session) readily create the illusion of a fuller head of hair by redistributing the hair in small skin units placed in random patterns. The more densely these units are placed, the better the illusion of fullness. To be effective, single- or two-hair graft transplants (recommended in persons with coarse, black hair and light skin) must be placed in massive quantities to make the impact financially and clinically practical and aesthetically pleasing. Often twice the number of hairs is required to achieve the same bulk in persons who have fine hair compared with persons who have hair of normal bulk. The finer (and lighter in color in light-skinned persons) the hair, the greater the number of hairs per graft can be used without the risk of producing a "picket fence" appearance. Three-hair grafts are best performed in an "average" person with light-brown, medium-weight, wavy, soft-character hair. In persons with higher hair bulk, the number of hairs per graft should be reduced; this becomes even more important when there is a high contrast between

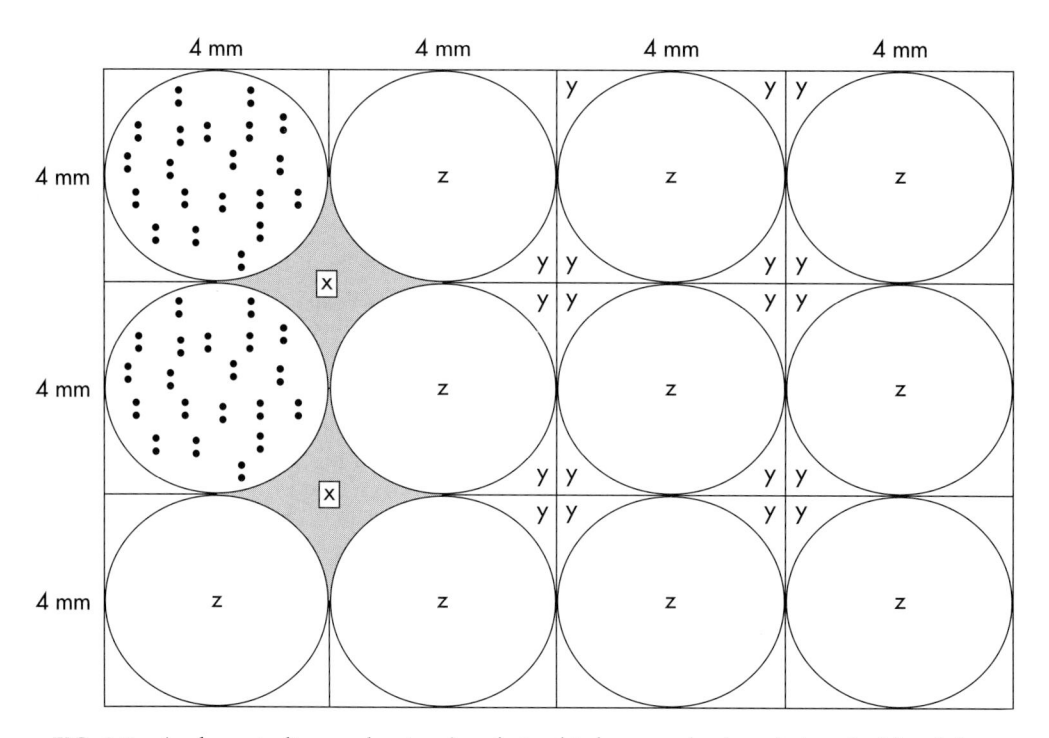

FIG. 6-2 A schematic diagram showing the relationship between the dense hair grafts (z) and the spaces between the grafts (x or $4 \times y$), which are always present under ideal conditions. It is important to note that on the basis of geometrical configuration alone, large grafts leave spaces equal in areas to the size of the grafts, which produces a "pluggy" appearance.

hair color and skin color. The number of grafts transplanted in any one session is limited by the size of the donor strip, not by the blood supply in the recipient area. In persons with very high donor site hair density, it is possible to transplant as many as 4000 grafts per session (averaging three to four hairs each). Patient satisfaction in such patients is extremely high (Fig. 6-3).

Fig. 6-4 reflects the actual placement of grafts with a dense packing technique used routinely in my surgical practice. The graft quantities (and the very close packing of those grafts) used with the patient portrayed in Fig. 6-4 should not be used in patients with advanced hair loss but should be reserved for use only in patients who will not lose significant amounts of hair. The case of the patient in Fig. 6-4 demonstrates that dense packing of grafts in large numbers and with small spaces between the grafts not only is possible but also does not produce a blood supply problem as commonly thought. If

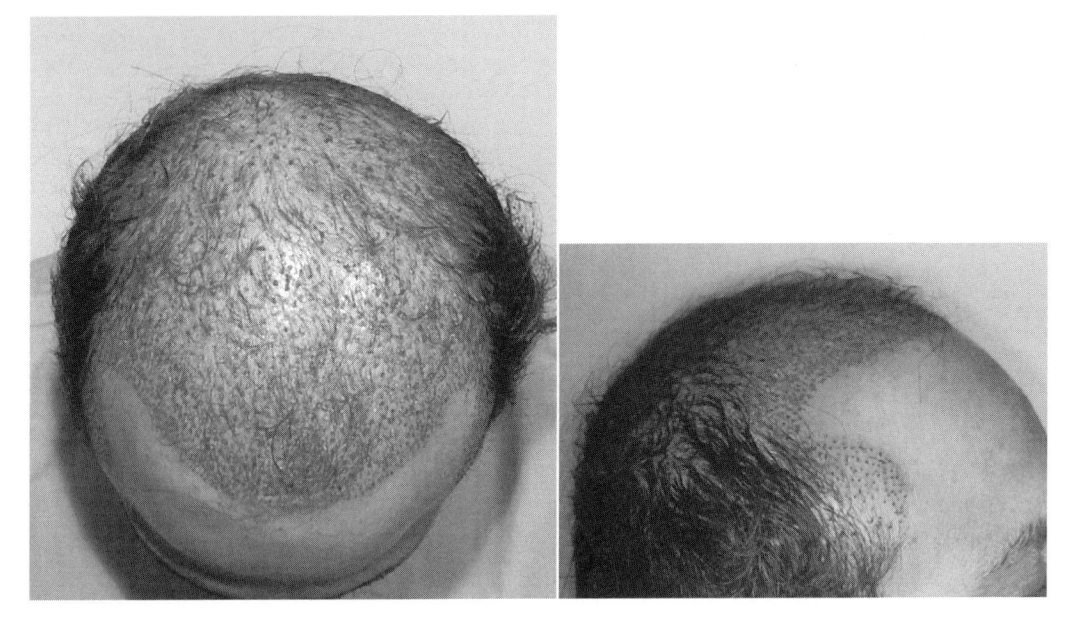

FIG. 6-3 Side and top views of a patient with a Norwood type VII pattern immediately after receiving 1691 grafts. Hair density from the donor area measured over 3 hairs/mm^2, which allowed such a high number of grafts. The donor strip, which measured over 7 square inches, was taken from the sides and back of the head.

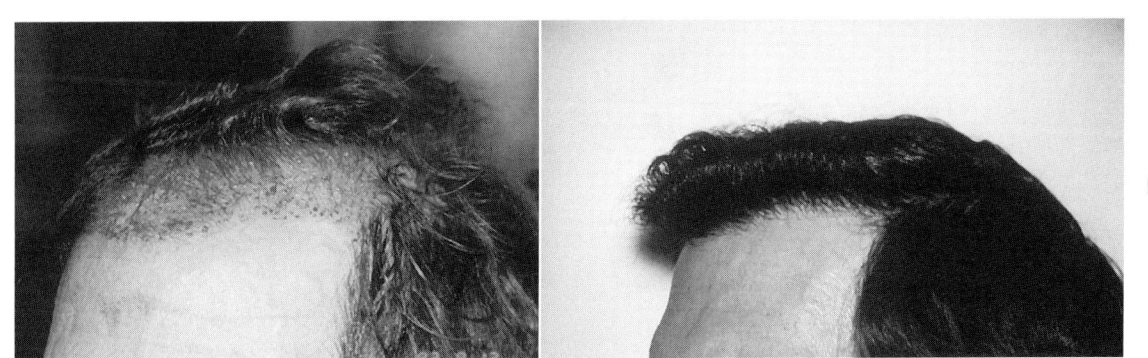

FIG. 6-4 A, Patient with a Norwood type IIIA-IVA pattern. Density of the donor hair measured 3 hairs/mm^2. This photograph was taken immediately after 570 three- and four-hair grafts were placed in 1 mm holes in the frontal hairline. These grafts were packed very close together for maximum density. **B,** The patient received an additional 690 grafts 3 weeks after the first procedure for a total of 1260 grafts. This photograph was taken 6 months after the first transplant.

dense packing of the grafts is used in patients with advanced hair loss, one must consider the possibility that an artificial appearance may result as the hair-loss pattern progresses.

In Fig. 6-5, on the other hand, a person with light-brown, curly hair with a Norwood type V A pattern of hair loss is shown after 5 months of hair growth (a total of 1331 four-hair grafts were placed in two sessions 3 weeks apart). The use of megatransplant sessions performed close together affords a significant advantage by telescoping a hair restoration that might normally take multiple procedures and years to complete into one or two procedures in a period of no more than 1 month.

The patient in Fig. 6-6, classified as having early Norwood type VI hair loss, received 1750 grafts in a single session. It is important to note that the results here were obtained in a 7-month growth period. The fast-track approach, in which up to 4000 grafts are transplanted in a single session, allows all the needed surgery to fit into an active person's lifestyle with minimum disruption.

Technical and Aesthetic Nuances

As with the development of any new technology, the recognition of subtle nuances that are often overlooked by the novice evolve with experience. This list is not meant to be exhaustive but it presents useful insight into discrete situations frequently encountered.

BLEEDING

Bleeding is clearly the most important aspect that differentiates the traditional hair transplantation session from the megasession. The perimeter surface area of the recipient area grafts in megatransplants is significantly larger than that of traditional transplants. Because more blood vessels are severed, more bleeding occurs. The use of graded epinephrine dosage keeps blood loss at acceptable levels. When epinephrine is properly mixed with anesthetic agents, not only is the bleeding controlled, but the effectiveness and duration of action of the anesthetic agents increase.

SCALP COMPLIANCE IN MULTIPLE SURGERIES

In some patients who have undergone previous procedures, the skin of the scalp loses compliance. As fluid builds up below the skin envelope during transplantation, a pressure gradient is created in the noncompliant scalp. Maintaining the position of the grafts in patients with this problem can be a technical challenge.

This complication can be diagnosed and averted by testing grafts in their recipient sites in quantities reflective of the intended graft distribution. If graft extrusion occurs, less dense packing will reduce the problem significantly. In the most extreme situations the use of surgical glue may be the only method available for obtaining stable graft positioning.

DENSE PACKING OF GRAFTS: BENEFITS AND LIABILITIES

With the smaller footprint of small grafts and the rich circulation of the scalp, grafts can be placed closer and closer to each other. The denser the packing of these grafts, the more hair can be placed.

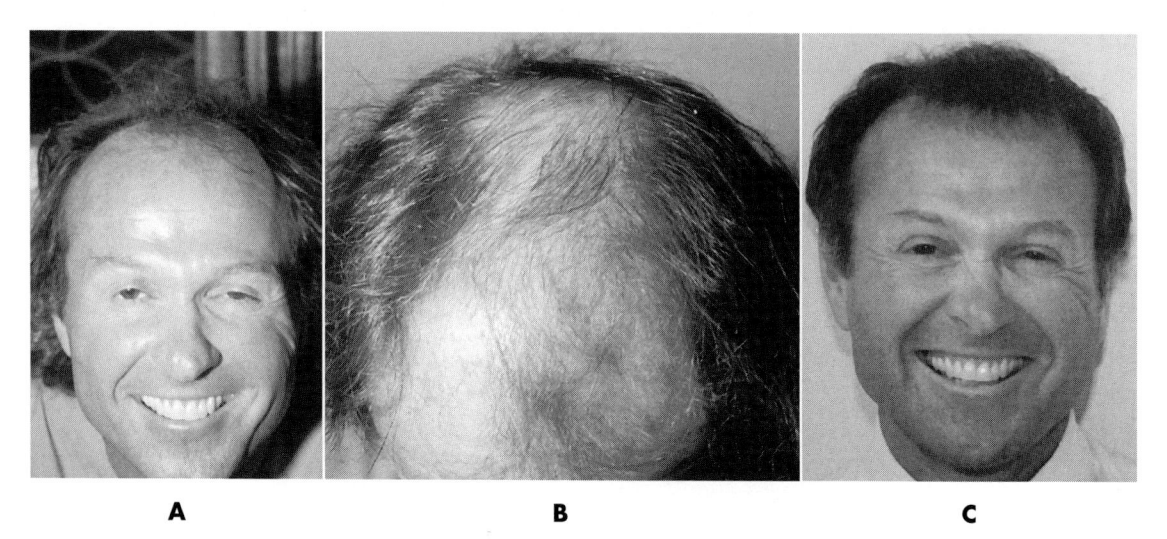

A   **B**   **C**

FIG. 6-5 **A** and **B,** Patient with a Norwood type V A pattern before hair transplants. Patient has light-brown, curly hair with a donor hair density of 2.8 hairs/mm^2. Two procedures were performed 3 weeks apart for a total of 1331 four-hair grafts. **C,** Result 5 months after the first procedure. Hair length does not exceed 2 inches and it is naturally curly, increasing the appearance of fullness.

The Art and Science of Small-Graft Hair Transplantation 157

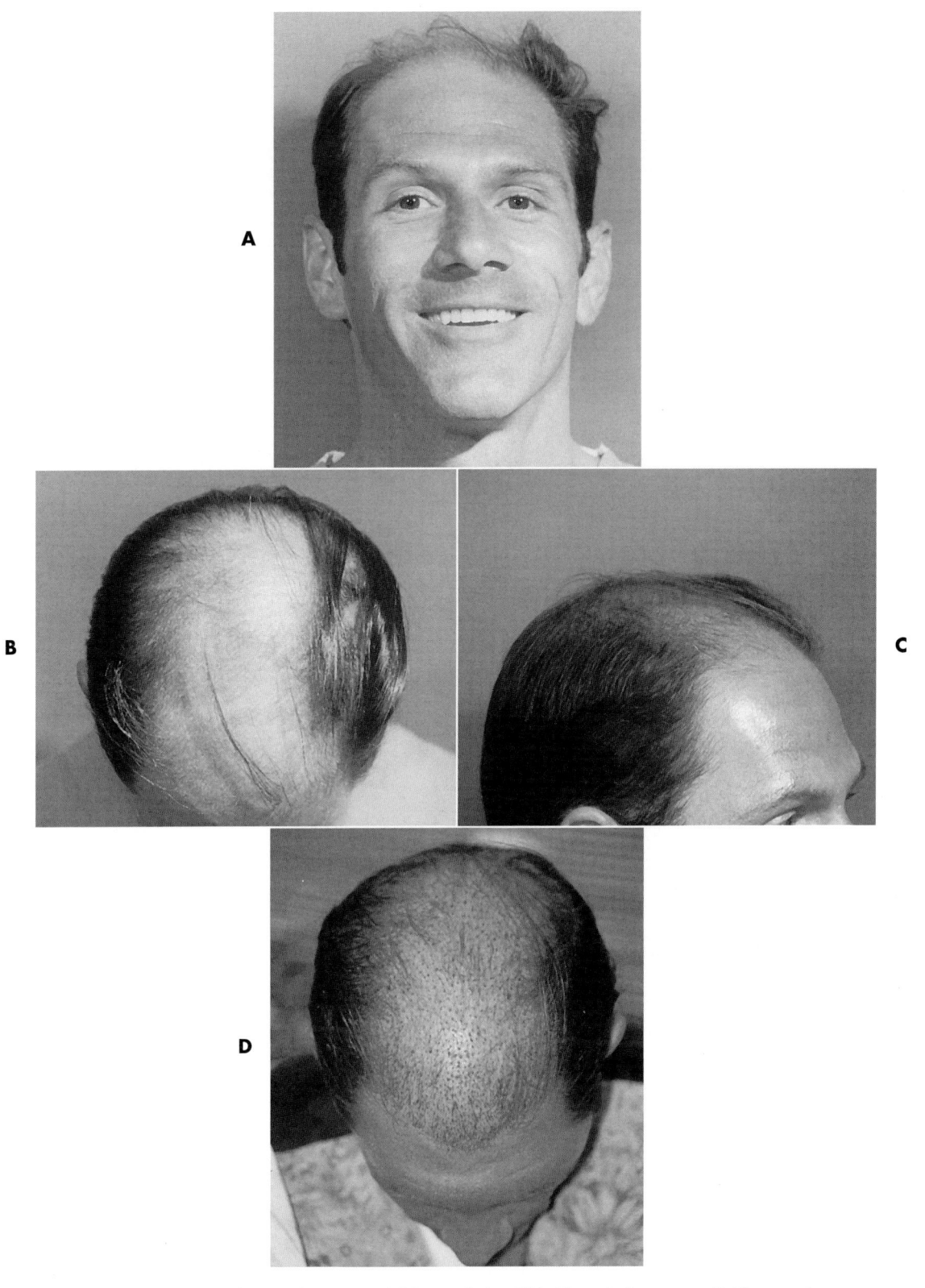

FIG. 6-6 **A,** Frontal view of patient with Norwood class VI baldness before surgery. **B,** Top view before surgery. **C,** Right lateral view before surgery. **D,** Day of surgery after transplantation of 400 single-hair grafts and 1350 two- and three-hair grafts.

Continued.

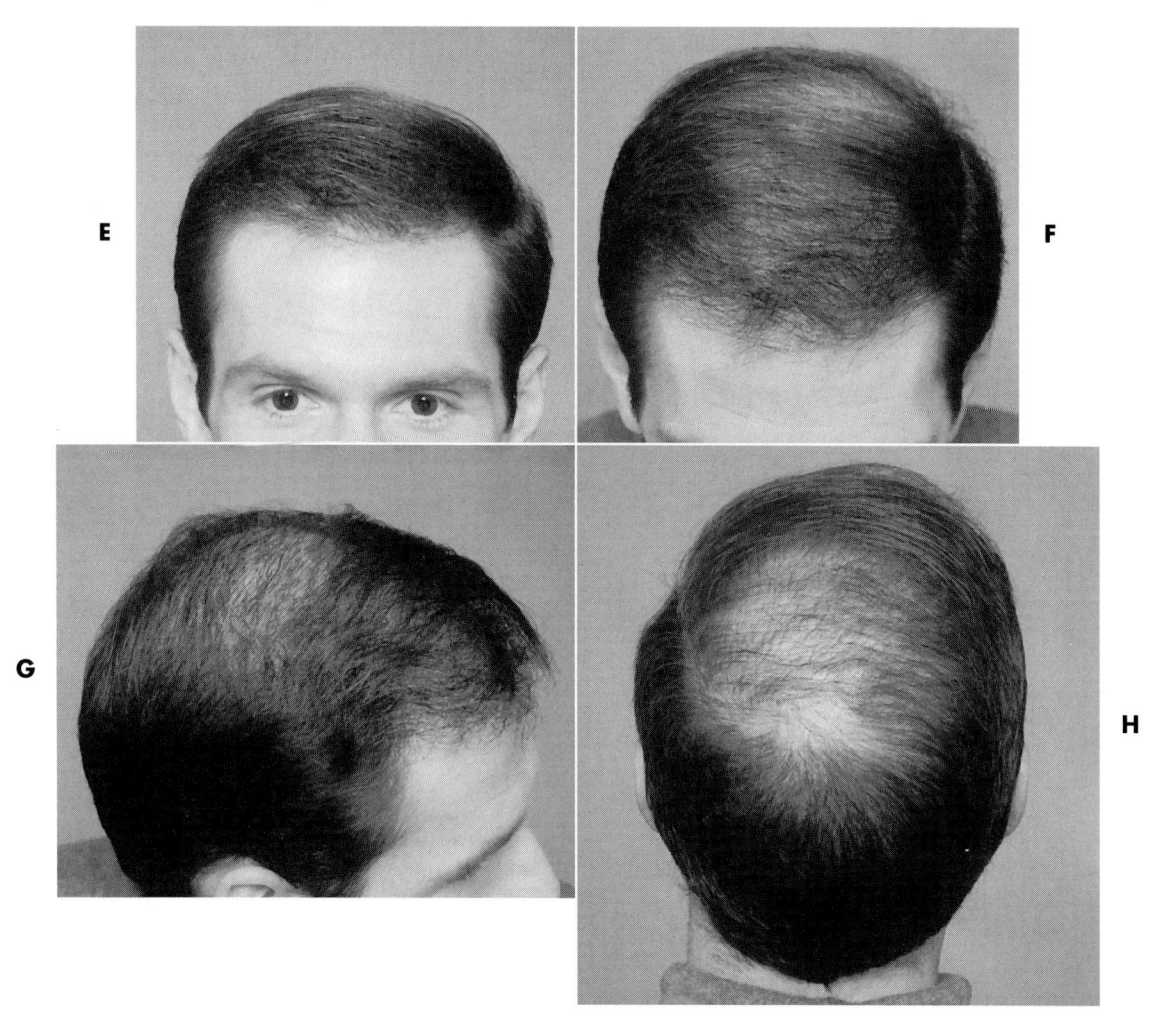

FIG. 6-6, cont'd **E,** Frontal view of patient after 7 months. **F,** Top view after 7 months. **G,** Right lateral view after 7 months. **H,** Crown view after 7 months.

Consequently, fewer surgeries will be required. From a patient's perspective, the problems with many repetitive surgeries that, at 100 grafts per session, may take years to complete have been solved. The only liabilities associated with dense packing of grafts are the staffing and technical needs associated with delivering the service; no negative side effects or complications have been manifested in the hundreds of patients who have undergone this procedure in the experience of Limmer, Swinehart, Stough (personal communications) or myself.

ESTIMATION OF THE NUMBER OF GRAFTS REQUIRED
Table 6-1 reflects an estimate of the grafts required on the basis of the Norwood classification of hair loss. The table is based on a three-hair graft standard. When two-hair grafts are used (often when the hair type is black, straight, and coarse), these numbers must be adjusted appropriately to the differential in bulk. The use of single- and two-hair grafts in building the transition zone in frontal or side hairlines is not calculated in these estimates. These estimates reflect the amount of work required to meet reasonable expectations in 50% of patients.

ESTIMATION OF THE AMOUNT OF DONOR SKIN NEEDED TO PRODUCE DESIRED HAIR TRANSPLANT RESULTS
Calculations of hair density are critical in estimating the number of grafts required. If the desired number of grafts required in any one session is 1000, then a person with a density of 1000 hairs per square inch should provide the required grafts in 4 square inches of donor skin. Waste, variable densities, and cutting techniques must be taken into account when these calculations are made.

TABLE 6-1 Estimation of Number of Grafts Needed According to Norwood Classification

NORWOOD TYPE	TOTAL NO. OF GRAFTS
III	500-1000
IV	800-1400
V	1200-3000
VI	1800-3500
VII	2000-5000

TABLE 6-2 Hair Density and Number of Grafts

HAIR DENSITY (NO. OF HAIRS/MM^2)	NO. OF THREE-HAIR GRAFTS	TOTAL NO. OF HAIRS
1.5	1500+	6000
2	3000+	12,000
2.5	4500+	14,000
3	6000+	18,000
3.5	8000+	24,000
4	10,000+	30,000

MATCHING THE NUMBER OF RECIPIENT SITES TO THE NUMBER OF GRAFTS

Matching the number of recipient sites to the number of grafts becomes a major personnel "management" problem. Careful, experienced technicians can produce between 100 to 200 grafts per hour in an unscarred scalp. On average, 150 grafts per hour is a reasonable estimate for staffing purposes. Careful accounting is critical, and the coordination of people becomes more of a problem than would be expected. Statistical sampling techniques may be incorporated to accurately estimate the final graft count so the number of holes does not exceed the number of grafts, thus permitting the design of the recipient sites to proceed expeditiously. Mathematical calculations alone do not suffice. After the removal of more than 8 square inches of donor scalp and estimation of the number of grafts on the basis of hair density, modification of those projections are best exploited with a computer-assisted statistical sampling program easily built with conventional spreadsheet software. The design of the recipient array of grafts requires accurate estimates of the number of grafts, and such a program will produce the needed accuracy for projections in the shortest period.

DEVELOPING A MASTER PLAN
Progressive Hair Loss

It is critically important to recognize that the hair-loss process will continue after the initial reconstruction is complete. The surgeon must project a "worst case" hair-loss pattern and imagine, both before and after transplantation, a head void of all remaining hair in the anticipated hair-loss pattern.

All too frequently, frontal hairlines are produced "out of balance" with the final hair-loss pattern. As recession continues after transplantation of the frontal area, the transplanted grafts will be viewed from the rear, and as such they may become visible. If large grafts are used behind the hairline because they are covered by the hair further behind them, this cover will disappear as the natural hair-loss process continues. For this reason, graft size and location must be designed with an understanding of the progressive nature of hair loss. When no long-term view of hair loss is included in the master plan, the end results may not reflect a natural appearance because the hair-loss process overtakes the initial benefits of the reconstruction all too quickly.

In the Norwood Type VI or VII Patient, How Many Grafts Are Needed?

Generally speaking, the balder the patient, the lower the expectations. Usually patients with a complete Norwood type VI or VII hair-loss pattern do not expect to fully recover what they have lost. Therefore expectations are usually modest. Once the hair density is determined, the potential number of grafts can be calculated.

The limitations of the donor area in supplying grafts reflect the measured hair density. The theoretical number of grafts available for transplantation can be calculated by subtracting the number of hairs left behind to maintain donor area coverage (approximately 12,500 hairs in a person with average hair bulk) from the calculated hair population of the donor area (25% of the original hair population). These calculations are rounded and presented in Table 6-2.

The impact of hair density in these persons should be obvious from Table 6-2. When expectations have been correctly established, two reasonable design options can be offered to a Norwood type VI or VII patient: (1) a frame to the face can be built, with more hair placed in the front and less or none in the crown or (2) a balanced, thinner look can be obtained with hair spread front to back, weighted to the front. All the facts should be presented to the patient and the design decisions should reflect the available number of grafts, the patient's budget, and common sense.

What Will I Look Like?

"What will I look like?" is the question most frequently asked and most difficult to answer. This question touches on the issue of adequate informed consent, which is not only a legal problem but also a moral issue. It is difficult for patients to visualize their appearance with a different hair distribution and density. The best way to help the patient to visualize the results is to introduce the prospective patient to another patient with similar hair color, hair type, and hair-loss pattern. When such a meeting is not possible, the prospective patient can perform the following experiment to help to visualize the benefits of transplantation. We approach the problem in writing as follows:

> I am often asked, "How much hair do I need?" or "Will a certain number of hair grafts be enough?" There are no simple answers to these questions, and as your physician, I can only make suggestions that you alone must evaluate and act on. Each person is different and has his/her own distinct expectations. Hair color, bulk, density, and character can have a substantial impact on the final result of hair transplantation. The visual effect of hair restoration can therefore vary according to the differentiating characteristics of each person's hair.
>
> To assess the impact for yourself, try a simple experiment. Take a cutting of your hair so that you have approximately 100 hairs with a length of 1 inch. Line them up on a table side by side (like a fence) and place clear tape directly over the hair on both sides. Move the tape to the area you want to consider transplanting. In this way you can determine what 100 hairs would look like. These 100 hairs will be like 100 small transplant grafts. Larger grafts contain more hair and will have a density magnified by the number of total hairs they contain. The longer the hair and the more the hair curls on itself, the greater the effect of the hair in acting as a visual barrier.
>
> This experiment has its limitations. In a real patient, the appearance of the added density is a composite of various hair characteristics in the existing hair located in and around the transplanted grafts. The expectations of each patient are also vastly different in many ways. What makes one person happy may not satisfy another person. Try this experiment to determine the impact of additional bulk in covering the balding areas you are considering for transplantation and see if this appearance meets your objectives. If not, transplantation may not be for you.

Management of the Low Forelock

What does the surgeon do with a low forelock that persists in being longer and lower than the hair behind it? Traditional answers to this question have produced two hairlines; the transplanted one, which is often too evident, is placed significantly higher than the persistent low forelock. The two hairlines by themselves produce an artificial look that is obvious to everyone, even if the new hairline itself is soft and graded naturally. To understand the problem posed here, one must recognize that the low forelock often persists for years, even when the balding pattern advances significantly into the crown.

I believe that the low forelock must be included in the master design of the hairline. If it is very low, a wispy, thinner low forelock may be required so an unbalanced hairline is not created. Because the use of small grafts does not intrinsically produce the artificially dense hairline that traditional grafting techniques would create, the wispy look can be exploited, preserving the low forelock, which, more frequently than not, is loved and cherished by those who have it.

Placement of the Hairline

Placement of the hairline is the principal topic of discussion at most transplant seminars. Rules that govern the placement of the hairline have developed over many years as physicians have learned the transplantation process. However, rules may be broken, particularly when numerous, very small grafts are used. The traditional rule of threes (the distance from chin to nose, nose to eyes, and eyes to hairline being three equal thirds) does not reflect ethnic background, actual hair-loss patterns, or the desire of the patient and therefore should not become the standard formula for hairline placement. The actual placement of the hairline should be a decision that reflects the goals of the patient, what ethnic background might dictate, and age. Younger men usually want lower hairlines, whereas older men will often accept a higher, receded hairline. Keep in mind that younger men will become older men; thus although the hairline can be placed in its normal position ($1/2$ inch above the last crease of the wrinkled brow), if the hairline is balanced and graded properly with a delicate transition zone, it will look natural for the rest of the patient's life, even if the hair behind this area thins or recedes. Filling in behind a delicate frontal hairline is not a difficult or expensive process.

With the density and distribution achieved with small grafts used in large quantities, the limitations of the older techniques no longer must restrict the placement of the hairline to the opinion of the hair transplant surgeon alone. Despite this radical departure from traditional thinking, there is one rule that cannot be ignored; since the hairline cannot be moved back, do not err by placing it too low.

Management of the Cowlick

Like the frontal hairline, reconstruction of the cowlick is one of the more difficult problems encountered because of the change in hair direction and the resultant swirl that draws the eye to the details of the reconstruction. Straight hair reflects a series of converging lines, which, as in art, draws the eye of the viewer to the point of convergence. I generally preserve the cowlick in straight-haired people and use less stringent standards in altering nature's original master plan as the hair becomes more wavy or curly. Large grafts in the cowlick can become an eyesore; therefore similar grafting techniques, as used in frontal hairline restoration, apply to the silver dollar–sized area of the swirl. Less than 5% of patients have a cowlick in the midfrontal area. These cowlicks are difficult to deal with, and each patient must be evaluated carefully and individually when the reconstruction of the frontal hairline is considered.

Management of the Blond Patient

In many cases, blond hair does not stay blond. Blond hair often turns brown as patients grow older. Some hair turns brown seasonally as sun exposure decreases in the winter. Dark roots are not uncommon. If the blond status lasts, in many cases the hair turns white beyond the fifth and sixth decades. When hair reconstruction of a blond patient is being designed, for safety's sake, the work must be planned as if the hair color were brown, not blond.

Side Hairline: A Value Long Overlooked

The impact of balding patterns on the frontal edge of the permanent rim of hair is similar to the impact they have on the frontal hairline. Side hair recession is almost always present with advanced hair loss. The aesthetic impact of a balder appearing person is reflected in the wider and higher forehead. A higher hairline appears less dramatic if the side hairline is moved medially.

Side hairline restorations offer great impact because the hairs, like the tiles on a roof, shingle one on another. A wispy appearance can be obtained with use of single- and two-hair grafts, and the restoration can often be completed in one surgical session. Great care must be taken to position the hair in the proper direction (inferior and posterior) and to grade the change from side hairline to frontal hairline at the junction area to place the hair correctly. Technically placement of the side hairline is more difficult than placement of the front hairline, but the results from the patient's perspective are usually outstanding.

How Should the Pluggy Look Be Treated?

Thousands of patients, especially those who were pioneers in hair transplantation, have a pluggy appearance. These pioneers frequently have two problems. The first is evident in the chief complaint with a "pluggy" focus. The second reflects a depletion of donor hair, which directly dictates what can or cannot be done. Small grafts placed in significant quantities can camouflage large grafts. As a general rule, effective camouflage can be obtained with the following ratios (with use of a wavy hair character as a baseline):

Hair Color	Ratio of Small Grafts to Large Grafts
Black	4:1
Medium brown	3:1
Blond or white	2:1

CASE EXAMPLE: A.T. is a Norwood type VI patient (color, black; texture, wavy; density, average; hair bulk, average) who received 350 grafts that contained from 10 to 16 hairs each. These large grafts became more noticeable when extensive compression developed. Successful reversal of the pluggy look was accomplished in two sessions that used a total of 1000 grafts containing three to four hairs each in the front, top, and crown and 400 grafts containing one to two hairs each in front of the hairline.

CONCLUSION

Although hair restoration procedures do not truly give the patient a full head of hair, in some cases they give the illusion of a full head of hair. To balance illusion and reality it is necessary to blend art and science, and the relationships between the various attributes of the patient's hair loss, character, density, bulk, and color must be carefully considered. Each and every element must be tied together with a master plan created by the surgeon on careful consideration of all of the qualitative and quantitative variables associated with each patient's hair in conjunction with an understanding of the patient's final hair loss pattern. Proper graft spacing in substantial graft numbers avoids the appearance of plugginess. The use of small grafts will minimize cobblestoning and donutting. The process produces results that more closely approximate the "natural-appearing" expectations of the patient. Ultimately a uniform distribution of small grafts in very large quantities, in which the spaces between the grafts themselves more closely approximate the spaces between growing hair groups, gives the natural appearance of normal hair. Therefore this approach may be the ideal solution to the hair restoration process.

REFERENCES

1. Gibbons RD and others: Quantification of scalp hair—a computer-aided methodology, *J Invest Dermatol* 86:78-82, 1986.
2. Gibbons RD, Fiedler-Weiss VC: Computer-aided quantification of scalp hair, *Dermatol Clin* 4:627-639, 1986.
3. Norwood OT, Shiell RC: *Hair transplant surgery*, ed 2, Springfield, Ill., 1984, Charles C Thomas.
4. Pecoraro V, Astore IPL: Measurements of hair growth under physiological conditions. In Orfanos CE, Happle R, editors: *Hair and hair diseases*, New York, 1989, Springer-Verlag.
5. Rassman WR, Pomerantz MA: The art and science of minigrafting, *Int J Aesthetic Rest Surg* 1:27-36, 1993.

6. Unger WP, Nordstrom REA: *Hair transplantation*, ed 2, New York, 1988, Marcel Dekker.
7. Van Neste D, Dumortier M, DeCoster W: Phototrichogram analysis: technical aspects and problems in relation to automated quantitative evaluation of hair growth by computer-assisted image analysis. In Van Neste D, Lachapelle JM, Antoine JL, editors: *Trends in human hair growth and alopecia research*, Boston, 1989, Kluwer.
8. Van Neste D: Dynamic exploration of hair growth: critical review of methods available and their usefulness in the clinical trial protocol. In Van Neste D, Lachapelle JM, Antoine JP, editors: *Trends in human hair growth and alopecia research*, Boston, 1989, Kluwer.
9. Frechet P: Micro and mini hair grafting using the standard hair implantation procedure, *J Dermatol Surg Oncol* 15:533-536, 1989.
10. Ferriman D: *Human hair growth in health and disease*, Springfield, Ill., 1971, Charles C Thomas.
11. Szabo G: The regional frequency and distribution of hair follicles in human skin. In Montagna F, Ellis RA, editors: *The biology of hair growth*, New York, Academic Press.
12. Alt TH: Evaluation of donor harvesting techniques in hair transplantation, *J Dermatol Surg Oncol* 10:799-806, 1984.
13. Alt TH: Scalp reduction as an adjunct to hair transplantation: review of relevant literature and presentation of an improved technique, *J Dermatol Surg Oncol* 6:1011, 1980.
14. Bouhanna P: The advantage of phototrichogram in hair surgery. Presented at the International Advanced Hair Replacement Symposium, Birmingham, Ala.: Feb. 1982.
15. Marritt E: *Hair Trans Forum Int* 1(3), 1991.
16. Nordstrom REA: "Micrografts" for improvement of the frontal hairline after hair transplant, *Aesthetic Plast Surg* 5:97, 1981.
17. Stough DB III, Nelson BR, Stough DB IV: Incisional slit grafting, *J Dermatol Surg Oncol* 17:53-60, 1991.

Editor's Note

This discussion by Dr. Rassman is very informative because it addresses technical nuances of the use of extensive quantities of small grafts. Will small grafts in large quantities still appear "pluggy"? Dr. Rassman cautions that the end results are still strongly influenced by hair and skin color, as well as by hair texture, density, and bulk. The quantifiable aspects of hair transplantation are often spoken about but seldom recorded in journal articles or textbooks. These quantifiable aspects are skillfully addressed in this discussion. Readers should appreciate the clarity and the distinction between hair contrast, hair bulk, and the character and strength of each hair follicle.

Do megatransplant sessions have adverse consequences? It appears that the megatransplant sessions have now been time-tested. Perhaps we have not identified a subgroup of patients in whom problems or poor growth develop as a result of small grafts in extensive quantities, but the vast majority of patients seem to do well.

The temporal fringe, or side hairline, has long been recognized as an area of recession. However, attempts to perform transplantation in this area in the past have been met with poor results. Dr. Rassman has noted good results with side hairline restoration when small grafts are used in extensive quantities. The overwhelming concern with this approach lies in the absolute need for further graft sessions as this area continues to recede after transplantation. The worst-case scenario would involve a person in whom a bald zone has developed posterior to the transplanted hairline. Time alone will be the judge and jury for this concept.

Many physicians deserve credit for studies regarding hair density measurements. However, the clinical application of hair density in regard to hair transplantation was pioneered by Drs. Rassman and Pomerantz. Due credit should be bestowed.

B. Aspects of Artistic Craftsmanship When Performing Small-Graft Hair Transplantation

Manfred Lucas

Initially, progressing baldness is accompanied by only gradual, creeping changes in a person's physique. However, because hair plays a decisive role in shaping our face and, consequently, our personality, we often observe not only physical but psychological changes in those who are affected by baldness. Unlike their unaffected peers, these persons must often contend with a feeling of loss.

If we as physicians are to provide optimal therapy for patients confronting this loss and the fear thereof, we must first understand how and why a face is so decisively changed by the loss of hair. It is only in so doing that we can, within the narrow possibilities of our art, achieve ideal results that remain acceptable for the remainder of a patient's life despite the changes that will come in the time after the transplantation.

PHYSICAL CHANGES THAT OCCUR WITH BALDNESS

The face is undoubtedly the most important aspect of the personality with which we identify ourselves, and hair is an integral part of the face. Depending on the hairstyle, the features of a face, be it male or female, can either be highlighted or softened. Hair thus makes it possible to give individual form to the face, a quality that is increasingly reduced by progressive hair loss.

Instead of combating this growing limitation, some men choose to take the bull by the horns. They completely renounce any possibility of styling the hair they have left and simply shave all of the hair (Fig. 6-7, A). The head in this case becomes

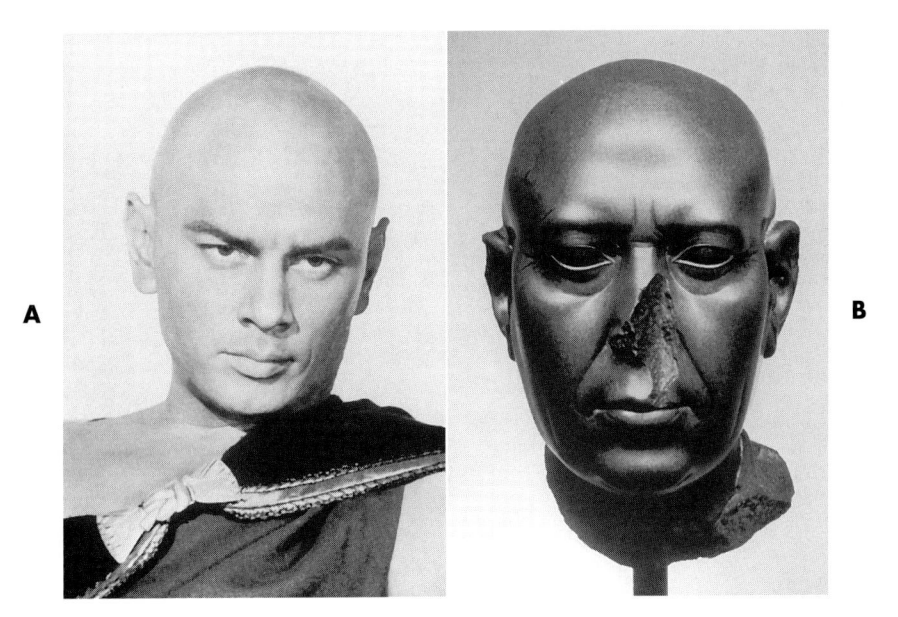

FIG. 6-7 A, Rather than fighting impending baldness, actor Yul Brenner shaved off all of his hair for the role of the King of Siam in *The King and I*. He continued this practice until his death. **B,** The pure form of the bald scalp can take on the appearance of a finely crafted sculpture. (From Interphoto, Munich.)

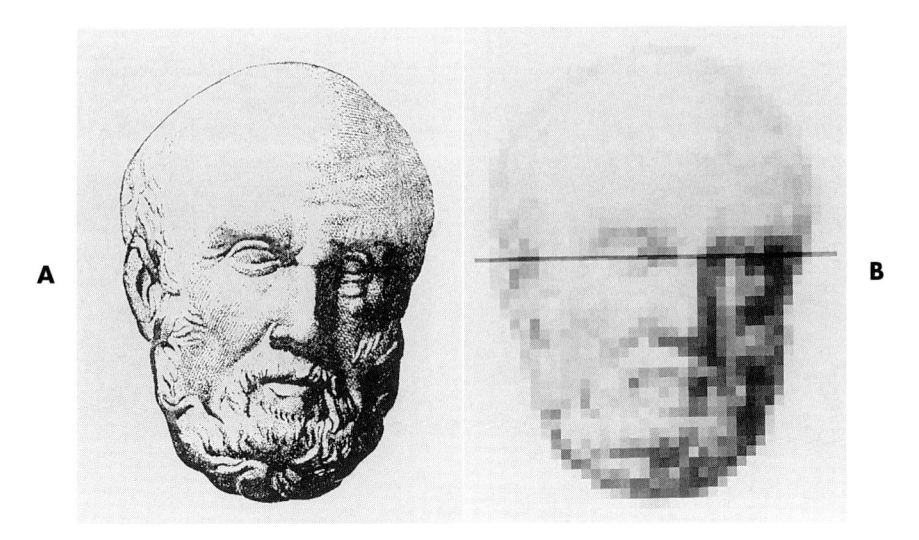

FIG. 6-8 A, Illustration of sculpture of the head of Hippocrates; the lower portion of the face is accentuated as the balding process continues. **B,** The head of Hippocrates distorted by computer. (From Interphoto, Munich.)

somewhat like a sculpture (Fig. 6-7, *B*). In such cases it is desirable to have a pleasantly shaped skull—a prerequisite with which not every soul has been blessed. Complete baldness is a style that seems most suitable for men with a high degree of self-confidence who have found their place in life.

Because typical baldness affects only the upper part of a person's head, the lower part of the face is increasingly accentuated as the balding process continues. We associate this change in proportions with the term *old*, as displayed by Hippocrates (Fig. 6-8). Some men unknowingly intensify this effect by growing beard or neck hair in hopes of compensating for the baldness. As a result, however, the lower part of the face is emphasized even more and, with it, the association with being "old" (Fig. 6-9).

Then again, hundreds of thousands of men take the opposite path: they try to compensate for

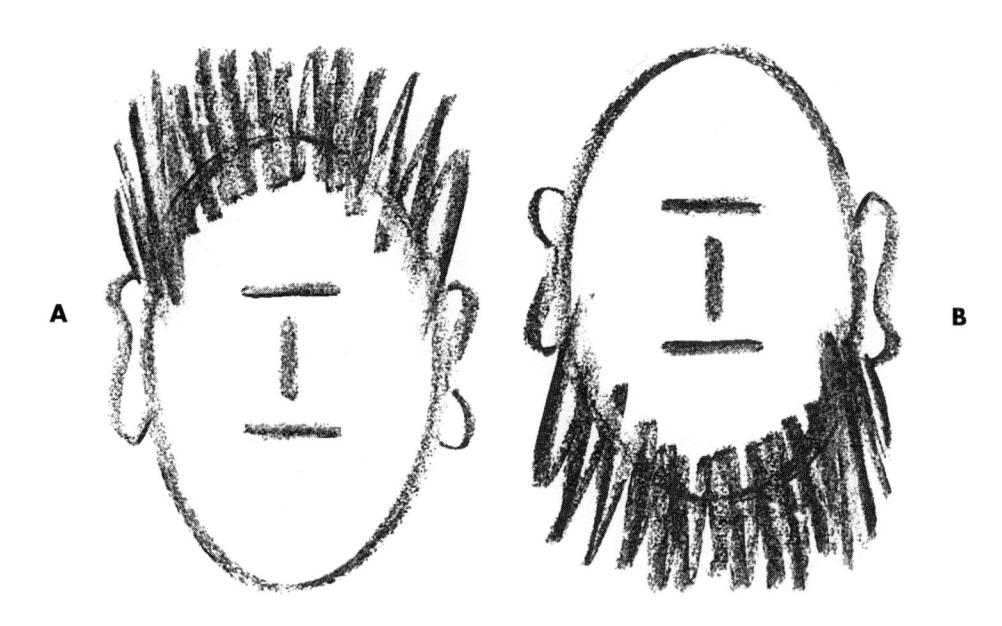

164 Technique—Small-Graft Hair Transplantation

FIG. 6-9 A, Youth is associated with a full head of hair. **B,** On the other hand, when the lower part of the face is emphasized, the perception is associated with old age. (Copyright Manfred Lucas, M.D.)

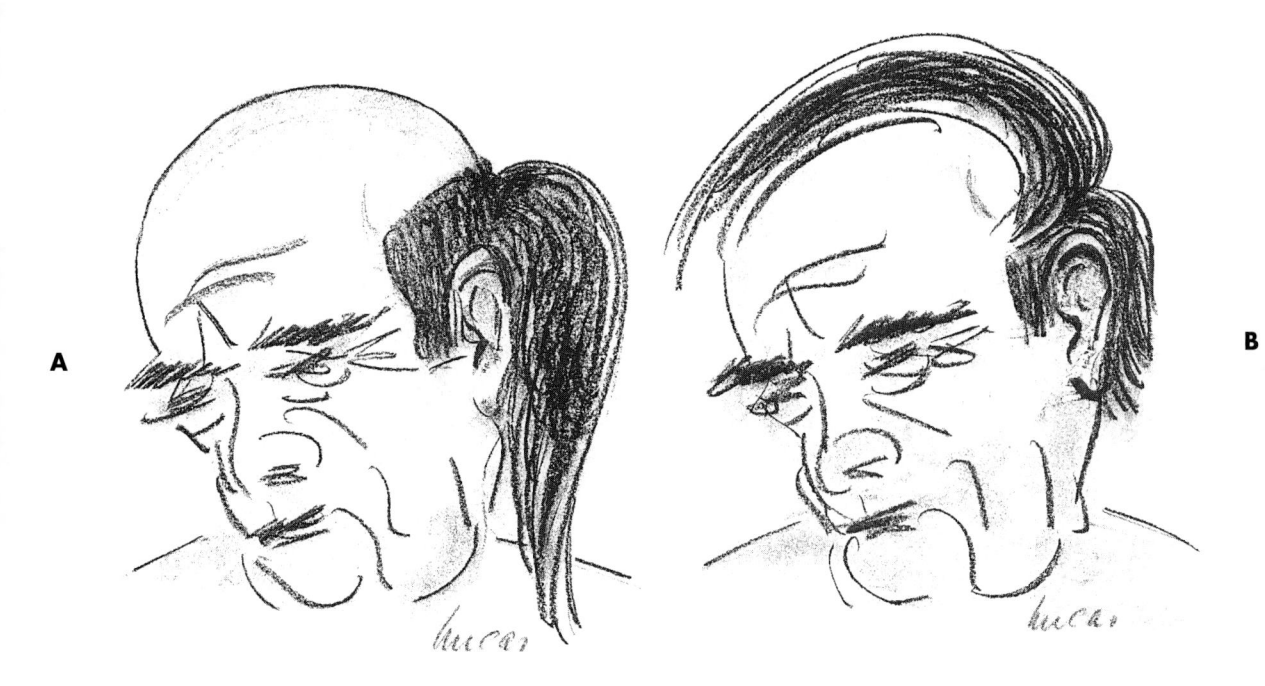

FIG. 6-10 A, "Hermes' wing" effect with long strands of hair along the side of the head. **B,** To compensate for hair loss, the "Hermes' wing" can be combed (or blown) forward, a style often used to depict a caricature of the classic balding older man. (Copyright Manfred Lucas, M.D.)

frontal hair loss by taking long strands of hair grown on the side of the head and plastering them over the forehead. A minor gust of wind quickly turns this masterpiece into a flying carpet. Everybody, even those who have this hairstyle themselves, sees it as comical. Comical though it may be, this hairstyle is far from becoming extinct because it restores predominance to the upper part of the face, an aspect that is a subconscious sign of *aging* when it is lacking (Fig. 6-10). This "youth-giving" effect is apparent even in "stick people" representations (Fig. 6-11).

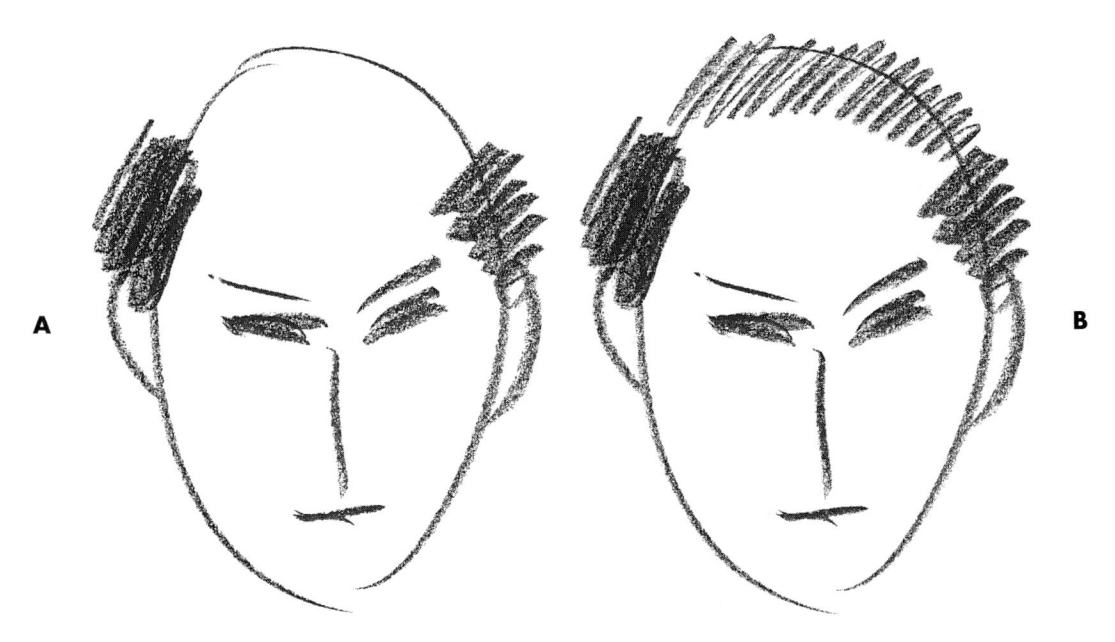

FIG. 6-11 A, One of the characteristics of an older man is baldness even when drawn simplistically. **B,** The "stick figure" drawing of a young man simply includes the addition of hair. (Copyright Manfred Lucas, M.D.)

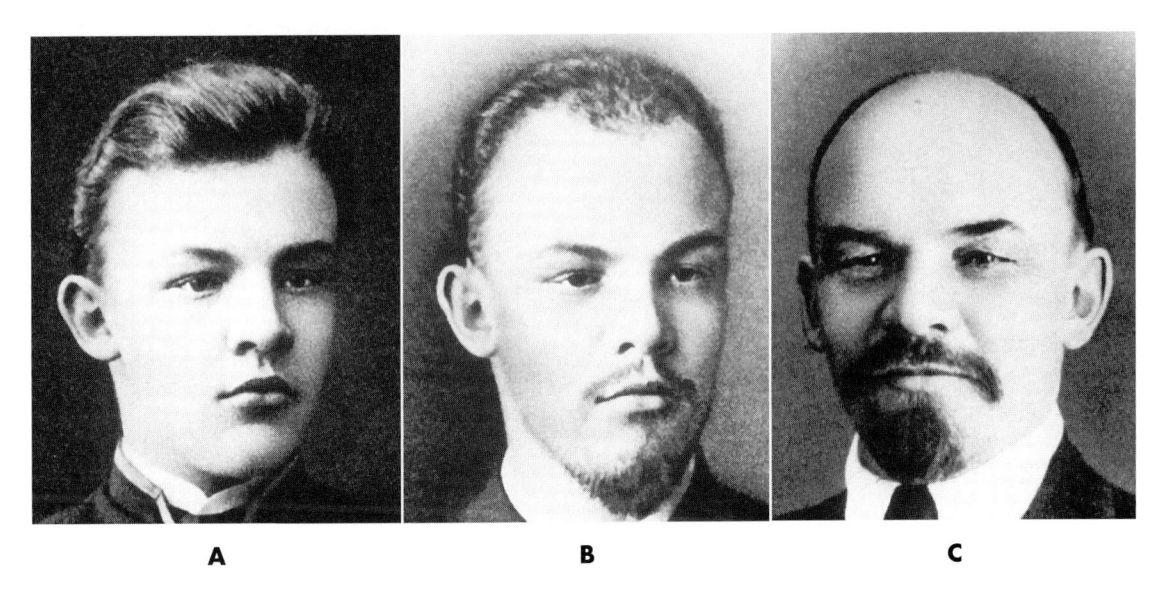

FIG. 6-12 The hairline of Lenin as an 18 year old (**A**) in comparison with his hairline at 38 years (**B**) and at 58 years (**C**). The physician/artist should consider which hairline will best suit the patient's purposes throughout his lifetime, not just during youth. (From Interphoto, Munich.)

A youth-giving effect can be reproduced much more efficiently when the physician places hair taken from a wig, in the appropriate form and color, on the patient's head. Later in this discussion I explain the importance of this procedure in detail.

The key to hair transplantation from the therapeutic point of view lies in restoring the emphasis to the upper part of the head. And now emerges one of the biggest—in my opinion *the* biggest—problem in hair transplantation: we cannot produce new hair; we can only realize a partial redistribution of what remains of it.

Three irrefutable facts should always be kept in mind: (1) the donor site is shrinking, (2) the recip-

166 Technique—Small-Graft Hair Transplantation

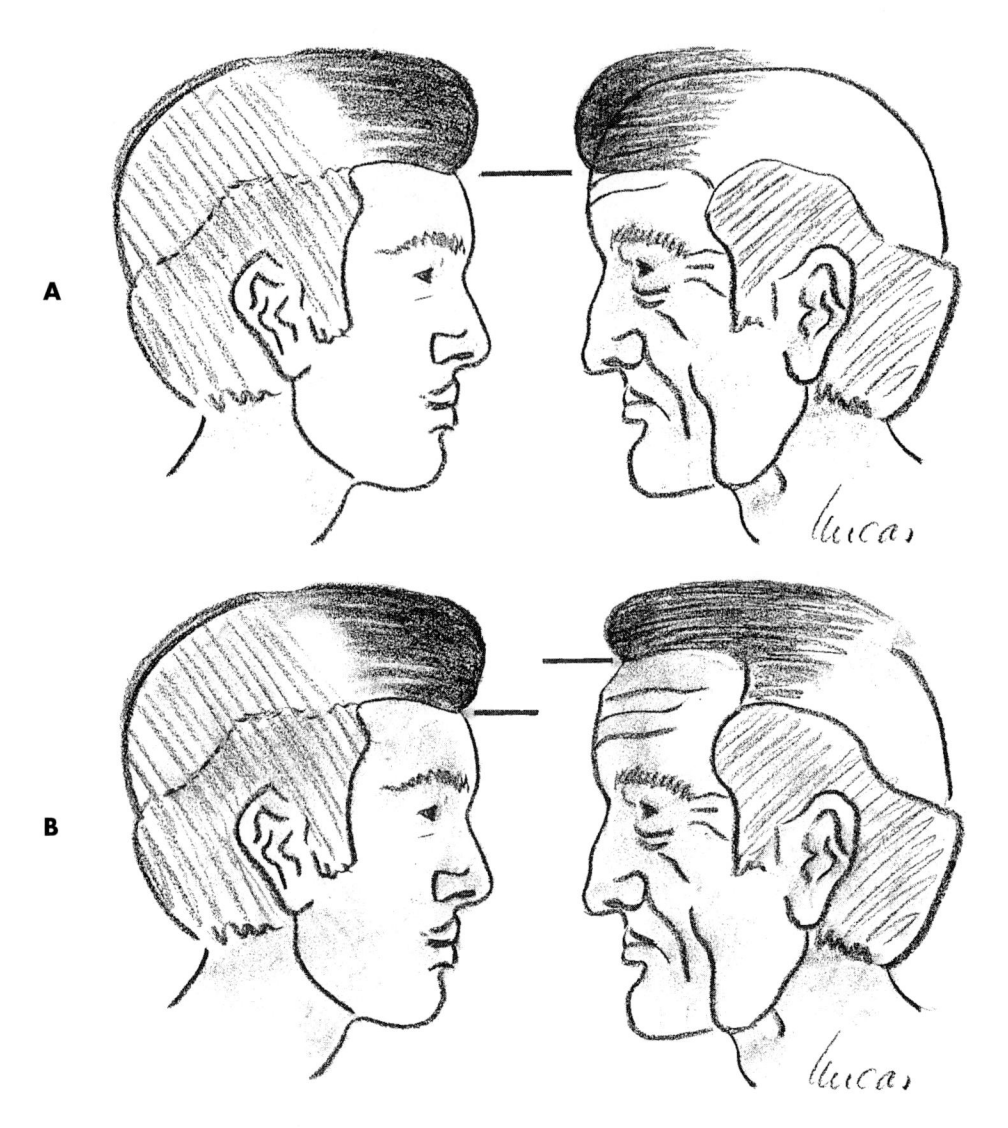

FIG. 6-13 A, If available hair is transplanted in a limited amount only to the place where the original hairline was, an unaesthetic relation between the forehead and the remaining bald area will develop with time. **B,** If, on the other hand, the transplantable amount of hair is placed where the hairline of a middle-aged man would be, an aesthetic result that will last for the remainder of the patient's life can be expected. (Copyright Manfred Lucas, M.D.)

ient site is growing, and (3) the transplanted hair will stay where it has been placed for the remainder of the patient's life. In younger patients these factors must be incorporated into a treatment plan that may extend for the next 40 years.

What other people notice most after a hair transplantation and what must consequently be accorded the greatest priority is the newly created hairline. Let us review the various stages of a human face. Which hairline can and may we restore—that of an 18-year-old teenager, a 38-year-old man, or a 58-year-old individual? This problem can be demonstrated by using the example of Lenin. How would his transplanted forehead have looked at the height of his power? Would he have ever dared to take the platform again (Fig. 6-12)?

Should we all be more cautious, especially when young patients come to us with the request that the hairline of a teenager be restored to their foreheads? On one hand, hair restoration surgeons can be happy that the transplanted hair will grow for the rest of the patient's life; on the other hand, many patients have suffered because that very hair has continued to grow for the rest of their lives in the wrong place. Fig. 6-13 illustrates this important problem.

INCORPORATION OF THESE CONSIDERATIONS IN SMALL-GRAFT HAIR TRANSPLANTATION

Hair transplantation took a major step forward with the introduction of micrografts and minigrafts some 10 years ago. Originally conceived as a hairline refinement after an Okuda-Orentreich operation, this treatment concept is becoming more and more an autonomous method. I heartily welcome this development and have been consistently pursuing it since 1986.[1,2]

Four approaches are currently available for preparing the recipient area for transplantation with minigrafts and micrografts: (1) dilators, (2) slits, (3) holes, and (4) a hollow needle (Choi transplanter).

In my opinion, once the hair has begun to grow it is not possible to tell whether the hair has been transplanted with use of a steel pin, a slit, a 0.7 mm diameter hole, or a Choi transplanter. The only prerequisite is that the surgeon perfectly master his/her method and find his/her own way with the operating team. My team and I prefer to use holes with punches between 0.7 and 1.4 mm primarily because this approach is the only one of the four methods that actually removes the bald skin instead of preserving it.

I abandoned use of standard grafts in 1986 and have used minigrafts and micrografts exclusively since then for two essential reasons:

1. Logically speaking, there is no way to restore original hair density by redistributing the remaining hair once hair loss has set in. Micrografts and minigrafts come the closest to achieving that natural "early thinning look." Flaps, for example, create a completely dense appearance, but this density is unfortunately restricted to the area of the flap.
2. In most cases the baldness formation is still progressing. Gaps that subsequently develop between the hair rim and the already transplanted areas can only be given a soft transition with use of minigrafts and micrografts.

When a patient requests hair transplantation, the following factors must be taken into account: age, hair structure, hair color, hair density, shaft thickness, size of the donor area, and family history. All of these elements play a vital role in the decision-making process. The desired hairstyle must also be considered.

As with any craftsman or artist, we surgeons first have an idea—an image. However, the patient also has an idea, which is more or perhaps less realistic—and thus begins the wrestling match regarding what is feasible. We must make our idea visible to the patient, who can then modify it within the limits of our capabilities. Alternatively, if this potential result is not acceptable, the patient can refuse surgery.

The use of hairpieces, a resource that I introduced, is very helpful in this process. Discarded (and, of course, cleaned) hairpieces can be obtained from any hair stylist in all possible colors and structures. I simply take this hair, cut off the amount I intend to transplant, and put it on the patient's head. In the place of a drawn hairline there is now a living, realistic image. Patients can then integrate their wishes within the limits of what is feasible and aesthetic. A look in the mirror may tell them that they would rather have their receding temple hairline covered a bit less and the midforehead area covered a bit more (Fig. 6-14).

The aspect of emotion is touched on here and must never be underestimated. The patient is looking, so to speak, into his "hairy" future and realizes what a positive change even a little hair can produce.

It is not only the patient who benefits from this imaging effect. Even the experienced surgeon can further train his/her eye by placing hair on a future patient's head; however, this method is of special significance for the beginner, because this practice is how he/she will develop a feeling for the infinite multiplicity of the human face and afterward will never even think of using stencils. After all, every human face is an original, and that it should remain.

Every face is also asymmetrical. Consequently, after drawing the forehead line, the surgeon should look at the patient not only from the front but also with the patient into the mirror. In this way the surgeon can double-check and "reflection-check" the forehead line that has been drawn and avoid the risk of having drawn the hairline too deeply on one side.

We must also make the distinction between the forehead line and the forehead. We see the forehead as the light section of skin between the eyebrows and the darker hair. For this reason it is important to ask patients how they intend to style their hair. If a patient wants to comb his hair toward the back, the drawn hairline comes together with the upper limit of the forehead when the hair begins to grow. In such cases I draw the hairline somewhat lower. If, on the other hand, the patient intends to comb his hair toward the forehead, this hair will later form the optical limit of the forehead, and the hairline can be drawn somewhat higher. This hairstyle allows the transplant "investment" in the forehead area to be reduced. The aforementioned wig hair has proved to be of great use in this decision as well, because it can help the patient understand and consequently accept the more highly

FIG. 6-14 **A,** Hairline on a bald forehead. **B,** Some hairs from a hairpiece make the forehead look higher. The patient wants to comb back his hair later. **C,** Some hairs from the hairpiece make the forehead look lower. The patient wants to comb his hair forward.

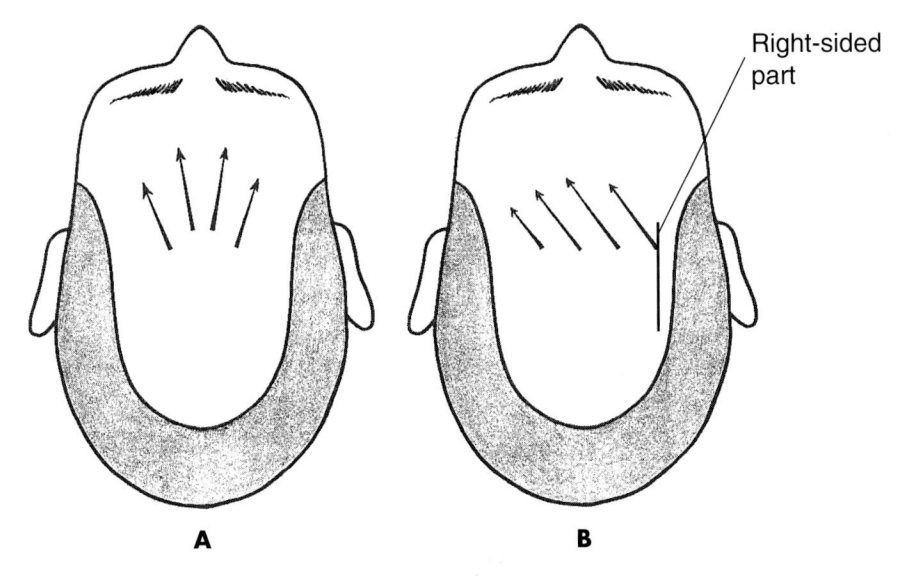

FIG. 6-15 **A,** Natural hair growth extends in a fanlike formation toward the forehead. **B,** With a planned right-sided part, the grafts are inserted in an angle from right to left. (Copyright Manfred Lucas, M.D.)

drawn hairline. Furthermore, it is important to remember that the hairline can always be moved forward in subsequent transplantations but never backward!

Combing hair toward the front or the back is not the only aspect to consider in planning. Where the hair will later be parted also plays an important role.

Seen from the cowlick, natural hair growth extends in a fan formation toward the forehead. We must transplant the hair in this pattern if the patient wishes to subsequently comb the hair toward the back without a part (Fig. 6-15). If, on the other hand, a part in the hair is requested, I no longer adhere to nature's model but orient the transplanted hairs in the desired direction of growth. In other words, on the entire area of the upper head I take the side part in the hair into account by transplanting the hairs slanting away from that part (Fig. 6-16).

Another good tip to remember when creating a side part in the hair is that this part generates asymmetry. The hair near the part will cover more baldness later than the hair further away from the part. The logical conclusion is that we should transplant more hair into the area near the part to make the best use of this "scarce commodity" (Fig. 6-17).

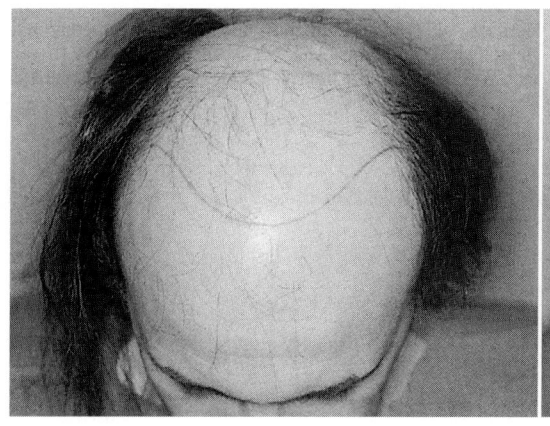

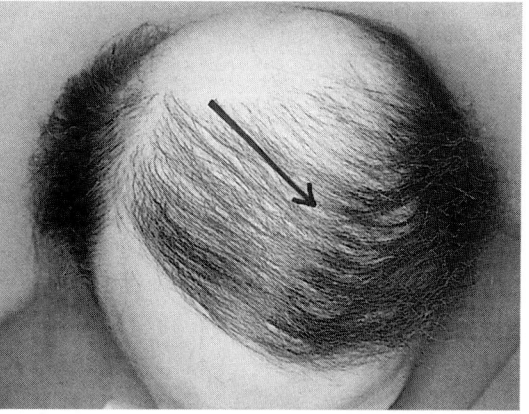

FIG. 6-16 A, Patient with hairline marked. **B,** Same patient with right part. The grafts were angled from the right to the left. (Copyright Manfred Lucas, M.D.)

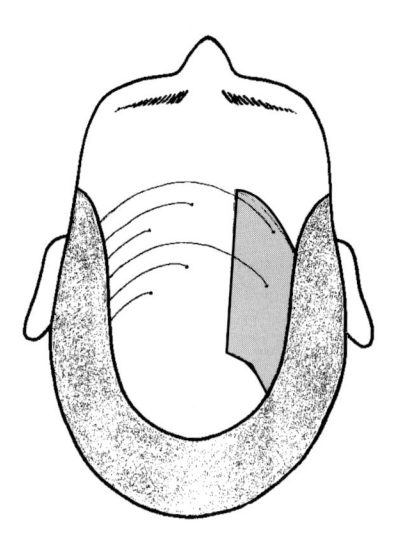

FIG. 6-17 Asymmetrical transplanting of the "scarce commodity." Shaded area represents the zone in which more hair is transplanted. (Copyright Manfred Lucas, M.D.)

The greatest problem zone, as we all know, is the forehead line. In actuality this line is not a line at all but a "no-line," similar to the edge of a forest where the transition from meadow to trees is gradually interspersed by smaller and larger bushes. We realize just how ugly an abrupt transition can be when we see a path that has been chopped and mowed through a forest. Norwood refers to this concept of a soft transition zone as a "no-line hairline." Stough depicts the creation of a deliberately irregular feathering zone to describe a transplanted hairline that is actually a zone and not a stark, abrupt line of grafts.

Micrografts and minigrafts were developed to make the abrupt transitions in hair transplantation less extreme. Just as in nature, it is only logical to transplant micrografts in the front rows and minigrafts in the area behind the front rows. Nonetheless, I do not follow a rigid scheme because the subsequent result still strongly depends on hair color, density, structure, and shaft thickness. If the hair color is dark, for example, the contrast between the scalp and the hair is naturally greater than it would be with blond hair, and wavy hair provides better coverage than straight hair. Consequently, with thick, black hair (which might also be combed toward the back later), it can be best to transplant micrografts exclusively. On the other hand, if a patient has white hair, the best solution can be to use minigrafts exclusively, which in this case does not produce a visible bunch effect.* Finding a happy medium between these two extremes can be learned only through consistent, critical observation of different results.

CONCLUSION

A comprehensive understanding of this subject calls for considerable investment of time and commitment. However, the responsibility for the appearance of a human face during the next 30 or 40 years lies in not only our manual capabilities but also our creative talent. Should this fact alone not be encouragement enough to make us forget all the effort?

REFERENCES

1. Lucas M: The treatment of male baldness exclusively with mini-grafts, Z Hautkr 62:1735-45, 1987.
2. Lucas M: The use of minigrafts in hair transplanting surgery, J Dermatol Surg Oncol 14:1389-1392, 1988.

---

*The use of the terms *micrograft* and *minigraft* in this discussion is consistent with the standardized terminology presented by Knudsen in Chapter 2, Part D; however, I consider five hairs as the upper limit for a minigraft.

Editor's Note

If a picture is worth a thousand words, the drawings by Dr. Lucas should be studied and reflected upon. Dr. Lucas combines literary and artistic talents to demonstrate the benefits of hair and the ill consequences that occur when hairlines placed seemingly appropriately in one's youth display an unnatural effect with age. Furthermore, Dr. Lucas makes a strong argument for a departure from nature's model of hair direction to a unidirectional growth pattern that takes into account the style and direction in which the patient plans to comb his hair. Dr. Lucas gives his advice concerning the placement of the frontal hairline or, properly stated, the placement of a "no-hairline hairline."

C. Hairline Placement

Dow B. Stough

Appropriate hairline placement has been debated for decades.[1] My views have been formed by careful evaluation of thousands of patients who have undergone hair transplantation. Many of these patients underwent hair transplantation in the early 1970s, and a few had hair transplants performed in the late 1960s.

These cases have allowed us to reevaluate previous attempts at hairline restoration. The progressive, relentless nature of alopecia now mandates that hairlines be placed in a position that antici-

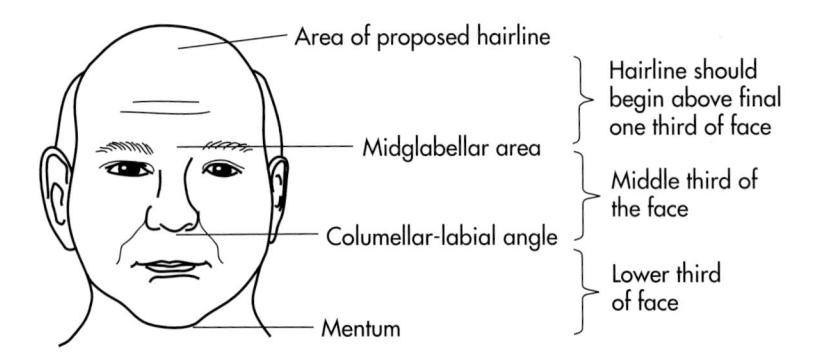

FIG. 6-18 A transplanted hairline will generally begin 7 to 11 cm above the midglabellar area. The exact placement will vary with facial features. Following the rule of thirds will result in a hairline placed too low.

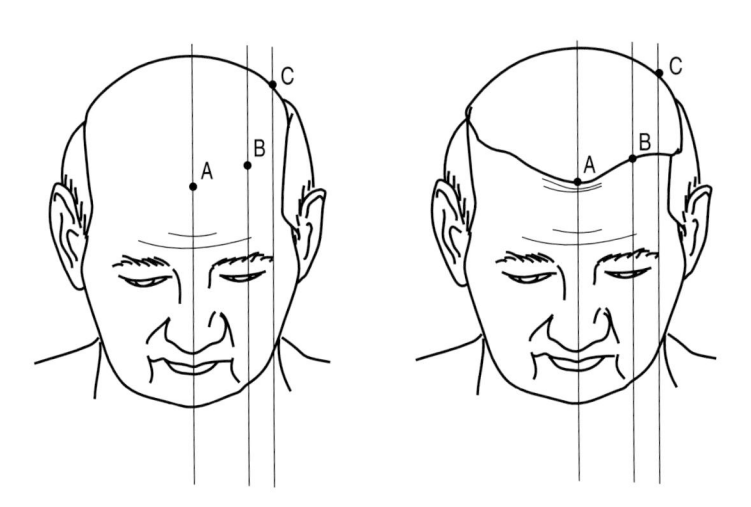

FIG. 6-19 Three points should be drawn, A, B, and C. Point A is midline and represents the hairline starting point. Point B indicates the start of the temporal recess. Point C is the highest area of the temporoparietal fringe. These points should be joined in a horizontal line. The horizontal line will be adjusted and tapered for the area of the frontal recess. This design avoids the bowl-shaped hairlines common in the 1970s. See Appendix D for more detailed instructions.

Hairline Placement **171**

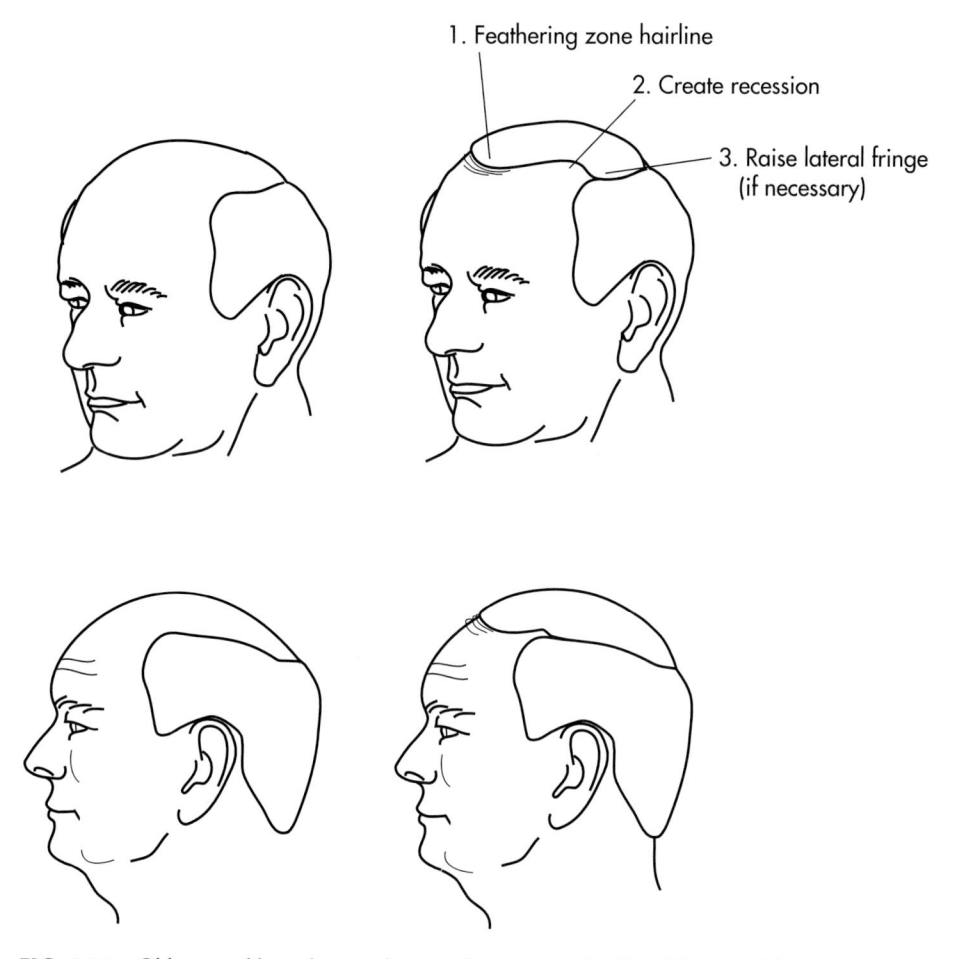

1. Feathering zone hairline
2. Create recession
3. Raise lateral fringe (if necessary)

FIG. 6-20 Oblique and lateral views showing the proposed hairline. The lateral fringe can be raised 1 to 2 cm if needed. Low temporoparietal fringes may be best managed with a frontal forelock as suggested by Marritt in Chapter 1, Part F.

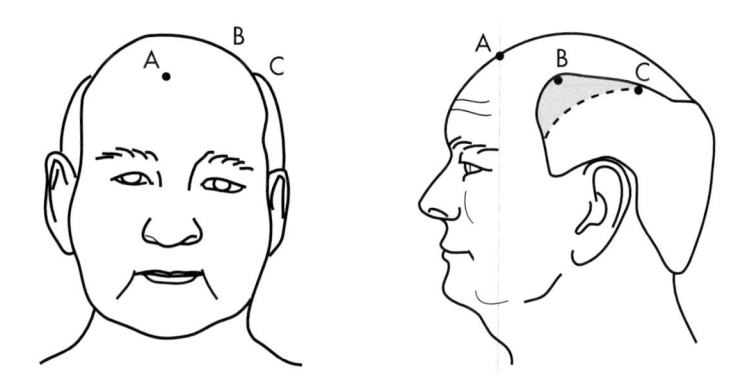

FIG. 6-21 As hair loss progresses, a horizontal line from point *B* to point *C* will be transplanted. No attempt is made to transplant into the shaded area below this horizontal line. Hair transplantation in this region may result in an unnatural appearance as a result of further hair loss posterior.

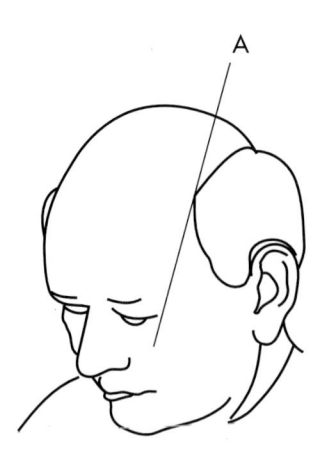

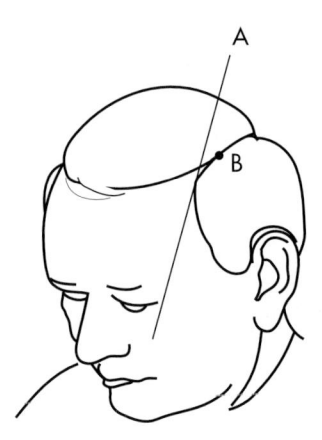

FIG. 6-22 Line A represents a line from the lateral eyebrow to the lateral fringe. Patients with fringes below point B can still undergo transplantation without undergoing scalp reduction. Hair transplantation is achieved by joining hair from one parietal fringe to the other and creating a midfrontal bridge pattern.

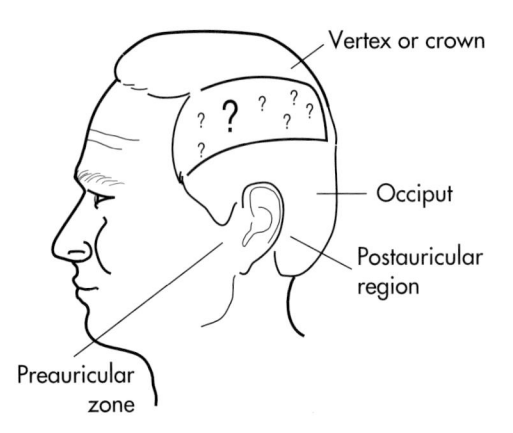

FIG. 6-23 The eventual height of the temporoparietal fringe represents the primary focus of concern with regard to the long-term risks of hair transplantation. An unnatural result may ensue if this fringe area drops in height because of progressive alopecia. This long-term risk is minimized with the skillful placement of small grafts.

pates future hair loss (a subject further addressed by Lucas in Chapter 6, Part B). A hairline that is pleasing to a 30 year old may become disfiguring by 60 years of age. Thus all rules and guidelines must be flexible enough to accommodate the changes expected with aging. The following remarks should be taken only as a general guideline to the placement of the hairline. Appendix D provides more detailed instructions.

Unique facial features will influence decisions to some degree in all patients. Assume that all patients will progress to at least a Norwood type V pattern with complete frontal alopecia. In some patients the hair loss will progress further, but the general principles outlined in Figs. 6-18 to 6-23 will apply. These comments and guidelines do not apply to scalp-lifting procedures.

REFERENCE

1. Norwood OT: Patient selection, hair transplant design, and hairstyle, J Dermatol Surg Oncol 18:386-394, 1992.

D. The Punctiform Technique with the 1000-Graft Session

Carlos Oscar Uebel

Before 1980, choices for surgical treatment of baldness were fairly limited.[1] In 1982, having been influenced by Marritt[2] and Nordstrom,[3] I introduced a procedure called the *punctiform technique*. The term *punctiform* originates from the Latin word *punctum*, which means "point," and refers to the many small pointed incisions that are made in the recipient area. The technique allows the surgeon to transplant 1000 to 1500 micrografts and minigrafts (equivalent to approximately 2500 to 4000 hairs) in one session during a 3-hour period. The outcome is a harmonic frontal hairline with a very natural appearance. Dilators, punches, and hand engines are not needed. Complications are negligible. This procedure is indicated for both young patients with incipient baldness and older patients with more advanced hair loss. Women with alopecia are also prime candidates. Although not all patients receive 1000 grafts per session, our goal is to transplant very large numbers of small grafts in all patients. This technique has been used for the past 12 years with hundreds of patients.[4]

METHOD

The procedure is office based. The patient is sedated with intravenous administration of midazolam (0.3 to 0.5 mg/kg) and fentanyl citrate (1.5 to 2 mg/kg). A long-acting local anesthetic is administered by local infiltration of 0.5% bupivacaine mixed with 1:200,000 epinephrine. We block the supraorbital branches and the coronal circumference of the trigeminal nerve 1 cm beyond the frontal hairline, extending posteriorly to encircle the surgical site (Fig. 6-24).

Donor hair is obtained from the occipital scalp by excising an ellipse that measures 8 to 12 cm long by 1.5 to 2.5 cm wide. After removal of this donor tissue, the wound is closed with sutures. A section of scalp this size typically contains 2500 to 4000 hairs, yielding approximately 1000 to 1400 micrografts and minigrafts (Fig. 6-25). Next the elliptical donor section is cut into strips 2 to 3 mm thick

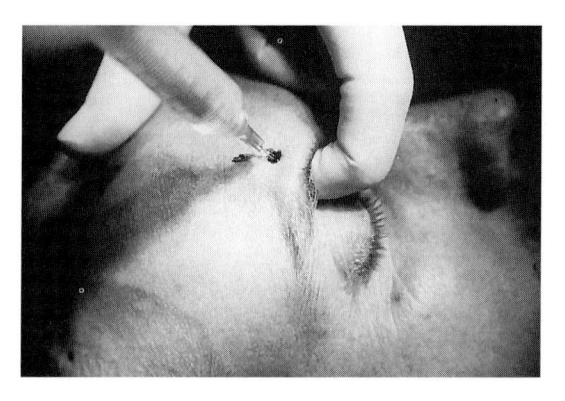

FIG. 6-24 Nerve block of the supraorbital nerve.

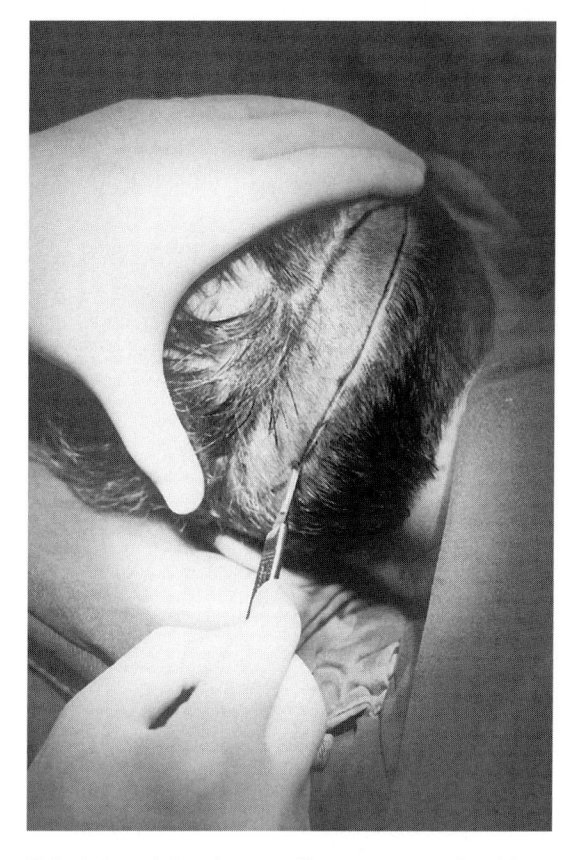

FIG. 6-25 A hair-bearing ellipse measuring 8 to 12 cm in length and 1.5 to 2.5 cm in width is harvested with a single blade.

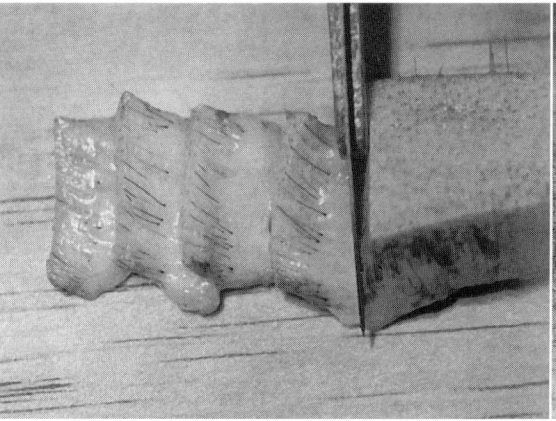

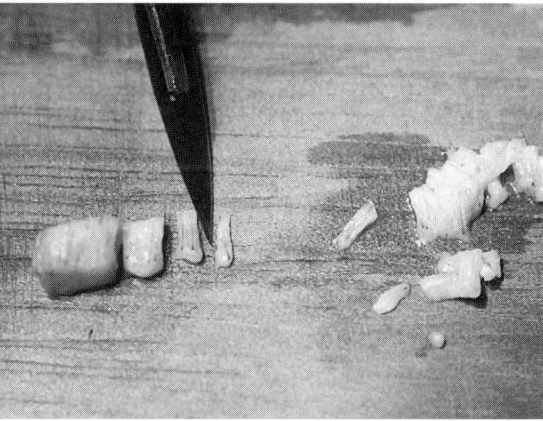

FIG. 6-26 **A,** With the donor section on a hard surface, the ellipse is sectioned into several strips 2 to 3 mm thick. The epidermis and dermis are left intact. **B,** The grafts are sectioned in two groups: micrografts containing one or two follicles and minigrafts with three to five follicles. (**A** from Unger WP: *Hair transplantation,* ed 3, New York, 1995, Marcel Dekker.)

over a hard surface of wood or acrylic (Fig. 6-26, A). The subcutaneous tissue is removed, whereas the epidermis and dermis are left intact. The strips are then divided into grafts, with micrografts containing one or two hairs and minigrafts containing three to five follicles (Fig. 6-26, B).

In an attempt to lessen the bleeding and create tumescence, the recipient area is copiously infiltrated with a solution of 0.25% lidocaine mixed with 1:160,000 epinephrine 20 minutes before the procedure. We call this maneuver "scalp ballooning" (Fig. 6-27). It is very important to wait briefly after the local infiltration of epinephrine for the maximal vasoconstrictive effect of the drug to take place. We typically start the implantation of grafts at the posterior margin of the area to be treated and then move anteriorly over the vertex toward the frontal region. A No. 11 blade is used to make the incisions in the posterior and vertex regions for the larger minigrafts that contain three to five hairs. A Beaver miniblade is used to make the punctiform incisions in the frontal areas (Fig. 6-28). The punctiform incisions hold the single- and two-hair micrografts.

GRAFT DIRECTION AND INSERTION

The incisions are angled obliquely forward in the frontal scalp and directed vertically in the vertex and posterior regions. An incisional depth of 2 to 3 mm is recommended, with care taken to not violate the galea aponeurotica.

Next, with the use of microsurgical forceps with 45-degree angled tips, the grafts are carefully grasped by the subcutaneous tissue and introduced into the incisions. Gently opening the orifice of the incision with the assistance of a blade helps to insert the graft (Fig. 6-29).

At the beginning of this procedure, micrografts should be implanted at 0.5 to 1 cm intervals to avoid possible graft extrusion. After 20 to 30 minutes, additional grafts can be intercalated in the previously transplanted areas. The grafts in these areas should be settled and securely held in place by the formation of fibrin by this time. The final distance recommended between grafts is 3 to 4 mm.

When the surgery is completed, the grafts are inspected for depth and direction. We do not recommend the topical use of creams postoperatively because they may macerate the follicles. Instead, we apply a compress with physiological saline solution and wrap the scalp region with an elastic turban bandage. This type of bandage applies moderate compression and should remain in place for 48 hours after which time the patient may take a shower and use antiseptic shampoo.

Thirty days after surgery, topical application of 2.5% minoxidil is recommended. In my opinion the continued application of this drug for 3 months may increase hair growth during this phase. Alternatively, a 20% solution of jaborandi can be applied. Jaborandi is a natural substance used extensively in Brazilian herbal medicines for the treatment of balding, seborrhea, and excessive oiliness of the skin. Micrograft survival with the punctiform technique is estimated to be 90%. Graft sessions are spaced 8 months apart.

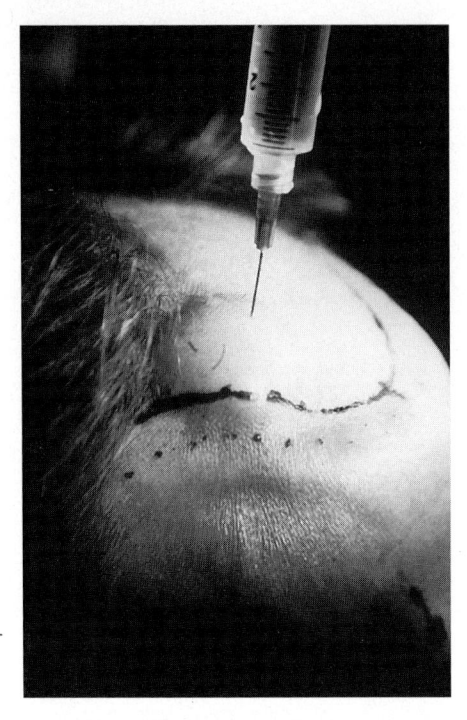

FIG. 6-27 Scalp ballooning. The bald area is copiously infiltrated with a solution of 0.25% lidocaine mixed with 1:160,000 epinephrine. It is important to wait 20 minutes for vasoconstriction before starting the procedure.

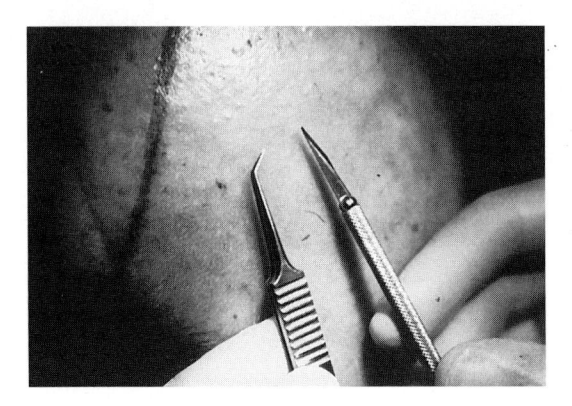

FIG. 6-28 Microsurgical instruments used: a Beaver miniblade (*right*) and an angular sharp-point forceps (*left*).

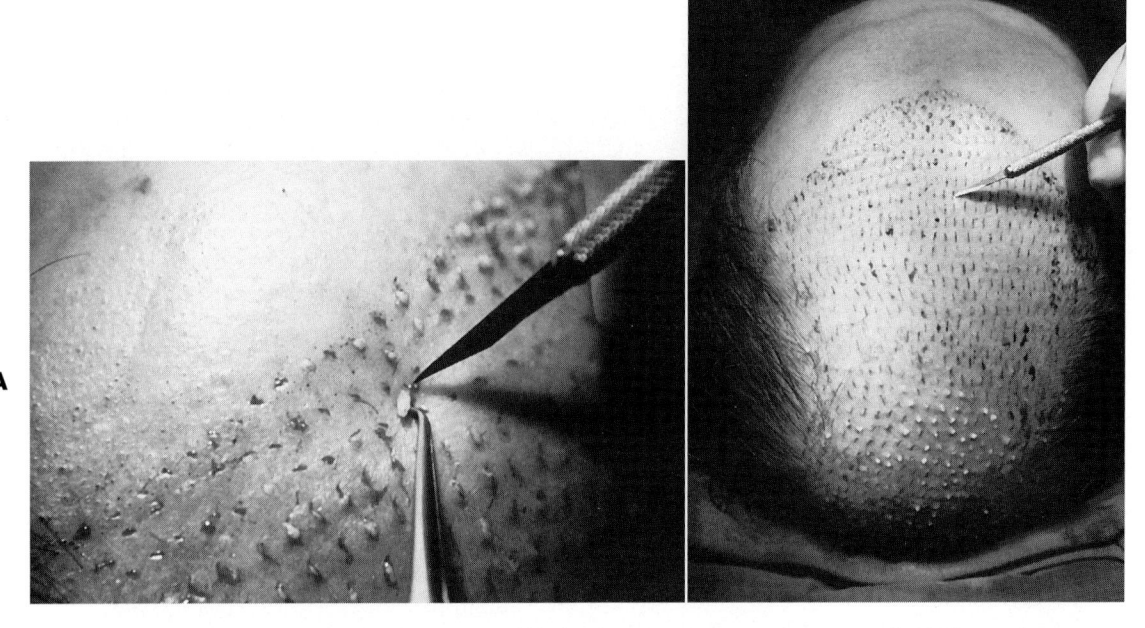

FIG. 6-29 **A** and **B,** With a microsurgical blade, the punctiform incisions are made. With angular sharp-point forceps, we gently introduce the micrografts and minigrafts. We use micrografts (one or two hairs) on the forehead and minigrafts (three to five hairs) on the crown. In this patient approximately 1000 grafts were placed.

During the early stages of developing this technique, micrografts were inserted much deeper into the scalp than they are now. Incisions were originally made down to the galea aponeurotica and follicles were buried completely. This deeper implantation of grafts made for more difficult outgrowth of hair. In these instances the hairs showed a tendency to become curled inside the follicles and often formed cysts. This complication occurred more frequently in patients with thick, tough scalps. With the evolution of this technique, micrografts are now placed more superficially in the scalp, that is, above the galea and closer to the orifice of the incision.

In some patients with excessive oiliness and seborrhea, the formation of small pustules or retention cysts is common. Treatment consists of opening these cysts with a small needle.

Vascular malformation such as arteriovenous fistulas may occur in some patients. Treatment of these vascular anomalies consists of either incision and compression or placement of a nonabsorbable mattress stitch at the fistula site for 2 weeks.

RESULTS

Although the punctiform technique can be used in patients with almost any type of baldness, this procedure is particularly recommended for patients who have bitemporal recessions (Fig. 6-30). Optimal results can be achieved with these patients because follicles can be added whenever hair fallout appears. This technique allows for the transplantation of as many hair follicles as are needed at intervals of no less than 8 months. Patients who have Norwood type II or III baldness will require two to three surgical procedures.

CONCLUSION

Although it appears that the definitive surgical solution for alopecia does not yet exist, we believe that large numbers of small grafts, artistically distributed on the scalp, offer the most natural appearance (Figs. 6-31 to 6-33). The punctiform technique offers patients the opportunity to receive more than 1000 micrografts and minigrafts in a single session with no apparent scarring. Patients are informed that the density of transplanted grafts can be increased in incremental stages depending on the number of sessions desired. No dilators, punches, or mechanical engines are needed.

REFERENCES

1. Alt TH: Evaluation of donor harvesting techniques in hair transplantation, *J Dermatol Surg Oncol* 10:799, 1984.

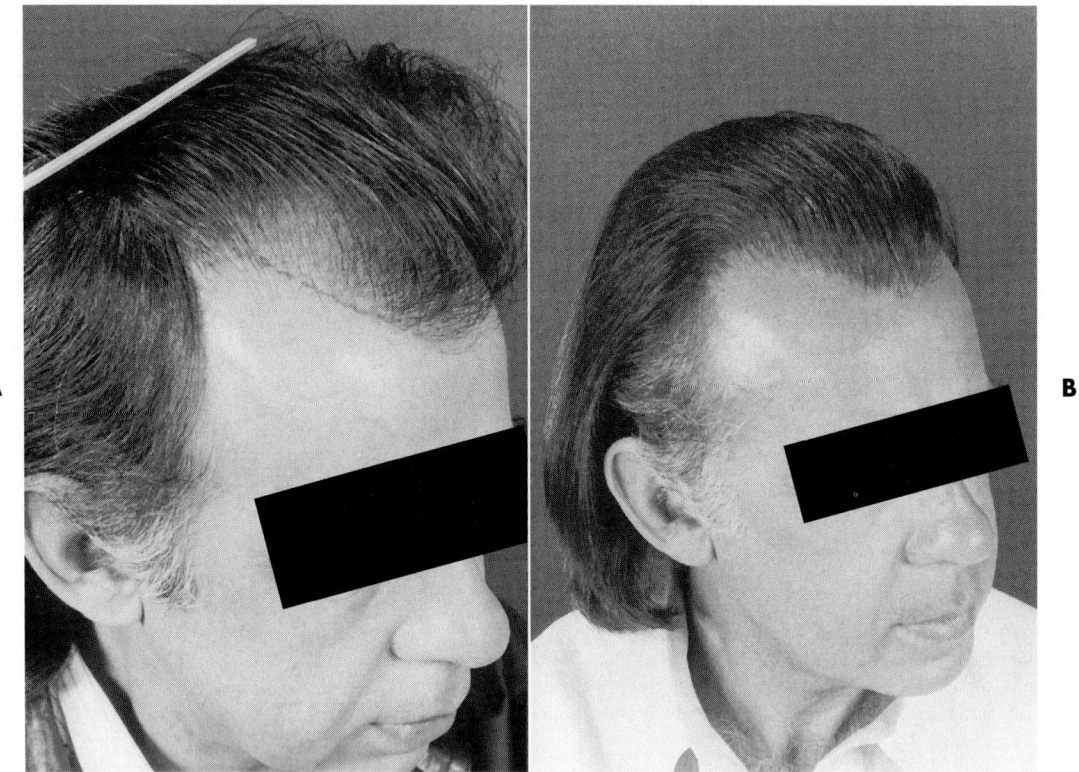

FIG. 6-30 **A** and **B,** This 52-year-old patient underwent one procedure with micrografts and minigrafts. (From Unger WP: *Hair transplantation*, ed 3, New York, 1995, Marcel Dekker.)

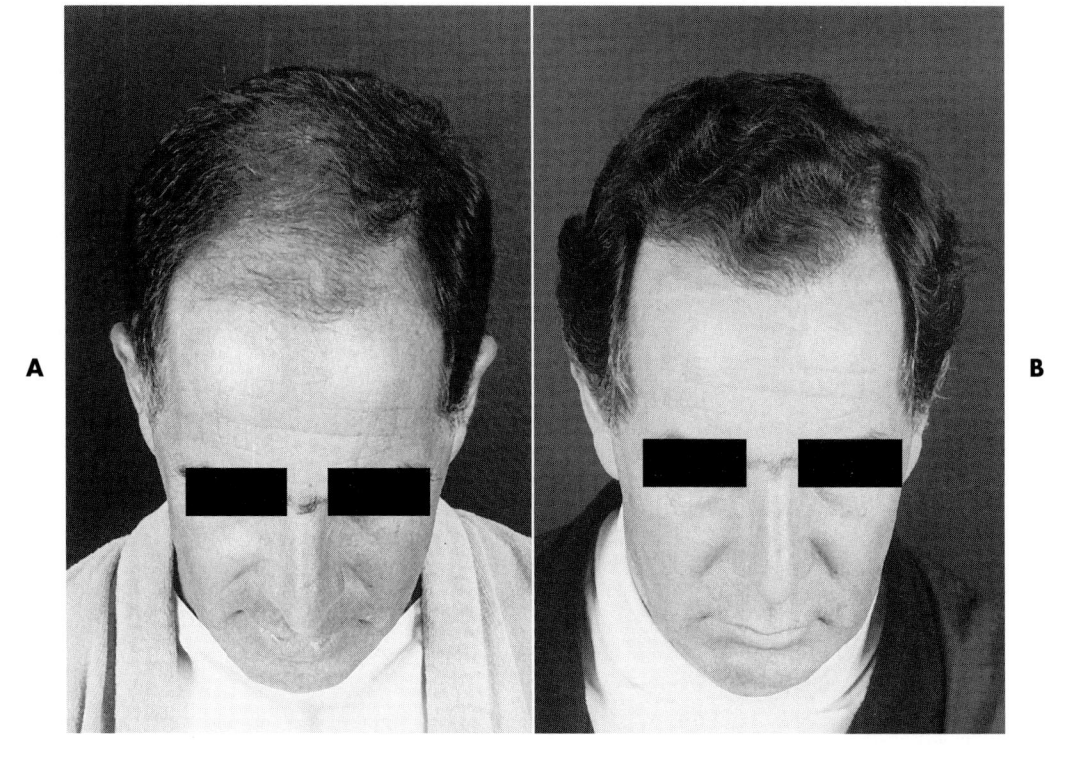

FIG. 6-31 **A** and **B,** Patient who underwent one replacement procedure.

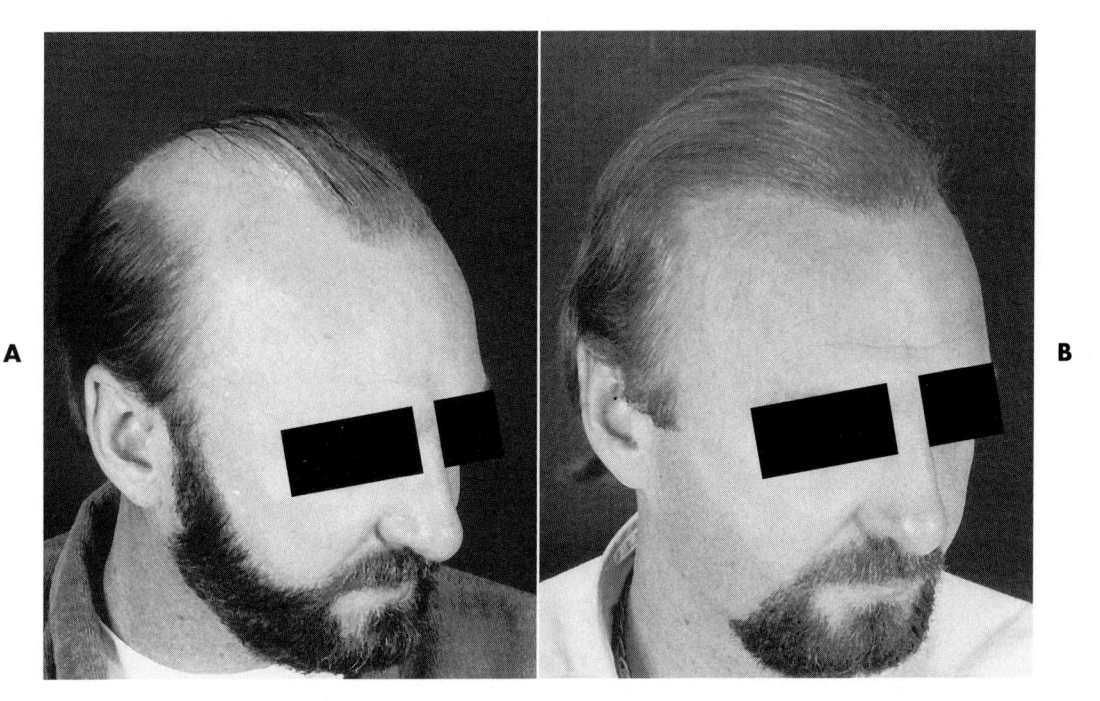

FIG. 6-32 A and **B,** This man is an ideal patient with thin, blond hair. He underwent two replacement procedures at 12-month intervals. (From Unger WP: *Hair transplantation*, ed 3, New York, 1995, Marcel Dekker.)

2. Marritt E: Single hair transplantation of hairline refinement: a practical solution, *J Dermatol Surg Oncol* 10:962, 1984.
3. Nordstrom REA: Micrografts for the improvement of the frontal hairline after hair transplantation, *Aesthetic Plast Surg* 5:97, 1981.
4. Uebel CO: Improvement of the frontal hairline with the angular flap and micrografts. Presented at the International Advanced Hair Replacement Symposium, Birmingham, Ala.: Feb. 1982.

Editor's Note
Dr. Uebel's discussion of the punctiform technique brings forth a wealth of experience in micrografting. The following items bear special consideration:

- Dr. Uebel began to use this technique in 1982 and deserves credit as the originator of the megatransplant session.
- Like most hair restoration surgeons who make extensive use of small grafts, Dr. Uebel's team has achieved the ability to transplant very large numbers of grafts in a very short period. His sessions generally do not last beyond 3 hours.
- A close inspection of the photographs presented in this discussion reveals the artistic quality that is a common thread between all of the authors of Chapter 6. Specifically, hairlines are not drawn and shaped in a rigid predetermined fashion; instead they are created with some degree of deliberate irregularity and scatter.
- The presence of cysts continues to plague those who perform extensive micrografting.
- Dr. Uebel removes no tissue at any time. It is evident from his photographs that this technique of incision slit grafting does not push hairs apart as commonly stated at meetings. His results speak for themselves and appear to have a far superior cosmesis than those of traditional round grafting.
- A compress using physiological saline solution in a turban wrap may eventually prove to be superior to antibiotic ointment. Finally, what of the herbal medicine, jaborandi? Perhaps this substance will be the second-generation treatment to Rogaine!

E. Combination Micrografting with Strip Harvesting for Male Pattern Baldness

Edmond I. Griffin

DEFINITION

Combination micrografting is defined as transplanting small grafts, each containing from 1 to 10 hairs, into both round and incisional recipient sites. No standard "traditional" round autografts (3 to 4.5 mm) are used. Therefore this definition encompasses micrografting, minigrafting, and slit grafting.

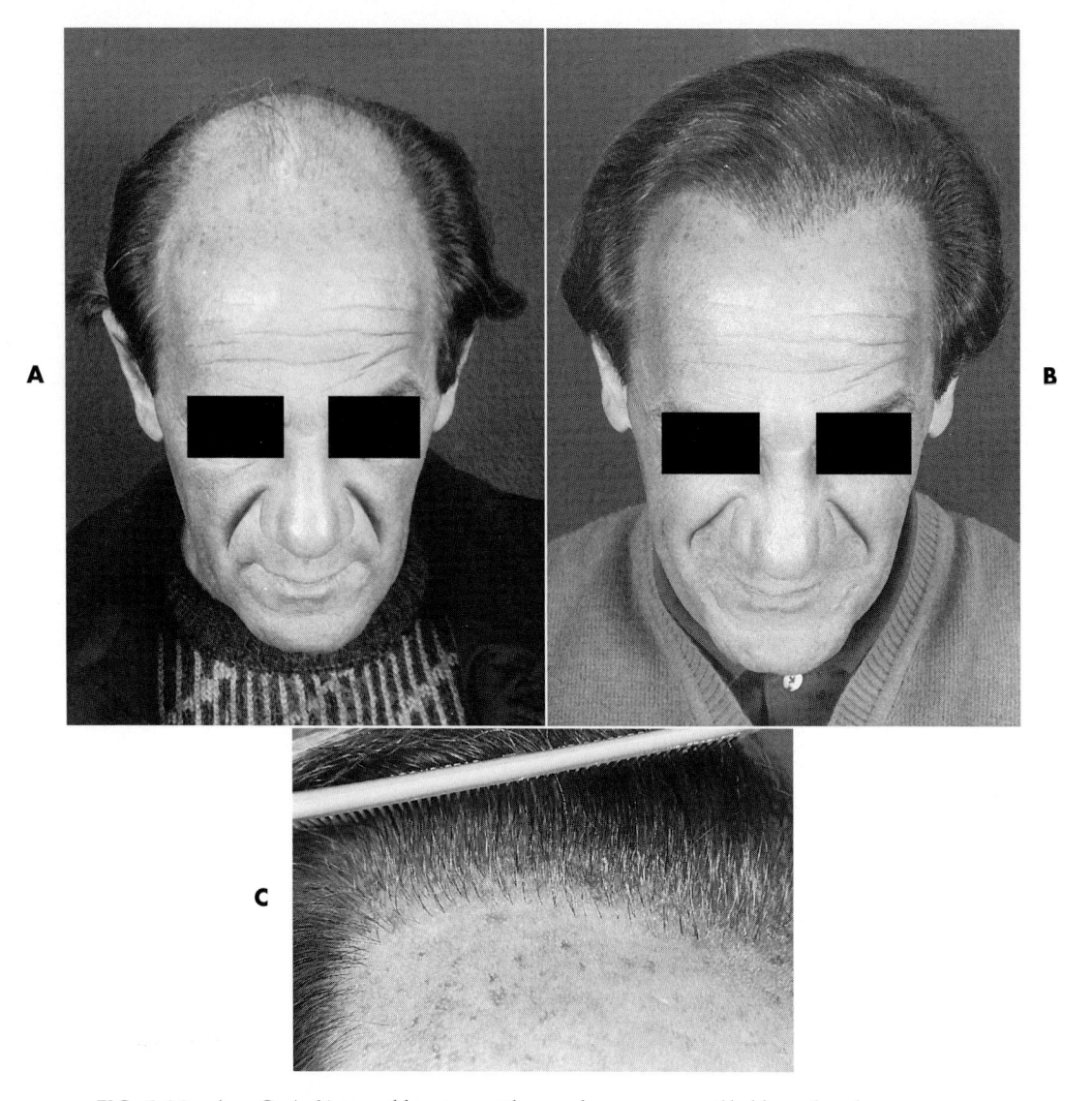

FIG. 6-33 **A** to **C**, A 64-year-old patient with a moderate pattern of baldness for whom we recommended two "megapunctiform" procedures. The resultant transplant can be combed in a variety of styles. (**A** and **B** from Unger WP: *Hair transplantation*, ed 3, New York, 1995, Marcel Dekker.)

This nomenclature is similar to that proposed by Knudsen in Chapter 2, Part D, who also defined micrografts by the number of hairs each contained. Combination micrografting best achieves the main goal of an undetectable hairline and maximizes density and coverage with greater flexibility. Patients with almost all varieties of hairstyles, hair colors, and hair textures can be treated with this method. Combination micrografting has applications in women with androgenic alopecia and helps to transform marginal hair transplant candidates into acceptable ones.[1] This technique can be combined effectively with reductions, lifts, flaps, expanders, and extenders to hide scars and improve the final results.

Combination micrografting is not just a stop on the continuum from single-hair grafts to punched standard grafts. In this discussion, techniques specific to combination micrografting are outlined, with an emphasis on greater flexibility in dealing with varying hair types and characteristics, which distinguishes this approach from standard grafting (see box on p. 179).

BACKGROUND

Early artists carved shapes without detail, with the form gradually evolving into lifelike sculptures. Refinements in any endeavor are a natural evolution of art and a science. Hair transplantation evolved

CRITICAL OBSERVATIONS ON COMBINATION MICROGRAFTING

1. Combination micrografting allows flexibility for a variety of hairstyles, hair colors, and hair textures.
2. Strip harvesting techniques are the cornerstone of combination micrografting.
3. If the scalp is loose and the hair is light and fine, compression is not a problem. Compression occurs with dark, coarse, dense hair and tight scalps.
4. Donor closure may be difficult in patients who have undergone multiple procedures because of tension produced by scarring of the previous procedures. Subcutaneous sutures with 2-0 Vicryl may be used if excessive tension is noted on closure.
5. Staples are superior to sutures.
6. All grafts should be graded, which offers the benefit of an improved cosmesis of the hairline (see text).
7. Removal of the epidermis minimizes complications commonly seen with incisional grafting.
8. Limited-depth incisions may prevent telogen effluvium from damaging adjacent hair follicles.
9. With the use of the fat that is located below the terminal of the hair follicle, grafts can be transplanted into small recipient sites without trauma to the follicles.
10. Some surgical assistants appear to have innate abilities with superior hand-eye coordination, which allows them to excel in the total micrografting procedure.
11. Staff fatigue can be a definite disadvantage of this technique.

slowly during the first several decades of its existence. In contrast, during the past decade there has been an exponential increase in new ideas and more refined techniques credited to many individuals who have been working toward a similar goal of more natural-looking hair transplants.

Hairline

The most obvious problem of traditional hair transplants was the tufting of the hairline. Early techniques produced a thick hairline composed of dense 4 mm grafts from the midoccipital scalp that were usually transplanted over four sessions. Occasionally the results would appear normal. The hairline was the testing site to determine the best techniques for optimal aesthetics. Surgeons began placing smaller and more delicate grafts toward the front, with the standard punches being placed further and further back. A shift toward minigrafts and micrografts distinguished most progressive transplant surgeons.[2-6] The goal was a more natural hairline: "feathered edge," "invisible hairline," "graduated frontal line," and "leading soft edge." Reproduction of a natural hairline required the study of nonbalding men at different ages (Fig. 6-34). The first progress toward a more delicate hairline was made by obtaining hair that was not as dense or as coarse as the midoccipital hair. These finer hairs could be harvested from above and behind the ears or from low on the scalp. Grafts harvested from areas of greater density and coarseness were divided into halves, quarters, and eighths. With this approach the tufted appearance was drastically improved or eliminated. Thus the evolution of combination micrografting was initiated and is now being refined by hair transplant surgeons throughout the world.

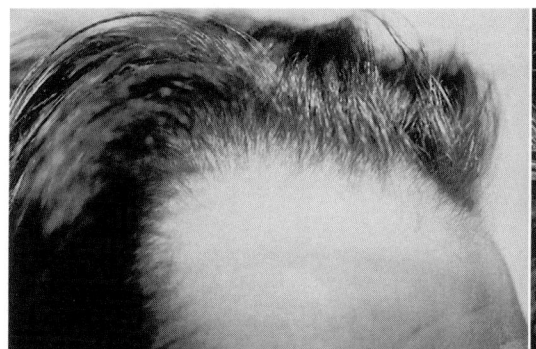

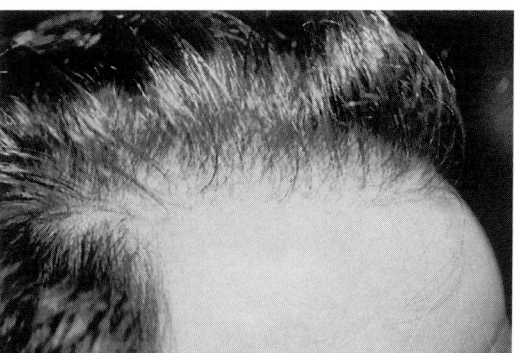

FIG. 6-34 **A,** A 35-year-old man with moderate hair loss. **B,** A similar-aged man after one combination micrografting session duplicating the natural look without tufting.

Vertex

Another area well-suited for combination micrografting is the vertex. The hairline is second only to the vertex in consuming an almost endless supply of grafts. Thickening the vertex with a whorl following the existing natural pattern is desirable[7] and requires artistic skill and attention to surgical details. With large grafts the hair tends to clump, especially when oily or sweaty. Combination micrografting improves coverage and provides more natural coverage with less clumping in fewer sessions. In younger patients who will continue to lose hair at both the hairline and the vertex, I urge a "limited" number of vertex sessions to ensure that an adequate donor area remains for use in future grafting sessions. Conservation of the donor area has been stressed by Marritt and continues to be a chief concern in combination micrografting.

Entire Balding Scalp

Once the hairline, vertex, and early balding areas are treated with the combination-sized grafts, it is difficult to return to standard punches for the remaining scalp.

Three factors are often cited in favor of standard punches: (1) increased bulk, (2) shortened surgical intraoperative time, and (3) the ability to hide large grafts with a shield of small micrografts placed anteriorly and posteriorly.

Combination micrografting uses the donor site more effectively and allows greater coverage with micrografts in areas where they are needed the

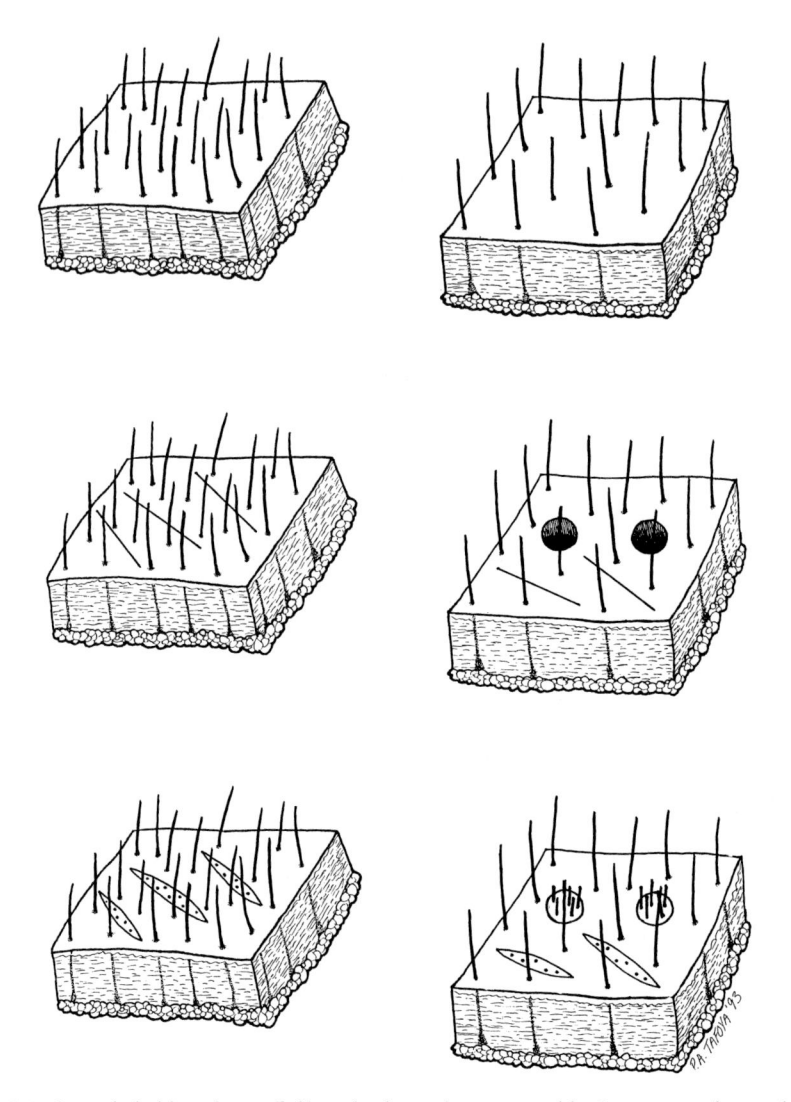

FIG. 6-35 In early balding fringe *(left)*, only slit grafting is possible. In a more advanced balding area *(right)*, both slit grafts and small round grafts can be used without removing any growing follicles.

most. Most important, these micrografts stand alone, blending nicely with the thicker hair but also looking less tufted as alopecia progresses[3,4,8] (Fig. 6-35). Prediction of hair loss in the balding fringes is impossible, even with family-tree studies.

Combination micrografting relies on obtaining large numbers of single- to 10-hair grafts from long strips of hair-bearing skin.[1,4,8-10] This strip-harvesting technique is the cornerstone of combination micrografting. Under direct vision, strip harvesting efficiently obtains large numbers and varied sizes of micrografts without excessive follicular damage. Limmer, Uebel, and Stough advocate strip harvesting for similar reasons.

PLANNING FOR THE SESSION SIZE

The surgeon determines the session size in advance so that the transplant team can use the target number and size of grafts to estimate the length of the strips needed (see Chapter 5, Part B). Unlike other surgeons in this text, I presently use the double-bladed nonangled Vallis knife (Robbins Instruments, Inc., Chatham, N.J.). This knife produces a single 5 mm strip from which 2.25 mm grafts, each containing 5 to 10 hairs, are produced. The angled triple-bladed knife designed by Brandy (Robbins Instruments, Inc., Chatham, N.J.) is useful for producing two 3 mm strips, ideal for two- to four-hair grafts inserted in slit incisions and in small, round 1.5 to 1.75 mm recipient sites. Angling of the handle helps the surgeon to keep the blades parallel to the follicles. Double and even triple strips yield the highest number of micrografts for "all-slit" sessions (Fig. 6-36).

The final graft yield depends on the number of hairs per graft. Proper matching of grafts to recipient sites is frequently necessary. At the beginning of the session, "template" grafts are sized to the recipient incisions or round holes for exact fit. These "template" grafts are used by the technicians as guidelines for sizing the grafts for that session. With this method, proper graft fitting is ensured.

AVOIDANCE OF COMPRESSION

Compression can be defined as an oversized graft being placed into a tight recipient site that squeezes the follicles closer together. Compression can also occur with proper graft fitting. Compression produces a clumped or tufted look. This "Indian filing" or "bouquet formation" is noticeable and must be avoided (Fig. 6-37, A). When single- and two-hair micrografts are used, neither texture nor color will be a concern, and compression will be avoided because of the grafts' small size (Fig. 6-37, B). Compression is worse in tight scalps, when donor density

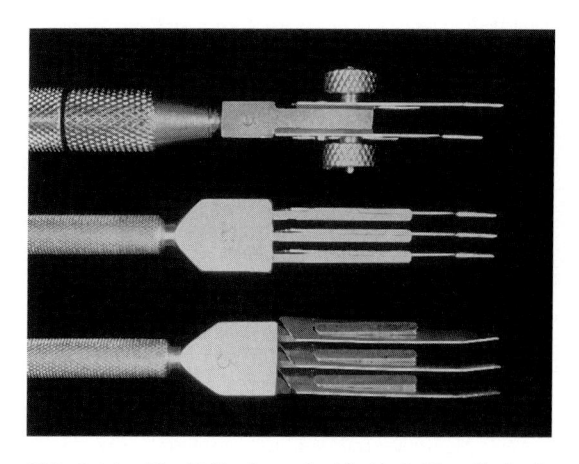

FIG. 6-36 The Vallis 5 mm double-bladed handle (*top*), the Brandy 3.5 mm triple-bladed scalpel handle (*middle*), and 3 mm beveled triple-bladed scalpel handle (*bottom*).

is high, and in patients with dark, coarse hair. When these factors are present, the recipient site must be exactly sized for the graft (i.e., round small circles [1.25, 1.5, 1.75 mm]) or dilated incisions should be used. If the scalp is loose and the hair is light and fine or the donor density is below average, compression is not a problem. In summary, compression is worse in the patient with dark, coarse, dense hair and may be avoided by decreasing the number of hairs per graft and by exact sizing of the graft to the recipient site.

HARVESTING THE STRIP

Before excision of the hair-bearing strip, normal saline solution is injected to stabilize the scalp. The incisions are made with an angled double- or triple-bladed scalpel. The separation of the blades varies from 5 mm on the double-bladed holder to 2.5 mm on the triple-bladed handles. Coated Personna Plus No. 15 blades glide easily and are crucial when multiple blades are used. The angle of the follicles may vary significantly in different areas of the scalp. After a short incision, the depth and angle of the follicles are evaluated. Special care is required to maintain the angle of the blades the same as the angle of follicles when the incision curves. The greater the number of blades, the greater the number of follicles severed if the angle is either too obtuse or too acute. It is precisely for this reason that Limmer advocates the use of the *single*-bladed approach. The occipital artery is avoided if possible. Keeping the incision more superficial by regulation of the downward pressure on the smaller No. 15 Personna Plus blades aids in this

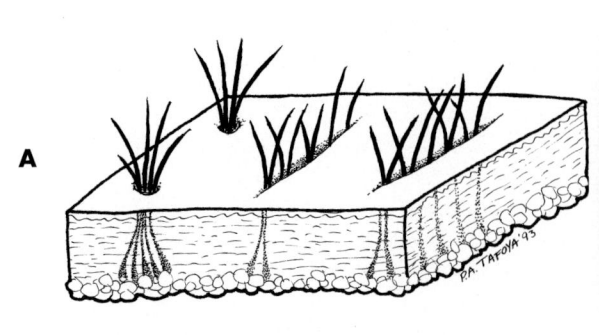

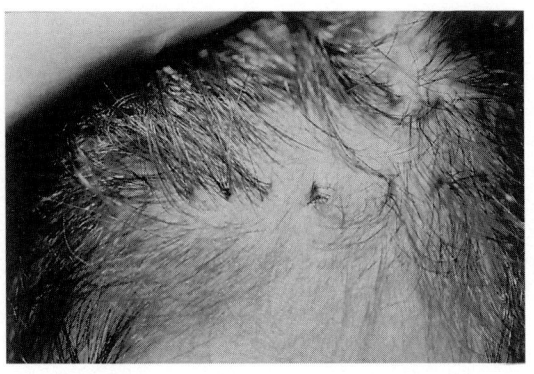

FIG. 6-37 **A,** Types of compression. Note Indian filing *(right)* vs. bouquet formation *(left)*. **B,** Patient with Indian filing compression with high donor-density grafts in tight incisions. The graft procedure was performed by another surgeon.

task. A strip length of 14 to 16 cm can provide approximately 200 grafts varying in size from single-hair grafts to 2.25 mm grafts.

CLOSURE OF THE DONOR SITE

The advantage of closure of the donor site has been stated in the past,[11-13] and there is no easier or smoother defect to close than that created by strip harvesting. Before closure, hemostasis is obtained with electrocautery. Undermining is rarely needed, and the linear defect left by the removal of one or two donor strips is closed without tension. The harvesting of the strip does not require a subgaleal plane unless the strip is especially wide or is harvested under tension. After multiple procedures, tension is more common because of fibrosis from previous procedures. Subcutaneous sutures with 2-0 Vicryl may be used if tension is noted. Two to four subcutaneous sutures may be used after minimal undermining.

I have used staples for many years. Staples efficiently close the incisions without compression of the hair follicles. Strangulation of the follicles is possible with running continuous sutures as a result of postoperative swelling. If additional grafts are needed, the staples can be quickly removed and again stapled for closure after a strip is taken freehand with a blade. If additional grafts are required in patients in whom subcutaneous sutures have been used, extending the length of the original incision is preferred. In a group of 10 patients who received sutures on one side and staples on the other, Stough observed that the patients had less pain and that healing time was decreased with use of staples. Final cosmesis was also superior on the stapled side (Stough DB: Personal communication, May 1993).

GRAFT GRADING

Although some curling or kinking is common, the donor hair generally retains its original qualities after transplantation. The qualities can be graded by the following characteristics: (1) hair texture and color (fine or coarse, dark or light), (2) number of hairs per graft (1 to 10), and (3) shape (slit, round, or stab).

Texture and Color

The fine-textured grafts are dissected from the section of the strip that was harvested from above or behind the ears or low on the neck. If the hair is fine and fair, greater density is desired, and grafts with more hairs are wanted. Compression is avoided by following the guidelines previously stated. In general, the finer hairs are reserved for the visible edges whether they are in the front or back.

Number of Hairs per Graft

Single- and two-hair grafts are designated for stab incisions, whereas grafts containing three to four, four to five, five to six, and six to ten hairs are used for the progressively larger incisions produced by the blades—Omnitome, Beaver No. 3764, and Personna No. 15. In a person with coarse hair, only the smallest grafts with the fewest hairs may be used. On the other hand, in the person with gray hair, no stab incisions are necessary unless the hair is especially coarse or has dark roots. In these patients larger grafts may be used.

Shape

Stab incisions are made for the single- and two-hair grafts regardless of texture. The incisions are sized for the number of hairs for each graft, that is, the

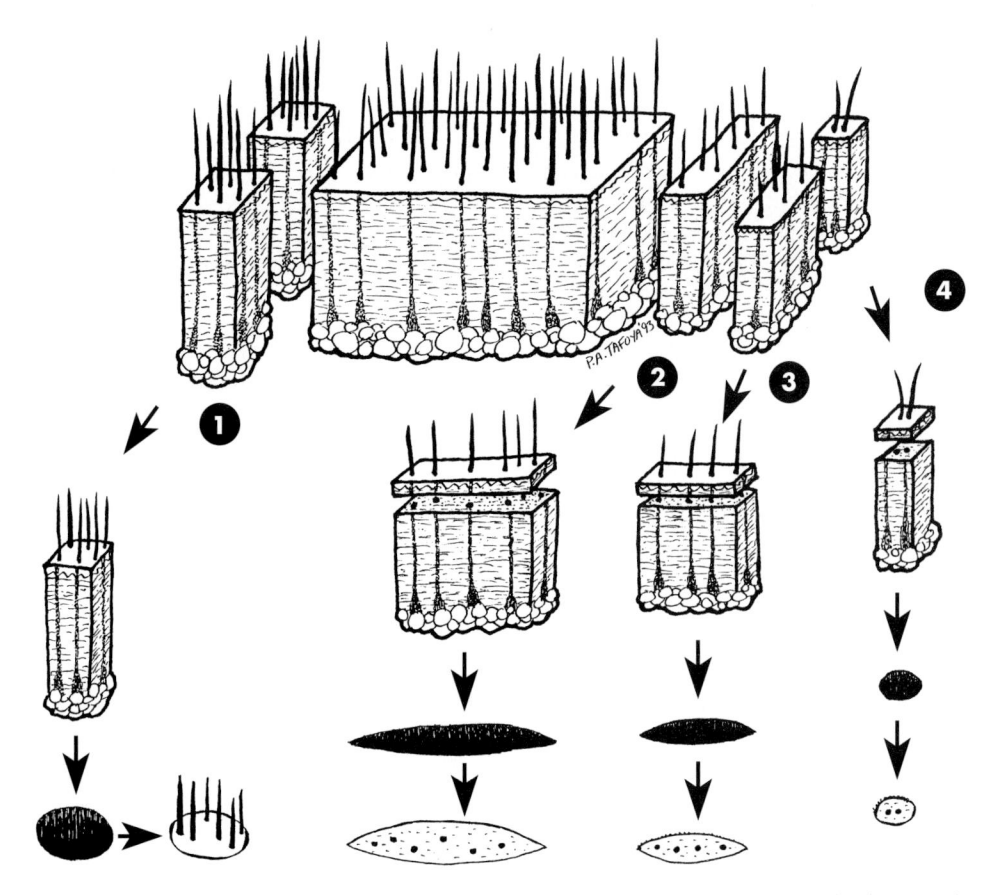

FIG. 6-38 Strip dissection into *(1)* micrograft for the round hole, *(2)* slit micrograft for the No. 15 incision, *(3)* delicate slit micrograft for the Beaver No. 3764 incision, and *(4)* single- or two-hair graft for the 16-gauge needle stab. Note the epidermis is removed from the last three types of grafts.

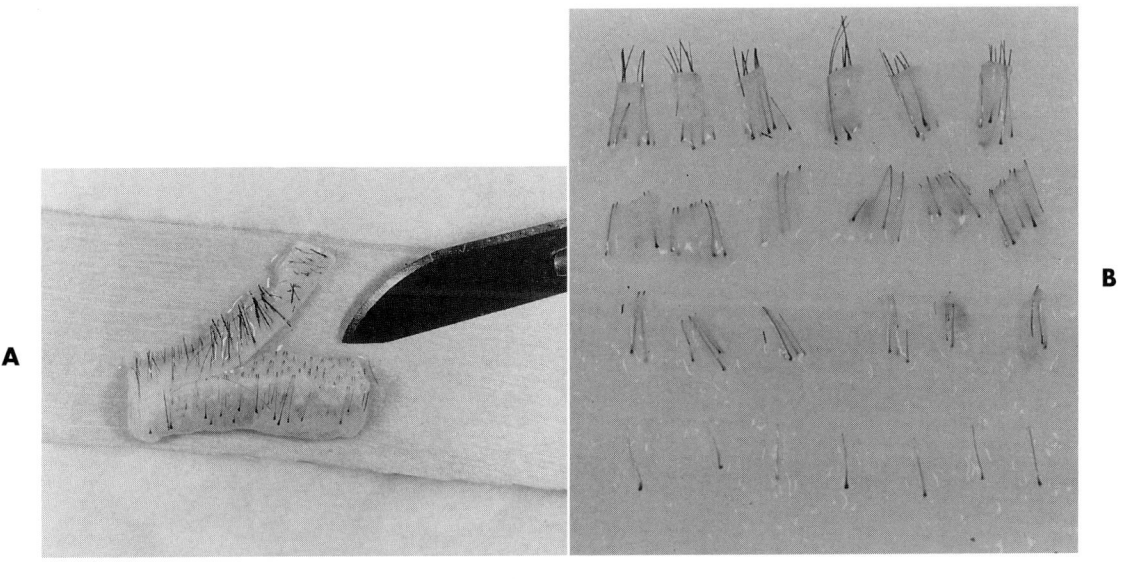

FIG. 6-39 A, Knife with a wooden surface used for stabilization of the cutting field. **B,** Petri dish with a lineup of the graded tufts. The top row of grafts is for round recipient sites. Note that the epidermis has been removed from the grafts in the second and third rows, which are for incision sites. The grafts in the last row are mainly single-hair grafts for stab incision recipient sites.

grafts with three to four and four to five hairs are inserted into the Beaver No. 3764 incisions, the five- to six-hair grafts are placed into the Personna No. 15 incisions, and the six- to eight-hair grafts inserted into the Personna Plus No. 15 incisions. The largest grafts from the donor areas that have the least density or the lightest-colored hairs are for the round sites. The darker and coarser the hair, the smaller the size of the graft, which results in fewer hairs per graft and less chance of tufting. Larger grafts having 6 to 10 hairs per graft are light and fine textured and come from areas with below-average donor density. These grafts may be placed either in No. 15 incisions in the loose scalp or in 2.25 mm round sites. The darker the hair, the more important there be fewer (one to five) hairs per graft with placement in the appropriately sized incision or 1.25 to 1.75 mm round recipient site.

PREPARATION OF GRAFTS

Dissecting a long hair-bearing strip into grafts is faster and easier than dissecting round grafts. Because the strip is flat on four sides, it will not roll like round grafts will. When grafts are being produced from a donor strip, a square cut rather than a round cut is made. This graft tends to contract to a rounder shape rather than remain square because of the dynamic elastic qualities inherent in skin. These square grafts are therefore well-suited for round recipient sites. Strip harvesting produces grafts ideal for slits or incisions; even the broader, more rectangular shapes become oval and fit snugly into the larger dilated incisions (Fig. 6-38). Stabilization of the cutting field is essential to the production of consistent high-quality grafts: A wooden block or a wooden tongue depressor is used as the cutting surface for this task (Fig. 6-39, A). All prepared grafts are graded as previously outlined. After dissection, the grafts are placed on filter paper moistened with physiological saline solution in petri dishes placed on ice packs (Fig. 6-39, B).

REMOVING THE EPIDERMIS—AN OPTION

Occasionally grafts slip below the surface and may produce swelling, epidermal cysts, follicular abscesses, and bouquet formation (in which several hairs appear to come from a dilated pore). The risk for cyst formation is greatest with slit grafts. This minor complication seems unavoidable in patients prone to cyst formation. As described by Nordstrom,[14] removal of the epidermis was intended to allow the deepithelialized grafts to be buried, thus permitting the follicles to grow through the scar. Removing the epidermis reduces but does not eliminate the incidence of these troublesome occurrences. This step requires minimal time and effort to perform. After the strips are divided into 3 to 4 cm segments, the epidermis is then removed from that entire strip (Fig. 6-40). If a small number of loosely placed micrografts are compared and checked and no graft is observed to slip beneath the surface, there is no benefit to removing the epidermis. With large micrografting sessions, however, an occasional micrograft slips beneath the surface. The epidermis is removed only from the small grafts that are planned for the slits and is not removed from any grafts planned for the round recipient sites. The direction of hair growth can still be determined if the epidermis is removed and will be dictated by the angle of the recipient site.

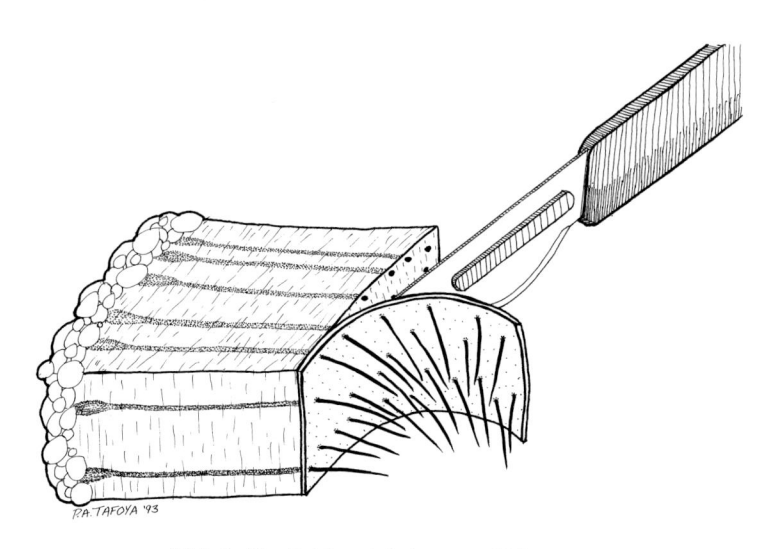

FIG. 6-40 Epidermis being cut off the strip.

THE NATURAL HAIRLINE

Grafts with the highest number of hairs and the coarsest hairs are placed posteriorly. As the hairline is approached, grafts with fewer and finer hair are chosen. With the preparation and grading of the grafts, the natural progression from the hairline backward can be achieved. The grafts that include one to two hairs are randomly placed in front of these multiple-haired grafts to mimic a natural hairline and produce a gradually thickening hairline. If one observes a normal hairline, there will be approximately 2 cm of gradually thickening hair. This appearance is mimicked with the placement of small grafts (1.5, 1.75, 2, and 2.25 mm) in either round punched-out sites or slits (incisions made by Beaver No. 3764 or No. 15 blades). The single- to two-hair grafts are placed anteriorly in stab sites produced with a large bore needle (No. 16 or No. 18 B-D or NoKor needles). The slits are dilated for ease and speed during transplanting; the round sites are not dilated (Fig. 6-41).

LIMITED DEPTH INCISIONS

"Limited depth" incisions is a concept I presented in 1990 at the Facial Plastic Surgery symposium in Birmingham, Ala., and is demonstrated in instructional videos.[15] A hemostat/needle driver can be used to prevent the No. 15 Personna Plus or Beaver No. 3764 blade from penetrating deeply to the galea, thus preserving blood vessel complexes and hair follicles. Dilators bluntly dissect and enlarge the space for the graft and are generally needed for limited-depth incisions.

USE OF DILATORS

As stated previously, dilators help with hemostasis, stretch the openings for the grafts, and assign sizes to each particular incision (dilators mark the sites of the finest, medium-, and coarse-haired grafts). Dilators atraumatically push aside the hair follicles so that shallow incisions can be used to produce a dilated, clot-free opening[5] (Fig. 6-42). Some technicians state that the use of dilators helps to speed the transplantating process by providing a dry field and a dilated recipient site that allows gentle, fast transplantation.

GRAFT INSERTION

The grafts are transplanted with use of the "pull-down" technique. The curved, smooth jeweler's for-

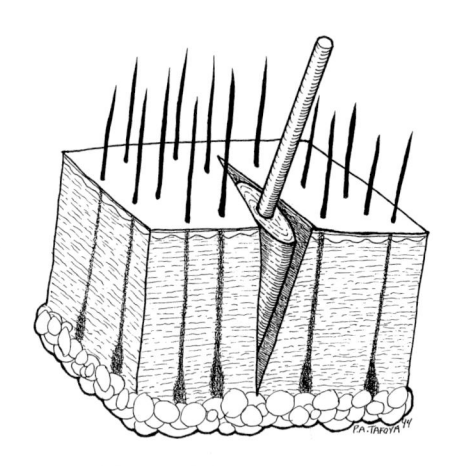

FIG. 6-42 Dilator within incision awaiting removal for insertion of micrograft.

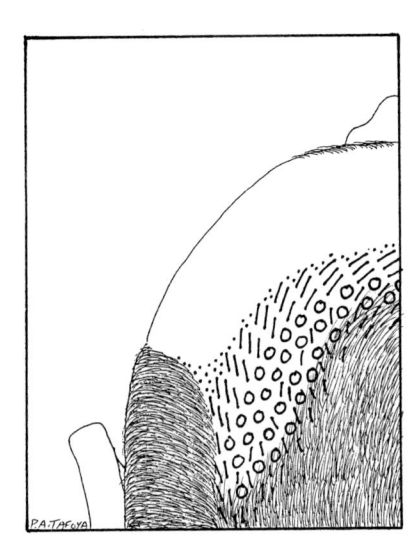

FIG. 6-41 Examples of hairline recipient sites using the graduated sizes from the hairline backward.

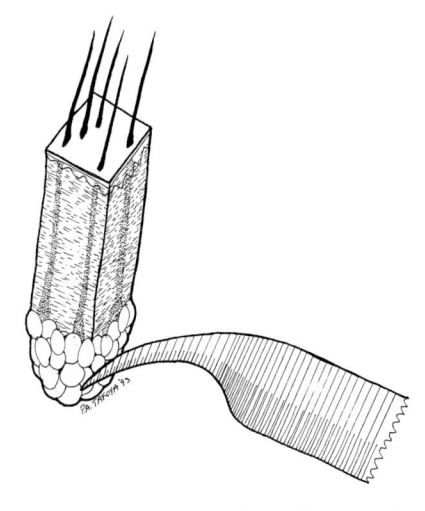

FIG. 6-43 Forceps grasping fat without touching the follicular bulbs.

ceps are used to grasp the fat and pull the graft down into the incision after the dilator is removed (Fig. 6-43). A moistened piece of gauze or a finger is used to hold the graft in place when it is released by the forceps. This technique results in less manipulation and trauma to the follicles, which in theory produces better growth.

ROLE OF THE SURGICAL ASSISTANT

The surgical assistant's role is crucial in combination micrografting. Dissecting the grafts from the strip into large numbers of specified sizes and textures demands special skills. Not all assistants will achieve the desired results or develop the speed and accuracy required. Only those with the best hand-eye coordination will excel in this role. Likewise, the placement of these small grafts requires above-average patience and skill. Staff fatigue in this lengthy procedure will also be more of a factor because of the large number and small size of the grafts.

CONCLUSION

Combination grafting sounds like a stopping point somewhere between all single- to two-hair grafts and standard 4 mm grafts, but it is neither. It uses the best of both grafting techniques and is a flexible situation that is hard to standardize. Multiple guidelines must be weighed and put into perspective according to a multifactorial equation in which the experienced physician's science is converted into art (see box).

REFERENCES

1. Cotterill PC, Unger WP: Hair transplantation in females, *J Dermatol Surg Oncol* 18:477-481, 1992.
2. Marritt E. Single-hair transplantation for hairline refinement: a practical solution, *J Dermatol Surg Oncol* 10:962-963, 1984.
3. Shiell RC, Norwood OT: Micrografts and minigrafts. In Norwood OT, Shiell RC, editors: *Hair transplant surgery,* ed 2, Springfield, Ill., 1984, Charles C Thomas, pp 107-110.
4. Nordstrom REA: "Micrografts" for improvement of the frontal hairline after hair transplant, *Aesthetic Plast Surg* 5:97, 1981.
5. Marritt E: Micrograft dilators: in pursuit of the undetectable hairline, *J Dermatol Surg Oncol* 14(3):268-275, 1988.
6. Lucas MWG: The use of minigrafts in hair transplantating surgery, *J Dermatol Surg Oncol* 14:1389-1392, 1988.
7. Goldman PM: Punch grafting the crown and vertex, *J Dermatol Surg Oncol* 11:2,138-142, 1985.
8. Brandy DA: Conventional grafting combined with minigrafting: a new approach, *J Dermatol Surg Oncol* 13:60-63,1987.
9. Swinehart J, Griffin EI: Slit grafting: the use of serrated island grafts in male and female-pattern alopecia, *J Dermatol Surg Oncol* 17:243-253, 1991.
10. Stough DB IV, Nelson BR, Stough DB III: Incisional slit grafting, *J Dermatol Surg Oncol* 17:53-60, 1991.
11. Unger WP: Suturing of donor sites. In Unger WP, editor: *Hair transplantation*, New York, 1979, Marcel Dekker, p 64.
12. Barnett J: Suturing of donor sites. In Unger WP, editor: *Hair transplantation*, New York, 1979, Marcel Dekker, p 172.
13. Sturm H: The benefit of donor-site closure in hair transplantation, *J Dermatol Surg Oncol* 10:987-990, 1984.
14. Nordstrom REA: Minisurgery: "micrografts," New York, 1988, Marcel Dekker, pp 329-332.
15. Norwood OT, editor: *Hair transplant forum video series*, 1992.

Editor's Note

Dr. Griffin's statement that "the strip harvesting technique is the cornerstone of combination micrografting" is noteworthy. It appears that strip harvesting, whether performed with a single-bladed or multibladed knife, has played a pivotal role in the evolution of total micrografting. Regardless of the specific technique used to obtain a strip, this method appears to be far superior to any harvesting techniques that use a motorized hand engine. Can compression be avoided? Perhaps a more critical assessment of tight scalps with high donor density is required. Dr. Griffin astutely describes patients in whom incisional slit grafting can be used with excellent results. Dr. Griffin has pioneered the use of staples in the scalp, which appears to be far superior to suturing. The efficacy of staples is now unquestionable. Finally, the box titled "Critical Observations on Combination Micrografting" will be of interest and perhaps a topic of controversy for all serious hair transplant surgeons.

COMBINATION GRAFTING

Advantages

Allows flexibility in dealing with different colors and textures of hair
Permits greater apparent density, especially in marginal donor areas
Allows options to fill in deficits completely and according to the size needed
Allows for filling of gaps left by standard 4 mm transplants
Requires fewer numbers of grafts and achieves greater density than single-hair grafting
Affords superior growth from the smaller grafts
Minimizes follicular damage
Avoids tufted appearance
Is ideal for the young patient and the female patient
Avoids dramatic changes in appearance

Disadvantages

Requires decision points and more careful planning of the grafting process
Requires that the staff track the numbers of each graft size and location
Causes greater staff fatigue with longer procedures
Requires specialized equipment
Requires talented support staff

F. The Origins of Single-Hair Grafting

Dow B. Stough and Shiro Yamada

In February 1943, Dr. Hajime Tamura published his second report on hair grafting.[1] In this report Tamura noted that "the grafting of a single live hair is possible, and the long-term results also attained a satisfactory level. In the case of single-hair grafting, the hairs must be separated into a single hair each with attached surrounding tissue. Circular holes produced by a thick injection needle suffice for single-hair grafting."

Tamura's article clearly indicates the previous discovery and use of single-hair grafting. Thus small grafts, minigrafts, micrografts, and single-hair grafts do not find their origins in modern transplantation. These terms simply define graft size and number more precisely. Fig. 6-44 is a photograph of the original *Japanese Journal of Dermatology and Venereology* in which Tamura's article was found. Fig. 6-45 is a translation of that article produced by Dr. Shiro Yamada. The first author (DS) has elected not to edit or change a single word of this English translation.

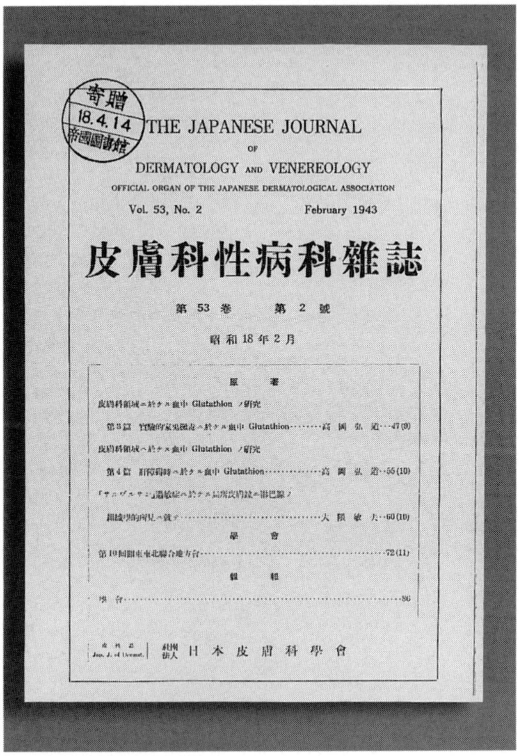

REFERENCE

1. Tamura H: Hair grafting procedure, *Jpn J Dermatol Venereol* [Japanese] 52(2):1943.

G. The Single-Hair Graft Technique for Advanced Male Pattern Alopecia

Dow B. Stough

SINGLE-HAIR GRAFTING

Hair transplant surgeons have now realized the importance of single-hair grafting in the creation of a natural hairline. In appropriate candidates the entire transplant procedure may be achieved with use of single-hair grafts. This approach involves the use of a large number of grafts (1500 to 4000) over four to six sessions (400 to 1000 grafts per session). The traditional method of round punch harvesting of donor hair from the occipital region presents logistical problems when the goal is to obtain a large number of single-hair grafts. Removing hair in thin strips with multibladed knives appears to be a superior method for obtaining single-hair grafts. This discussion focuses on the individual patients who are candidates for the single-hair graft technique as well as the mechanics of transplanting a large number of single-hair grafts.

FRONTAL HAIRLINE

For the past three decades, techniques of hair transplantation have revolved around the concept of building a "wall of hair" to create a frontal hairline. In some instances an unnatural appearance resulted from the abrupt nature of the interface between bald scalp and the hairline. In a departure from standard hair transplantation, the goal of single-hair transplantation is to build a "soft" zone of hair. No distinct sharp hairline is created. An essential element of single-hair follicle transplantation incorporates deliberate irregularity and scatter in hair placement. The appearance at the conclusion of grafting simulates a pattern of natural thinning. No attempt is made to create the density of a full head of hair. The fulfillment of this transplant goal requires multiple sessions, each involving the placement of 400 to 1000 hair grafts per session. There is no role for the standard round graft with this approach (Fig. 6-46).

FIG. 6-44 The issue of the *Japanese Journal of Dermatology and Venereology* in which Dr. Hajime Tamura published his article in February 1943.

```
Hajime Tamura

Hair grafting procedure (The second report)

In my first report, I stated about a method which uses shaved
hairs.  I reported not only that the results immediately after
operation with that method are good, but grafted hairs fall out
gradually but also that because the suppurative inflammation
and the accumulation of comedo like sebum often occur, the
long-term results are not good.  Therefore, afterwards I made
efforts for a method which grafts hairs with the tissue, and
improved referring to both the studies of Tomosuke Maeda and
Shoji Okuda, and, from 1937 on, tried this method on 130 cases
of atrichia vulvae and hypotricosis, 4 cases of cicatricial
baldness, 1 case of cicatricial alopecia of eyebrow and 1 case
of atrichia of hirci — a total of 136 cases, and finally
confirmed that the grafting of a single live hair is possible,
and the long-term results also attained the satisfactory level,
and therefore I submit the second report.  It is this procedure
that the scalp is excised in a ship-shape and the excised
portion is immediately sutured.  It is more convenient for
the following treatments to only cut hairs short to a length
of 3-4cm from the skin surface and never to shave hairs.  The
excised scalp is cleansed by a physiological saline solution
to remove blood, etc., and subcutaneous fat is excised, and
then is separated into small pieces of hair being donors with
scissors in parallel to the direction of hair shaft.  In case
of single hair grafting, the hairs must be separated into a
single hair each with attaching surrounding tissue.  And then,
these hair being donors are preserved in a physiological
saline solution.  On the other hand, the recipient site is
disinfected, and anesthesia is applied, and circular holes
are made with a "punch" of 1.0mm to 2.0mm or a thick injection
needle.  Circular holes by a thick injection needle suffice
for single hair grafting.  After all the necessary number of
such circular holes are finished, hair being donors are inserted
into the holes one by one.  Then, sterilized "gauze" soaked
with "olive oil" is put on the operated region and a bandage
is applied.  Afterwards, the region is disinfected every day
and the gauze is exchanged for a new one.  It is enough if
this is done for 1 week to 10 days.  The grafted hairs fall
out once in 2-3 weeks after the operation, but afterwards the
hairs regrow from the same region.  A donor is better if it is
as small as possible.  The reason is that if a donor is big,
hairs grow in a bundle from one donor, in a very unnatural
appearance.  Therefore, the best way is to conduct the single
hair grafting entirely, and the hairs grafted using this method
almost cannot distinguish from natural grown hairs.  But this
method is very complicated in manipulations, and therefore I
usually conduct using the method which uses a "punch" of 1.0mm
and the method of the single hair grafting, together.
```

FIG. 6-45 English translation by Yamada of the article published by Tamura in 1943 in the *Japanese Journal of Dermatology and Venereology*.

OBTAINING SINGLE-HAIR GRAFTS

A variety of techniques may be used to obtain single-hair grafts.[1-3] For more than 20 years, hair transplant surgeons have used trephines or punches to harvest round grafts in hair restoration procedures.[3]

Round punch grafts were sectioned to obtain smaller grafts, often called minigrafts. As smaller and smaller units were sought, micrografts were obtained by dissecting the minigrafts. As the use of these smaller grafts and the numbers needed for each transplant session increased, the need for a new, faster method of donor tissue harvesting became imperative. To this end several multibladed knives were developed that are capable of holding two, three, or four blades.[4] Chapter 4, Part B deals exclusively with multibladed knives. These instruments allow the removal of multiple long narrow strips of tissue. The thinness and relative ease in handling of the strips expedite the production of

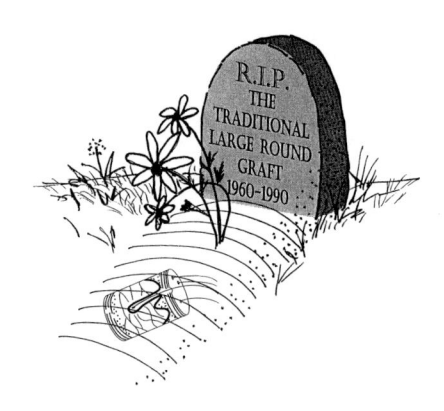

FIG. 6-46 When the single-graft technique for advanced male pattern alopecia is used, there is no role for the larger round traditional graft.

very small grafts, which is especially important in the dissection of single-hair grafts. Without a method for rapid removal and production of single-hair grafting, the technique would become too tedious and time-consuming. Our experience with strip harvesting involves hundreds of patients in a 3-year period and has led us to abandon traditional round-graft harvesting.

PROCEDURAL OUTLINE

Preliminary Preparation

- Perform the patient interview and selection
- Obtain a brief medical history
- Classify the pattern of baldness and hair quality
- Discuss the transplant design and expectations with the patient
- Plan the progression and timing of the sessions
- Obtain initial photographs and patient consent
- Explain the preoperative instructions to the patient
- Perform preoperative laboratory tests for hepatitis and HIV

Transplant Session

- Outline the proposed hairline
- Select and trim the donor hair region
- Estimate the length of the strip based on calculation charts
- Administer local anesthesia (10 ml 0.5% lidocaine with 1:100,000 epinephrine buffered with sodium bicarbonate)
- Harvest donor strips with multibladed knife
- Detach strips and place immediately in saline solution
- Close donor area with staples
- Trim and prepare strips into single-follicle grafts
- Anesthetize recipient site by nerve block
- Prepare recipient sites by stab incisions
- Implant prepared grafts
- Apply pressure bandage and provide instructions about hygiene and postoperative care to patient
- Twenty-four hours later, shampoo and inspect transplant area

SURGICAL TECHNIQUE*

The technical description and photographic illustration of the donor area are found in Chapter 5 (see Color Plates II through XIII). A 20 × 3 cm area of donor hair is trimmed in anticipation of producing donor strips 10 to 16 cm in size. It is important that the donor area be trimmed to expose a band that is 3 cm in width. Trimming facilitates rapid strip removal and closure. Ten minutes before surgery, approximately 10 ml of 0.5% lidocaine with 1:100,000 epinephrine is administered to the donor area. Sterile saline solution is injected for additional turgor. The triple-bladed knife is held at an angle of approximately 100 to 110 degrees. The knife is not held perpendicular to the skin because this positioning would result in hair-shaft transection. The precise angle of the incision is determined by the patient's hair-follicle orientation. Inspection of the incision after 1 to 2 cm progress has been made will reveal whether an adjustment needs to be made. The initial depth of insertion of the knife blade should be approximately 5 mm into the scalp. The incision should not be extended to the galea but should reach a depth of 1 to 2 mm below the terminus of the deepest hair follicle. A deeper incision risks the transection of arteries and therefore is not desirable. The incision is made in one smooth, pulling motion; sawing movements are avoided. After the incision is made, the ends are contoured with a single surgical scalpel to produce an elliptical pattern. The strips are then grasped with Adson's forceps and cut from their base with sharp scissors. Adequate depth to remove the strips is critical. If the cut is too superficial, hair follicles are sectioned, rendering the strips unusable. Good visualization during this stage is essential. Arterial bleeders are cauterized or tied with subcutaneous sutures. It should be noted that if the right depth of incision is achieved, few bleeders will be encountered. The wound is closed with 3M 25S staples. Keller suggested use of these particular staples to me (Keller G: Personal communication, April 1993). These staples differ from other brands in that they lie close to the scalp. Approximately 30 staples are required to close the incision after the removal of a 16 cm strip. Polysporin ointment is applied to the wound bed.

Triple-Bladed Knife

The triple-bladed knife with 2 mm spacers provides adequate donor tissue strips. A single pass with this instrument will produce two strips, each approximately 2 mm in width. With an incision length of 12.5 cm and average hair density, the dissection of two strips will result in approximately 500 single-follicle grafts. Table 6-3 provides a guideline for estimating graft numbers when the single-hair graft technique is used. This table assumes average density counts (18 to 22 hairs/4 mm field) measured with a trichoscope (see Chapter 5, Part B). Adjustments need to be made for density counts outside this range.

---

*The material in this section pertains to cases of single-hair grafting and differs slightly in approach to routine donor harvesting explained in Chapter 5.

TABLE 6-3 Estimation of Donor Strip Length for the Single-Hair Graft Technique*

NO. OF SINGLE-HAIR GRAFTS DESIRED	LENGTH OF DONOR STRIP (CM)
50	1.25
100	2.5
150	3.75
200	5
300	7.5
400	10
500	12.5
600	15
800	20

*Figures are based on the use of a triple-bladed knife with 2 mm spacers and average hair density.

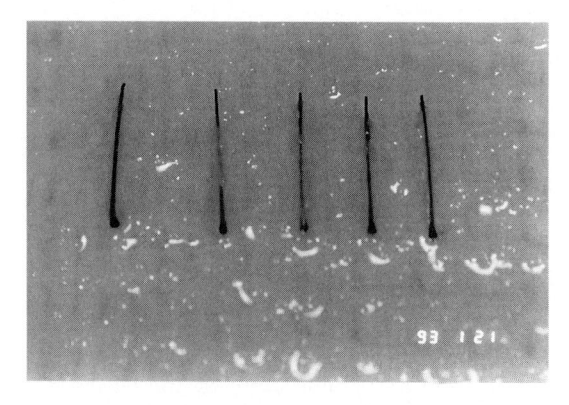

FIG. 6-47 A petri dish containing single-hair grafts produced from strips. Note that all excess tissue has been removed. The skill necessary to trim grafts to the degree shown is a requirement for the single-hair graft technique.

Spacer Sizing

When the single-hair graft technique is used, it is advisable to use blade spacers that are 1.8 to 2 mm in width. The larger spacers produce thicker donor tissue strips that are more difficult to section into single-hair grafts. We therefore favor small spacer size when the goal is to produce single-hair grafts.

Graft Preparation

The strips are separated from each other and immersed in saline solution. Surgical technicians then prepare the single-hair grafts by sectioning follicles from the strips, working toward the center of the strip. All grafts are sectioned with a Personna No. 10 surgical blade. The yield of grafts depends on the density of hair present in the donor tissue. Excess tissue may be trimmed from the single follicles if density is low (Fig. 6-47). The total number of single-hair grafts used varies from case to case, but virtually all cases average more than 400 grafts per session.

Recipient Site Preparation

The usefulness of dilators to aid in graft insertion has been the subject of debate. Some surgeons believe that dilators permit closer placement of grafts. However, dilators can be cumbersome and their use can be time-consuming. In contrast, a 18-gauge Yeh needle (Accuderm, Inc.), which has a solid tip, can be used to quickly and easily create large numbers of single-stab incision sites for slit grafting of the single-hair grafts.[5] One needle can be used in a sequential, nonstop fashion. No back-cut, twisting, or extension of the slit is required. Yeh needles are disposable and will stay sharp after hundreds of stab incisions. Chapter 4 deals exclusively with the recipient site preparation with use of the NoKor needle, which differs slightly from the Yeh needle. The NoKor needle has a sharper tip but tends to barb and dull with repeated incisions.

Graft Insertion

Skilled surgical assistants are indispensable when a large number of single-hair grafts are used. Surgical assistants can transplant a relatively large number of small grafts in a single session when equipped with the proper instrumentation. Single-hair grafts may be difficult to insert with use of the standard version of jeweler's forceps, even for assistants with experience. However, the finer version of jeweler's forceps, designed for microvascular surgery, has proved to be excellent for the insertion of single-hair grafts into small slit recipient sites (Fig. 6-48). It should be emphasized that the placement of tiny single-hair grafts into small, tight recipient slits is technique-sensitive. Considerable experience is needed to acquire the skill of rapid graft placement. Care is also required to avoid follicular damage.

DISCUSSION

Single-hair grafting represents a significant technical advance that contributes to the surgeon's ability to create hair transplants that have and will retain a natural appearance. It should be noted that the goals of this approach differ from the goals of the traditional approach. Specifically, no attempt is made to produce a distinct, sharply demarcated hairline. A soft feathering zone rather than a sharp, abrupt wall of hair is created.[6] This approach has also been advocated by others who use single-hair grafts, micrografts, and minigrafts. The best candi-

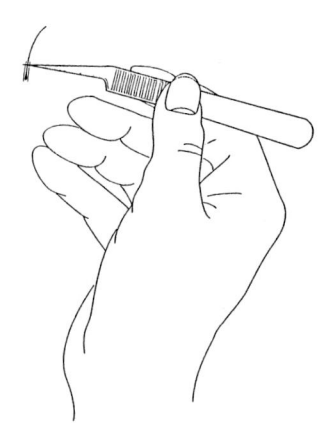

FIG. 6-48 Jeweler's forceps, designed for microvascular surgery, are a requirement for the insertion of single-hair grafts. Considerable experience is needed to acquire the skill of rapid placement. Gloves (not shown) should be worn by assistants.

dates for single-hair grafting are those with total alopecia of the frontal and/or crown region (Figs. 6-49 to 6-52). In these patients the results of this approach constitute a diffuse, thinned look. Patients with an ample quantity of retained native, nontransplanted hair may fail to notice any relative increase in volume and thus are less suitable candidates. This technique cannot create dense growth with thick hairlines. In patients with total frontal alopecia before transplantation, the single-hair graft approach can achieve acceptable density. Counseling regarding realistic expectations before transplantation is essential.

Single-hair grafting creates minimal to no visible scarring in the recipient bed. Inspection of patients who have undergone this technique shows little if any difference between the single-hair grafts and the native, nontransplanted hairs. This statement holds true only when single-hair grafts have

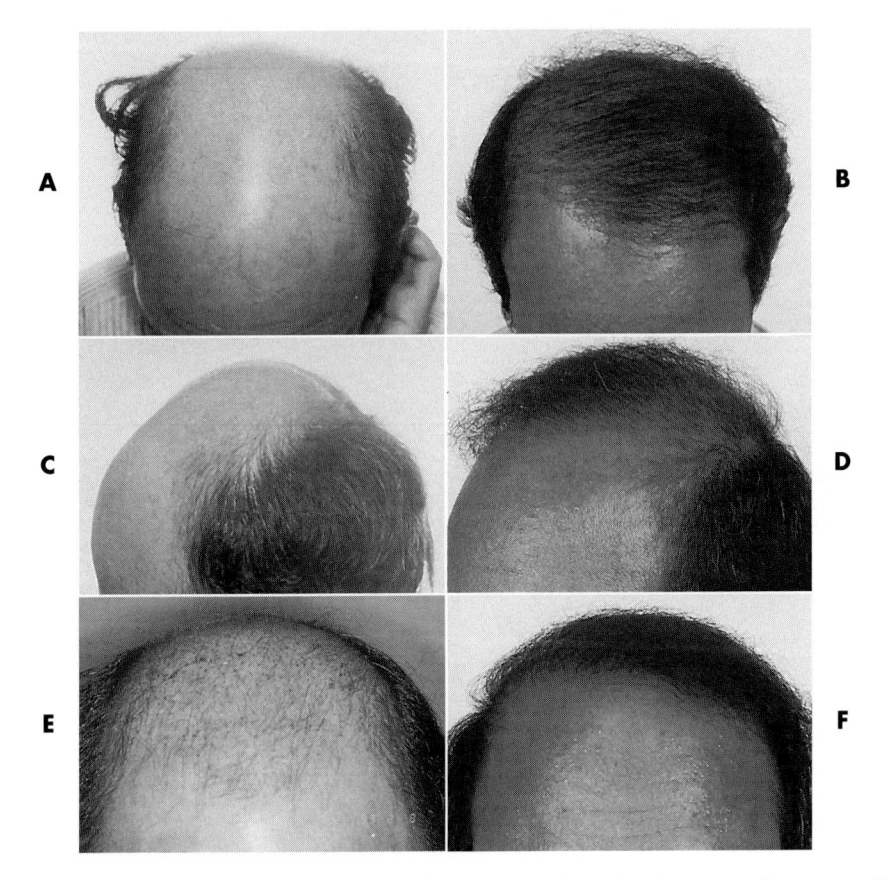

FIG. 6-49 A, This patient is classified as having Norwood type VI alopecia and is expected to progress to Norwood type VII alopecia. He is an excellent candidate for the single-hair graft technique. **B,** Result after six sessions of single-hair grafting. All grafts were placed into slit recipient sites produced with Yeh or NoKor needles. Each session involved more than 500 single grafts. **C,** Lateral preoperative view. **D,** Lateral view after six transplant sessions. **E,** Frontal view 3 months after the first session. **F,** Frontal view after six transplant sessions.

been transplanted into small recipient slits made with a 18-gauge Yeh needle (Fig. 6-53) or an 18-gauge NoKor needle. Slits made with a larger needle or by the removal of recipient tissue are more easily detectable as transplants and in some instances will create visible scarring.

Requirements

One disadvantage of single-hair grafting is the requirement for a minimum of two skilled technicians. With time and practice, transplant sessions that use 400 to 1000 grafts can routinely be completed within a 3- to 4-hour period.

Long-term Consequences

All forms of surgical hair replacement involve some long-term risk because the future extent of alopecia can never be predicted with certainty. Traditional techniques (larger 2 to 4 mm round grafts) can achieve acceptable results in many patients. However, even those who initially experience good results with traditional techniques can experience

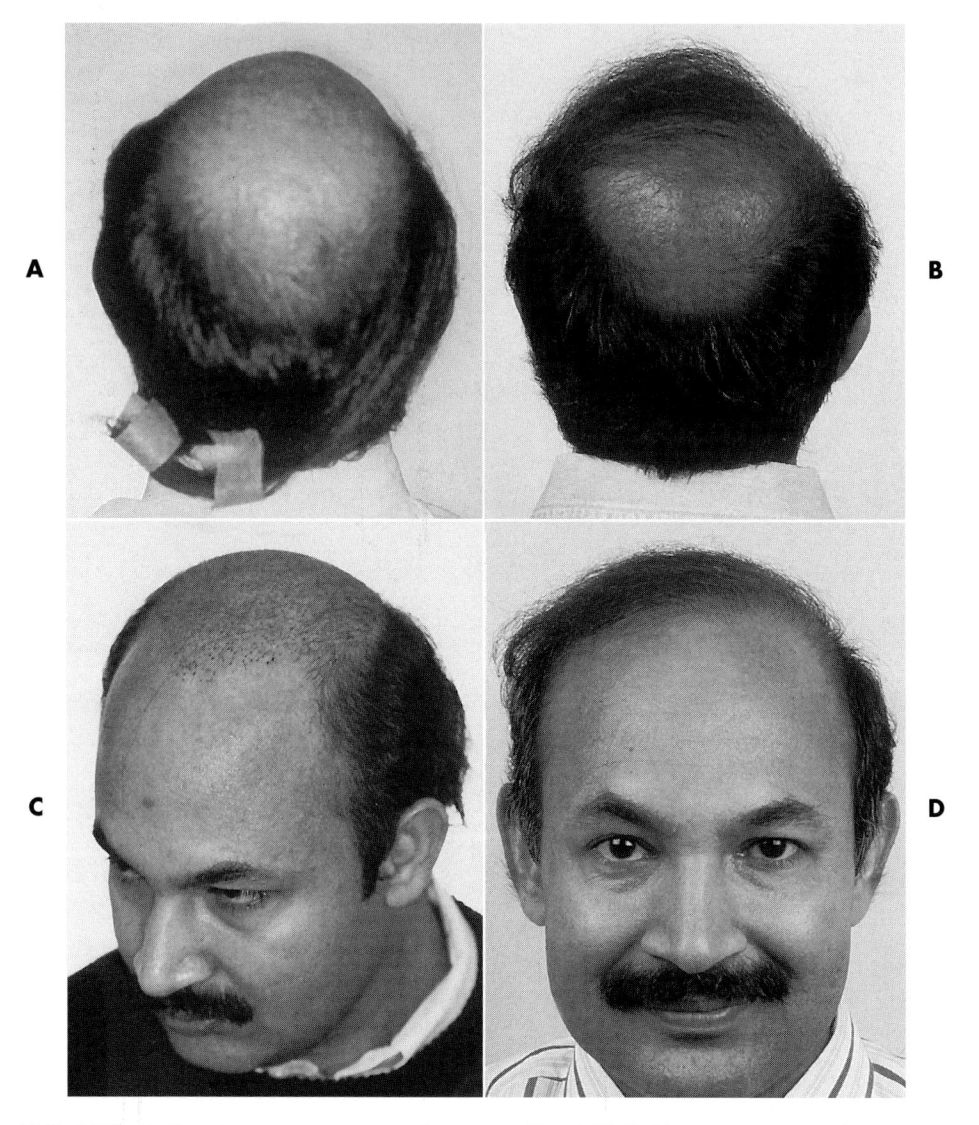

FIG. 6-50 **A,** Preoperative vertex view of patient in Fig. 6-49. **B,** No attempt was made to extensively transplant the vertex region. Single-hair grafts were placed in a pattern to simulate the natural vertex swirl. A complete restoration of the frontal and vertex region is not possible. **C,** One-day postoperative view after the placement of 886 single-hair grafts. All of these grafts were placed into recipient sites created with a 18-gauge NoKor needle. **D,** After six sessions, fair to good density was achieved.

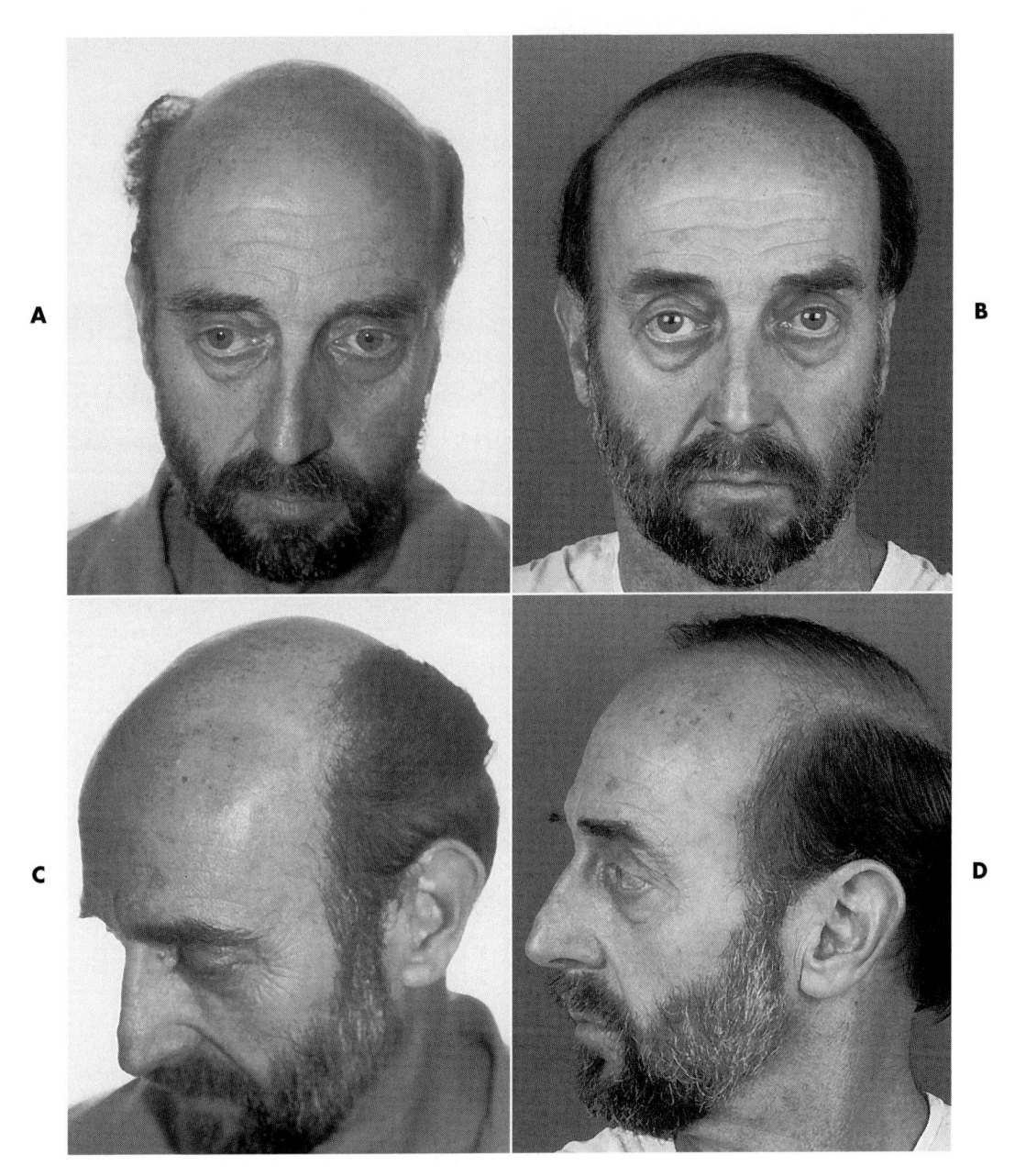

FIG. 6-51 A, Because of extensive alopecia, this 52-year-old man is an excellent candidate for the single-hair graft technique. **B,** Result after four sessions demonstrating the facial framing achieved by this technique. Note that no sharp hairline has been created. **C,** Preoperative oblique view. **D,** Lateral view after four graft sessions.

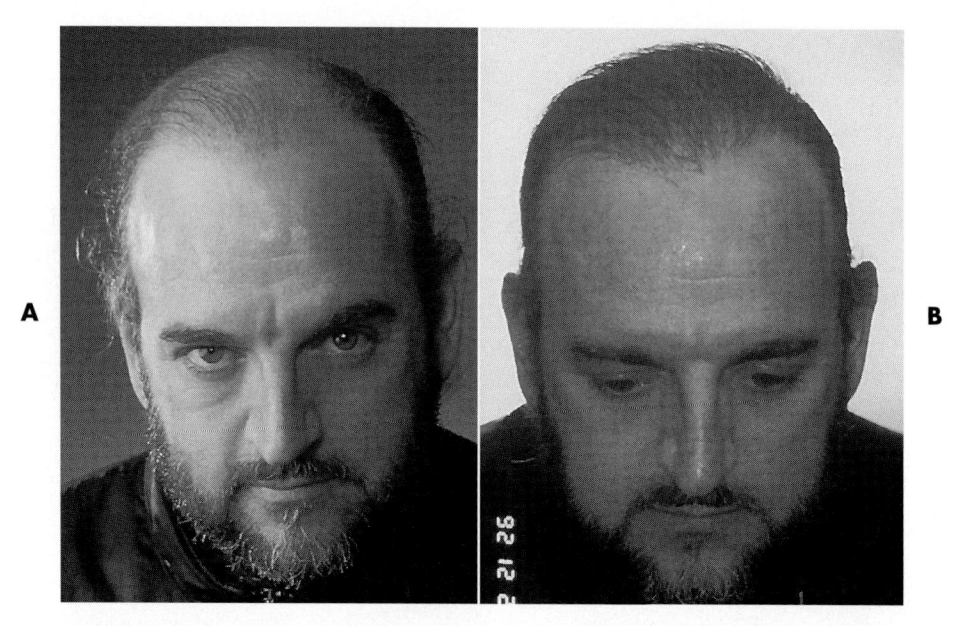

FIG. 6-52 **A,** A 45-year-old man with Norwood type V to VI alopecia. **B,** Result after five sessions of single-hair grafts in the frontal region. It should be noted that 1 mm grafts were used. These grafts contained up to three hairs.

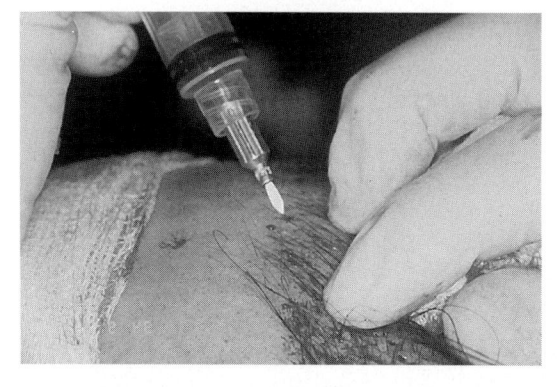

FIG. 6-53 The Yeh needle, a solid 18-gauge needle, provides consistent depth control and durability for sessions involving a large number of grafts.

SINGLE-HAIR GRAFT TECHNIQUE

Advantages
Provides superior cosmesis
Achieves facial framing
Permits a wide variety of styling possibilities
Allows a gradual change in appearance
Will not result in disfigurement if not all of the transplant sessions are performed
Minimizes the consequences of future hair loss

Disadvantages
Is time-consuming
Is labor-intensive
Requires skilled technicians
Creates a final result that mimics a thinning appearance
Requires multiple (four to six) sessions
Can be performed only on limited candidates (those with advanced alopecia)

severe hair loss in time, leaving the patient with an unnatural result. The concerns about the long-term consequences of hair loss are minimized with the single-hair graft technique. Parietal thinning and regression can occur and still leave the patient with a natural, albeit thin, look.

CONCLUSION

The new methodology using multibladed knives to obtain donor tissue strips represents a significant advance in hair restoration. Donor harvesting of strips can be used for the production of large numbers of single-hair grafts. Single-hair grafts can be inserted into slits produced with an 18-gauge needle similar to the technique first described by Tamura in 1943.[7] In appropriate candidates, hair transplant surgeons can now perform entire transplant procedures using only single-hair grafts. This method requires four to six sessions with the insertion of 400 to 1000 grafts per session. The grafts are often indistinguishable from native hair and are undetectable as transplants. Single-hair grafting represents a realistic option in the treatment of male pattern alopecia provided that candidates are carefully selected (see box on p. 194).

REFERENCES

1. Stough DB III, Nelson BR, Stough DB IV: Incisional slit grafting, *J Dermatol Surg Oncol* 17:53, 1991.
2. Swinehart JM, Griffin EI: Slit grafting: the use of serrated island grafts in male and female pattern alopecia, *J Dermatol Surg Oncol* 7:243, 1991.
3. Unger WP, Nordstrom REA: Quarter grafts: a technique for minigrafts. In Unger WP, Nordstrom REA, eds: *Hair transplantation*, ed 2, New York, 1988, Marcel Dekker, pp 333-351.
4. Brandy DA: A new instrument for the expedient production of minigrafts, *J Dermatol Surg Oncol* 18:487, 1992.
5. Jimenez FJ, Avram SR, Stough DB: The surgical pearl: the Yeh needle—a solid needle for single-hair recipient sites, *J Am Acad Dermatol* 32(6):1041-1042, 1995.
6. Stough DB IV: Hair transplantation by the feathering zone technique: new tools for the nineties, *Am J Cosmet Surg* 9:243, 1992.
7. Tamura H: Hair grafting procedure, *Jpn J Dermatol Venereol* [Japanese] 52(2):1943.

H. Vertical Strip Dissection for Graft Production

James Arnold

Sectioning of donor tissue into hundreds of required grafts is a bottleneck in the transplant procedure because it requires a large amount of time and effort. Each graft must be cut individually and precisely. To separate grafts, cuts must be made between hairs without injury to adjacent hair. Because the spacing between adjacent hairs is often less than 0.3 mm, obtaining the level of precision necessary for accurate cutting is a challenge and requires considerable experience.

Most techniques used to section donor tissue into micrografts and minigrafts use what I term a *knife and fork method*. The tools are large and are designed to be held by the hands. Movement of the hands and forearms provides motion to the knife. Whereas the knife and fork technique serves us well at the table, it lacks the precision and economy of effort needed for accurate, rapid cutting on the small scale required for cutting minigrafts. Even when smaller instruments such as a forceps and scalpel are used, their size requires gross hand movements to produce the cutting. Obtaining small grafts in this manner is slow and tedious.

I have developed a method of cutting small grafts that uses the fine motor skills of the fingers used for penmanship. With this technique, minigrafts, micrografts, and single-hair grafts can be cut more rapidly and accurately than has been previously possible. This technique can be quickly taught to technicians. When this method is used, minigrafts can be cut from 2 mm wide donor strips at a rate equivalent to 600 to 800 minigrafts per hour. Single-hair micrografts can be cut at a rate of 250 to 300 per hour. (The terminology used in this discussion is consistent with that defined by Knudsen in Chapter 2, Part D).

EQUIPMENT

2× Magnifiers

It is essential to be able to see the donor tissue clearly. The sectioning process requires placement of the cutting blade precisely between two adjacent hairs. Magnification can assist in the placement of the cutting blade and allows the subsequent cutting of the minigraft to proceed at a rapid rate.

Foerster Forceps

Foerster forceps (3⅜ inch) (A to Z Surgical, San Jose, Calif.) have octagonal rings that allow the forceps to be held and manipulated with just the thumb and forefinger of one hand (Fig. 6-54). The forceps are therefore "finger-sized" and function as an extension of the fingers. The forceps have curved, serrated tips and are used to move the minigrafts.

Tongue Blades Saturated in Saline Solution

Tongue blades serve two purposes in the cutting process. First, the tongue blade provides a firm cutting surface, which allows the actual cutting of the tissue to occur rapidly. Second, with the donor strip laid along the tongue blade, the strip can be moved or repositioned quickly by simply moving the tongue blade. In the cutting process the donor strip

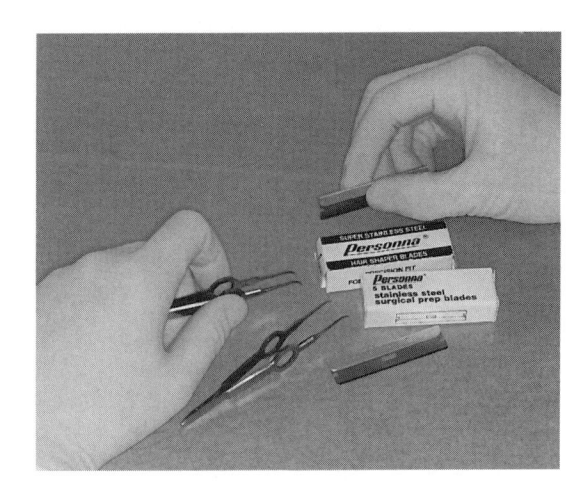

FIG. 6-54 Foerster forceps and surgical prep blades are "finger-sized" and easily manipulated by finger movements alone.

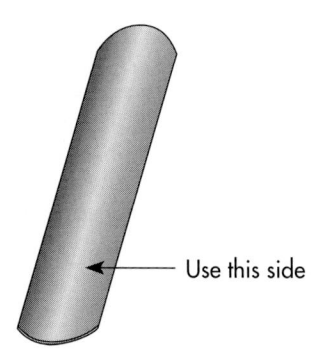

FIG. 6-55 After soaking in saline solution, a tongue blade may curve or "cup" along its length. The side that curves upward is used for cutting.

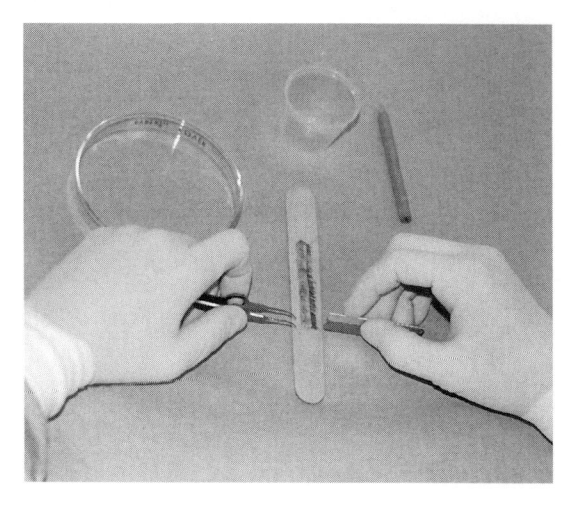

FIG. 6-56 In the cutting position, the hands rest comfortably on a solid surface to allow the fingers to move with minimal effort.

must be moved several times, and it is easier to move the tongue blade than the strip itself. The tongue blades should be soaked for 10 minutes in a shallow tray of saline solution. If not saturated with saline solution, the tongue blade will absorb moisture from the donor strips and quickly dry them out.

Hair-Shaper Blades (Surgical Prep Blades)

Hair-shaper blades originated as replaceable blades for an instrument similar to a straight razor used by hair stylists to cut hair. The same blade is sold as a surgical prep blade through a few surgical supply outlets (Fig. 6-54). Hair-shaper blades may be purchased from beauty supply outlets or as surgical prep blades. Hair-shaper blades, made by Personna, are sharp and durable. More important, they are the proper shape and size to be used by the fingers alone. Hair-shaper blades have an invisible coating of oil, and it is suggested that they be wiped with a dry sponge or cleaned with alcohol before use.

TECHNIQUE

The technique of using finger movement for sectioning minigrafts relies on three basic rules:

1. Only finger movements are used; the hands are relaxed and rest on a solid surface.
2. The tools used must be finger-sized. Tools that are designed to be held by the hands such as conventional scalpels and forceps must be abandoned.
3. The cutting motion used to section minigrafts should be a vertical (up-and-down) motion. Lateral, sawing movements of the cutting blade should be avoided.

The donor tissue used with this technique is obtained as 2 mm wide strips cut with a multibladed knife. Donor strips wider than 2 mm or single elliptical pieces of donor tissue require that the technicians divide them into multiple sections before individual minigrafts are obtained. In the interest of minimizing the time required to obtain the needed minigrafts, it is important to present the technicians with the donor tissue in the form of 2 mm wide strips.

A donor strip is placed lengthwise along the center of a tongue blade. If a donor strip is especially long, it can be divided into two halves that are sectioned separately. Excess fat can be trimmed from the donor strip after it has been placed on the tongue blade by using the hair-shaper blade in a careful manner.

Many tongue blades will warp or cup after soaking in the saline solution. If cupping occurs, the donor strip should be placed on the surface of the tongue blade that curves upward (Fig 6-55).

The tongue blade with the donor strip is oriented to a 90-degree angle in front of the technician (Fig. 6-56). The Foerster forceps and the hair-shaper blade are held by the fingertips while the weight of the hands rests on a solid surface. The hair-shaper blade is held in a comfortable position and the donor strip is oriented so the hair shafts are exactly parallel to the cutting blade (Fig. 6-57). Often the hair shafts in the donor strip emerge at an angle. It is easier to turn the tongue blade on which the strip is lying to get a parallel alignment than it is to move the strip itself or move the hand into an uncomfortable position (Fig. 6-58).

The technician views the end of the donor strip from above and places the cutting blade between two adjacent hairs. With use of a vertical guillotine-like motion, the blade is passed down through the donor strip, yielding a minigraft. The pressure

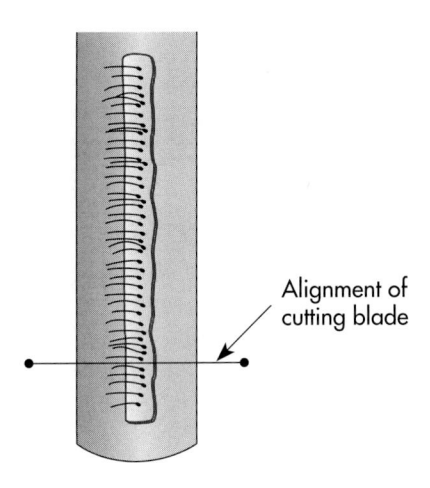

FIG. 6-57 The cutting blade is aligned parallel to the hair shafts of the donor strip.

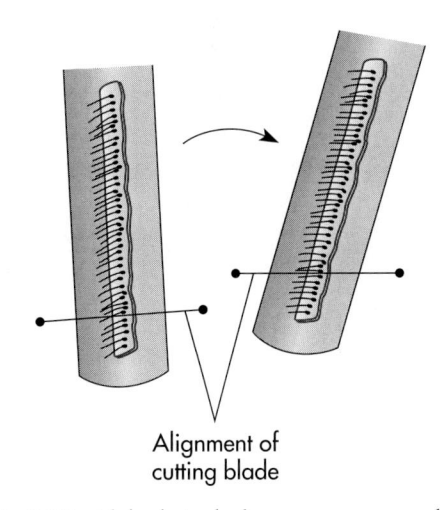

FIG. 6-58 If the hair shafts emerge at an angle, the tongue blade can be moved to obtain parallel alignment with the cutting blade.

needed for the blade to cut through the tissue is not great. The pressure allows cutting of the tissue but not the tongue blade. The cutting blade simply comes to rest on the tongue blade surface (Fig. 6-59). One reason for using a strictly vertical cutting motion is to prevent the cutting edge from being drawn across the surface of the tongue blade. Lateral motions against the wooden blade will quickly dull the cutting edge.

As soon as the minigraft has been separated, the Foerster forceps are used to draw the graft away from the blade (Fig. 6-60). Moisture on the grafts may cause several minigrafts to adhere to the forceps. For the sake of expediency, the presence of the adhering grafts should be ignored. The forceps will continue to function and the clump of grafts will eventually fall away. As the minigrafts are cut, the technician should count each one mentally to ensure an accurate tally at the end.

With the minigraft moved out of the way, the cutting blade is returned to its original position. Because the donor strip is 2 mm, the up-and-down movement of the cutting blade is only about 3 mm. Precise movement in this 3 mm range is easily accomplished with only finger movement. The next graft can be cut immediately if the alignment of the hair shafts is still parallel to the cutting blade. Maintaining this exact parallel alignment is the second reason for using a vertical cutting motion. Lateral, sawing motions of the blade tend to misalign the donor strip. The ability to immediately cut each subsequent graft is the key to generating minigrafts at a brisk rate. With the use of a vertical cutting motion, the parallel alignment is ensured, thus allowing a rapid sequence of cutting strokes (Fig. 6-61).

After 12 to 15 minigrafts have been cut, the fingers reach the end of their range of motion. The hand can again be moved to reach the end of the donor strip, or the tongue blade can be advanced to bring the strip back to the cutting blade. Each time a move is made, the proper parallel alignment of the hair shafts and cutting blade is adjusted. This rapid vertical cutting with the hair shafts exactly aligned with the blade is the essence of this technique.

GRAFT SIZE

The technicians are advised of the desired number of hairs per graft. Thirty or 40 grafts will be cut by counting individual hairs to determine the approximate size of the needed grafts. Once the size containing the correct number of hairs has been determined, all subsequent grafts will be cut to produce grafts of similar size. Technicians can proceed at a faster rate by aiming for uniform size rather than continuing to count hairs.

SINGLE-HAIR GRAFT DISSECTION

Single-hair micrografts can also be cut using this technique. Although this method will allow single-hair grafts to be generated more rapidly than most other methods, the rate of cutting single hairs is much slower than cutting multiple-hair minigrafts. Each single-hair graft requires a minimum of two cuts. A very precise cut must be made very close and exactly parallel to one side of the hair followed by an equally precise and exact cut on the opposite side. Whereas a minigraft requires a single cut to separate it from the donor tissue, the need for two very exact cuts results in a much slower rate of gen-

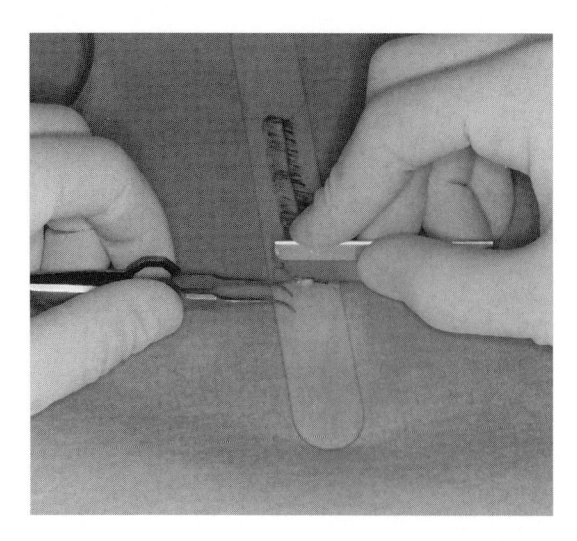

198 Technique—Small-Graft Hair Transplantation

FIG. 6-59 After the cutting blade is placed between adjacent hairs, a quick downward stroke produces a minigraft.

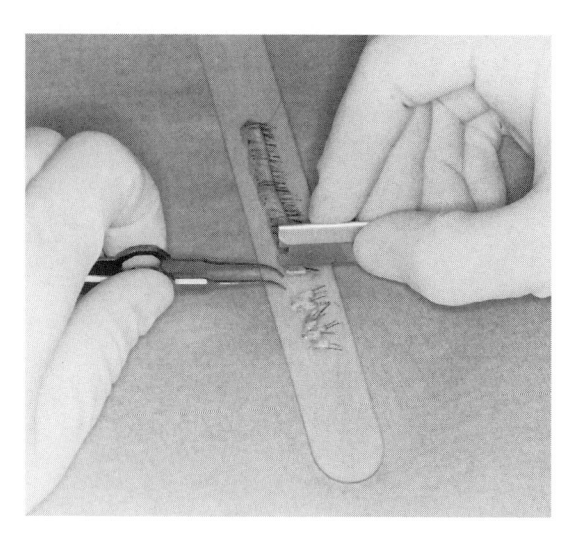

FIG. 6-61 Several minigrafts can be generated quickly by rapidly repeating the cutting cycle.

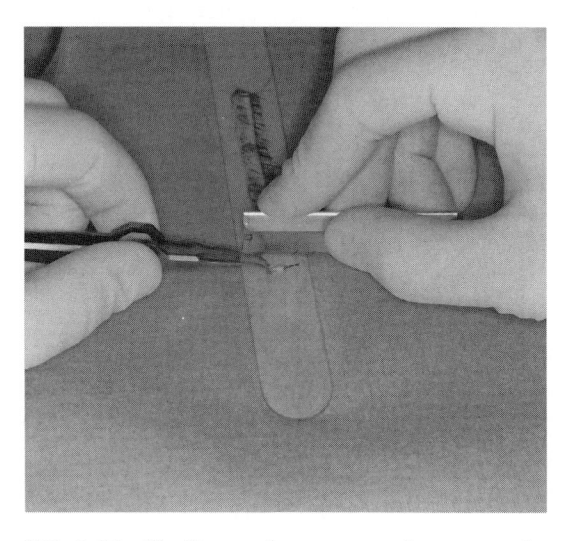

FIG. 6-60 The Foerster forceps are used to remove the minigraft from the cutting area.

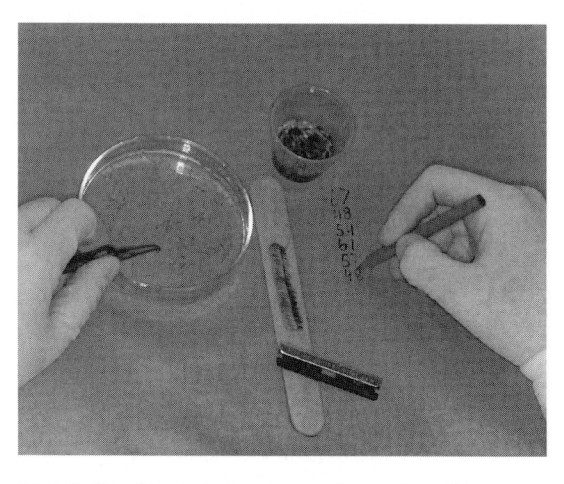

FIG. 6-62 Single-hair micrografts are floated in a petri dish. Minigrafts are transferred in groups to a holding cup. As each group is transferred, their number is recorded with a pencil to maintain an accurate tally.

erating single-hair micrografts. An experienced technician who is able to section multiple-hair minigrafts at a rate of 800 per hour is usually able to produce single-hair micrografts at a rate of only 250 to 300 per hour.

To minimize the time spent on cutting single-hair micrografts, technicians find it helpful to look for opportunities to obtain single-hair grafts while cutting minigrafts. Often a single hair will be at the edge of the donor strip, allowing a deft cut to quickly harvest it as a micrograft. Also, a few minigrafts will have single hairs along one edge that can be quickly cut into grafts. Some minigrafts will have a relatively wide spacing of individual hairs that the technician can separate quickly into micrografts. A petri dish with saline solution is placed close to the left hand to allow these single-hair micrografts to be moved quickly away from the cutting area (Fig. 6-62). Single-hair grafts obtained fortuitously during the cutting of minigrafts require a relatively small amount of invested time. When donor strips are cut specifically into single-hair micrografts, the need for multiple, exact cuts becomes evident with the relatively slow rate of graft generation. Technicians should be encouraged to seek out and harvest as many single hairs as possible while sectioning the larger minigrafts.

At the end of the cutting process, the technicians must be able to give the surgeon an exact count of both the single-hair micrografts and the minigrafts. Our technicians use a system of mentally counting each minigraft as it is sectioned from the donor tissue. After 60 to 80 minigrafts accumulate on the tongue blade they are transferred as a group to a 30 ml disposable medicine cup and kept moist with saline solution. The number of grafts transferred can be recorded on the work surface with a golf pencil. This method works well to keep an accurate count of the minigrafts as they are cut (Fig. 6-62).

CONCLUSION

This method of cutting minigrafts relies on an approach that differs from most techniques presently used by hair replacement surgeons. It is simple and straightforward, allowing technicians to learn the method quickly. Other, less precise methods of cutting minigrafts tend to be frustrating to technicians, whereas technicians express a feeling of accomplishment with their increased output when cutting micrografts by vertical strip dissection.

Editor's Note

The vertical strip dissection method for graft production represents a significant advance in training technicians to produce high-quality micrografts and minigrafts in a very short time period. It should be noted that in our clinic, my most experienced technicians still prefer the use of a No. 10 scalpel blade for the production of single-hair grafts. The surgical prep blades as described by Dr. Arnold are quite adequate for the production of all other sized grafts.

7
Special Categories

A. Hua Laan Chon Kan

Damkerng Pathomvanich and Dow B. Stough

History gives us very few examples of bald men who were appreciated and admired. One such example was the *Hua Laan Chon Kan* ("bald-headed fighting event"), which took place in Asia. What made this event unique was that only those with completely bald pates were allowed to compete. The *Hua Laan Chon Kan* originated in the Sukhothai Era (1238 to 1365). However, it was not until the Ayutthaya Era (1365 to 1782) that it peaked in popularity. This game was held to the cheers of spectators and contestants dressed in traditional costumes. Bald contestants crawled around quickly and bashed each other head-on with their bald heads. The *Hua Laan Chon Kan* continued until one of the contestants collapsed or was unable to knock heads any longer, usually a period of 10 to 20 minutes. Wagering was the key element to this event, and crowds would cheer contestants on fanatically.

This small bit of Thai history has now been preserved by the creation of fiberglass figures of bald men performing the *Hua Laan Chon Kan* (Fig. 7-1).

B. Hair Transplantation in the Asian Population

Damkerng Pathomvanich

No statistics indicating the percentage of Asians who are bald are available in medical literature. I believe that the percentage of Asians who are bald is lower than the percentage of whites who are bald. Asians with alopecia are as concerned about baldness as whites—perhaps even more so. Many Asians begin to wear hats with the inception of baldness, and most Asians consider themselves bald when they have slightly high hairlines or recessions of the frontotemporal angle. In comparison, minor thinning is well accepted among whites.

Despite the fact that the punch graft was created in Asia by Okuda[1] in 1939 and the micrograft by Tamura[2] in 1943, hair transplantation is not well

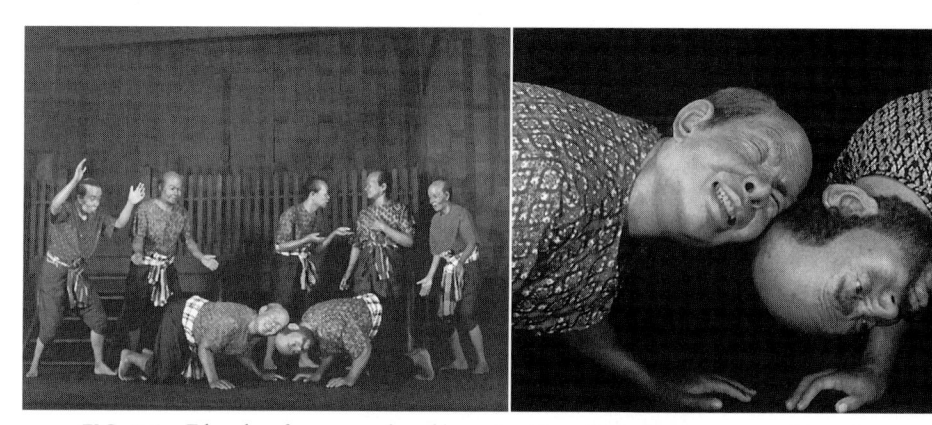

FIG. 7-1 Fiberglass figures, produced by artist Ajaan Duangkaew, preserve the ancient game of *Hua Laan Chon Kan* ("bald-headed fighting event"), which originated during the Sukhothai Era (1238 to 1365). (From Tripathid M: Male baldness: celebrated at last, *The Nation*, March 7, 1994. Photographs by Prathai Piriyasurawong.)

known or popular in Asia, even among physicians. Hairpieces are still the treatment of choice. Most physicians prescribe minoxidil and other medical treatments to treat baldness, probably because of rumors of unsuccessful results with hair transplantation.[3] However, the public can now see good results achieved with smaller grafts; the cornfield effect that occurs with standard round grafts has been eliminated.

In 1990 I opened the first clinic in Thailand totally dedicated to hair restoration surgery.

HAIR TRANSPLANTATION IN ASIANS— THERE ARE DIFFERENCES

In many respects hair transplantation in Asians is similar to that in whites.[4] However, there are several differences that need to be discussed.

Hairline

Asian culture and customs vary from nation to nation. These varying cultures lead to different hairline preferences among ethnic groups. The skull of the Oriental appears round and wide compared with the long, narrow skull of the white person (Fig. 7-2). The facial structure of Asians is also different. Typically Asians have round faces with flat noses, single eyelids, small palpebral fissures, slightly receding chins, high cheek bones, and prominent mandibular angles.[5] These characteristics create difficulties in hairline design. Most Asians want low hairlines and round frontotemporal angles or straight hairlines across the forehead. In short, one must negotiate with the patient and modify the desired hairline to produce good cosmetic results.[6]

Hair Density

Whites have a greater hair density than Asians. Trichoscope counts in Asians generally are below 20 hairs per 4 mm field. Asian hair caliber is big, coarse, and straight, usually with low density counts. Therefore to obtain the same number of grafts per session, a larger donor area is required.

Hair Color, Skin Color, and Hair Character

Asians have black hair except for those who are of mixed heritage; however, skin color varies from white to dark (e.g., Japanese and Chinese tend to have white skin, whereas Malaysians and Indians tend to have dark skin). The degree of contrast between skin color and hair color can be challenging for the hair transplant surgeon.

Scarring

Asians, like blacks, tend to form keloids or hypertrophic scars. However, these scars are formed to a much lesser extent in Asians than in blacks but probably at a higher rate than in whites. Scars respond well to intradermal cortisone injections (triamcinolone acetonide [Kenalog] 10 mg/ml).

PREOPERATIVE EVALUATION IN SELECTING THE ASIAN PATIENT FOR HAIR TRANSPLANTATION

Asians have high expectations and reluctantly accept alopecia on the vertex. Asians generally want a full head of hair. The patient must be well informed of the realistic achievements in hair transplantation surgery. As with whites, future hair loss is of great concern to Asians.

The Problem of Minoxidil and Foltene

My research and experience have indicated that of patients who decide to have surgery, 14.5% previously used minoxidil. Many patients used both oral and topical minoxidil in an attempt to grow hair. Foltene, another hair growth product from France, is claimed to be very potent for hair growth and is popular in the Orient. It is notable that all patients who use Foltene before surgery experience heavy bleeding, which results in increased operating time and a requirement for more local anesthetic. After the operation these patients may experience oozing for several days, which results in a stormy postoperative course and an unhappy patient. We now instruct our patients to discontinue the use of Foltene for 4 months before surgery. Patients who took minoxidil orally with an average dose of 10 mg/day and also used topical minoxidil also bled profusely. In a small study of six patients, three stopped taking oral minoxidil 3 weeks before surgery whereas the other three continued its use. There was no difference in bleeding. In conclusion, oral Foltene and minoxidil must be discontinued at least 2 months before surgery.

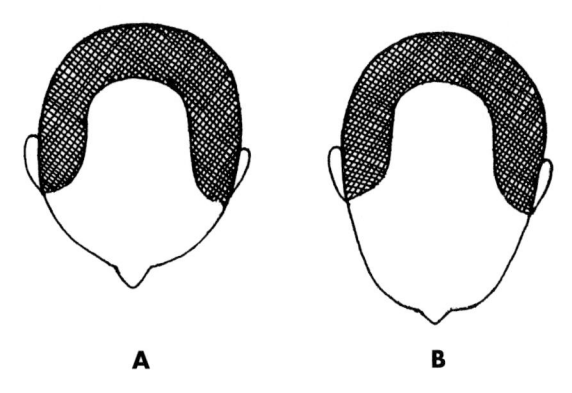

FIG. 7-2 The skull of the Oriental patient (A) appears round and wide compared with the long and narrow skull of the white patient (B).

Preoperative Laboratory Work

Routine blood tests for HIV and hepatitis surface antigen B, as well as a thorough patient history and physical examination, must be performed in all patients. Despite negative laboratory tests, all staff are required to wear goggles, gloves, and masks. In my practice, 6.5% of the patients have been positive for hepatitis B; only 0.5% have been HIV positive.

CURRENT TECHNIQUE FOR HAIR TRANSPLANTATION IN ASIANS

Scalp Reduction

Hair transplantation and scalp reduction went hand in hand until 1992. Since the advent of transplant megasessions (500 to 1000 grafts), the number of scalp reductions has been declining.[7] Scalp reductions in Asian patients often resulted in unhappy patients because of wide scars, slot effect, and stretchback. The success of this procedure in the Asian population is now in question.[7]

Hair-Bearing Flaps

Hair-bearing flaps often have an unnatural appearance, especially in Asians because the hair is strong and course. The flap hairline will invariably be directed opposite to the remaining hair on the back of the head. Furthermore, the donor scar and recipient scar can be obvious with depigmentation of the skin along the hairline.

Total Micrografting

For the past few years, minigrafts and micrografts have been used in all cases with good to excellent results. Consistent with the terminology used by Knudsen (Chapter 2, Part D), minigrafts contain three to five hairs and micrografts contain one or two hairs. Only micrografts are used in the frontal hairline. We routinely transplant 400 to 1000 grafts per session in a 4-hour period. We use a team of three technicians and one surgeon.

DONOR HARVESTING

Preoperative photographs are taken and a mutually agreeable hairline is drawn. Preoperatively, 10 mg of oral diazepam (Valium) and up to 15 mg of intravenous midazolam are administered. Most patients will not remember the session because of amnesia from the midazolam. Pulse oxymetry is used throughout the procedure. Antibiotics are administered to the patient preoperatively and are continued 3 days postoperatively. The donor area is chosen and trimmed to a length of 2 mm with a mustache trimmer. An elliptical area is then marked in the donor area with gentian violet; the length and width of the ellipse depend on the number of grafts to be transplanted. A single blade is used to produce a wide ellipse. The skin is undermined if needed and bleeders are cauterized. The wound is closed with 3-0 monofilament nonabsorbable sutures, which are removed in 10 days.

Since I have abandoned the punch graft and begun employing a single-bladed knife, wound healing is much improved, with the results demonstrating a fine linear scar. I find that when I use the wide ellipse technique, the length of the

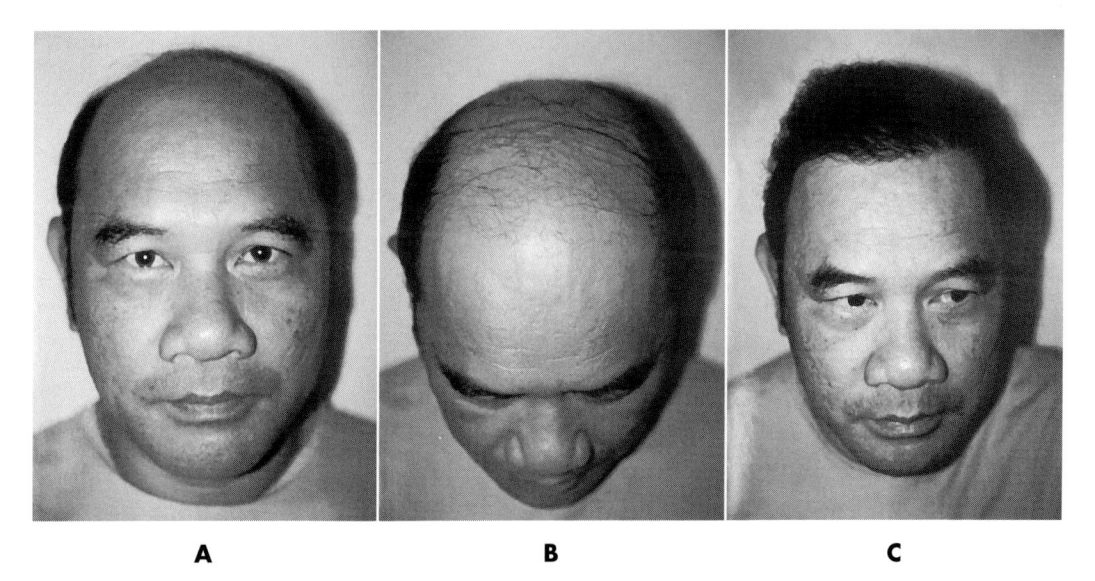

FIG. 7-3 **A,** Preoperative frontal view of a patient with Norwood type VI to VII alopecia. The patient had excellent hair density. **B,** Preoperative top view. **C,** Postoperative view 1 year after two sessions in which 1150 minigrafts and micrografts were transplanted.

FIG. 7-4 A, Staphylococcus infection on postoperative day 17 with pustules involved in 80% of the grafts. **B,** Five-month postoperative view with about 60% hair growth. **C,** One-year postoperative view after two sessions. The hair grafts survived well without any infection and minimal scarring.

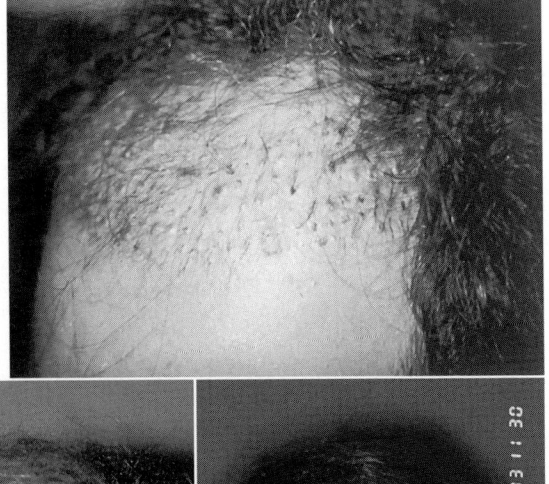

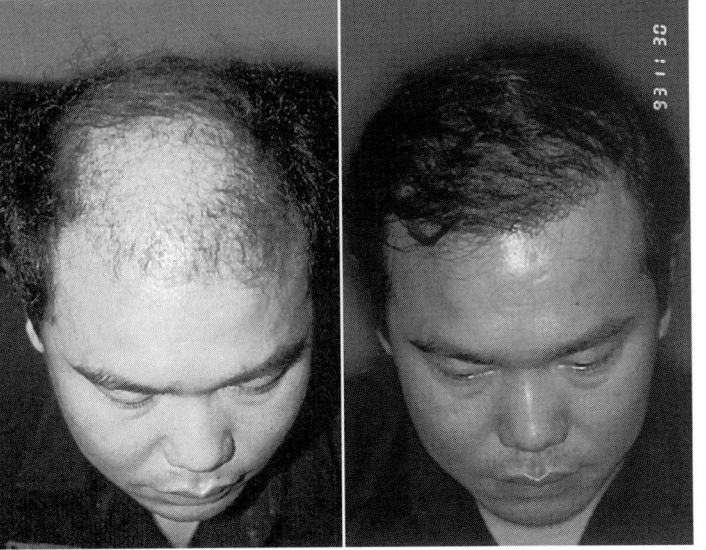

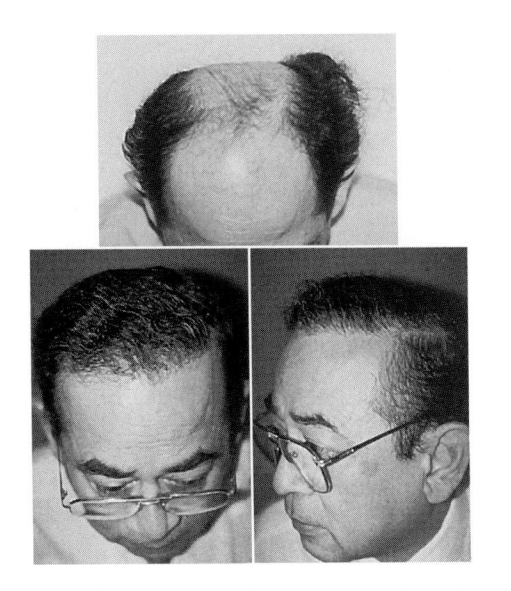

FIG. 7-5 Preoperative and postoperative views of a patient with type VII alopecia. The result is shown 1½ years after five sessions of minigrafts and micrografts.

scar is shorter at no expense of graft count. Similar to Uebel and Limmer, we favor the ellipse technique using a single-bladed knife over the triple-bladed knife. The latter results in a longer scar in the donor region.

RECIPIENT SITE TRANSPLANTATION

Supraorbital and supratrochlear nerve blocks using 2% lidocaine with epinephrine are routinely performed. Additional infiltration with 1:50,000 epinephrine solution is administered, which makes the operative field appear dry and decreases the amount of lidocaine required. We favor small recipient holes except in patients who have existing hair. In these patients we use recipient slits.

Compared with whites, Asians require larger numbers of micrografts for the hairline. Behind the hairline, 1.25 mm and 1.5 mm recipient holes are used, depending on hair quality. On the vertex only 1.25 mm and 1 mm holes are used.

No dilators are used throughout the procedure. Antibiotic ointment and dressings are applied

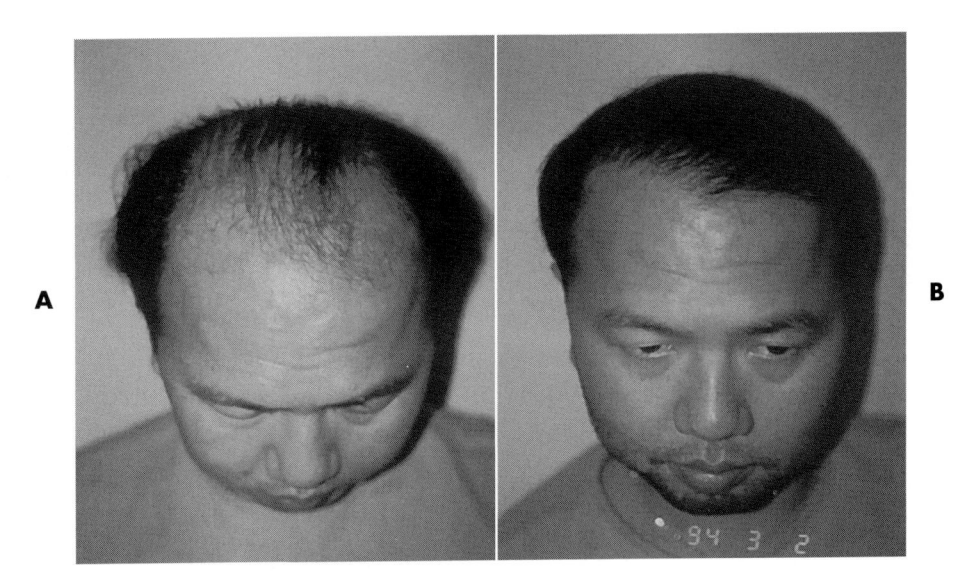

FIG. 7-6 **A,** Preoperative view. **B,** Result 10 months after only one session of 700 minigrafts and micrografts.

postoperatively. The patient returns the following day for shampooing. Sessions are spaced 4 months apart. In subsequent sessions, the previous scar is harvested as described by Stough and Haber in Chapter 5, Part A. This technique will leave the patient with only one scar.

When small grafts are transplanted in megasessions, most patients are satisfied with the results after only two or three sessions (Figs. 7-3 to 7-6). We use this approach with patients who have varying degrees of alopecia. Even Norwood type VII patients with good density are acceptable candidates for hair transplantation (Fig. 7-3).

Finally, tattooing the scalp reduction scar or between the grafts will help to improve the final outcome. Although this practice is not commonly used in the West, it aids in creating the illusion of density so critical to the aesthetic goals of the Asian patient.

COMPLICATIONS AND UNTOWARD EFFECTS

A common complaint among Asians is the inability to cope with society for a few weeks because postoperative appearance is prominent. However, swelling subsides by the eighth day. We have experienced one case of fungal infection and three cases of staphylococcus infection, all of which responded to treatment with antifungal agents or antibiotics (see Fig. 7-4).

REFERENCES

1. Okuda S: Clinical and experimental studies of transplantation of living hairs, *Jpn J Dermatol* 46:235-238, 1939.
2. Tamura H: Pubic hair transplantation [Japanese], *Jpn J Dermatol* 53:76, 1943.
3. Zappacosta AR: Reversal of baldness in patients receiving minoxidil for hypertension, *N Engl J Med* 303:1480-1481, 1980.
4. Unger WP, Nordstrom REA, editors: *Hair transplantation,* ed 2, New York, 1988, Marcel Dekker.
5. Pathomvanich D: Current hair transplantation in Asians [Thai], *The Medical News,* February 1992.
6. Norwood OT: Patient selection, hair transplant design, and hairstyle, *J Dermatol Surg Oncol* 18:386-394, 1992.
7. Pathomvanich D: Scalp reduction in Asians [Thai], *The Medical News,* February 24-March 1, 1992.

C. Hair Restoration in Blacks

John Karl Randall and Dow B. Stough

Hair restoration in black patients involves many of the selection criteria, surgical techniques, and sequelae as in white patients. Nevertheless, several unique characteristics differentiate hair restoration in black patients.

A major consideration in hair restoration surgery in the black patient is the characteristic curl and the associated curvature of the hair follicular unit (Fig. 7-7). The diameter and elliptical cross section of hair shafts in blacks contribute to the degree of curl.[1] The extreme follicular curl found in hair in black patients makes donor harvesting difficult. Hair-shaft transection can occur with a greater frequency in blacks than in whites.

To minimize complications, the donor area should be well infiltrated with saline solution to achieve very firm turgor. The firmer the donor area, the greater the likelihood of straightening the hair follicles and the lesser the risk of hair-shaft transection.

DONOR HARVESTING

The optimal technique for harvesting donor hair in black patients is a subject of debate. One of the authors (JKR) believes that power-driven punches will result in a higher hair yield with less hair-shaft transection.[2] With the punch method, an arcing motion of the power-driven punch is required to prevent transection of the follicles. Often test grafts will be required, and the angle of the arc may need to be altered as harvesting proceeds (Fig. 7-8). Recommended trephine sizes are within the range of 3 to 5 mm. The other author (DS) prefers strip harvesting.

Other surgeons advocate the use of a multibladed knife with spacer sizes varying from 2 to 3 mm (see Fig. 7-8). It appears that regardless of the harvesting technique, a small group of patients still present the surgeon with difficulties in removing donor hair with an acceptable number of intact follicles. For such patients, harvesting the donor area as a large ellipse as described by Limmer, would theoretically obtain the highest yield[3,4] (see Chapter 5, Part C).

GRAFT SIZES

Micrografts, minigrafts, and larger grafts can be used for hair transplantation depending on individual patient hair characteristics and the patient's goals (Fig. 7-9). Independent of graft size, the curly nature of the hair will give the aesthetic appearance of greater coverage.

COMPLICATIONS

Before any hair restoration procedure, a history of keloid formation, hypopigmentation or hyperpigmentation, and pseudofolliculitis barbae should be obtained.

Hypertrophic scarring and keloid formation are more common in blacks than in whites. Because keloid formation can be catastrophic, some surgeons perform a test graft before alopecia correction.[5] At a minimum, a thorough history should be obtained and observation of existing scars should be carried out.

Postoperative hypopigmentation and hyperpigmentation also occur at a higher incidence in the black population.

Black men who have a history of either pseudofolliculitis barbae or acne keloidalis nuchae can have severe problems with ingrown hairs, particularly after hair transplantation with small grafts. If

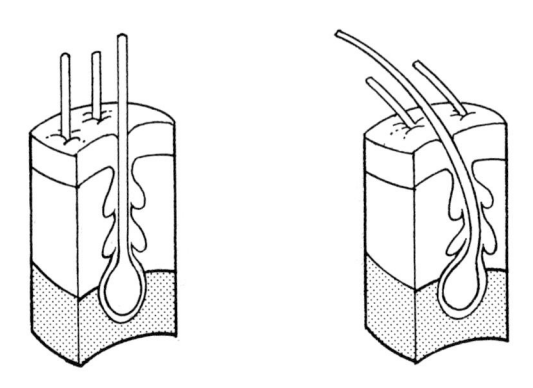

FIG. 7-7 Hair follicles from blacks (*right*) and whites (*left*).

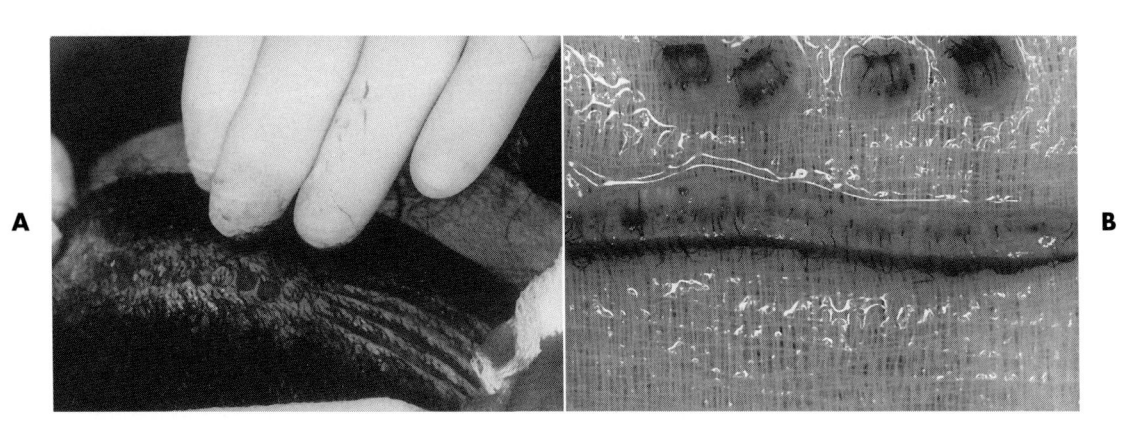

FIG. 7-8 A, Donor sites in a black patient in whom multibladed knife strips (2.5 mm wide) and standard punch grafts (4.5 mm diameter) were taken. **B,** Closeup view of harvested 2.5 mm linear strip and 4.5 mm tissue cylinder grafts. Note the extensive transection of peripheral follicles, particularly with the 2.5 mm strip.

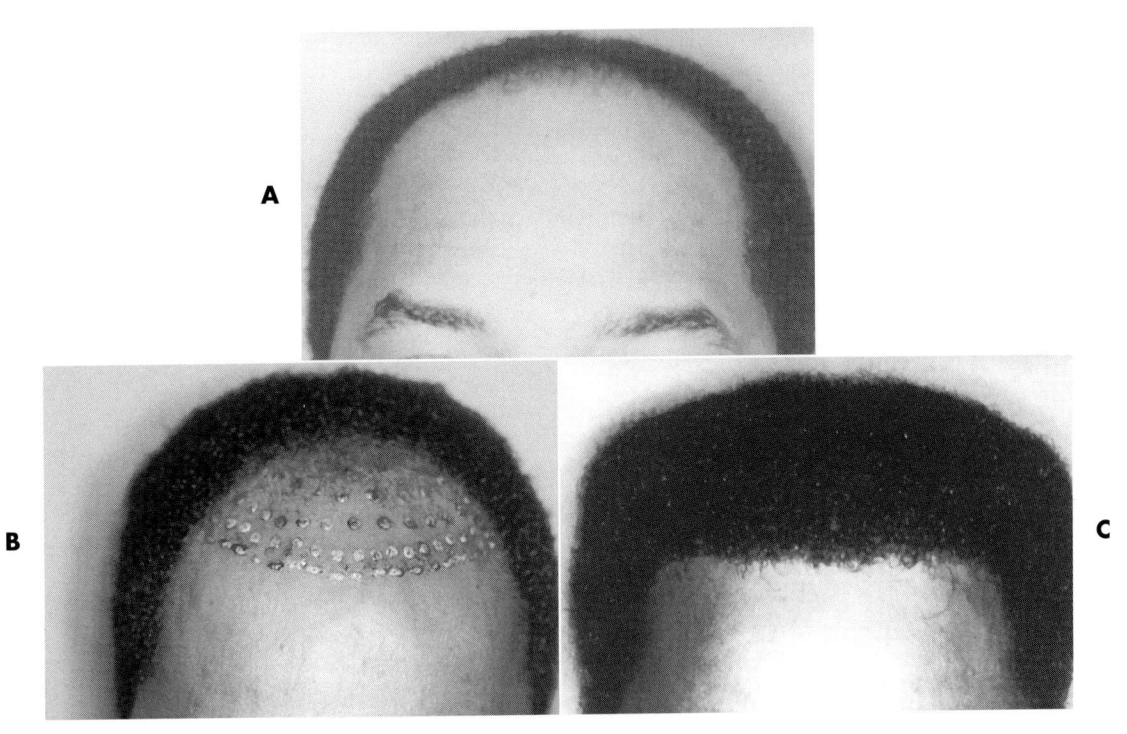

FIG. 7-9 A, Preoperative view of 30-year-old black man. **B,** One-day postoperative view. The patient underwent transplantation with 4 mm traditional punch autografts and slit grafts. This photograph was taken in 1988 and represents older techniques. **C,** Postoperative view. The patient has undergone multiple grafting sessions, mostly incision-slit grafting.

the patient history is positive for either disorder, the patient should fully understand the risk of surgery or the performance of a test graft should again be considered.

CONCLUSION

A respect for patient selection criteria and sequelae that are unique to the black patient is a requirement for hair restoration surgeons involved with this patient population. Hair restoration surgeons must also be cognizant of the amount of hair curvature encountered in a particular patient to do quality alopecia correction.

REFERENCES

1. Wecht CH: *Forensic sciences*, Vol 2, New York, 1991, Matthew Bender, pp 37A-22–37A-29.
2. Randall JK, Schauder CS: Current concepts in alopecia correction in the black patient, *Am J Cosmet Surg* 10(3):173-178, 1993.
3. Norwood OT: The elliptical method. In Norwood OT, editor: *Hair Transplant Forum International* 2:6 July/August 1992.
4. Limmer BL: Using micrografts as a total approach to male pattern alopecia. Presented at the International Society of Hair Surgeons World Congress. Dallas: April 30-May 2, 1993.
5. Unger WP: Hair transplantation in blacks. In Unger WP, Nordstrom REA, editors: *Hair transplantation*, ed 2, New York, 1988, Marcel Dekker, p 300.

D. Hair Transplantation in the Genetically Male Transsexual

Richard C. Shiell

DEFINITION

Transsexualism has been defined as the adoption of a social sex role opposite to that of the biological sex. It is characterized by a persistent and irreversible conviction that one does not belong to one's biological sex but rather to the opposite sex.[1] It is important to stress the difference between transsexuals and homosexuals, who are not distressed with their biological sex but prefer to express their sexuality differently than heterosexuals.

The adult man who rejects his gender and desires sexual reassignment is a rare, although increasingly common, phenomenon. The present incidence is estimated to be from 1:5000 to 1:50,000, and although most who receive medical attention are men, Swedish studies suggest that the sex incidence is almost equal.[2] Some of these persons have gained considerable publicity and notoriety, but from my experience the vast majority wish to remain anonymous and pass silently from being a man to being a woman without fanfare or fuss.

Unfortunately such a luxury is rarely permitted because transsexuals have parents, siblings, or even wives and children, all of whom must confront this issue. Their reaction is generally predictable and is one of shock, hurt, and outrage that their son/brother/husband/father could humiliate the family in such a manner. As a result, many of these persons, in addition to the distress of feeling "like a woman trapped inside a man's body," have the problems of rejection by those whom they love most. On rare occasions a wife or parents may accept the man's desire for gender reassignment with sympathy and understanding, and they may even continue to live under the same roof.

Transsexuality encompasses quite a spectrum of behavior, from a man who enjoys putting on women's clothing in the privacy of his apartment to the man who likes to shop and socialize while dressed as a woman. Later the individual may gain the courage to commence living and working full time as a woman and taking hormone therapy to soften the skin and increase breast development. The final phase, which is sought by only a small percentage of transsexuals, involves surgical removal of the male genitalia and construction of a functional vagina.

At any stage in this progression the individual may seek cosmetic surgery for a variety of feminizing procedures such as breast augmentation, removal of a prominent jawline, augmentation of cheekbones, and removal of a prominent cricoid cartilage ("Adam's apple"). In addition, the older patient may seek surgical correction of wrinkles, baggy eyelids, and "turkey neck" to appear younger.

Male pattern baldness is particularly distressing because it not only is extremely aging but also emphasizes the very attribute that the individual is trying to deny, namely masculinity. For this reason the plastic surgeon or hair transplant specialist is frequently asked for assistance by the genetically male transsexual.

ROLE OF THE PHYSICIAN

The transsexual patient requires empathy and understanding. It is not the physician's place to be critical or judgmental about the patient's choice of lifestyle. That decision was made years earlier, and the patient has often paid for it dearly with loss of old friends, family, and associates. Our role should be to provide sympathy, understanding, support, and an honest assessment of what is and is not possible with regard to hair replacement. If the surgeon is unable to feel comfortable with this situation, these cases should be referred to a more sympathetic colleague.

HAIRLINE DESIGN

The male transsexual is generally seeking to acquire a frontal hair zone that is as near to that of a genetic female as possible. It must be pointed out to the patient that there is a variety of "normal" female hairlines and that some compromise from his ideal may be necessary, depending on the extent of the baldness and the available donor hair.

There are distinct differences between the hairline of the male transsexual and a genetic female with thinning hair. The latter generally retains the hairline and thins immediately behind this region.

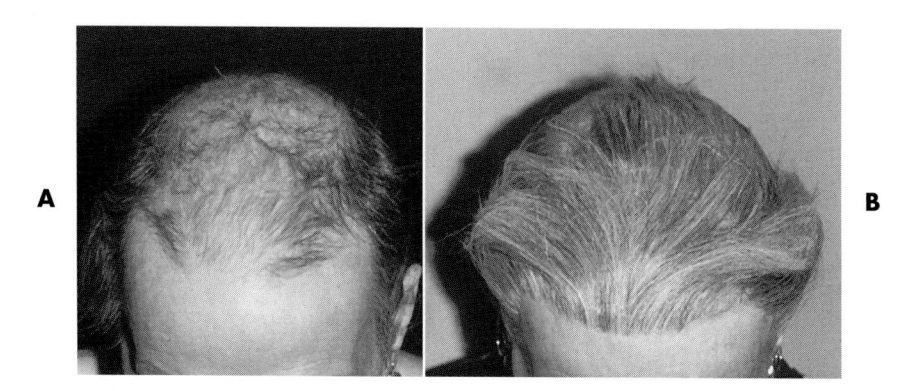

FIG. 7-10 A, Preoperative view of a transsexual patient undergoing hair restoration surgery with a transposition flap. **B,** Postoperative view after completion of a transposition flap.

The transsexual male has male temple recession or more advanced balding of the typical Norwood patterns as shown in Chapter 1, Part C (Fig. 7-10).

TYPE OF TRANSPLANT PROCEDURE

All types of hair restoration surgery are valid for the transsexual, but consideration must be given to the degree of baldness present and the patient's wishes. For well-established baldness of Norwood type V to VII, reduction of the bald area is essential, whereas for smaller degrees of baldness, reconstruction of the frontal hair zone by flap, graft, or minigraft are all very successful if carefully and artistically executed.

There are many variables to consider when advising the patient about the best possible course of action. First, these patients are generally very good at hairstyling and thus can often get by with minimal surgical interference and clever styling. This fact is important because these patients are frequently in financial difficulty as a result of loss of regular employment and divorce and have much other cosmetic surgery to undergo in addition to hair restoration. Second, the site of the donor scars is very important. Most patients want the option of being able to wear their hair up as well as down, so scarring at the lower hair margins is unacceptable.

Most patients want a hairline that is low and rounded at the temples. This is feasible in most cases, but occasionally in middle-aged transsexuals the temple hair has receded too far to allow such a hairline. However, if the surgeon does his/her best, the patient is usually grateful for the extra hair and can usually work miracles with artful hairstyling (Fig. 7-11).

PROGRESSION OF BALDNESS

The male transsexual seeking hair restoration is almost invariably undergoing estrogen therapy and is taking antiandrogens; as a result, progression of the baldness is very slow unless she is required to cease therapy. In this case it is not uncommon for hair loss to begin rapidly and continue until estrogen therapy is resumed. Some older transsexuals have attained Norwood type V or VI baldness before seeking therapy, and these individuals provide the biggest challenge to the hair transplant surgeon because the available donor hair is so limited. It may be best to advise these patients to wear wigs because even after a lengthy series of operations the cosmetic results would still not pass as a convincing female hairstyle.

USE OF SURPLUS FACE-LIFT SKIN

It is common for the older male transsexual to undergo meloplasty for the removal of facial wrinkles and a sagging neck. Modern face-lift procedures attempt to conceal the posterior scars within the parietal hair-bearing zone instead of placement at the posterior hair margin as in older procedures. This scar placement allows the patient to "wear her hair

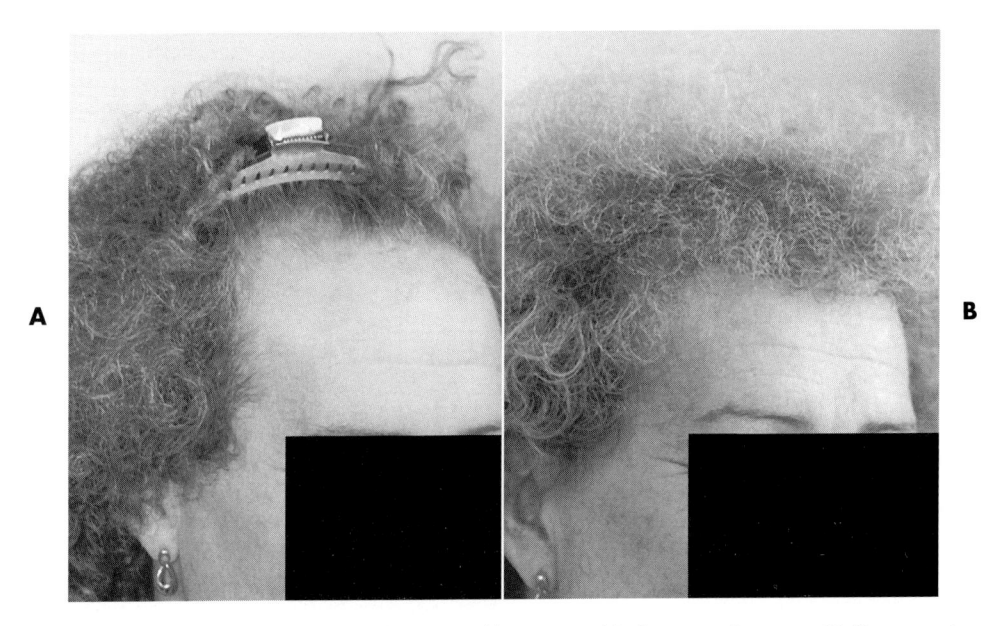

FIG. 7-11 A, Preoperative view of 50-year-old transsexual before transplantation. **B,** Postoperative view after transplantation and hair bleaching.

up" and thus increase the variety of hairstyles that are possible.

When the scar is placed in the parietal zone, much good hair-bearing skin is excised, whereas in the older procedure bald skin or hair of inferior quality on the nape of neck was removed. It is essential that the hair transplant surgeon work with the cosmetic surgeon to utilize these precious hair follicles, as well as those from the surplus temple skin. Occasionally the plastic surgeon is skilled at hair transplant procedures, but generally after a 4- to 5-hour meloplasty with upper and lower blepharoplasties, he/she is in no mood to proceed with a further 1 to 2 hours of hair transplantation. He/she would be well advised to seek the assistance of a skilled hair transplant team at this point.

COORDINATION OF EFFORT

In my experience, cooperation between the two surgeons makes the transplant a simple add-on procedure to the face-lift. The transplant surgeon can time his/her arrival to whenever the cosmetic surgeon estimates he/she will have removed the first section of hair-bearing skin. This donor section is then dissected into whatever size grafts are to be inserted, and the grafts are kept moist in cool saline solution. The skin from the contralateral side will be available shortly thereafter and is similarly dissected and stored. As soon as the plastic surgeon has finished the meloplasty, the hair transplant surgeon gains access to the patient's scalp. Because the patient is usually under general anesthesia, analgesia is no problem, but it is advisable to infiltrate the recipient zone with the usual mixture of saline solution and epinephrine to gain optimum vasoconstriction before graft placement. If this procedure is followed, anesthetic administration need not be prolonged for more than 1 hour and the plastic surgeon can be enjoying a well-earned rest or commencing another case while the transplant surgeon utilizes the otherwise-discarded hair follicles.

REFERENCES

1. Walers WAW: Transsexualism and abdominal pregnancy, *Dev Health Field Bioethical Implications*, 11:12-26, 1990.
2. Walinder J: Incidence and sex ratio of transsexualism in Sweden, *Br J Psych* 119:195-196, 1971.

E. The Treatment of Female Pattern Alopecia by Hair Transplantation

Edmond I. Griffin

Hair loss in women is culturally unacceptable and is not sexually appealing as it may be for some men. Women do not adjust to hair loss as many men do, even if other family members also have hair loss. Most women go to extremes to conceal and treat their hair loss; they use a broad array of creative camouflaging and hair-thickening cosmetic techniques to hide their balding condition. Unfortunately, women experience psychological problems that are even more severe than those experienced by men when their balding process begins. In Chapter 1, Part A, Cash's data show that 70% of balding women were very upset and 52% were extremely upset by their alopecia, whereas only 25% of balding men exhibited this high level of distress because of their alopecia.

Successful treatment of female pattern alopecia is within reach today more so than in the past as a result of three time-intensive refinements: micrografting, strip donor harvesting, and slit grafting. When these techniques are used, both the physician and the patient should be pleased with the results.

These improvements in hair transplantation require that surgeons reexamine their approach to balding female patients who may have been rejected for hair transplants in the past or who would have been dissatisfied with the results of the earlier hair transplant procedures. What distinguishes the improved techniques is that they thicken the thinning hair while avoiding damage or removal of any existing hair follicles. They produce a more natural and delicate appearance by decreasing the sizes of grafts into minigrafts and micrografts, and they conserve the donor area. They minimize both the donor and recipient site scars.

DIAGNOSIS OF FEMALE ANDROGENIC ALOPECIA

Workup

The approach to the balding woman involves a more involved and time-consuming workup than in men. This workup can be facilitated by an appropriate referral to a dermatologist, who will direct the evaluation. The woman with diffuse hair loss may incur significant expense to obtain the necessary biopsy and hormonal testing. To simplify matters, women who suffer a particular pattern of hair loss as described and classified by Ludwig[1] do not need to undergo the barrage of testing required by women who do not fit into this pattern of hair loss. With experience, one can categorize the pattern of hair loss in a woman almost as easily and with as much skill as in a man (as classified by Hamilton[2] or Norwood[3]). When there is any doubt about the classification of the female patient who has the diffuse generalized variety of hair loss, initial testing with a complete blood count, ferritin, and thyroid studies (T3, T4) can be performed. An extensive medical, drug, and family history must also be obtained. If the patient's review of systems suggests a hormonal abnormality, additional testing with serum and free testosterone, dehydroepiandrosterone sulfate, and possibly prolactin, sex hormone–binding globulin, luteinizing hormone, and follicle-stimulating hormone can be performed.[4] Most women with nonscarring alopecia have no evidence of abnormal androgen production.[5] A scalp biopsy may be necessary to complete the workup and to help to confirm the diagnosis.

Progression of Alopecia in Women

In women, hair loss is usually on the central scalp rather than being bitemporal as it is in men (Fig. 7-12). After menopause, additional bitemporal loss is noted. Venning and Dawber,[6] in a survey of normal premenopausal women, reported a Ludwig pattern in 87% and a Hamilton type in 13%. Data of Olsen[7] show that in 5% of women with androgenic alopecia there is a global decrease in scalp hair density. Balding occurs in women at an older age and the progression is usually not complete as in men. Complete loss is rare in women, and if present, an underlying androgen excess should be investigated.

Important Cosmetic Questions for the Female Patient

The desires and goals of women with baldness are different from those of men. The following questions should be considered: How has the patient styled her hair? Is she willing to change her hairstyle, curl, and/or color? Is she now dyeing her gray hair a dark color? Would she consider possibly a frosted shade of brown? If genetically her hair is dark black and coarse as found in Asians (in which case color change is difficult and culturally unacceptable), would she consider curling her hair? Many women limit styling options. Would she consider wearing a hairpiece or hairweave if she wants the thick, high-fashion appearance? Have extenders been used or considered as an option? Does she participate in athletic activities in which heavy perspiration is usual?

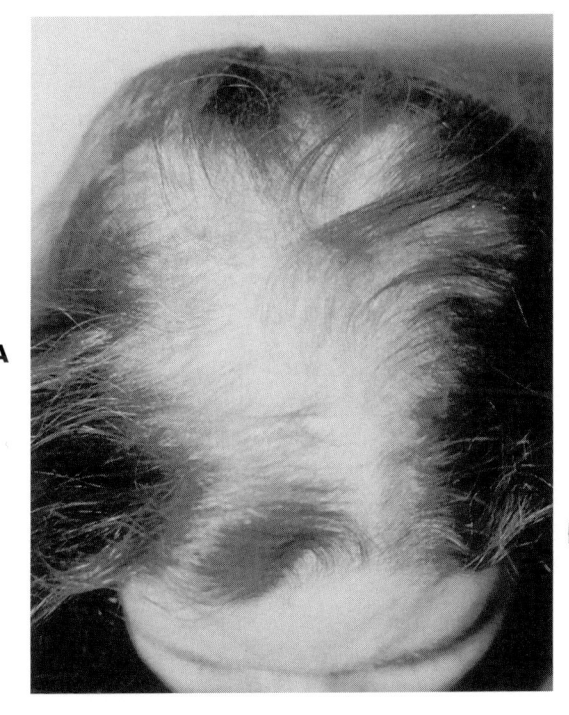

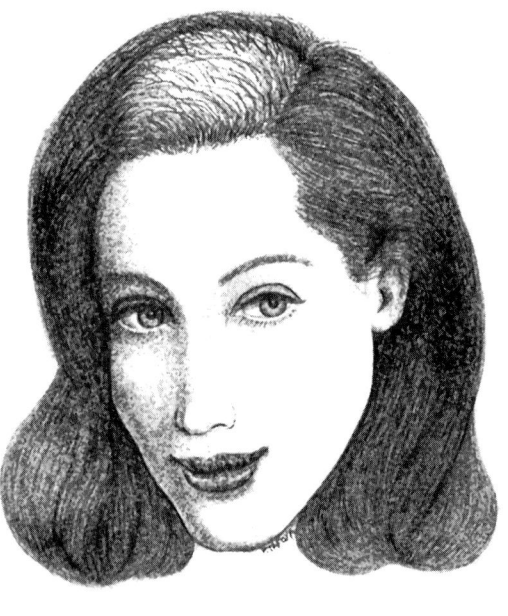

FIG. 7-12 Photograph of typical patient (**A**) and artist's drawing (**B**) demonstrate Ludwig-type female baldness in which there is preservation of the frontal rim with central hair loss.

EVALUATION OF THE FEMALE PATIENT WITH PATTERN HAIR LOSS

Patient Assessment

Evaluate the hair characteristics, including color (black, brown, red, blonde, or gray); texture (coarse, medium, or fine); skin-to-scalp contrast (high-contrast black hair on fair skin, low-contrast red hair on ruddy skin or medium-contrast brown hair on olive skin); and level of curl (kinky, curly, or straight). These four hair characteristics play an important role in determining the patient's suitability for transplantation and represent four of the six major factors. According to Norwood,[8] density and the amount of donor hair represent the other two major factors for the proper patient selection. Cotterill and Unger[9] approach suitability for transplantation by combining these factors into ratios of donor:recipient area and donor:recipient hair density (modified by hair quality and color).

Evaluate the extent of alopecia and assess the percentage of loss. The patient should be classified as having a Ludwig grade I, II, or III pattern. Next, evaluate the level of bitemporal loss as described for men by Hamilton. Search for the third type of hair loss, which is the diffuse loss of discrete areas. Identify the areas of loss that most concern the patient. How much loss can be anticipated for the future? Evaluate the donor area, which must be large enough and have the necessary density of hair follicles to cover the area of alopecia. The greater the density of donor hair, the more grafts that can be produced from a given donor area. With below-average density of fine black hair, more than four sessions may not sufficiently thicken the area of alopecia to the satisfaction of the patient. If the patient needs grafts to correct frontal loss, the total grafts remaining to treat the area of Ludwig pattern hair loss will be significantly reduced because of the large number required to produce a restored frontal hairline. The middle-aged woman with Ludwig grade II central hair loss with the preservation of a thick, wide donor fringe may be an excellent candidate, especially if her hair is gray, light brown, blonde, or red. In contrast the premenopausal patient with a similar loss pattern who has a narrow, thinned donor fringe with dark, fine hair may be a poor candidate for grafting. The relative significance of each of these parameters relies on the judgment and experience of the hair transplant surgeon, who must weigh each factor for the individual patient at that point in time. Future loss both in the donor and recipient areas must be considered if multiple initial transplant sessions are planned.

Evaluate the potential for additional hair loss. Age, family history, and hormonal status are all factors that may help to estimate possible future hair loss. If a 20-year-old patient with familial alopecia is losing her hair, she may experience extensive balding in the future. This patient should be warned about the unpredictable and progressive course of androgenic baldness as it affects both men and women. A low estrogen–high progesterone birth control pill may precipitate hair loss. Changing the type of birth control pills the patient uses may slow the loss, as suggested by Olsen.[10] If the patient continues to lose hair despite medical intervention, estimate the donor area left in the "bank" after the planned sessions.

Role of Scalp Reductions or Flaps in Women

Scalp reductions with or without expanders or extenders are considered mainly for patients with traumatic localized loss or loss resulting from cosmetic surgery (coronal lift or rhytidectomy). For these postsurgical areas of alopecia, the multiple small-graft technique satisfies the patient's need to cover her scars. Scar lines can be transplanted, producing the desired camouflage. Flaps, scalp-lifting, and scalp reductions are rarely treatment options in women with Ludwig androgenic alopecia. The patient has a broad, central area of loss and possibly a thinned donor area. Women may have thinning in the lateral regions, making any additional scars a liability. Female styling requirements dictate that as few scars as possible be created. For women with the less common bitemporal loss, a feathered hairline can be created with the delicate transplanted grafts with the fewest risks.

INFORMED CONSENT

Satisfaction is sometimes impossible to achieve in the patient with unrealistic expectations. Another unknown in the equation of satisfaction is the opinion of the family member, close friend, and especially hairstylist. These outsiders may be the final judge of the hair transplant surgery. The prudent physician must take the time to assess what the patient and "friends" will accept for final thickness and coverage and the number of sessions required to reach her goal. The balding woman approaches hair transplantation and what she will accept as the outcome differently than her male counterpart. In general, she is harder to please, more demanding, and less forgiving. Sometimes, questioning the patient reveals that she did not hear what you said or understand what you meant. Time well spent before the process may save time in the long run.

TESTING, MEDICATIONS, AND POSTOPERATIVE INSTRUCTIONS

Blood tests and preoperative and postoperative medications do not differ for the female patient. Coverage after the procedure is less of a problem than in men because of the existing hair. Patients must be encouraged to shampoo their hair regularly and are allowed to use gentle shampoos with cream rinses, styling gels, and unscented hair sprays, allowing them to return to normal activities. As with men, they may restart Rogaine application 1 week after surgery.

ANESTHESIA

Women are similar to men in their requirements for local anesthesia. Women seem to have less initial anxiety, and their overall tolerance of the procedure is better. The majority of the local anesthesia is provided by 0.5% lidocaine (Xylocaine) with 1:200,000 epinephrine. Supraorbital blocks with fringe blocks with long-acting anesthetics help to sustain the anesthesia for these lengthy procedures.

DONOR SITE

Selection of the donor site in women is influenced by their hairstyling preferences in addition to the hair loss pattern. In general, the most commonly selected site is the midoccipital area. Use of this site avoids possible future loss while avoiding a site low on the neck, where both styling and future loss are important considerations. The location of the highest density of hair is the central occipital area. The parietal areas over the ears are frequently thinned in women but can be harvested as in men if the finest hairs are needed for the hairline in women with bitemporal loss.

STRIP HARVEST TECHNIQUE

The strip harvest technique is used exclusively for harvesting donor grafts because of the ease of obtaining a large quantity of high-quality hair grafts. After a narrow band of hair is trimmed, the remaining hair is combed away from the incision site with the help of a water-based gel lubricant (Surgilube). Women's hair strands can be kept free from the surgical area with use of small rubber bands. Immediately before the strip is harvested, a solution of normal saline solution is injected to stabilize the hair follicles, making them stand upright so that the incisions produce less follicular damage. Injection of this solution improves hemostasis, resulting in a drier operative field with overall decreased surgical time. The strip is harvested with either a double- or triple-bladed scalpel, and the resulting defect is closed with surgical stainless staples, which are especially favored in scalp surgery in women without the use of subcutaneous sutures. They create fine surgical scars without compromising the remaining hair follicles due to compression from edema postoperatively. The comfort level is comparable to that with running horizontal mattress sutures (unpublished data, E.I. Griffin).

RECIPIENT SITE

Many hair follicles in the female patient will remain for the rest of her life. Many follicles will not involute completely as they may in the aging man. Balding women will not become totally bald, and they need to preserve every possible hair. This be-

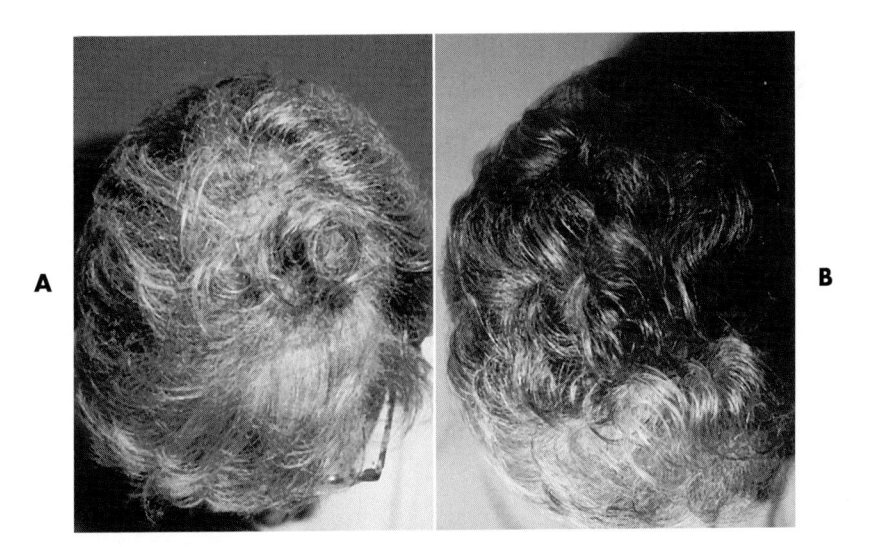

FIG. 7-13 **A,** Graying older woman with Ludwig grade I loss with central scalp thinning. **B,** Postoperative view after two micrografting sessions.

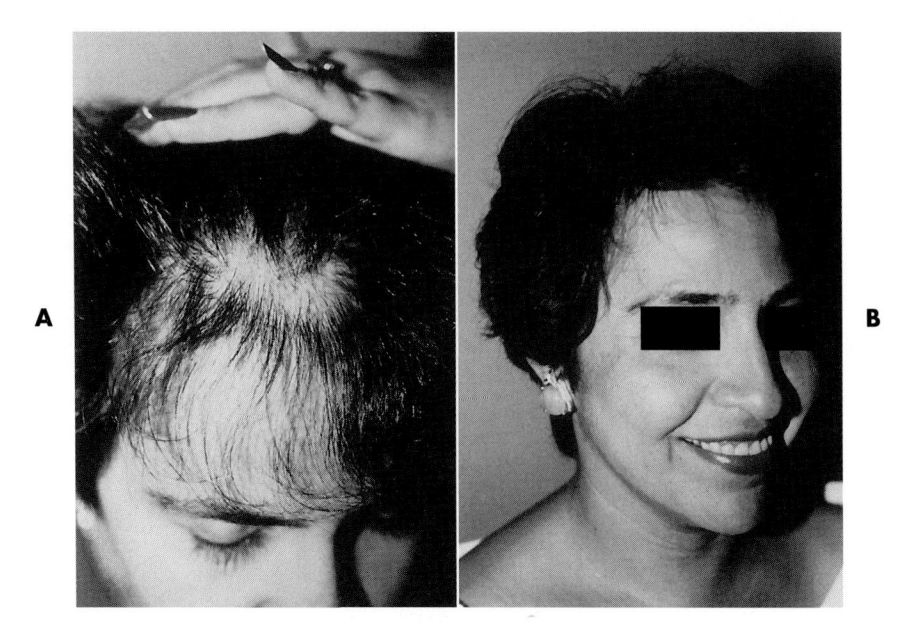

FIG. 7-14 A, Dark-haired woman with a white scalp, which is difficult to disguise as hair loss increases. **B,** Increased hair density after two micrografting sessions allows for easier styling.

comes especially important in the woman with thinning hair whose hair in the donor site is also below average density. In the past this type of patient was dissatisfied with the hair transplanting process. The treatment goal for the woman with pattern hair loss is to not damage or discard any follicles because all are needed.

TRANSPLANTING THE RECIPIENT SITES
Women with Ludwig Grade I To III Pattern Loss

The Ludwig grade I to III pattern applies to most of the women whose frontal hairline persists (Fig. 7-13). The transplanting process begins behind this natural hairline. In this hairline several thinning areas may be noted, which are corrected with the appropriately sized graft. In women the transplanted grafts start 5 to 10 mm behind the hairline. Along this edge the first rows of incisions are made with the Beaver No. 64 blade for the grafts containing two to three lighter, finer hairs. The B-P No. 15 blade makes the slits for grafts containing four to five, five to six, or six to eight hairs. (In general, darker, coarser hair should have fewer hairs in each graft, whereas lighter, finer hair may have a higher number of hairs per graft, up to six to eight hairs.) Again, the hair characteristics and the balding patterns dictate what type of grafts will be used. Round recipient holes from 1.25 to 2.25 mm are used to avoid compression and provide the perfect-sized site for the grafts. If no round patches of baldness exist at the time of transplantation, no round grafts are used (Fig. 7-14).

Women with Bitemporal Loss

For the small number of female patients who have the male type bitemporal loss, the transplant approach is like that used with men (Fig. 7-15). The feathered, irregular, soft natural edge is the goal. Created with the lightest, finest, and most delicate grafts, the hairline is started with single-hair grafts, into which are progressively intermingled the grafts with two to four, four to six, and finally six to eight hairs as one progresses further back. Occasionally the balding area may require small, round recipient sites.

TECHNICAL CONSIDERATIONS
Alopecic Scalp vs. Thinning Regions

ALOPECIC SCALP. Look for areas of complete baldness that can be removed (Fig. 7-16). A water-based gel (Surgilube) helps to expose these bald areas and prevents hair from tangling in the hand engine. Remove the bald areas with a 1.25 to 2.25 mm round punch. If the patient has dark coarse hair, select the smaller sized punches (1.5 mm accommodates a three- to four-hair graft, and 1.75 mm accommodates a four- to six-hair graft). If the hair is fair or fine, the larger size punches (2.25 mm) are selected. No dilators are necessary for any round recipient sites because the size of the graft placed

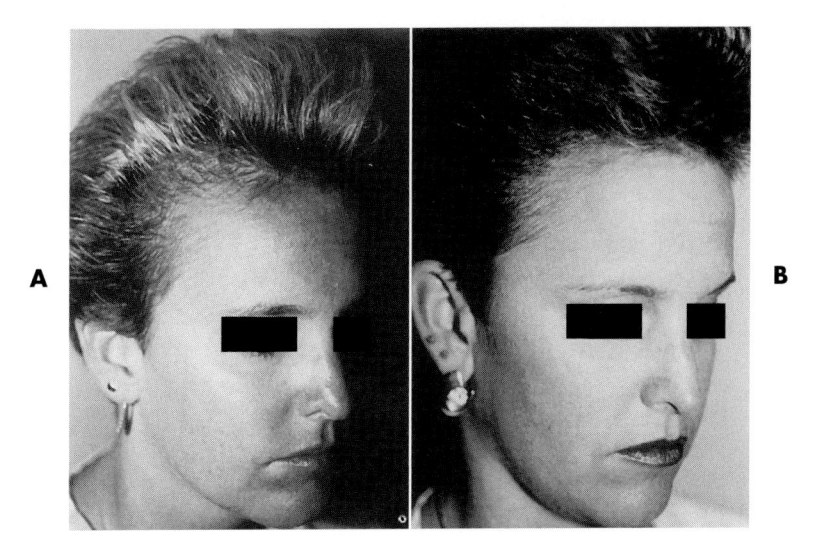

The Treatment of Female Pattern Alopecia by Hair Transplantation 215

FIG. 7-15 **A,** Temporal thinning in young female patient who lightens her hair to hide thinning. **B,** Patient with her natural dark hair after two micrografting sessions in the temporal zone.

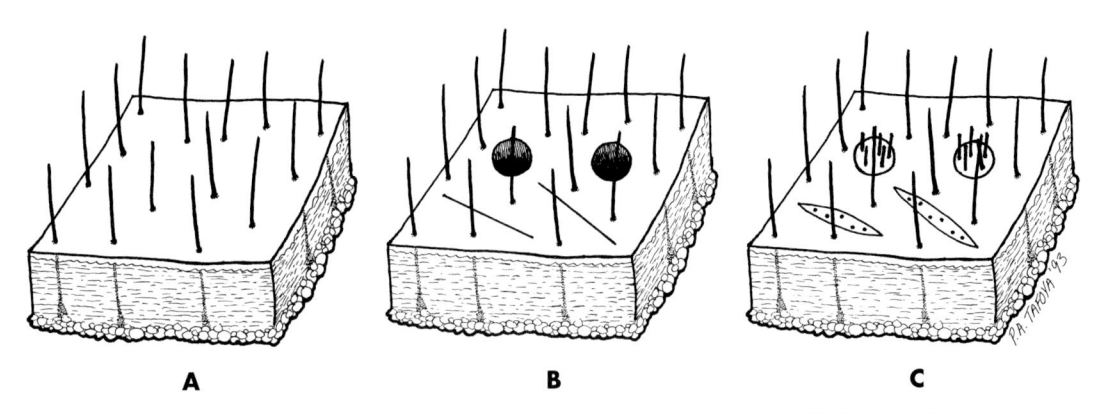

FIG. 7-16 **A,** Alopecia with totally bald areas. **B,** Round punch excisions of bald areas where possible and incisions in other areas. **C,** Placement of incisional and round grafts.

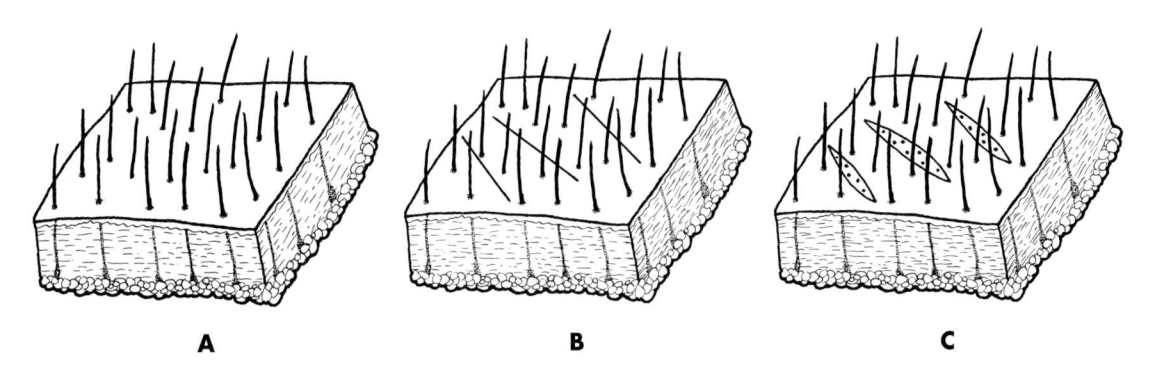

FIG. 7-17 **A,** When there is less thinning in the fringe area and there are no totally bald areas (and thus bald skin could not be removed without damaging or removing follicles), then only slit grafts are placed **(B). C,** Incisional grafts in place.

into it will be sized for the best results, and it is unlikely that the graft will slip below the epithelial surface.

THINNING REGIONS. Thinning regions should be transplanted with slit grafts as opposed to round punches (Fig. 7-17). The usefulness of slit grafts has been pointed out in the past.[11,12] Thinned hair in which there are no areas of total baldness are ideal areas for the slit grafts. To avoid damaging any follicles,[13] incisions for the slit grafts are placed between hair follicles at the same angle and direction as the follicle. It has been my impression that the "shallow incision" damages fewer follicles and avoids the deeper vascular plexus.[14] Because it is not deep enough to make an adequate pocket for the graft, a blunt dilator pushes through the follicles without injury and makes the graft pocket.[15] This is analogous to a liposuction cannula that pushes around nerves and blood vessels.

CONCLUSION

Women are indeed candidates for hair transplantation. The workup and approach used with women differs considerably from that used with men. Expectations of the surgical outcome and the need for a more detailed, female-oriented informed consent are stressed. Properly selected female patients with both Ludwig and bitemporal loss patterns have undergone micrografting and have been pleased with the outlined techniques.

REFERENCES

1. Ludwig E: Classification of the types of androgenetic alopecia (common baldness) occurring in the female sex, *Br J Dermatol* 97:247-254, 1977.
2. Hamilton JB: Patterned loss of hair in man: types and incidence, *Ann N Y Acad Sci* 53:708-728, 1951.
3. Norwood OT: Male pattern baldness: classification and incidence, *South Med J* 68:1359-1365, 1975.
4. Fiedler VC, Hafeez A: Diffuse alopecia: telogen hair loss. In Olsen EA, editor: *Disorders of hair growth*, New York, 1994, McGraw-Hill, pp 241-255.
5. Futterweit W and others: The prevalence of hyperandrogenism in 109 consecutive female patients with diffuse alopecia, *J Am Acad Dermatol* 19:831-836, 1988.
6. Venning VA, Dawber RPR: Patterned alopecia in women, *J Am Acad Dermatol* 18:1073-1077, 1988.
7. Olsen EA: Androgenetic alopecia in disorders of hair growth. In Olsen EA, editor: *Disorders of hair growth*, New York, 1994, McGraw-Hill, pp 258-259.
8. Norwood OT: Patient selection, hair transplant design, and hairstyle, *J Dermatol Surg Oncol* 18:386-394, 1992.
9. Cotterill PC, Unger WP: Hair transplantation in females, *J Dermatol Surg Oncol* 18:477-481, 1992.
10. Olsen EA: Androgenetic alopecia in disorders of hair growth. In Olsen EA, editor: *Disorders of hair growth*, New York, 1994, McGraw-Hill, pp 257-279.
11. Swinehart JM, Griffin EI: Slit grafting: the use of serrated island grafts in male and female pattern alopecia, *J Dermatol Surg Oncol* 17:243-253, 1991.
12. Stough DB IV, Nelson BR, Stough DB III: Incisional slit grafting, *J Dermatol Surg Oncol* 17:53-60, 1991.
13. Stough DB and others: Hair transplantation by incisional slit grafting in women with androgenic alopecia, *J Cutan Aging Cosmet Dermatol* 1:233-247, 1991.
14. Griffin EI: Hair Transplantation in the Female. Presented at the American Academy of Facial Plastic Surgery Course on Hair Transplantation, Birmingham, Ala.
15. Marritt E: Micrograft dilators: in pursuit of the undetectable hairline, *J Dermatol Surg Oncol* 14:268-275, 1988.

F. Hair Transplantation of the Eyelashes and Eyebrows

Jung-Chul Kim and Yung-Chul Choi

The eyebrows remain an important cosmetic asset of the face; when eyebrows are absent, individuals may suffer significant distress over their appearance. The cause of an eyebrow defect or loss may be a burn, trauma, complications resulting from tattoos, alopecia areata, or leprosy. Most patients who need eyebrow transplantation, especially Asians, have patchy eyebrow growth. Reconstruction of eyebrows by using micrografts of various sizes usually yields good results.[1-3] We have developed the single-hair transplantation technique for reconstruction of the eyebrows with the Choi hair transplanter.[4]

EYEBROW ANATOMY

The normal direction of eyebrow hair demonstrates an upward direction of the hairs in the medial region. The middle and lateral eyebrow hairs grow toward each other with a central convergence (Fig. 7-18). The second distinctive feature of the eyebrow is the flat angle of growth as the hairs emerge from the follicular orifice (Fig. 7-19).

Successful reconstruction of the eyebrow depends on the surgeon's ability to reproduce the di-

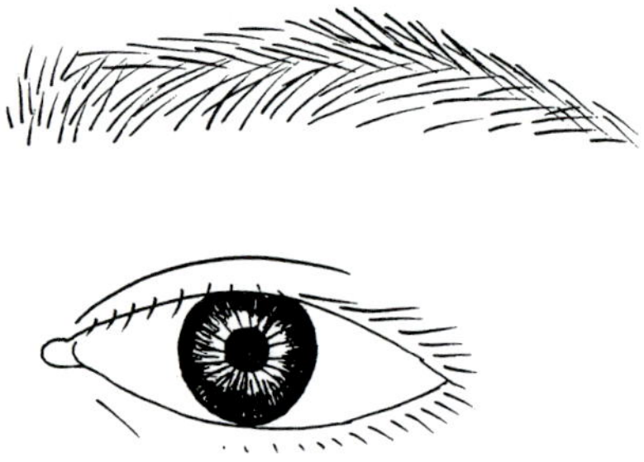

FIG. 7-18 Eyebrow hairs grow toward each other and converge centrally.

rection and angle of a normal eyebrow with the use of single-hair grafts.

EYEBROW TRANSPLANTATION

All sites requiring grafts are marked with an indelible pen. Patients assist in drawing the outline of their eyebrows. After the site is anesthetized with 1% lidocaine, an ellipse of hair-bearing scalp is taken from the lower occipital region. The donor area is then closed with suture.[5] The hair-bearing strip is sectioned into several segments with a No. 20 scalpel blade; the blade must be carefully positioned between the visible hair follicles. Further sectioning produces single-hair grafts (Fig. 7-20). Once again, great care must be taken to cut between and at the same angle as the hair follicles. Excess epidermis, dermis, and fat are trimmed away (Fig. 7-21). Grafts are sectioned on a block of birch wood. Normally no magnification is required, but some nurses prefer to cut under a 4× magnification lens positioned on the instrument trolley. It is not desirable to remove the epidermis from the grafts. The epidermis aids in graft positioning and orientation. Extensive pitting is unusual with single-hair grafts.

The hair shaft of the single-hair graft is grasped with fine forceps and inserted onto the needle of the hair transplanter (Fig. 7-22). The operator now inserts the needle into the skin at the desired angle and pushes the plunger. The needle is automatically withdrawn, leaving the hair follicle neatly tucked under the skin. It should be noted that the ring around the needle holds the single-hair graft in place while the needle is withdrawn. Once the graft is in place, gentle pressure is applied with a swab while adjacent hair grafts are inserted. No dressing or bandage is required. Although we use the Choi transplanter, similar results can be achieved with single-hair grafts placed into small, 18-gauge needle recipient sites or small slit incisions.

The advantages of this method are as follows:

1. One can complete work on the eyebrow with one operation by close graft placement. We transplant approximately 600 single-hair grafts for the reconstruction of both eyebrows in a single operation.

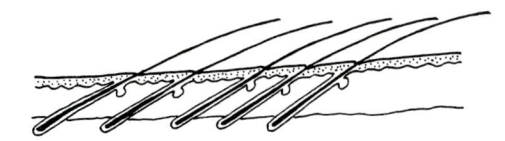

FIG. 7-19 Hairs of the eyebrow emerge at a flat angle from the follicular orifice.

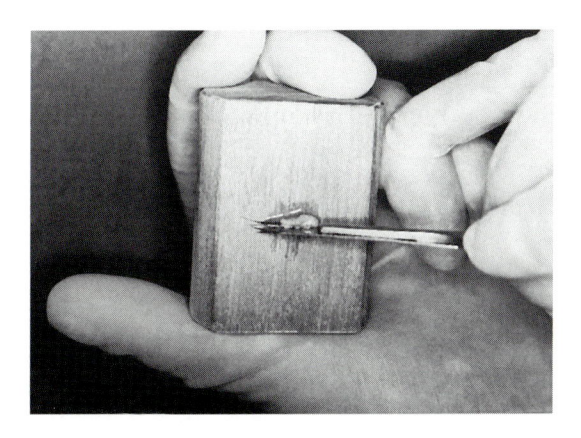

FIG. 7-20 Separation of single-hair grafts.

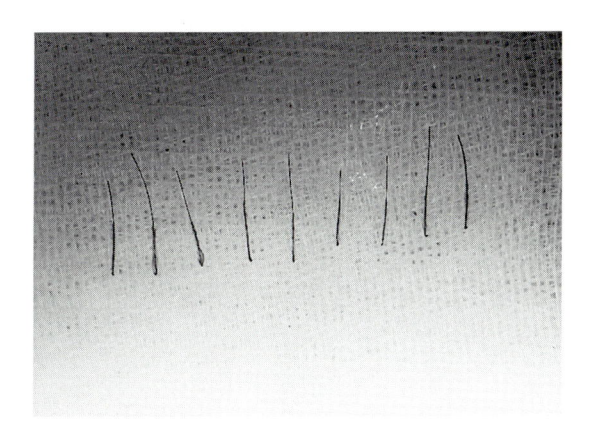

FIG. 7-21 Single-hair grafts.

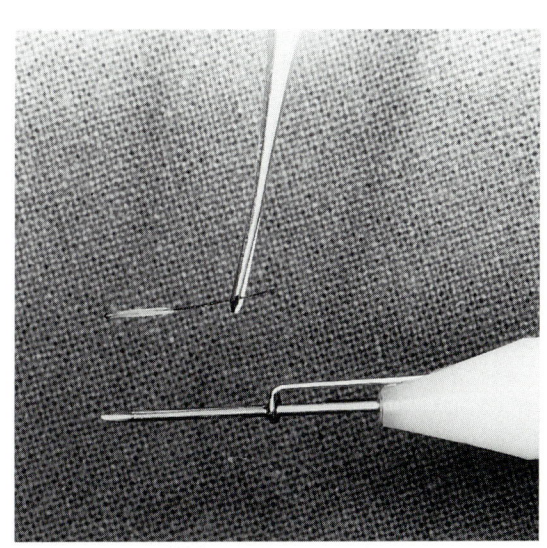

FIG. 7-22 Choi hair transplanter with single-hair graft.

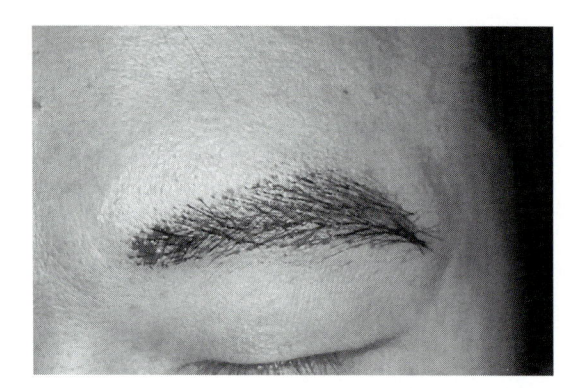

FIG. 7-23 Natural hair direction of reconstructed eyebrows.

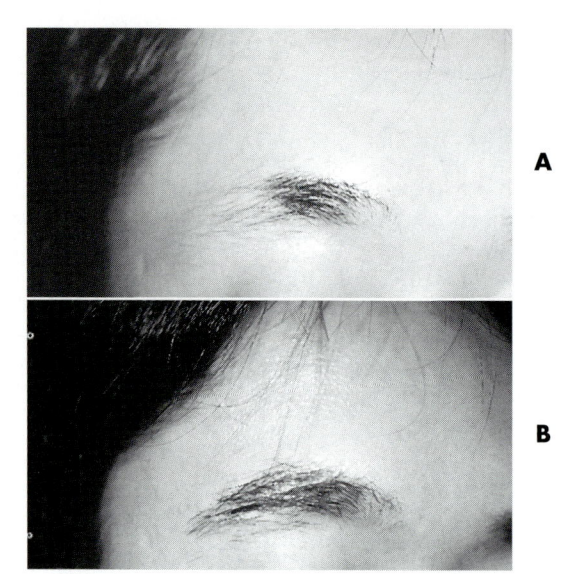

FIG. 7-24 **A,** Preoperative view. **B,** Ten-month postoperative view after eyebrow reconstruction.

2. It is necessary to both reconstruct and mimic the flat angle of the hairs against the skin in the normal eyebrow, the upward direction of growth in the medial part of the brow, and the convergence of the lateral part as normally seen in eyebrows. However, experience has shown that the medial segment of the transplanted eyebrow should be reconstructed with a convergent and more lateral direction as opposed to the normal upward growth (Fig. 7-23). This modification is needed because the transplanted hair is thicker than normal eyebrow hair. Transplanting hairs in an upward direction in the medial part produces growth that may be unnatural.
3. This method can be used to correct partial failures resulting from other methods of eyebrow reconstruction.
4. Almost 100% of the transplanted hairs in the grafts survive, generating a dense growth of hair in the new eyebrow (Fig. 7-24).

EYELASH TRANSPLANTATION

With slight modification, the technique we use for eyelash transplantation is similar to that described for eyebrow reconstruction. The inferior nape is chosen for the donor site. To obtain fine single-hair grafts, excess epidermis, dermis, and fat are trimmed away. The epidermal segment is not required for eyelash transplantation.

After the eyelid is anesthetized with 1% lidocaine with 1:100,000 epinephrine, a flat metal eyeshield is placed under the eyelid to protect the cornea. A single-hair graft is placed onto the needle of the hair transplanter (Choi hair transplanter, type S–21 gauge) with fine jeweler's forceps. The operator now inserts the needle of the hair transplanter into the eyelid and pushes the plunger while the left finger steadies the eyelid. The hair follicle will remain in the eyelid while the needle is withdrawn. Approximately 50 single-hair grafts are inserted for reconstruction of both eyelids in a single session. No dressing or bandage is required. Some surgeons use a special ophthalmologist's eyelid holder during the recipient site lancing and insertion of the single-hair grafts.[6] We find this instrument cumbersome and have noted grafts popping with its use. Because the needle of the Choi hair transplanter type S (21 gauge) is sharp, gentle pressure on the eyelid is adequate to maintain the lid position upright while the single-hair graft is inserted. The eyelashes must be trimmed regularly to prevent them from growing unnaturally long.

REFERENCES

1. Arkawa I: Simple hair transplantation for eyebrow, *Jpn J Plast Reconstr Surg* 8:8, 1965.
2. Ishiko S: Repair of eyebrows: single hair transplantation using Kanazashnis needle, *Jpn J Plast Reconstr Surg* 8:11, 1965.
3. Nordstrom RE: Eyebrow reconstruction by punch hair transplantation, *Plast Reconstr Surg* 60:74, 1977.
4. Choi YC, Kim JC: Single hair transplantation using Choi hair transplanter, *J Dermatol Surg Oncol* 18:945-948, 1992.
5. Hitzig GS: Pulley suture, utilization in scalp reconstruction surgery, *J Dermatol Surg Oncol* 18:220-222, 1992.
6. Unger WP, Nordstrom REA: *Hair transplantation*, New York, 1988, Marcel Dekker.

8
Wound Healing

A. Wound Healing in Hair Restoration Surgery

David J. Margolis

Wound healing is the final event of almost every surgical procedure. In hair restoration surgery at least two distinct areas of the patient's scalp, the donor site and the graft recipient site, need to heal. Although scar formation is the final outcome of most wounds, tissue regeneration is the ideal outcome for injured tissues. Many of the physiological processes involved in acute wound healing have been well described in the past. In recent years studies have focused on the biochemical events in acute wound healing and on methods to minimize the time to complete healing, maximize the strength of a scar, and improve the overall cosmetic acceptability of a scar. These advances concern both bandaging techniques and altering the tissues and messengers involved in acute wound healing. Because very few of these studies have been directed toward hair replacement surgery, this chapter attempts to provide the reader with a basic understanding of wound healing so that a curious and thoughtful physician may be able to improve his/her surgical and postoperative techniques, thereby maximizing graft success. Excellent reviews on wound healing have been published in the past several years.[1-4]

WOUND HEALING

A wound is the disruption of normal anatomical structure and function in living biological tissue.[5] An acute wound proceeds through an orderly and timely process that results in a sustained restoration of anatomical and functional integrity.[5] Acute wounds are present in both the donor and recipient sites during hair restoration surgery. Porcine and murine species are most commonly used for acute wound studies. Although both of these species are hair-bearing animals, very few studies have focused directly on hair appendages during wound healing. Although it is believed that wound healing in these animals mimics the events that take place in humans, this is not always true. For example, wound contraction is much more important in murine than in human acute wound healing; the chronic wound cannot be adequately mimicked in either porcine or murine species. In general, animal studies indicate that wound healing occurs in three overlapping phases: inflammation, proliferation, and remodeling[6] (Fig. 8-1).

Inflammatory Phase

The inflammatory phase of wound healing begins with tissue injury. The injury in hair restoration surgery results in the disruption of the epidermis, dermis, and dermal blood vessels. These events result in altered vascular permeability, exudation of plasma components and blood into the surrounding tissues, activation and aggregation of platelets, and activation of the coagulation and fibrinolytic cascades.[6-8] Many of these cascades are initiated by the release of cellular mediators as a result of disruption of tissue and cellular integrity. Vasoconstriction occurs shortly after the disruption of the blood vessels. Platelet aggregation and activation are promoted by the exposure of the blood vessel wall collagens—type IV and V collagen[9]—to platelets and by the release of cytokines from damaged cells. These events initiate the formation of a fibrin plug within both the vessel and the surrounding tissue. These early steps also trigger several cascades that result in the migration and activation of neutrophils, macrophages, monocytes, and lymphocytes into the wound area.[7,8,10] The goals of this phase are to establish hemostasis; remove wound contaminants; establish a provisional extracellular matrix, which will act as the scaffolding for the next two phases of wound healing; create a proper environment for granulation tissue formation and epithelization; and activate and accumulate the cells required for the proliferative phase. The monocyte or macrophage may be the most pivotal cellular element for the passage from the inflammatory phase to the proliferative phase of acute wound healing.[10,11]

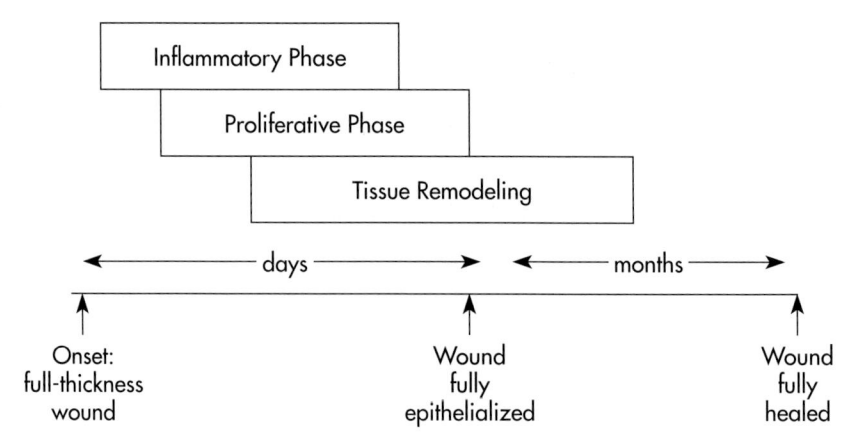

FIG. 8-1 The overlapping phases of acute wound healing.[1]

Proliferative Phase

The proliferative phase, or the beginning of new tissue repair, begins shortly after establishment of the inflammatory phase. The proliferative phase occurs within the dermis and epidermis. Dermal repair is equated with granulation tissue formation; this requires the repair of both blood vessels and dermis. This phase is probably most closely modulated by cytokines, which are protein agents responsible for the migration, maturation, and mitogenesis of the cellular components required for tissue repair. The initial release of these factors is from platelets, macrophages, other cells involved in the inflammatory phase, cells injured in wounding, and other constituent parts of the dermis. Fibroblasts, which are essential to dermal repair, undergo migration into the wound. Several different fibroblast phenotypes are needed in wound healing.[12] This process appears to be modulated by the extracellular matrix[13] and by cytokines released primarily by platelets, macrophages, and injured cells. As the fibroblast population is reestablished in the wound, fibronectin is produced,[14] which acts as an early scaffolding on which the extracellular matrix is formed.[13] Wound contracture also occurs during this phase. Wound contracture is an effective method of wound closure that probably has a greater role in murine than in human acute wound healing. Wound contracture is controlled by fibroblasts and is both a function of fibroblast movement and a true tissue contraction. It is governed by a phenotypically distinct fibroblast that contains actin microfilaments.[15]

Angiogenesis, the creation of new blood vessels, also occurs in the dermis during the proliferative phase. This process requires the migration and proliferation of endothelial cells, which seldom divide once formed in a vessel.[16] In response to angiogenic stimuli, new vessels begin as outgrowths from existing vessels.[17,18] The stimulus for angiogenesis is from cytokine growth factors and from dermal constituents, which include oxygen, platelets, macrophages, mast cells, heparin, and fibronectin.[19] The origin of the stem cell line for fibroblasts and endothelial cells has not been established.

The repair of the epidermis is called *epithelialization*. It is part of the proliferative phase and begins shortly after wounding. The wound healing process is often incorrectly noted to be completed when a wound is fully epithelialized. Unlike the dermal cellular components, the epidermal cells are continually replenished in the nonwounded state. The stem cell or transient amplifying cell of the epidermis is located in the basal cell layer.[20] As cells from the basal cell layer mature, they undergo extensive phenotypic alteration until they become fully keratinized, mature epidermal cells.[21] In acute wound healing, the migration of the new keratinocytes seems to be directed from any epithelial source on the wound edge or from within the wound such as the infundibulum of the hair.[22,23] Cell movement probably does not occur by individual cells but by sheets of keratinocytes.[24,25] The stimulus for keratinocyte migration is probably modulated by the loss of contact inhibition and the local production of cytokine growth factors. The basement membrane that is required to reestablish the dermal epidermal junction is not established until after epithelial cell migration is complete.[1]

Cytokine growth factors are protein mediators involved in cell-to-cell interactions. Many cytokine growth factors are involved in wound healing.[26,27] The discovery of novel cytokine growth factors and new activities for previously described cytokine growth factors occurs several times a year. Their exact role in acute wound healing has not been precisely determined. The most studied growth factors are epidermal growth factor, fibroblast growth fac-

TABLE 8-1 Commonly Reported Cytokine Growth Factors

CYTOKINE GROWTH FACTOR (ABBREVIATION)	EFFECTOR SITES	COMMENTS
Epidermal growth factor (EGF)	Epithelium	Shares TGF-α receptor
Transforming growth factor–α (TGF-α)	Epithelium, fibroblasts, inflammatory cells	
Fibroblast growth factor (FGF)	Endothelium, fibroblasts	Not normally secreted by cells
Platelet-derived growth factor (PDGF)	Fibroblasts, endothelial cells	Two distinct receptors
Transforming growth factor–β (TGF-β)	Epithelium, fibroblast, endothelial cells	May modulate other factors

tor, transforming growth factor–α, transforming growth factor–β, and platelet-derived growth factor (Table 8-1). These factors are often produced by both the injured cells and the cell types involved in the healing process. A deficiency of a growth factor does not always indicate deficient healing. For example, mice deficient for transforming growth factor–α heal normally but have a hair abnormality.[23,28] Although growth factors are frequently linked to one aspect of healing (e.g., fibroblast growth factor is angiogenic), many of the cells involved in the healing process may be influenced by several different cytokine growth factors for finite periods of time.

Tissue Remodeling Phase

Tissue remodeling is the final phase of acute wound healing. This phase occurs mainly in the dermis and begins when the extracellular matrix is first produced during the proliferative phase. Tissue remodeling continues for several months after the wound is fully epithelialized. It is essential for the orderly progression of healing[13] and ultimately for the development of wound tensile strength. When most acute wounds first clinically appear to be fully epithelialized, they have regained only 20% of their tensile strength. The wound reaches its maximum tensile strength in several months and is equal to less than 80% of the unwounded skin's tensile strength.[29] The early matrix formation is dependent on fibronectin, hyaluronic acid, and proteoglycans. As the healed wound matures, the early matrix is replaced in an orderly process with type III and then type I collagen.[1] The remodeling phase is ultimately dominated by the production and destruction of type I collagen. Both of these processes are required for the remodeling of collagen into more tightly cross-linked collagen bundles. These activities are controlled by proteinases and cytokine growth factors.[13,30] In reality this scheme may be an oversimplification because as many as 13 genetically distinct collagens have been found in a repairing wound.[31] Cutaneous appendages are seldom regenerated and are often absent in the healed full-thickness wound.

The Future

As a greater understanding of the modulation of wound healing by growth factors and cellular interactions is gained, tissue regeneration may be possible. Recent studies have indicated that the renewable cell for the hair follicle is present in an area of the outer root sheath called the bulge.[20,32] These bulge cells may be responsible for the production and proliferation of matrix required for hair formation[20,32] (Fig. 8-2). Practitioner-instigated hair regeneration may occur if research on the bulge region can successfully navigate this area through anagen, telogen, and catagen phases of the normal hair cycle. This research may allow for either tissue regeneration of the hair bulb or more likely the restoration of the hair cycle and hair growth.

WOUND DRESSINGS

The function of a wound dressing is to facilitate the dynamic process that occurs as an acute wound heals. A report of the first experimentally successful attempts to accelerate acute wound healing was published in 1962 by Winter,[33] who decreased by 50% the time it took for an acute wound to heal in a pig by occluding the acute wounds with polyurethane film, thereby preventing wound crusting. This phenomenon has since been described in both nonprimate species and humans.[34] Moist wound healing probably has its greatest effect during the proliferative phase of healing. In addition, occluded wounds are less painful and may heal with a smaller, more cosmetically acceptable scar.[35] The method of achieving wound occlusion is probably less important than its capability of keeping the wound in a continuously moist state. The minimal amount of time that an acute wound in a human should be occluded and still receive some of the benefits of wound occlusion is probably 48 hours.[35]

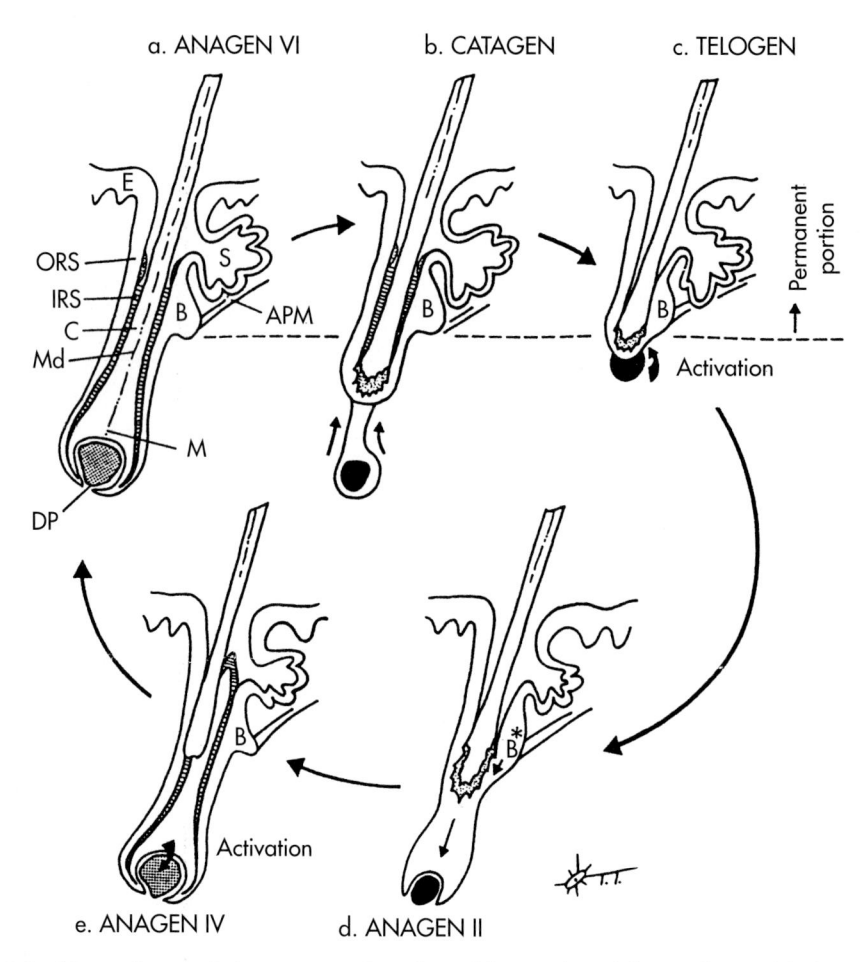

FIG. 8-2 Hair cycle—the bulge activation hypothesis. Illustrated are different phases of the hair cycle, including (a) anagen VI, (b) catagen, (c) telogen, (d) anagen II, and (e) anagen IV. Different structures are labeled, including the arrector pili muscle (APM), bulge (B), cortex (C), dermal papilla (DP), epidermis (E), inner root sheath (IRS), matrix (M), medulla (Md), outer root sheath (ORS), and sebaceous gland (S). B and B* denote quiescent and activated bulge cells, respectively. Follicular structures above the dashed line form the permanent portion of the follicle; keratinocytes below the bulge degenerate during catagen and telogen and are therefore dispensable. This model defines four major elements involved in controlling the cyclic growth of hair follicles: activation of the bulge by dermal papilla (c), activation of mesenchymal papilla by the growing matrix (e), limited proliferative potential of matrix cells as transient amplifying (TA) cells (a), and upward migration/movement of the dermal papilla (b). (From Cotsarelis G, Sun TT, Lavker RM: Cell 61:1329-1337, 1990.)

An occlusive dressing is any material or combination of materials that covers the wound, protecting it from the external environment. The application of an occlusive dressing will alter the transmission of liquids and gases from the wound surface to the external environment. More than 100 types of bandages (see box), pastes, powders, ointments, and solutions will occlude wounds. Obviously, some of these agents create a moister, less vapor-permeable barrier than others. The bandages can be arbitrarily categorized as fabrics, hydrogels, hydrocolloids, polyurethanes, and composite/foams. In addition, bandages are often impregnated with other materials. The choice of dressings depends on the wound being treated. Factors that may alter dressing selection include cosmetic acceptability, presence of wound exudate, need for wound debridement, true tissue infection, and need for wound manipulation or observation.

Grafted tissue has very special requirements. These requirements are the same as those of an acute wound, but the graft also requires the rapid institu-

> **DEFINITION OF COMMON DRESSINGS**
>
> **Fabric:** Dressing manufactured by weaving a man-made or natural fiber such as cotton or seaweed. Often impregnated with other materials such as petroleum jelly.
>
> **Hydrocolloid:** Gas-impermeable and usually opaque dressing. Basis of dressing may vary with manufacturer but is often composed of carbohydrate compounds. Can be left on a wound for several days.
>
> **Hydrogel:** Hydrophilic polymer absorptive dressing. Often complexed to a rigid backing. Usually transparent and nonadhesive.
>
> **Polyurethane film:** Transparent polymer-based dressing with variable vapor permeability. Not absorbent and will allow fluid accumulation.
>
> **Composite/foam:** Dressings that usually combine a thin nonadherent layer of hydrocolloid with a polyurethane sponge.

tion of a provisional blood supply. This blood supply is very fragile during the early phases of healing and is maximized by graft immobility. Therefore it is essential that the dressing material maintain tissue moisture, be nonadherent, and minimize external shear to the grafts.[36,37] Attempts have been made to diminish external shear by the use of cyanoacrylates,[38,39] tissue pins, and gentle external pressure. Because hair restoration surgery is performed on the scalp, cosmetic acceptability is also essential.

There are no randomized controlled studies that indicate the best postoperative method for dressing the wound of a patient who has undergone hair restoration surgery. Requirements for the ideal dressing depend on the wound site (i.e., the graft recipient site or the graft donor site). The donor site should be either closed primarily or, if it is to heal secondarily, covered with an occlusive dressing. The graft recipient site should be covered by an occlusive dressing and then with material that will immobilize the graft sites. These dressings should be left undisturbed for at least 48 hours and preferably longer. Neovascularization in split-thickness grafts is still very fragile even 1 week after grafting.[36] An example of a technique that is compatible with these statements is presented in Chapter 8, Part B by Haber and Stough. Although I am aware that many hair restoration surgeons oppose the use of bandaging and dressings after hair transplantation surgery, thus creating a postoperative environment that is dry and not protected from external shearing forces, this approach is not supported by the available literature on acute wound healing.

REFERENCES

1. Clark RAF: Cutaneous tissue repair: basic biologic considerations. I. *J Am Acad Dermatol* 13:701-725, 1985.
2. Clark RAF: Mechanisms of cutaneous wound repair. In Westerhof W, editor: *Leg ulcers: diagnosis and treatment*, Amsterdam, 1993, Elsevier, pp 29-50.
3. Cohen KI, Diegelmann RF, Linblad WJ: *Wound healing: biochemical and clinical aspects*, Philadelphia, 1992, WB Saunders.
4. Kirsner RS, Eaglstein WH: The wound healing process, *Dermatol Clin* 11:629-640, 1993.
5. Lazarus GS and others: Definitions and guidelines for assessment of wounds and evaluation of healing, *Arch Dermatol* 130:489-493, 1994.
6. Ross R: Wound healing, *Sci Am* 220:40-55, 1969.
7. Snyderman R, Phillips JL, Mergenhagen SE: Biological activity of complement in vivo: role of C5 in the accumulation of polymorphonuclear leukocytes in inflammatory exudates, *J Exp Med* 134:1131-1143, 1971.
8. Tonnesen MG, Smedly LA, Henson PM: Neutrophil-endothelial cell interactions: modulation of neutrophil adhesiveness induced by complement fragments C5a and C5a des Arg and formyl-methionyl-leucyl-phenylalanine, *J Clin Invest* 74:1581-1592, 1984.
9. Legrand YJ and others: Activation of platelets by microfibrils and collagen, *Lab Invest* 54:566-573, 1986.
10. Diegelmann RF, Cohen IKH, Kaplan AM: The role of macrophages in wound repair: a review, *Plast Reconstr Surg* 68:107-113, 1981.
11. Leibovich SJ, Ross R: The role of the macrophage in wound repair: a study with hydrocortisone and anti macrophage serum, *Am J Pathol* 78:71-91, 1975.
12. Assoian RK and others: Expression and secretion of type β transforming growth factor by activated human macrophages, *Proc Natl Acad Sci U S A* 84:6020-6024, 1987.
13. Haralson MA: Extracellular matrix and growth factors: an integrated interplay controlling tissue repair and progression to disease, *Lab Invest* 69:369-371, 1993.
14. Brotche H, Wakefield D: Fibronectin: structure, function and significance in wound healing, *Australas J Dermatol* 31:47-56, 1990.
15. Rudolph R, Vande Berg J, Ehrlich HP: Wound contraction and scar contracture. In Cohen IK, Diegelmann RF, Linblad WJ, editors: *Wound healing: biochemical and clinical aspects*, Philadelphia, 1992, WB Saunders, pp 96-114.
16. Hobson B, Denekamp J: Endothelial proliferation in tumours and normal tissue: continuous labelling studies, *Br J Cancer* 49:405-413, 1984.
17. Dudar TE, Jain RK: Microcirculatory flow changes during tissue growth, *Microvasc Res* 25:1-21, 1983.
18. Sandison JC: Observations on the growth of blood vessels as seen in the transparent chamber introduced in the rabbit's ear, *Am J Anat* 41:475-496, 1928.
19. Whalen GF, Zetter BR: Angiogenesis. In Cohen IK, Diegelmann RF, Linblad WJ, editors: *Wound healing: biochemical and clinical aspects*, Philadelphia, 1992, WB Saunders, pp 77-95.
20. Lavker RM and others: Stem cells of pelage, vibrasse, and eyelash follicles: the hair cycle and tumor formation. *Ann N Y Acad Sci* 642:214-225, 1991.
21. Cooper D, Schermer A, Sun TT: Classification of human epithelia and their neoplasms using monoclonal antibodies to keratins: strategies, applications and limitations, *Lab Invest* 52:243-256, 1985.
22. Lenoir MC and others: Outer root sheath of human hair follicle are able to regenerate a fully differentiated epidermis in vitro, *Dev Biol* 130:610-620, 1988.
23. Mann GB and others: Mice with a null mutation of the TGF-α gene have abnormal architecture, wavy hair, and curly whiskers and often develop corneal inflammation, *Cell* 73:249-261, 1993.

24. Krawczyk WS: A pattern of epidermal cell migration during wound healing, *J Cell Biol* 49:247-263, 1971.
25. Vaughan RB, Trinkaus JP: Movement of epithelial cell sheets in vitro, *J Cell Sci* 1:407-413, 1966.
26. Falanga V: Growth factors and wound healing, *Dermatol Clin* 11:667-675, 1993.
27. Sporn MB, Roberts AB: Peptide growth factors and inflammation, tissue repair and cancer, *J Clin Invest* 78:329-332, 1986.
28. Luetteke NC and others: TGF-α deficiency results in hair follicle and eye abnormalities in targeted and waved-1 mice, *Cell* 73:263-278, 1993.
29. Levenson SM and others: The healing of rat skin wounds, *Ann Surg* 161:293-308, 1965.
30. Overall CM, Wrana JL, Sodek J: Independent regulation of collagenase, 720kd progelatinase, and metalloendoproteinase inhibitor expression in human fibroblasts by transforming growth factor-β, *J Biol Chem* 264:1860-1869, 1989.
31. Miller EJ, Gay S: Collagen structure and function. In Cohen IK, Diegelmann RF, Linblad WJ, editors: *Wound healing: biochemical and clinical aspects*, Philadelphia, 1992, WB Saunders, pp 130-151.
32. Cotsarelis G, Sun TT, Lavker RM: Label retaining cells reside in the bulge area of pilosebaceous unit: implications for follicular stem cells, hair cycle, and skin carcinogenesis, *Cell* 61:1329-1337, 1990.
33. Winter GD: Formation of the scab and the rate of epithelization of superficial wounds in the skin of the young pig, *Nature* 193:293-294, 1962.
34. Nemeth AJ: Eaglstein WH: Wound dressings and local treatment. In Westerhof W, editor: *Leg ulcers: diagnosis and treatment*, Amsterdam, 1993, Elsevier, pp 325-334.
35. Nemeth AJ and others: Faster healing and less pain in skin biopsy sites treated with an occlusive dressing, *Arch Dermatol* 127:1679-1683, 1991.
36. Branham GH, Thomas JR: Skin grafts, *Otolaryngol Clin North Am* 23:889-896, 1990.
37. Netsher DT, Marchi M, Wigoda P: A method for optimizing skin graft healing and outcome of wounds of the penile shaft and scrotum, *Ann Plast Surg* 31:447-449, 1993.
38. Elliott RM, Thomas RA, True RH: Advanced use of tissue adhesive in hair transplantation, *J Dermatol Surg Oncol* 19:853-858, 1993.
39. Kamer FM, Joseph JH: Histoacryl: its use in aesthetic facial plastic surgery, *Arch Otolaryngol Head Neck Surg* 115:193-197, 1989.

B. Postoperative Dressings

Robert S. Haber and Dow B. Stough

There are as many approaches to the postoperative dressing as there are hair restoration surgeons, and a variety of techniques will achieve the primary goal, which is the protection of the grafts during their most vulnerable period. Postoperative dressings run the gamut from bulky turban wraps left on for several days, to an ointment dressing with no overlying wrap, to spray-on adhesives, to application of cyanoacrylates.[1,2] Many surgeons advocate a "no bandage" approach after hair transplantation.

In our experience with hundreds of patients we have found that patients do not mind wearing a dressing the day after surgery, and the theoretical benefit of being able to offer a patient a "dressing-free" procedure is far outweighed by the risk of graft loss as a result of desiccation or trauma. As discussed by Margolis in Chapter 8, Part A, wound healing studies convincingly demonstrate that the most favorable conditions for healing exist in a moist environment.[3,4]

Our postoperative dressing is simple, rapidly applied and well tolerated. It is secure enough to remain on overnight and yet is easily removed the next morning. A list of required items is presented in Table 8-2.

STEP 1. Visually inspect recipient and donor sites to confirm secure graft placement and adequate hemostasis.

STEP 2. Apply Polysporin-coated Telfa pad (Kendall Co., Mansfield, Mass.) with attached Reston foam backing (3M Health Care, St. Paul, Minn.) over donor site. Secure to head with tape, using folded gauze to prevent contact of tape with hair or forehead, except for the attachment area in center of forehead (Fig. 8-3).

TABLE 8-2 Supplies Needed for Postoperative Scalp Dressing

ITEM	MANUFACTURER
Three 3 × 8 inch Telfa pads	Kendall Co., Mansfield, MA 02048
Polysporin ointment	Burroughs Wellcome, Research Triangle Park, NC 27709
Reston self-adhering foam, trimmed to 2 × 8 inch	3M Health Care, St. Paul, MN 55144
Supply of 1-inch flesh-colored Micropore paper tape	3M Health Care, St. Paul, MN 55144
Supply of 4 × 4 inch gauze	Various suppliers
One 11 ft roll of 3-inch Kling	Johnson + Johnson, Arlington, TX 76004
Supply of 6-inch tubular stockinette bandages cut into 20-inch lengths, folded in half alongside itself	Abco Dealers, Milwaukee, WI 53218 (list # 1560M, medium support)

STEP 3. Apply folded gauze below first piece of Telfa pad and secure in place (Fig. 8-4).

STEP 4. Apply Polysporin-coated Telfa pads to frontal recipient site and secure with tape (Fig. 8-5).

STEP 5. Apply a sagittal strip of tape over the entire scalp, again preventing contact of tape with hair using gauze (Fig. 8-6).

STEP 6. Using a roll of Kling (Johnson & Johnson, Arlington, Tex.), first secure the dressing to the scalp by encircling the scalp from the mid forehead to below the nuchal ridge. Without cutting the roll, traverse the scalp from side to side and from back to front, again secure the wrap by encircling the scalp, and tape in place (Fig. 8-7).

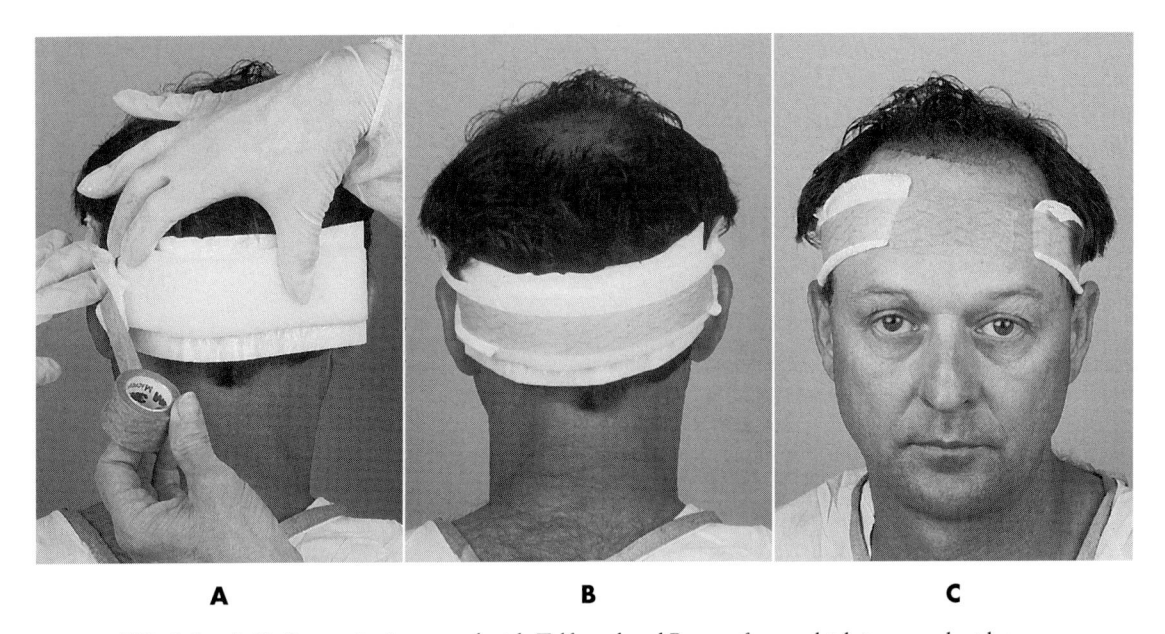

FIG. 8-3 A-C, Donor site is covered with Telfa pad and Reston foam, which is secured with tape.

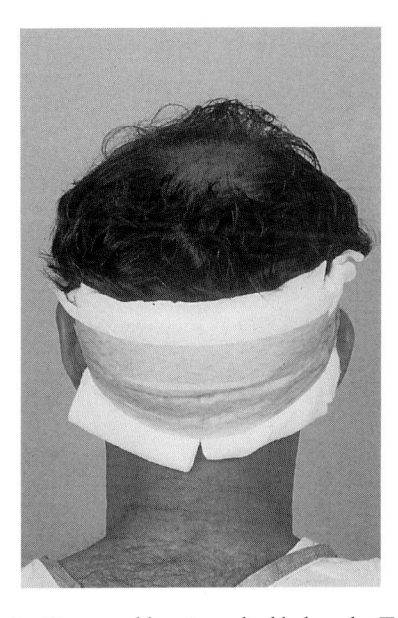

FIG. 8-4 Gauze padding is applied below the Telfa pad and secured with tape.

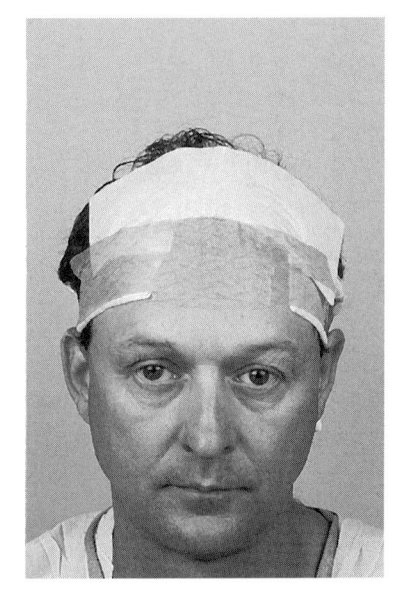

FIG. 8-5 Telfa pads coated with Polysporin are secured over the recipient site.

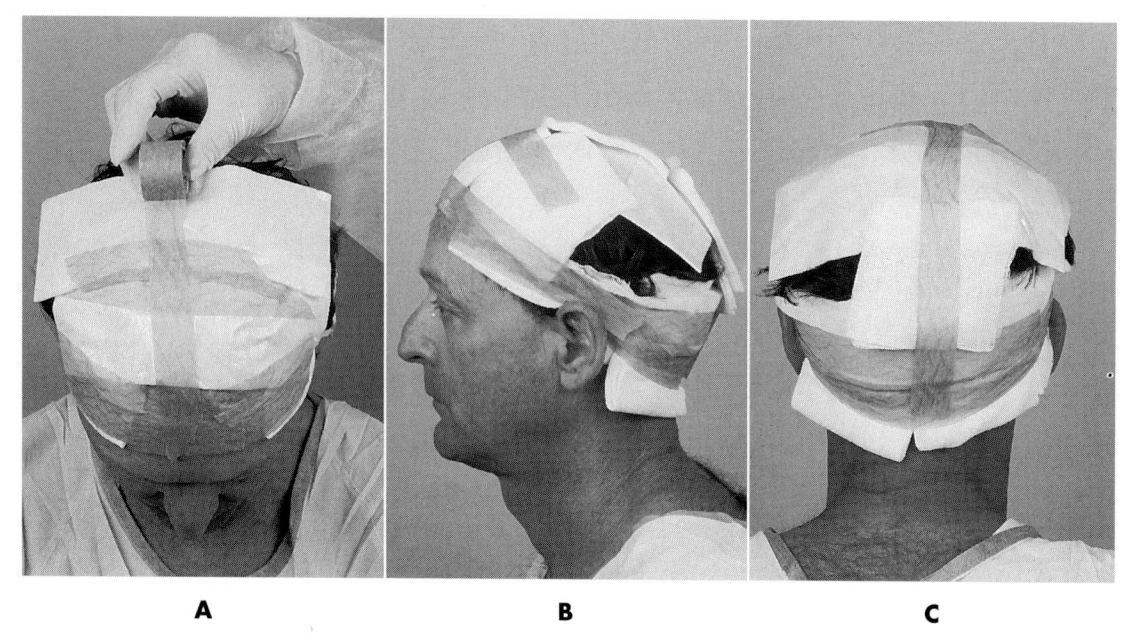

FIG. 8-6 A-C, Sagittal strip of tape is applied from front to back, taking care not to contact the hair with tape.

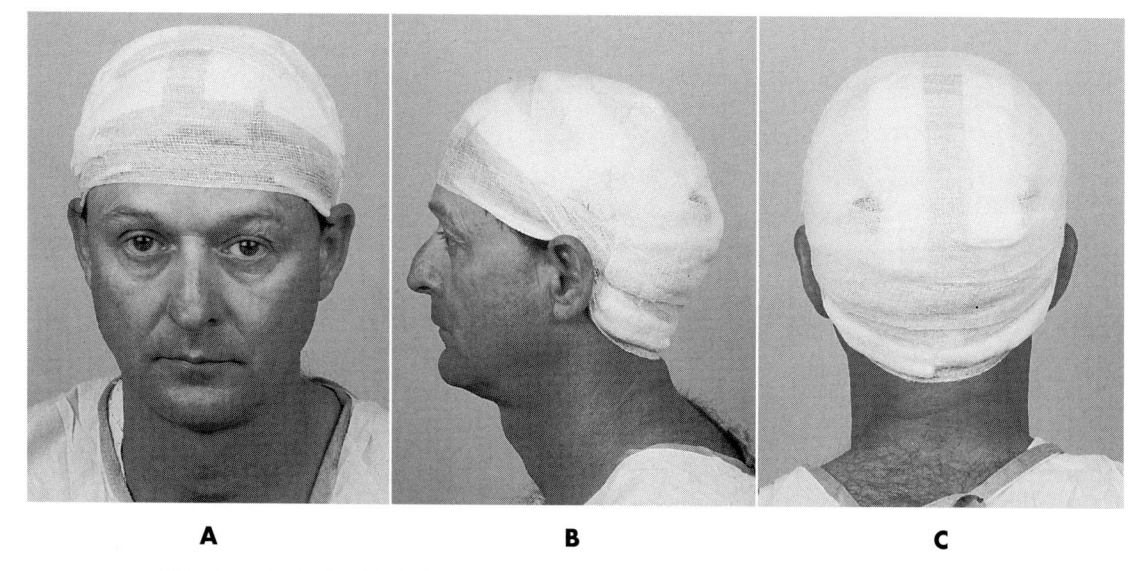

FIG. 8-7 A-C, A roll of Kling is used to wrap the entire scalp and is secured with tape.

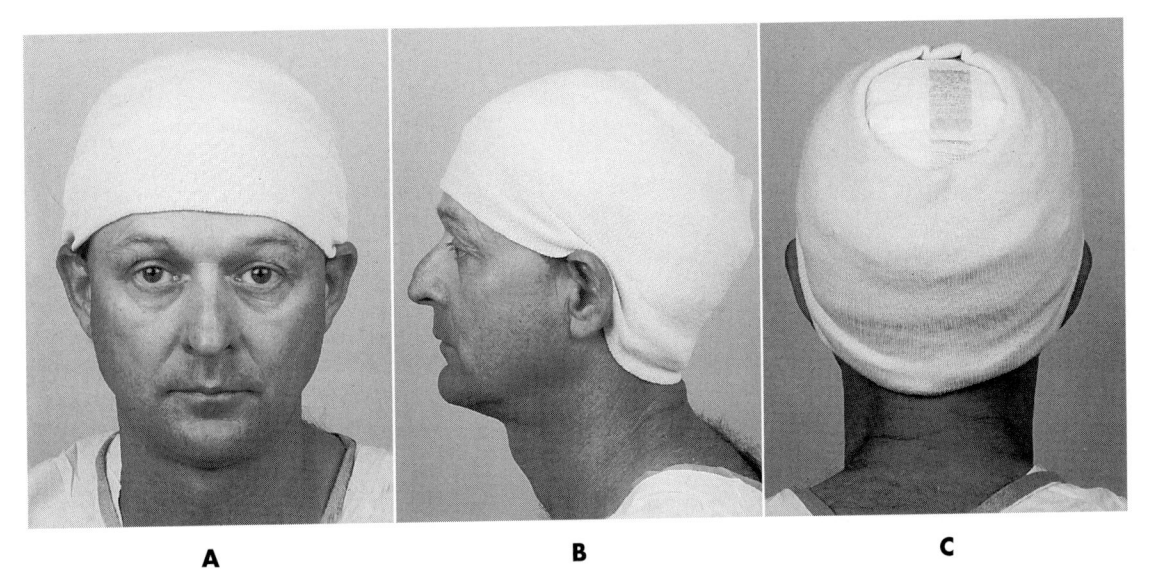

FIG. 8-8 A-C, A length of tubular stockinette bandage is gently stretched over the gauze bandage.

STEP 7. Finally, gently stretch a length of tubular stockinette bandage over the gauze bandage to cover all but the vertex (Fig. 8-8).

STEP 8. To remove the dressing, simply lift the dressing up gently from the nuchal ridge and the entire bandage will lift off. Gently separate the tape from the forehead contact zone, and the donor and recipient sites are ready for inspection and cleansing.

REFERENCES

1. Elliott RM, Thomas RA, True RH: Advanced use of tissue adhesive in hair transplantation, *J Dermatol Surg Oncol* 19:853-858, 1993.
2. Kamer FM, Joseph JH: Histoacryl: its use in aesthetic facial plastic surgery, *Arch Otolaryngol Head Neck Surg* 115:193-197, 1989.
3. Branham GH, Thomas JR: Skin grafts, *Otolaryngol Clin North Am* 23:889-896, 1990.
4. Netscher DT, Marchi M, Wigoda P: A method for optimizing skin graft healing and outcome of wounds of the penile shaft and scrotum, *Ann Plast Surg* 31:447-449, 1993.

9

Scalp Reductions and Scalp-Lifting

A. Scalp Reductions

Paul M. Straub

Scalp reduction, also known as alopecia reduction, is an excision of portions of the bald skin before grafting. It can effectively diminish or even eliminate bald areas on the top or back.

The Blanchards,[1] Sparkuhl[2] and the Ungers[3] made early contributions.[4] During the 1980s, large numbers of scalp reductions were performed. In recent years the popularity of scalp reductions has declined and many hair restoration surgeons who previously performed scalp reductions have ceased to use this method of hair restoration. The reason scalp reductions have diminished in popularity is that they were used without discrimination in selecting suitable patients and circumstances. I do not perform as many scalp reductions as I did at one time. Scalp reductions are not performed in patients with tight scalps. Whether to perform a scalp reduction on a patient with thinning hair is a difficult clinical decision.

PATIENT SELECTION

Patients can be divided into three categories: (1) patients who should not have scalp reductions, (2) patients who can get satisfactory results with or without scalp reductions, and (3) patients who, if denied scalp reductions, will not get as good a result.

Patients Who Should Not Have Scalp Reductions

Patients with too much hair or patients with too little hair should not undergo scalp reductions. Some of the greatest abuses of scalp reductions occurred when performed on younger patients with mild thinning. Following the procedure the patients had less hair than before plus unsightly scars on the head. The surgeon often rationalized that the patient would eventually have lost this hair anyway.

In addition, scalp reduction should not be performed in patients who have or eventually will have too little hair to obliterate the scar. No one can precisely predict how much hair will eventually be lost, so one should always err on the conservative side. However, a properly designed incision closed under minimal tension in a patient who heals normally requires much less hair to obliterate the scar than a poorly planned procedure.

Patients with tight scalps should not undergo scalp reductions unless either a tissue expander or a Frechet extender is used adjunctively.

Patients Who Can Get a Satisfactory Result with or without Scalp Reductions

There is a large group of patients in whom satisfactory hair restoration can be obtained with or without scalp reduction but the final results will look different.

The hairline should be as wide as the eyes. If the sides are pulled high enough that future hair loss will not recede below a line extended vertically from the lateral canthus, the patient will always have a cosmetically acceptable hairline. If it recedes below this line, a space will develop between the frontal forelock and the sides. New grafts can be placed in this area, widening the hairline, or a lateral scalp reduction can be carried out at that time. In this event at least the anterior end of the scalp reduction scar must be grafted. Often the patient looks best at this stage if the gap is left ungrafted and the hair is combed back. Scalp reductions performed earlier may prevent this gap from forming. Also the hair on the back of the head can be made denser if the scalp is narrowed before the last few centimeters are grafted.

Patients Who, If Denied Scalp Reductions, Will Not Get As Good a Result

In patients with a flexible scalp and a totally bald area in the crown, scalp reduction can be easily and satisfactorily performed. One can argue that an abuse equal to that of excessive scalp reductions is being committed by failing to reduce the crown before grafting. The grafted area will not be as dense as the surrounding hair, but a posterior whorl constructed with grafts over a width of 3 to 4 cm may be superior to a whorl constructed 10 to 12 cm wide.

Usually two scalp reductions are enough. If the goals have not been accomplished with two scalp reductions, it is rare that more than two will improve the situation.

The two greatest problems that have turned the hair transplant community against scalp reductions are disfiguring scars that cannot be obliterated by grafts and the change in hair direction that occurs when the temporal hair is pulled to the top. Both of these problems can be eliminated with proper technique. Usually when scalp reduction is properly done, little to no evidence remains of a scar after hair grafting is performed. However, with a sagittal midline scar, camouflaging the scar is rarely possible.

SCALP REDUCTION WITH MINIMAL SCAR VISIBILITY AFTER GRAFTING

In the following discussion I describe the procedure as it is performed in our office presently.

Scalp reductions, just as hair transplantation, should be customized and individualized to the circumstances and the patient. Just as a hair restoration surgeon should have mastery of a wide variety of transplanting techniques, so also should he/she use many different varieties of scalp reductions and match each to the circumstances. In addition, the surgeon should be innovative in special cases such as previously grafted areas that may need to be saved or moved to another area.

The patient must demonstrate average or better-than-average healing (Fig. 9-1).

Zigzag Scalp Reduction

The most common incision used in our office today is a zigzag incision with an inverted-Y posterior incision. This design is sometimes called a Z-plasty, but that term is a misnomer because in a true Z-plasty the points are transposed prior to closing. In the zigzag scalp reduction no change in the relationship of the points occurs but the pieces of excised bald skin are shaped like a Z or several Zs on top of one another (Fig. 9-2).

ADVANTAGES

The zigzag incision has many advantages over the midline incision:

1. The eye does not follow the zigzag line as easily as the straight line.
2. The zigzag line is much longer than the straight line, thus the tension per unit length (centimeter or inch) is much less. Since scarring and grooving is dependent on the tension per unit length, the reduced tension results in a scar with little or no indentation.
3. The force on the zigzag line is a sliding force rather than a force at 90 degrees to the line, which tends to pull the line apart (Fig 9-3).
4. If the temporal hair is pulled to meet in the middle (a condition that I do not recommend), the hair is directed laterally away from the scar. With a zigzag incision, misdirected hair is less of a problem (Fig. 9-4).

Options After Sagittal Midline Scalp Reduction

I believe that the most natural hair restoration occurs if the side hair is not brought to meet in the midline. It is preferable that two to three fingerbreadths of scalp remain to be grafted. In this grafted section the natural direction of the hair can be reestablished. Occasionally a patient presents after a scalp reduction with a sagittal midline incision in which hair from the sides was brought to meet in the center of the head. There are three possible treatments: (1) conversion of the sagittal mid-

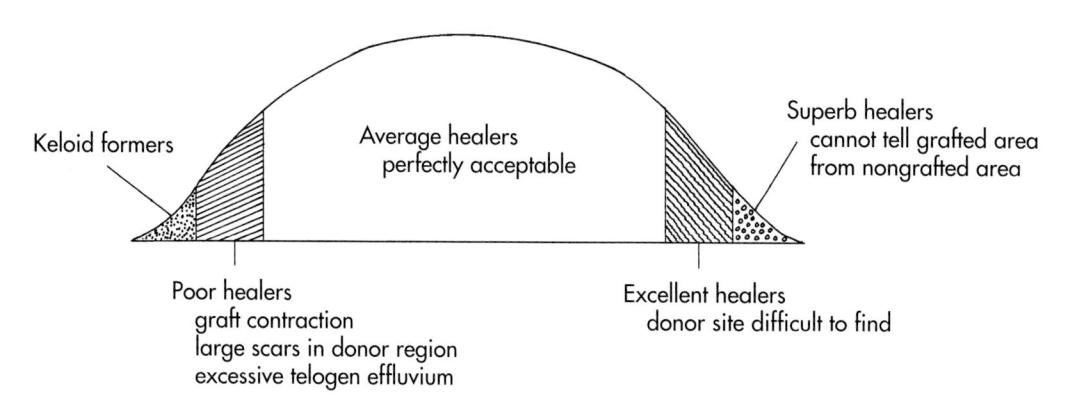

FIG. 9-1 Patient healing. It is important to try to determine the patient's pattern of wound healing preoperatively by asking about how he heals and inspecting previous surgical or traumatic scars.

Scalp Reductions **231**

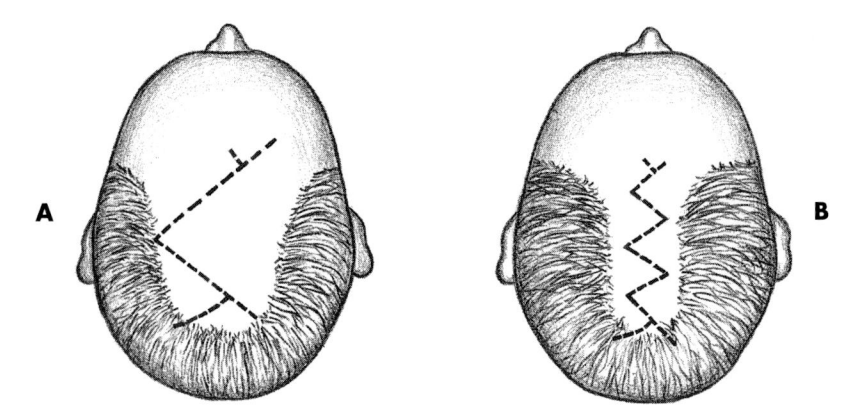

FIG. 9-2 Z-plasties. **A,** This design has a single Z (as seen in a mirror) with several extensions to remove dog ears. This Z-plasty design is used for a wide bald area. **B,** This Z-plasty design has several Zs on top of each other and is used for a narrow bald area.

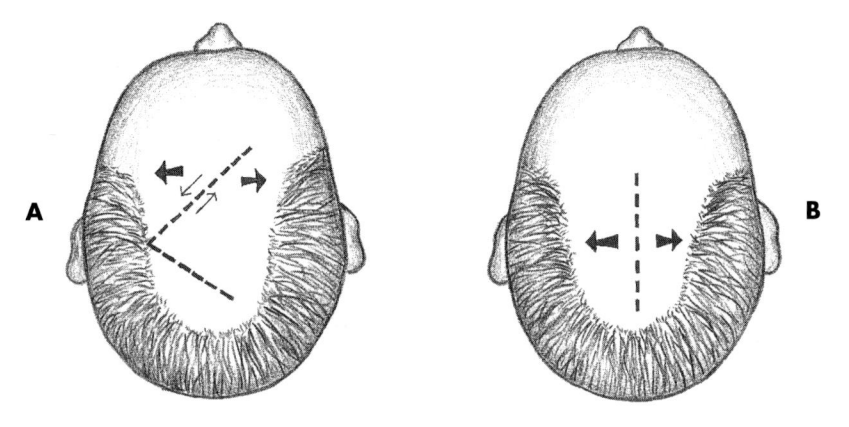

FIG. 9-3 A, Sliding force on a Z-plasty. **B,** The force on a sagittal line is at 90 degrees.

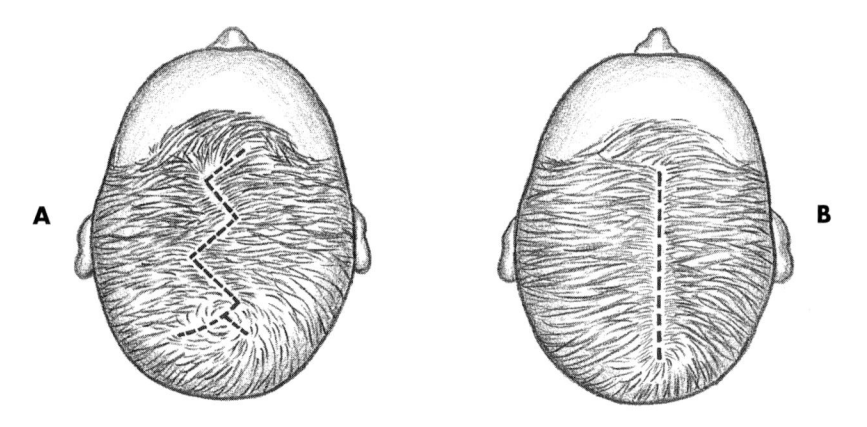

FIG. 9-4 Hair direction if temporal hair meets in the midline. Pattern in **A** has distinct advantages over that in **B.**

line incision to a zigzag incision; (2) if the incision extends far enough posterior that it forms a posterior slot, use of a Frechet flap; and (3) grafting. However, attempts to graft in this situation are rarely satisfactory for the following reasons:

1. The follicles of the side hair extend farther medially than the exit point of the hair[5] (Fig. 9-5).
2. Hair growth in scar tissue frequently is not as productive as in nonscarred skin.

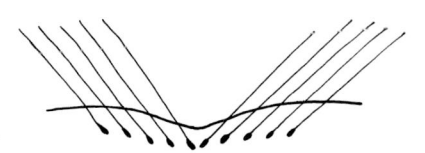

FIG. 9-5 Cross section of scalp when hair is brought to meet in the midline after a midline reduction. Nordstrom[5] described a double bevel incision that supposedly minimized this problem. I used this double bevel incision for many years, but now I believe the finest scar line is produced by meticulously following the direction of the hair shafts with the scalpel.

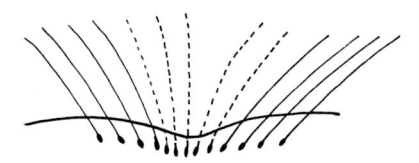

FIG. 9-6 Comparison of hair within a reduction scar (*dotted lines*) and hair that falls outside of scar (*solid lines*). Nongrafted side hair (100 hair/cm^2) is layered and appears denser than grafted hair (100 hair/cm^2) because of the fan effect caused by the angle changes.

3. Even if one is successful in growing hair to a density that would be adequate in other areas, it will appear thin because of the fan effect caused by the angle changes (Fig 9-6).

No grafting technique produces an excellent result under these circumstances, but the best technique is a herringbone pattern using five- or six-hair grafts in No. 15 Bard-Parker scalpel incisions. Scalpel incisions are less likely to damage adjacent follicles than punch holes (Fig. 9-7).

Conversion to Zigzag Scalp Reduction After Sagittal Midline Scalp Reduction

STEP 1. If possible, determine from the medical records the width of the previous excision. If this is not possible, estimate the amount that can be excised based on the flexibility of the scalp using the method I devised in 1980, which was reported by Bosley and associates.[6]

STEP 2. Estimate the amount that can be excised without excessive tension on closure.

STEP 3. Draw a zigzag line across the sagittal incision (Fig. 9-8). The distance B-D is the estimated width of the excision. The angles are drawn at 90 degrees. The final angle will be less than 90 degrees. Use as many zigzags as length allows.

STEP 4. Make an incision along the zigzag line, keeping the scalpel blade parallel to the hair shafts, that is, forward in the front and top and posterior in the back section.

STEP 5. Control bleeding by conservative electrocauterization. As little as possible should be cauterized near hair follicles and a needle-tip cautery is

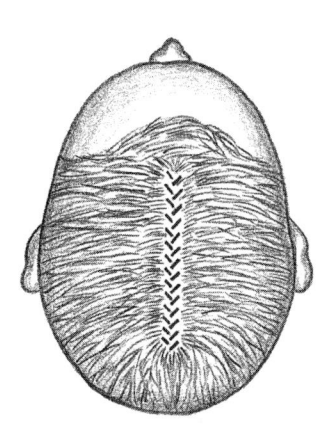

FIG. 9-7 To make the best of a midsagittal reduction scar, a herringbone pattern can be used for grafting the midline incision. This pattern is the most useful for transplanting midline reduction scars.

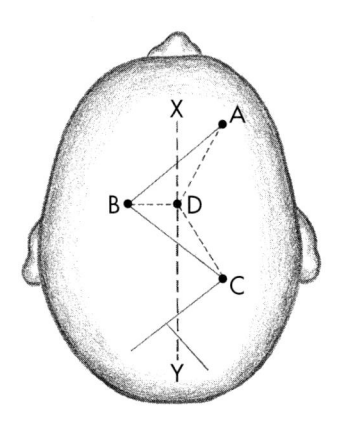

FIG. 9-8 Design of a zigzag scalp reduction. Distance B-D is the estimated width of the excision.

used so that individual vessels can be cauterized while causing minimal damage to the surrounding tissue. I recommend avoiding the Shaw hot blade for cauterization.

STEP 6. Begin at the point that will have the maximal excision. That is, the incision begins in front if the maximum excision width is to be in front or it begins in back if the maximal excision width is to be in back.

STEP 7. Push a needle through the skin at point D and push the sides together such that the needle at point D meets the incision at point B. The tension is judged, and the needle is moved closer or farther from the zigzag incision to determine the maximal excision that will still close under only mild tension.

STEP 8. Make incisions with the needle from point D to point A and from point D to point C. Naturally these incisions are parallel with the hair shafts. This step excises an arrowhead-shaped piece of bald skin (A-B-C-D-A).

STEP 9. Place a buried interrupted 2-0 Maxon or Dexon suture at closing points B and D.

STEP 10. Move anteriorly or posteriorly to the next point, which will be on the opposite side of the midline. Repeat steps 7, 8, and 9. Continue until all the points have been closed.

STEP 11. Place interrupted sutures in the galea at any other points that gap.

STEP 12. Make the final epithelial closure with a finely stitched continuous suture of 3-0 Maxon. This suture catches the epithelium above the hair follicles so as not to embarrass the blood supply. Patients appreciate the less noticeable Maxon suture more than Prolene, which is blue, or skin clips. Although Maxon is an absorbable suture, it should be removed since the reaction of absorption makes a less desirable scar and may damage hair follicles adjacent to the line. I advise leaving in skin sutures for scalp reductions and closed donor sites for 14 days. I believe the scars are wider if sutures are removed prior to 14 days because the tensile strength of the wound is insufficient.

FAILURE TO CLOSE

If the needle at point D must be moved to the left side of the sagittal scar line X-Y, there will remain a triangular-shaped piece of bald skin totally surrounded by scar tissue. Because of poor blood supply, grafts may not grow well in this triangle (Fig. 9-9), so it is better not to create this avascular triangle of skin. Instead the entire area A-B-C-D-A should be excised. The wound will be difficult to close without special measures (Fig. 9-10). The surgeon converts the lazy-V closure into a lazy-Y closure with one suture between points F and G and closes the wound normally (Fig. 9-11).

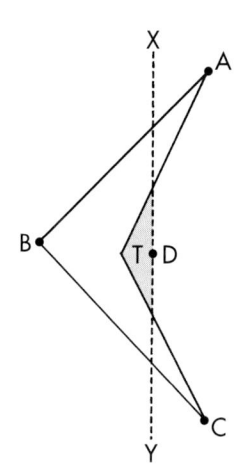

FIG. 9-9 Failure to excise all of an older reduction scar. Closure would leave a triangular area (T) totally surrounded by scar tissue. There is little to no growth from grafts placed in this area.

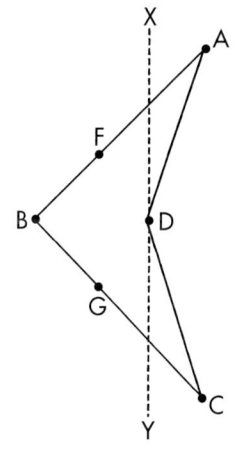

FIG. 9-10 Conversion of a midline reduction pattern by the creation of a lazy-V incision. This pattern is advisable over that in Fig. 9-9. However, the wound may not close until transformed into a lazy-Y incision as shown in Fig. 9-11.

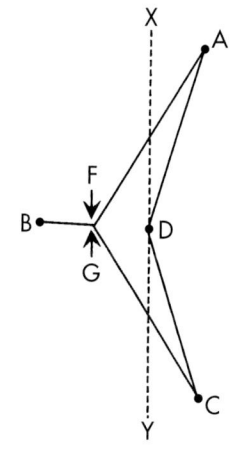

FIG. 9-11 Conversion of design shown in Fig. 9-10 into a lazy-Y incision. With a suture joining points F and G, the wound closes easily with little tension.

INVERTED-Y POSTERIOR INCISION

Extensive thought must be given to the design and placement of the inverted-Y posterior incision. These considerations also should include planning the grafting. Scalp reductions cannot be considered separately from the grafting process.

Points of Consideration

1. Frequently the best place for the convergence of the Y is at the center of the patient's original whorl. Except in the baldest patients some fine hair can be used to locate it. It is usually to the right of the midline.
2. Because the confluence of the Y is not in the midline, the two arms of the Y are usually of different lengths.
3. The arms sometimes are easier to conceal if one is slightly curved. This curve can be directed anteriorly or posteriorly but no part of the curve should be vertical (Fig. 9-12).
4. One arm of the Y is usually easy to conceal because the hair is directed in the same posterior direction on both sides of the incision.
5. On the other side, particularly if one is successful in pulling the posterior flap a significant amount superiorly, the hair changes direction. The hair below the incision is directed inferiorly, and the hair above the incision is directed anteriorly. This arm often looks better curved.
6. There are two alternate locations for the confluence of the Y:

   - High on the head: This placement creates a large posterior flap. Undermining continues posterior to the nuchal ridge. This frequently is the best location in the very bald patient. The scar is kept small to ensure that there will be enough donor hair to obliterate it (Fig. 9-13).
   - Low on the head: This technique requires careful planning in the very bald patient (Fig. 9-13). Although the arms of the Y are easily covered since all hair is directed posteriorly, the long incision line requires a large number of grafts to obliterate it. Before this design is attempted, be sure that (1) the scalp is very flexible so as to make the scalp reduction worthwhile, (2) the patient is a very good healer, and (3) the surgeon is very experienced in obliterating the scars with grafts.

• • •

To understand how to properly shape an inverted-Y posterior incision, the surgeon must look at the natural direction of the hair in the whorl, which can vary from patient to patient. The whorl is most often to the right of the midline and most often has a clockwise direction. The further from the center of the whorl, the more the hair direction turns centrifugal. To further clarify, the whorl is artificially divided into two concentric areas (even

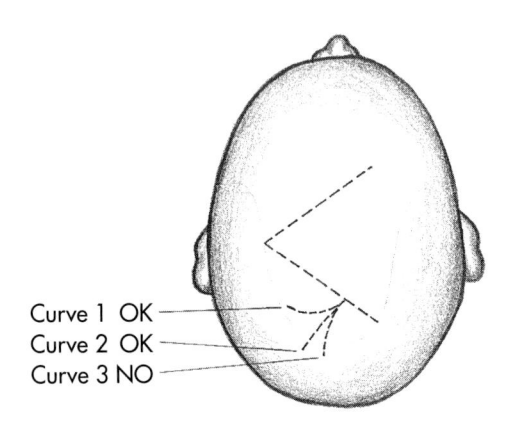

FIG. 9-12 Hair tends to hang away from any vertical portion of the incision. An incision at curve 3 would result in a vertical scar, which may become cosmetically noticeable.

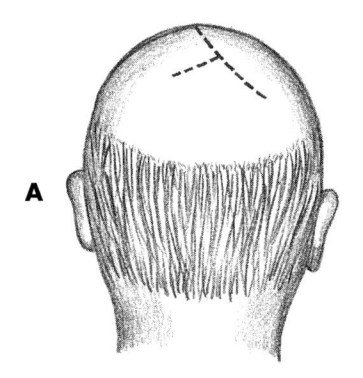

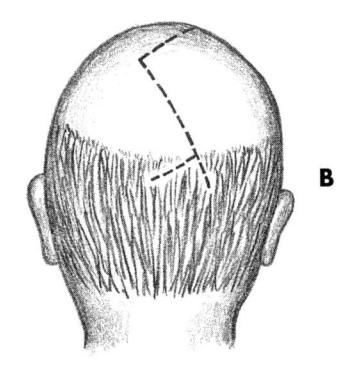

FIG. 9-13 Frequently the best plan for the convergence of the Y is at the center of the patient's original whorl. Alternatives include the high-Y incision **(A)** and low-Y incision **(B).** All the donor hair is directed posteriorly.

though there is actually a gradual transition from one direction to the other) (Fig. 9-14).

The incision a-b does not present a problem. The hair on both sides of the line is directed posteriorly, as in a closed donor site. If the incision is continued for a long distance (i.e., b-c), it is best to curve the incision slightly anteriorly to provide coverage.

The incision a-d is more likely to show because the anterolateral hair below the line is much less likely to cover the line.

The incision d-e is in the same direction as the hair, so it is likely to show. The incision a-d-e is less likely to show if it is curved anteriorly or posteriorly. In this case it will tend to be covered with hair. However, the surgeon should avoid a downward curve until it becomes vertical as this shows more than any other incision.

The area to be excised is a-b-c-f-e-d-a. Note that in the outer circular area (area B), the wider the excision, the more the hair is directed away from the incision, producing an effect as shown in Fig. 9-5. To avoid this hair misdirection, the arms of the Y incision should be slightly curved and not made too long.

BROWLIFT COMBINED WITH SCALP REDUCTION

Whenever a patient who is a candidate for a scalp reduction also wishes to have forehead wrinkles removed, a sagging brow elevated, and/or crow's-feet lateral to the eyes removed, a browlift can be combined with the scalp reduction.

Traditional browlifts have several possible incisions. The coronal incision sacrifices hair and moves the hairline upward. This outcome is acceptable with bald patients who will later undergo hair transplantation since the scar will eventually be concealed with grafts and a new hairline will be established.

An incision at the hairline is sometimes used to avoid elevating the hairline and sacrificing hair. This scar can be improved with micrografts but is rarely satisfactory.

An incision following a forehead crease does not elevate the hairline or sacrifice hair. Sometimes the scar is satisfactory and occasionally it is not.

The incision for a combined scalp reduction–browlift is shown in Fig. 9-15. A short anterior sagittal portion allows the two sides to be sutured together to form a bridge. This produces a firm platform to which the front can be sutured. Otherwise the middle of the brow will not stay elevated as the entire scalp is undermined. A second benefit of this straight section is that it avoids the creation of an acute angle that would otherwise be formed between the anterior coronal incision and the zigzag incision. An acute angle in this area may be subject to necrosis.

Undermining

In addition to the usual scalp reduction undermining, which should continue to within ½ inch of the hairline laterally and to or just over the nuchal ridge posteriorly, the forehead is undermined to the brow. The galea aponeurotica ends near the hairline and is continuous with the anterior belly of the occipitofrontalis muscle. The simplest method of dissecting under this muscle is with the iconoclast (Fig. 9-16).

The iconoclast is passed down to the lateral corner of the eyebrows on both sides, and the instrument is opened. This maneuver produces two wide tunnels. These tunnels are then joined with Metzenbaum scissors. The iconoclast is also used to undermine lateral to the orbit (Fig. 9-17). In this re-

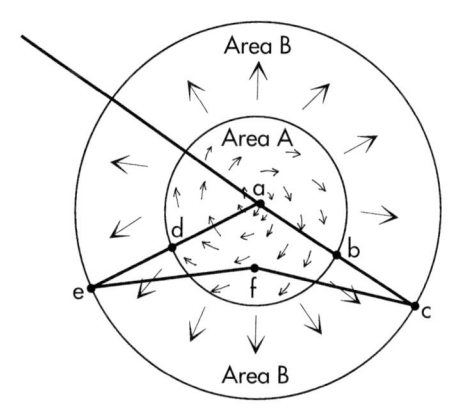

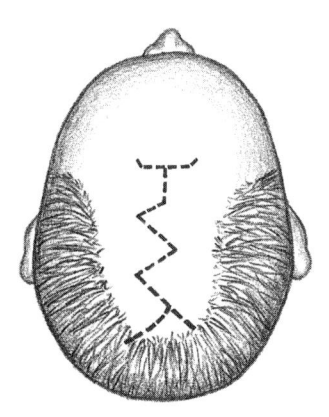

FIG. 9-14 In *area A*, the hair spirals around the center. In *area B*, the direction of the hair growth is centrifugal. This growth pattern will make coverage of incision line a-d more difficult.

FIG. 9-15 The incision for a combined scalp reduction–browlift.

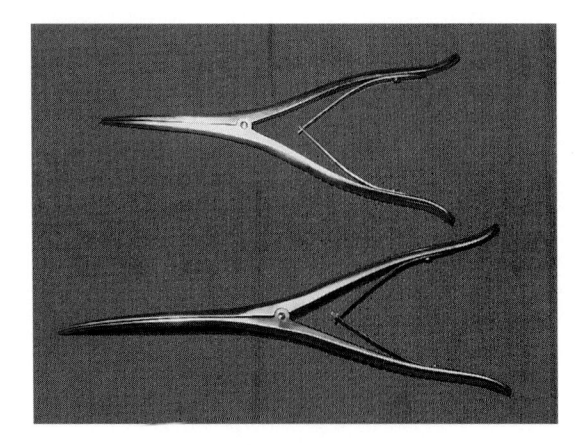

FIG. 9-16 Two sizes of iconoclasts.

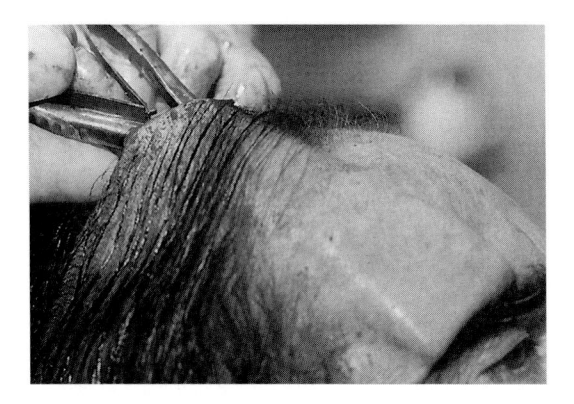

FIG. 9-17 Undermining a scalp reduction–browlift with the iconoclast.

gion the temporal branch of the facial nerve is found. Gentle blunt dissection rarely damages the nerve, which is the motor nerve for wrinkling the forehead and raising the eyebrows. The patient should be informed preoperatively that occasionally there is some temporary paralysis of the forehead. In my experience this function has always returned within a few weeks to a few months. Should movement of the forehead not return after a long period of time, the standard treatment is to cut the frontal branch of the facial nerve on the other side, which makes the face symmetrical.

Closure

The right and left sides are pulled up to overlap at the anterior straight sagittal portion. The amount of overlapping is marked with a needle, and the overlapping portion is excised. This section is then sutured at the galea using interrupted 2-0 Maxon with buried knots. This suturing forms a stable bridge to anchor the forehead lift.

The midportion is then pulled upward, the point of overlap is marked with a needle, and the excess is excised.

The dog ears at both ends of the anterior coronal incision are excised.

The remainder of the excision and closure is the same as for any other zigzag incision. The epithelium is sutured with a continuous 3-0 Maxon or Dexon suture.

A disadvantage of the combined scalp reduction–browlift is that the undermining cannot be carried out over the orbital rim. With traditional browlifts some surgeons extend the undermining; others do not. In addition, subperiosteal browlifts are being advocated by some. The combined scalp reduction–browlift is more effective for lateral crow's-feet and lateral brow sagging than medial brow sagging; nevertheless, it raises the medial brow effectively.

To its advantage, the combined scalp reduction–browlift is a simple operation, well within the limits of any surgeon who can perform a scalp reduction, and it accomplishes two goals with one procedure.

SCALP REDUCTION AFTER HAIRLINE GRAFTING

In general, the best head of hair is produced if scalp reductions are completed before grafting is performed. However, sometimes the front will be grafted first, and scalp reductions are carried out later. This sequence can occur when the patient prefers to begin restoration in the front or when hair loss has occurred only in the front and, after it is grafted, then sometime later hair is lost on the back of the head.

There are two ways of handling this situation. The hairline can be grafted wider and later narrowed to the final hairline with scalp reductions. At first this option may appear the best choice because a younger man may look good with a wider hairline and the narrowing that occurs later as a result of scalp reductions appears to be a natural consequence of aging. However, the hairline narrowing achieved with scalp reductions occurs primarily at the corners. Natural narrowing results in a more pointed widow's peak (Fig. 9-18).

It would be possible to produce the ideal hairline after the hairline has been narrowed with scalp reductions by following the pattern shown in Fig. 9-18, *D*. Unfortunately this hairline does not look good until it is narrowed later. Most patients prefer not to have this unnatural hairline for the period until it is narrowed with scalp reductions.

Natural temporal recession, as Unger and Nordstrom[7] pointed out, occurs on a line extending su-

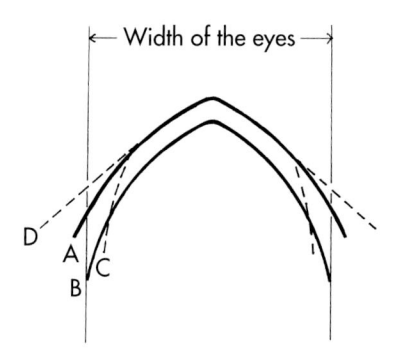

FIG. 9-18 A, Younger hairline; B, Natural narrowing; C, Narrowing of scalp reductions; D, Shape required for natural look after scalp reductions.

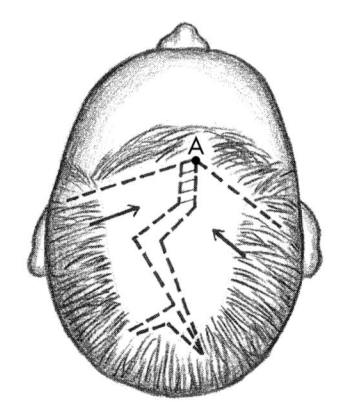

FIG. 9-19 Scalp reductions on a patient whose hairline has been previously grafted will result in a narrowed hairline. The anterior stabilizing incision forms two advancement flaps. This method is beneficial since it prevents narrowing of the hairline.

periorly from the lateral canthus. Recession of the sides occurs simultaneously with recession of the front. When a scalp reduction is carried out, the temporal recession is pulled medially out of this normal relationship.

If a scalp reduction is carried out at the same time as a grafting session, the scalp reduction should always be performed first because the hairline is altered. It is best not to perform scalp reductions and hair transplantations on the same day. A well-performed scalp reduction is widely undermined. Thus a closed donor site has a pull on it against the sutures. Undermining results in a wider donor site scar. In addition, round recipient sites are pulled into an oval shape resulting in graft popping and cobblestoning, and scalpel incision recipient sites also have forces acting on them, resulting in difficulty placing grafts.

A second method of approaching a previously grafted hairline is to fix it in place with a stabilizing incision. I presented this method at the International Society of Hair Restoration Surgery, Dallas, Texas, April 1992.

To prevent narrowing of a grafted hairline by a scalp reduction, an anterior stabilizing incision is made (Fig. 9-19).

The area in front of the incision will not be affected by the pull of the scalp reduction, so the hairline will not be narrowed. To fix the hairline, the incision must extend into the side hair well beyond the temporal recession similar but not quite as low as the incisions of Brandy[7] and Marzola.[7] Otherwise the hairline will be narrowed. The incisions anterior and posterior are parallel, forming two advancement flaps. These flaps have the advantage of pulling the temporal hair forward as well as upward in the manner of Marzola and Brandy.

The incision posterior from point A in Fig. 9-19 extends for 2 to 3 cm in the midline before the zigzag is started. This design prevents the creation of a sharp point at A, which may necrose because of a poor blood supply.

Closure proceeds as follows. A section of bald scalp 2 to 2.5 cm wide (hatched area in Fig. 9-19) is excised parallel to the midline incision. The flaps overlap more than 2.5 cm but not more than 2.5 cm should be excised.

A tack suture of 2-0 Maxon is placed at point A, joining the two advancement flaps with the anterior skin edge. No undermining is carried out anterior to the stabilizing incision. This tack suture is not at the junction of the angle in the stabilizing incision because resection of bald skin occurs only from one advancement flap. This resection moves the short sagittal section away from the midline. Once the tack suture is in place, the stabilizing incision is closed with intermittent 2-0 Maxon sutures to the galea and either skin clips or continuous sutures to the skin. The wound is then converted to a zigzag incision and is closed as previously described.

UNDERMINING IN SCALP REDUCTION

Quality results with a scalp reduction, as with a face-lift, depend on adequate undermining. Most of the undermining occurs in the adipose layer under the galea aponeurotica and above the periosteum. This layer is relatively avascular, having only a few perforating vessels. Laterally the galea is attached more firmly at the temporal line. After the temporal line the undermining continues between the galea, which becomes thinner, and the temporal fascia, which covers the temporalis muscle. This soft tissue is easy to dissect, but blunt dissection is

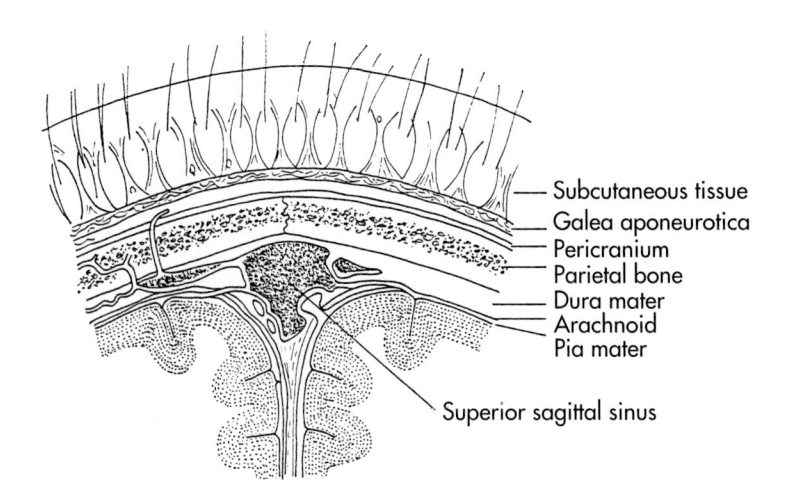

FIG. 9-20 Cross section of the scalp and skull. Note the veins passing through the skull joining the subaponeurotic veins with the superior sagittal sinus. These veins are potential pathways for intercranial infection.

recommended because the superficial temporal vessels lie in this region.

Over the mastoid, several vessels may be encountered. Many of these veins connect via the mastoid foramen to the sigmoid sinus. Also a small branch of the occipital artery enters through the mastoid foramen to supply the dura mater. Thus the potential for intracranial infection exists (Fig. 9-20).

Sharp dissection using scalpel and/or scissors must occasionally be used to start the undermining. In addition, sharp dissection is occasionally necessary in the occipital and parietal regions because of previous surgery. Otherwise blunt dissection is recommended. In general, blunt dissection can be easily performed using the fingers, Metzenbaum scissors in a spreading motion, or an iconoclast. The end of the iconoclast usually is easily pushed in the desired plane. When the iconoclast is opened, a wide tunnel is formed. A number of these tunnels are formed, and the entire region is undermined except for bands between the tunnels. The surgeon's fingers are placed in the dissection, and the scalp is pulled away from the skull. The remaining bands can now safely be cut with Metzenbaum scissors. If the iconoclast does not push easily in the plane, as can occur at the temporal line, the Metzenbaum scissors are pushed in and opened. After this maneuver, the iconoclast passes in easily and, when opened, enlarges the tunnel.

Some scalps can be undermined by blunt finger dissection. If a single layer of gauze is placed over the finger that does the pushing, the vessels are crimped and the field usually remains dry. Perforating vessels in the occipitoparietal and mastoid regions can bleed and usually respond to electrocau-

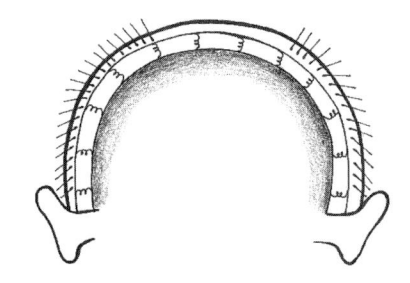

FIG. 9-21 Schematic cross section of the scalp and skull showing fibroelastic bundles (or "springs") between periosteum and galea.

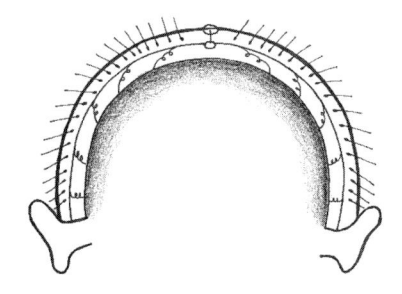

FIG. 9-22 Scalp reduction with inadequate undermining. Only the bald skin has been undermined. The hair-bearing skin has been pulled upward but no undermining has been performed. The fibroelastic bundles between the periosteum and galea are under tension and stretch-back will occur.

terization. Should electrocauterization fail to control bleeding from these vessels, bone wax (Ethicon) which should be available in the operating room, can be used.

An instrument should be passed from temple to temple via the occiput to demonstrate that the entire area is undermined. The undermining should extend posterior to the nuchal ridge and to within ½ inch of the hairline above the ear and over the mastoid bone. Undermining in front of the ear should extend at least to the level of the external auditory meatus.

Undermining the bald skin in front of the temporal hairline results in the temporal hairline being pulled posteriorly on closure. Hair direction will also change after scalp reduction (Fig. 9-21 to 9-24).

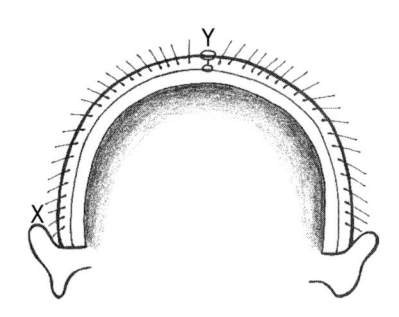

FIG. 9-23 Scalp reduction with adequate undermining to the inferior hair margin. The fibroelastic bundles are all broken down. They will reattach themselves in their new positions. No stretchback will occur. The skin acts like a rubber band stretched between the lower hair margin (X) and the suture line (Y). Although the skin will relax and after a time will no longer be as tight as immediately after the scalp reduction, it will relax equally in the bald areas and in the hair-bearing areas, and the upper hair border will not change.

GRAFTING AFTER SCALP REDUCTION

Scalp reductions cannot be considered separately from the grafting of the top and the back of the head. The goal of scalp reduction and grafting is to produce a head of hair that is as undetectable as possible. All scalp reduction incisions should be planned with careful consideration of hair grafting in the most natural manner and direction. When the scalp reduction portion of the hair restoration is complete, the surgeon should be able to create the new head of hair in the direction that hair normally grows. With improvements of minigrafting and micrografting techniques, hair restoration is less detectable in the front than in the back.

There are several ways to minimize or avoid detectability. The Frechet flap successfully converts a posterior slot into posterior-directed hair (Fig. 9-25). This flap is a major improvement over a posterior slot, but there are some disadvantages. Frequently a fairly large scar is created inferior to the third flap. This problem is not too serious since the hair from the first and largest flap covers it. The second problem is more serious. Continuing hair loss can occur in the flaps, eventually exposing the scars. A third problem is that above the Frechet flaps, if the sides are brought to meet in the midline, the "parting of the Red Sea" look continues.

I believe that all old posterior slots should be corrected using the Frechet technique. One problem with this approach is that Frechet flaps should be performed before any grafts are harvested from the donor region. If grafts have been harvested prior to the Frechet flap procedure, there is a marked increase in the probability of necrosis of the flaps. Most patients who underwent posterior slot procedures also had grafts removed from the donor region. If a Frechet flap procedure is to be carried out,

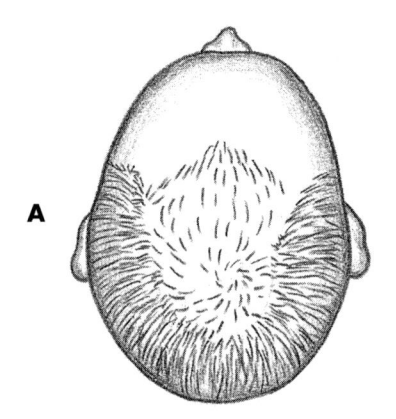

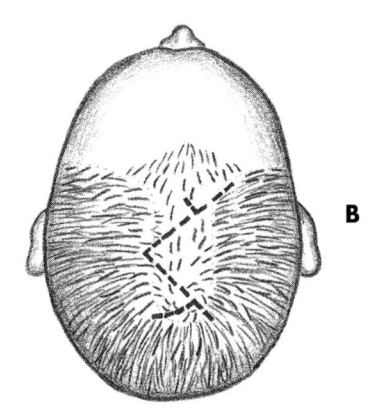

FIG. 9-24 **A,** Typical direction of hair and vellus hair prior to scalp reductions. **B,** Hair direction after two scalp reductions and grafting.

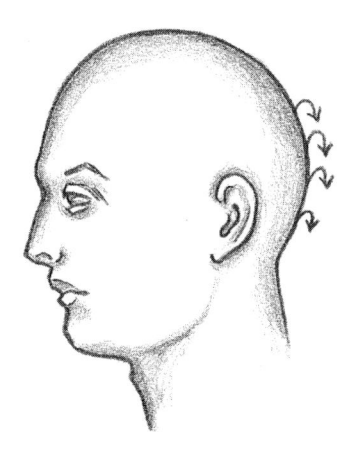

FIG. 9-25 Correcting posterior slot formation is advisable. Forward-facing grafts will help to conceal scalp reduction scars and the base of the grafts. However, even these grafts will not always conceal scalp reduction scars. Unless there is no laxity of the scalp in back, the Frechet flap is more appropriate.

it should be part of a planned program. Grafting is begun after the Frechet flaps have healed. It is possible that later the Frechet extender will prove so efficient at pulling the side hair superiorly that slot correction may become more desirable.

The best method to create an undetectable crown of hair is to carefully choose the shape and location of the scalp reduction incisions, being careful that all incisions are parallel to the hair shafts and are closed under minimum tension.

The whorl is constructed of minigrafts placed in No. 15 Bard-Parker incisions. The optimum number of hairs per graft in a patient with black hair and light skin is three or four. Often five- or six-hair grafts are used because of economics since using grafts of this size requires only half as many grafts. This method produces a slight tufted effect that is not obvious when the hair is styled. One or two hairs can be added to each graft size for light brown or blond hair.

The incisions are begun at the the center of the whorl as tightly as possible. In addition to placing the incisions as close as possible, the blade is canted in the direction of the spiral. Thus the grafted hair tends to cover the spaces between grafts. The grafts are smaller than the incisions, and the center grafts are pushed in the incisions toward the center of the spiral. As the grafting pattern gradually progresses away from the center of the spiral, the direction of the incisions gradually turns centrifugal. In general, the incisions match the direction of the remaining fine vellus hair.

After the first session the surgeon tries to graft between the previous incisions, but if a second graft is placed on top of a previous one, this is not a serious problem because the hair in the previous graft will be separated just as thinning hair would be separated.

Incisions remove no bald skin, and small areas of white skin remain between the incisional grafts. If desired, after the incisional grafts grow, these areas can then be grafted with small punch grafts, usually 1.5 mm in size, removing enough of this skin to rid the last vestige of a grafted look in the crown. There remains a small bald circle at the center of the whorl. This can be grafted with single-hair or two-hair grafts using NoKor needles. Punch grafts are not recommended for this area because the follicles of the surrounding grafts may extend into this area.

With this technique, the hair on the top, back, and whorl is not as dense as the patient would wish, but most patients retain no vestige of a scalp reduction scar.

The remaining part of the head and the scalp reduction scar are grafted following the natural direction of the hair using minigrafts in either small punch holes or incisions. Small punches produce the best result in a hairless area because they remove a small amount of bald skin and are less likely to show compression. But if some thin hair remains that can be saved, incisions are preferred since they remove no hair. The application of 2% minoxidil (Rogaine) beginning on the 10th postoperative day appears to diminish telogen effluvium.

When grafting the entire head at one sitting, I begin in front and then graft the whorl as tightly as possible. All remaining grafts are placed in the top.

An older method of grafting the back of the head and concealing scars was to place all grafts facing forward. Those grafts in the back then grow up and fold backward, elevating the hair from the scalp and concealing the base of the graft (see Fig. 9-19).

ANESTHESIA AND OPERATIVE PROCEDURE FOR SCALP REDUCTION[8]

After signing the operative consent form, the patient is given 20 mg diazepam orally. Preoperative photographs are taken and the patient dresses in an operating gown. The patient lies supine in a dental chair that has been modified with a Timo headrest. An IV drip is started, and electrocardiograph and pulse oximeter are connected. Meperidine (25 mg) and diazepam (5 mg) are administered intravenously. Other drugs, including midazolam (Versed) are used successfully in other offices. A mixture of 50% nitrous oxide and 50% oxygen is used as inhalant anesthetic for most patients while local anesthetic is being injected. A mixture of 20 ml of 1% lidocaine with 1:100,000 epinephrine and 10 ml of 0.25% bupivacaine (Marcaine) is prepared. This produces 30 ml of the mixture, which is sufficient for most scalp reductions.

A Dermajet filled with 2% lidocaine with epinephrine is used to make a pericephalic ring of blebs just anterior of the frontal hairline, across the temple to just in front of the external auditory meatus, above the ears, over the mastoid to the occiput just below the nuchal ridge. If the patient is breathing nitrous oxide, a No. 25 needle is used. If the patient is not breathing nitrous oxide, a No. 30 needle is used and the lidocaine mixture is injected more slowly. The needle is passed into each of the blebs and advanced under the skin anteriorly, posteriorly, and inferiorly. Each time a small amount of the mixture is injected. In the general area of the occipital nerves on both sides, a larger amount is injected. A small amount of the mixture is injected near the lambdoid suture since many patients have perforating vessels and nerves at this site. This method provides adequate anesthesia to perform a scalp reduction with wide undermining painlessly in most cases. Occasionally some discomfort is felt and 1% lidocaine with epinephrine is added during the procedure.

Blocking the supraorbital and supratrochlear nerves is effective for providing anesthesia to the frontal area, but because patients do not like it, it is seldom used in my office except when a scalp reduction–browlift is performed. Blockade of these nerves is carried out as follows. With the finger the surgeon palpates the supraorbital rim. Approximately 0.5 cm lateral from the nasal bone one and sometimes two notches will be felt. Over these notches the surgeon raises a bleb of 2% lidocaine with a Dermajet and injects 1 ml of 2% lidocaine through this bleb into the periosteum. When applied bilaterally, this injection provides excellent anesthesia for the middle two thirds of the frontal hairline and the region posterior to it. Since this method requires less anesthetic than a ring block, it may be preferable for patients who are hypersensitive to lidocaine (see Chapter 3, Part B).

The scalp reduction procedure should be carried out under operative sterile conditions. Masks, gowns, and standard operating room procedure should be used. Although infections are rare because of the copious blood supply in this region, the surgeon should be aware that the perforating veins are directly connected to the superior sagittal sinus and sigmoid sinus and that any contaminant has only 1 to 2 cm to travel via the perforating veins to produce an intracranial infection.

EXPECTED WIDTH OF EXCISION

In 1980, I devised a classification of scalp laxity. If two dots are placed 10 cm apart across the proposed excision and the skin between the dots is compressed, approximately two times the amount of the compression can be excised.

Class One: < 0.5 cm compression between the dots. Scalp reduction is not recommended.
Class Two: 0.5 to 1 cm compression between the dots. No wave in the compressed skin.
Class Three: 1 to 1.5 cm compression between the dots. This is the most frequent finding. With average mobility, about 3 cm width of excision can be expected. A double wave is formed in the compressed skin.
Class Four: 1.5 to 2 cm compression between the dots. The sides of the wavelike pattern meet and form shallow furrows.
Class Five: > 2 cm compression between the dots. Expect the need for a large excision. The compressed skin forms deep furrows.

COMPLICATIONS OF SCALP REDUCTIONS[9]
Stretchback

The subject of stretchback is a source of heated debate among hair transplant surgeons.[10-12] Unger's study[7] with tattoo marks demonstrated that a properly performed scalp reduction does not stretch back. However, some surgeons adamantly believe that stretchback can occur. I believe that stretchback is primarily the result of inadequate undermining. A face-lift that is inadequately undermined will rapidly revert to its previous position. Similarly, a scalp reduction carried out without adequate undermining will be subject to stretchback. There are fibroelastic bundles between the periosteum and the galea (see Fig. 9-20). If these bundles are stretched, they tend to pull the skin back to its previous position, resulting in stretchback (see Fig. 9-21). If they are broken down by undermining, they will reattach themselves at the new, higher position and there is no stretchback (see Fig. 9-22).

Infection

As a result of the abundant blood supply, serious infections are very rare. However, a purulent infection under the galea theoretically could be fatal since both the venous system and the arterial system are connected to the intracranial system.

Superficial infections most often occur at the sutures and are usually caused by dirty caps. Such infections could also be caused by necrosis if the sutures were placed too tight. Antibiotic ointments such as Neosporin applied to the suture line may prevent contact infections. The treatment for any infection is the administration of appropriate antibiotics chosen by culture and sensitivity.

Edema

Edema of the forehead and eyes occurs in approximately 25% of my patients, beginning on the third postoperative day and lasting for three or occasionally more days. We begin a Medrol Dosepak on the first postoperative day and, at the first sign of swelling, begin ice cold compresses 20 minutes on and then 20 minutes off.

Numbness

All patients undergoing scalp reductions and hair grafting should be forewarned that they have a 95% chance of suffering from some numbness of the scalp, lasting approximately 6 months.

Hair Loss

Telogen is frequent with scalp reductions, and permanent hair loss can occur. Hair loss may have been labeled as stretchback by some. The degree of hair loss that occurs shortly after surgery appears to be proportional to the amount of tension used when closing.

Late hair loss may appear more severe for the following reason: If the hairline on the sides of a patient's head was destined to drop 1 inch in the next 10 years and that 1 inch was stretched to 1½ inches, then the patient will lose 1½ inches of hair in the next 10 years.

Diminished Density of the Donor Region

Diminished hair density of the donor site is often cited as a negative, but I do not consider it so. Although it is true that a graft of any given size may contain fewer hairs, it is also true that a larger number of grafts can be harvested.

If the goal is to transplant the area as uniformly and as undetectably as possible, it is usually preferable to have a larger number of less dense grafts than a smaller number of denser grafts.

OTHER INCISIONS

Many incisions for scalp reductions have been suggested. A few of these incisions are shown in Fig. 9-26. All incisions eventually end up as midline incisions if carried to the extreme.

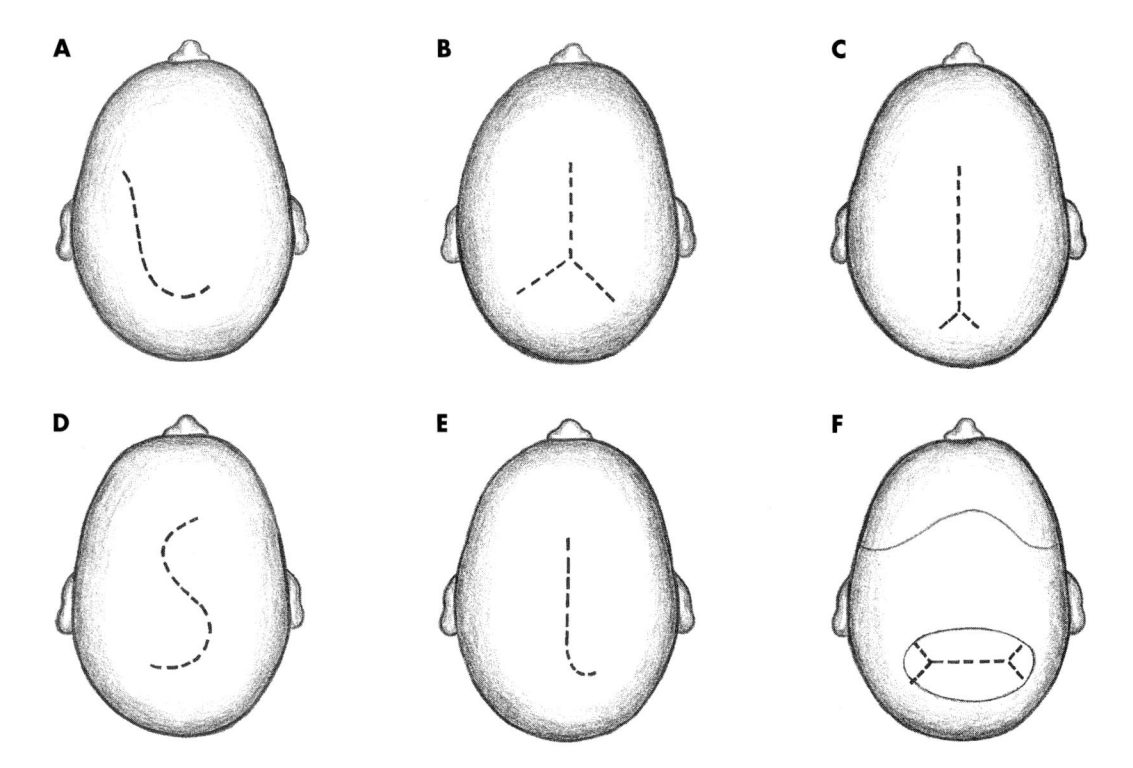

FIG. 9-26 Other scalp reduction incisions. **A,** Paramedian incision. This incision is promoted by Alt.[13] It has improved visibility and no posterior slot. **B,** Mercedes Benz incision. This incision is promoted by Unger.[7] There is no posterior slot and the back of the scalp can be elevated somewhat. **C,** Rocket ship incision. This incision is a modification of the Mercedes Benz incision. **D,** Lazy-S incision. This incision is promoted by Stough and offers a major improvement over the midline incision. A frequent problem at the back of the scalp is that the posterior curve is much greater than the curve to which it is sutured, resulting in bulging posteriorly. **E,** J-shaped incision. A whorl can be formed at the end of the J, but the "parting of the Red Sea" look continues in front. **F,** Horizontal incision. This incision is often tempting for wide bald spots but rarely is the surgery worthwhile because there is so little laxity of the scalp in the anteroposterior direction.

REFERENCES

1. Blanchard G, Blanchard B: Obliteration of alopecia by hairlifting: a new concept and technique, *J Natl Med Assoc* 69:639-641, 1977.
2. Sparkuhl K: Scalp reduction: serial excision of the scalp with flap advancement. Presented at the International Hair Transplant Symposium. Lucerne, Switzerland: February 4, 1978.
3. Unger MG, Unger WP: Management of alopecia of the scalp by a combination of excisions and transplantations, *J Dermatol Surg Oncol* 4:670-672, 1978.
4. Alt TH: History of scalp reductions and paramedian method. In Norwood OT, editor: *Hair transplant surgery*, ed 2, Springfield, Ill., 1984, Charles C Thomas, pp 221-244.
5. Nordstrom REA: Change in direction of hair growth, *J Dermatol Surg Oncol* 9:156-158, 1983.
6. Bosley LL and others: Reduction of male pattern baldness in multiple stages: a restrospective study, *J Dermatol Surg Oncol* 6:498-503, 1980.
7. Unger WP, Nordstrom REA: *Hair transplant*, ed 2, New York, 1988, Marcel Dekker.
8. Norwood OT, Shiell RC: *Hair transplant surgery*, ed 2, Springfield, Ill., 1984, Charles C Thomas.
9. Norwood OT, Shiell RD, Morrison ID: Complications of scalp reductions, *J Dermatol Surg Oncol* 9:828-835, 1983.
10. Nordstrom REA: "Stretch-back" in scalp reductions for male pattern baldness, *Plast Reconstr Surg* 73:422-426, 1984.
11. Nordstrom REA: Scalp kinetics in multiple excisions for correction of male pattern baldness, *J Dermatol Surg Oncol* 10:991-995, 1984.
12. Nordstrom REA: "Stretch-back" in scalp reductions for male pattern baldness, *Plast Reconstr Surg* 73:422, 1984.
13. Alt TH: Scalp reduction as an adjunct to hair transplantation, *J Dermatol Surg Oncol* 6:1011-1018, 1980.

PREREQUISITES FOR THE FRECHET FLAP

1. This procedure is used with midline elliptical scalp reductions only, preferably with extenders.
2. This procedure can be accomplished if no scars are present in the flaps or their bases.
3. Patients should massage energetically the postauricular and occipital scalp regions for 1 month before surgery.
4. Flap dimensions should be strictly followed.
5. The flaps should contain good permanent hair.

DIMENSIONS OF THE FRECHET FLAP

Length
B-C = 4 to 5 cm
G-i = 7 to 8 cm
D-H = 10 to 11.5 cm
C-J = 5.5 to 6.5 cm
C-i = 8.5 to 10 cm
D-i = 11 to 12 cm

Width
Flap 1 (upper flap)   2 cm
Flap 2 (intermediate flap)   3 cm
Flap 3 (lower flap)   3.5 cm

B. The Frechet Flap

Patrick Frechet and Richard C. Shiell

A common side effect of scalp reduction is the creation of a "slot" with hair growing in opposite directions from the scar. Overcoming the unnatural appearance of the slot has been a vexing problem in scalp reduction surgery.[1] None of the conventional corrective surgical techniques (e.g., Z-plasties, hair grafts) provide completely satisfactory aesthetic results.[2-5]

The Frechet flap is a triple transposition flap used for the correction of the slot defect secondary to scalp reduction surgery.[6-8] A number of conditions are necessary for a patient to be a candidate for the Frechet flap (see box).

PROCEDURE

A 1-month interval is recommended if scalp extension is performed and a 2-month interval is recommended after standard scalp reduction before performing slot correction.

Success depends on maintaining certain dimensions and relations between the different flaps (see box). In this way tension in the flaps may be avoided. It is essential that the right and left scalp borders of the slot oppose each other, and the inner border of the different flaps must contain terminal hair predicted to last for many years (Figs. 9-27 and 9-28).

All the undermining is performed in the subgaleal plane, similar to conventional scalp reductions. The undermining reaches the upper auricular sulcus and stops just above the nuchal ridge. This undermining is achieved after the lower incision of the inferior flap is made in order to have excellent surgical visibility of the area.

The following are key points of case selection and operative technique:

1. Scalp flap surgery requires a higher level of attention to surgical details than alopecia reduction surgery. Design of the incision line, skin edge approximation, skin tension, and hemostasis all must be meticulous.
2. There should be no scarring within the proposed flaps or within a 4 to 5 cm vicinity of the proposed flap bases.

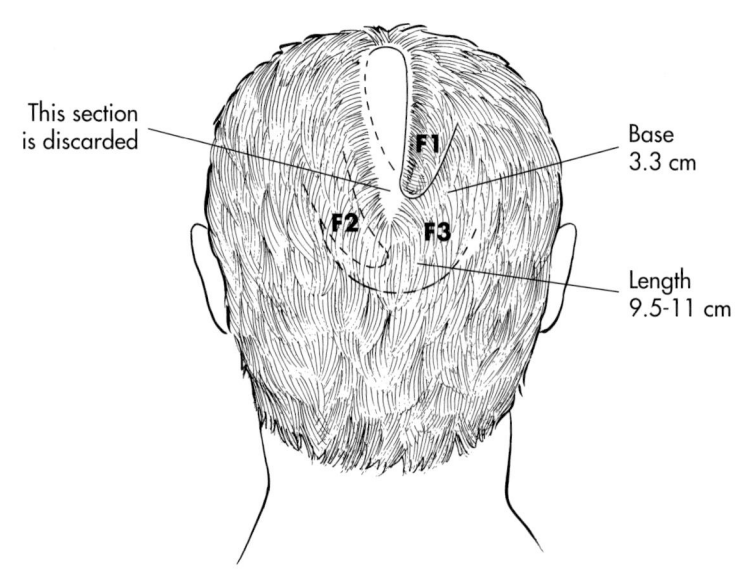

FIG. 9-27 Diagrammatic representation of the Frechet triple transposition flap. *F1,* flap 1; *F2,* flap 2; *F3,* flap 3. (Redrawn from Shiell R, *Hair Transplant Forum* 3(6):18-19, 1993.)

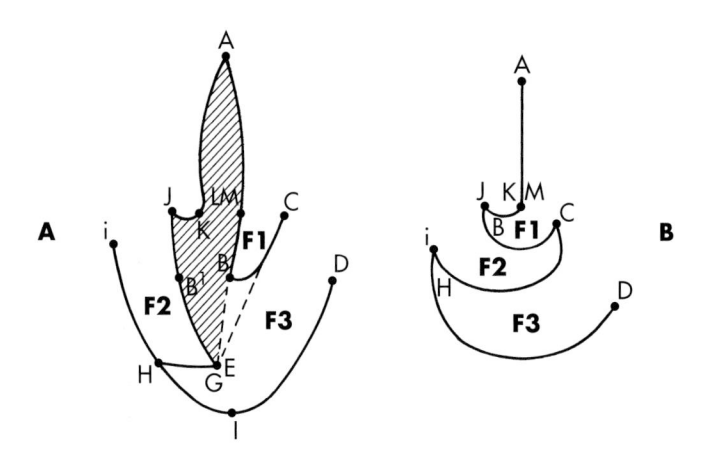

FIG. 9-28 Incision lines of the three hair-bearing flaps before **(A)** and after **(B)** transposition. *F1,* flap 1; *F2,* flap 2; *F3,* flap 3.

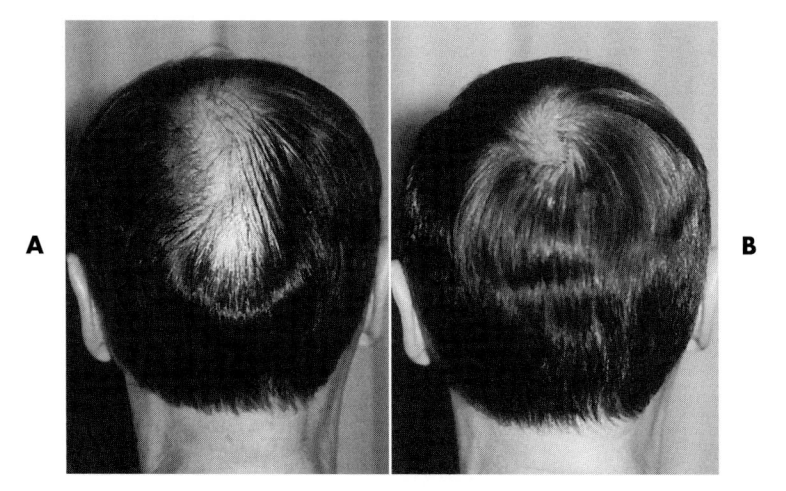

FIG. 9-29 A, Slot defect before treatment. **B,** Postoperative view after slot correction with the Frechet flap.

3. Patients with long scars passing through the temporoparietooccipital zones should not be selected for this surgery.
4. Patients who have had arterial ligation during lateral reduction operations seem to be at increased risk for necrosis and should be rejected.
5. The margins of the slot should be within 2 cm of each other and contain good-quality hair.

COMPLICATIONS

After performing 200 double hair-bearing scalp flaps, the first author (PF) has observed a total of three cases of tip necrosis <1 cm.[2] In a study of 60 triple hair-bearing flaps, only two cases of tip necrosis were noted. Twenty percent of patients experienced some degree of telogen effluvium, usually at the distal end of flaps 2 and 3. Working mostly with scarred patients, the second author (RCS) has observed a much higher rate of necrosis of all degrees.[9]

DISCUSSION

The previous technique involving two hair-bearing scalp flaps offered a very satisfactory aesthetic result. However, with three hair-bearing scalp flaps, the aesthetic results are further improved and there is seldom a need for further scar revision (Fig. 9-29). The Frechet technique provides a solution to the problem of concealment of the central slot that is unattainable by other means such as Z-plasties and minigrafting.

REFERENCES

1. Norwood OT, Shiell R, Morison I: Complications of scalp reductions, *J Dermatol Surg Oncol* 9:831-834, 1983.
2. Nordstrom REA: Change in direction of hair growth, *J Dermatol Surg Oncol* 9:156-158, 1983.
3. Frechet P: How to avoid the principal complication of scalp reduction in the management of extensive baldness, *J Dermatol Surg Oncol* 11:637-640, 1985.
4. Mayer TG, Fleming RW: Management of alopecia. Presented at the International Symposium on Hair Replacement Surgery. Los Angeles: March 17-20, 1988, p 89.
5. Unger W, Nordstrom REA: *Hair transplantation*, ed 2, New York, 1988, Marcel Dekker.
6. Frechet P: A new method for correction of the vertical scar observed following scalp reduction for extensive baldness, *J Dermatol Surg Oncol* 16:640-644, 1990.
7. Shiell R: Frechet's flap procedure: new treatment to correct central slot defect, *Hair Transplant Forum* 2(5):2-5, 1992.
8. Frechet P: Slot correction by a three hair-bearing transposition flap in combination with scalp reduction, *Dermatol Aesthetic Restor Surg* 2:27-32, 1994.
9. Shiell R: Care with choice of patients for Frechet flap procedure, *Hair Transplant Forum* 3(6):18-19, 1993.

C. Expansion Terminology

Dow B. Stough

MECHANICAL CREEP. A stretching response created by tension applied to skin for periods of minutes to hours is referred to as *mechanical creep*. The amount of stretch is minimal since it is a result of collagen fiber realignment. No tissue growth occurs.

BIOLOGICAL CREEP. A stretching response incited by tension applied to skin for periods of weeks to months is referred to as *biological creep*. Stretching may be maximal as a result of tissue growth.[1]

VOLUMETRIC EXPANSION. Both delayed and intraoperative scalp expansion may be accomplished by a volume of fluid injected into an expandable device known as a balloon. Thus any method that uses balloon-filled expanders is referred to as *volumetric expansion*.

NONVOLUMETRIC TISSUE EXPANSION. When the scalp is extended by means other than a balloon-filled device, this process is referred to as *nonvolumetric tissue expansion*. Examples include the Suture Tension Adjustment Reel (Miami STAR), towel clips, Sure-Closure (Life Medical Sciences, Inc., Princeton, N.J.), and the Frechet scalp extenders.[2] Nonvolumetric tissue expansion can be intraoperative or delayed.

INTRAOPERATIVE SCALP EXTENSION. Intraoperative scalp extension is a stretching response incited by tension of a nonvolumetric device applied only during the intraoperative period. Examples include the Miami STAR, towel clips, and the Sure-Closure device.

DELAYED SCALP EXTENSION. The Frechet scalp extender is a device that induces a nonvolumetric delayed scalp extension.[3] Prolonged scalp extension with the Frechet extender does not require balloon-filled expanders but uses a stretchable band placed below the galea under constant tension. The band remains below the galea for approximately 1 month and is then removed. The constant pressure causes the hair-bearing temporoparietal scalp to move into the scalp reduction defect.

INTRAOPERATIVE VOLUMETRIC SCALP EXPANSION. Intraoperative Silastic balloon expanders function on the same principle as stated for volumetric expansion but employ volumetric expansion techniques only during the intraoperative period.[4]

DELAYED VOLUMETRIC SCALP EXPANSION. Commercial balloon expanders are available in a number of shapes and all are designed to gradually increase their volume and create forces in which the scalp is "stretched."[5] This pressure can be applied over a prolonged period, resulting in "delayed" Silastic balloon expansion. The delayed (also known as prolonged) balloon expanders use injection ports that can be intermittently injected with saline solution. These ports are placed below the galea and allow for biweekly injections of fluid.

REFERENCES

1. Cohen BH: Navigating through tissue expansion terminology, J Dermatol Surg Oncol 19:614-615, 1993.
2. Cohen BH, Cosmetto AJ: The suture tension adjustment reel: a new device for the management of skin closure, J Dermatol Surg Oncol 18:112-123, 1992.
3. Frechet P: Scalp extension, J Dermatol Surg Oncol 19:612-622, 1993.
4. Lam AC and others: Decrease in skin-closing tension intraoperatively with suture tension adjustment reel, balloon expansion, and undermining, J Dermatol Surg Oncol 20:368-371, 1994.
5. Gibson T: The physical properties of the skin. In Converse JM, editor: *Reconstructive plastic surgery*, Philadelphia, 1977, WB Saunders.

D. Prolonged Scalp Extension

Patrick Frechet

In 1993, I published the first narrative report on scalp extension.[1] Scalp extension referred to a surgical technique that uses a thin sheet of a bioplastic extender. The extender is stretched and attached with hooks to the galea after a scalp reduction. Scalp expansion involves volumetric distention of the scalp. Scalp extension is a nonvolumetric procedure involving no expansile balloons.

The scalp extender consists of a thin sheet of bioplastic material, bearing a row of hooks at each end and affixed to the galea after it is stretched. Immediately after placement, the extender is stretched by 100%. Over the next month, the extender gradually returns to its resting position, and the hair-bearing scalp increases as a result of biological creep.

PROCEDURE

A standard midline scalp reduction is performed with the same width of bald scalp being excised as without the use of extenders. Before closure of the galea, the hooks of the extender should be approximated in the dense hair-bearing scalp as near as possible to the hair margin. The hooks are affixed to the underside of the galea and should penetrate into the deep adipose tissue. The extender is stretched to the contralateral side and again attached to the galea. The extender is left in place for approximately 30 to 40 days.

Before extender removal, the distance separating the two rows of hooks will be reduced considerably by the process of biological creep. The second operation is performed in a fashion similar to conventional scalp reduction surgery. The extender is removed by detaching the row of hooks. Special forceps are required for extender detachment. The scalp is again undermined up to the supraauricular and postauricular hair margin, just as in normal scalp reduction. The ellipse of bald scalp is excised.

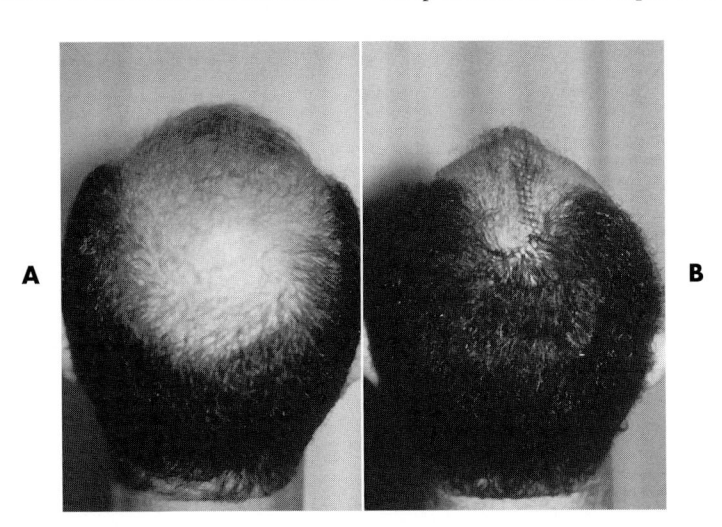

FIG. 9-30 A, Preoperative view. Vertex alopecia measures 15 cm in width. **B,** Postoperative view after two scalp extensions over an interval of 58 days. Slot correction was achieved using three transposition flaps.

Should any bald scalp remain, a second scalp extension can be performed under the same conditions as the first except that the extender used is shorter.

RESULTS

Scalp extension using the extender has been performed since 1990. Since the experimental phase, I have performed more than 110 scalp extensions. All patients with alopecia less than 10 cm wide have had the posterior and vertex baldness entirely reduced. One to two scalp extensions were required for this group. Those patients with more extensive alopecia (i.e., 10 to 17 cm) required two or three scalp extensions for complete closure. One patient with a 19.5 cm width of baldness underwent five scalp extensions to completely reduce the bald area. I use midline scalp reductions followed by a triple hair-bearing transposition flap procedure (see Chapter 9, Part B). These hair-bearing transposition flaps, or Frechet flaps, are used after the last extender is removed (Fig. 9-30). A small width of baldness may remain anterior to the vertex in some cases.

DISCUSSION

The use of extenders reduces the number of scalp reductions by one third to one half. The effectiveness of scalp extension increases progressively up to 6 weeks. After 6 weeks, minimal stretch occurs.

The time necessary to eliminate baldness has been shortened considerably and has varied from 1 to 3 months maximum for all bald areas less than 17.5 cm wide. In comparison, multiple reductions over a 1- to 2-year period were previously required to obtain the same results.[2] The results are secondary to the immediate and permanent pulling effects of the extender on the hair-bearing scalp (see box).

Compared with standard scalp reductions, temporal baldness can now be reduced significantly with extenders. Reduction design can be flexible. However, I prefer the midline elliptical scalp reduction.

COMPLICATIONS

The only complication reported has been a single case of infection. Only two incidences of hematomas have been reported and they occurred at the very beginning of the study. The risk of infection is probably the only "weak" point in using the internal device.

Patients' acceptance of scalp extension has been excellent. Postoperative pain and discomfort were noted to be greater with the extender than with standard scalp reductions. Most patients experience pain or discomfort for only a day. A few patients have had pain for as long as 10 days (see box).

STRETCHBACK

Stretchback does not appear to occur with scalp extensions. As seen in Fig. 9-31, B and C, patients experience compression of the bald area during the process of extension (Fig. 9-31).

WIDENING OF THE SCARS

Scars are minimal since no traction is placed on the wound at the time of closure. This is true even if the wound has been closed under maximal tension. The scars, which are being compressed under the effect of extenders, are now extremely narrow and barely perceptible. This observation underscores the need to close all reductions with minimal tension.

SLOT FORMATION

At the time the extender is removed, both wound edges of the lateral hair-bearing scalp are approxi-

---

RESULTS WITH THE FRECHET EXTENDER

1. Increases the amount of bald scalp removed by at least 50%.
2. Reduces total number of reduction procedures by as much as one half.
3. Decreases stretchback tendency and atrophic scarring.
4. Does not cause any appreciable postoperative hair loss.
5. Increases scalp laxity.
6. Causes earlier development of scalp laxity.

COMPLICATIONS AND SIDE EFFECTS OF THE FRECHET EXTENDER

1. Mild to severe pain during the first 24 hours, especially when sleeping on scalp overlying extender hooks
2. Some serosanguinous drainage through approximated wound margins for up to several weeks with some delayed healing
3. Hematoma or seroma formation over extender (occasionally)
4. *Staphylococcus aureus* infection overlying extender (one case)

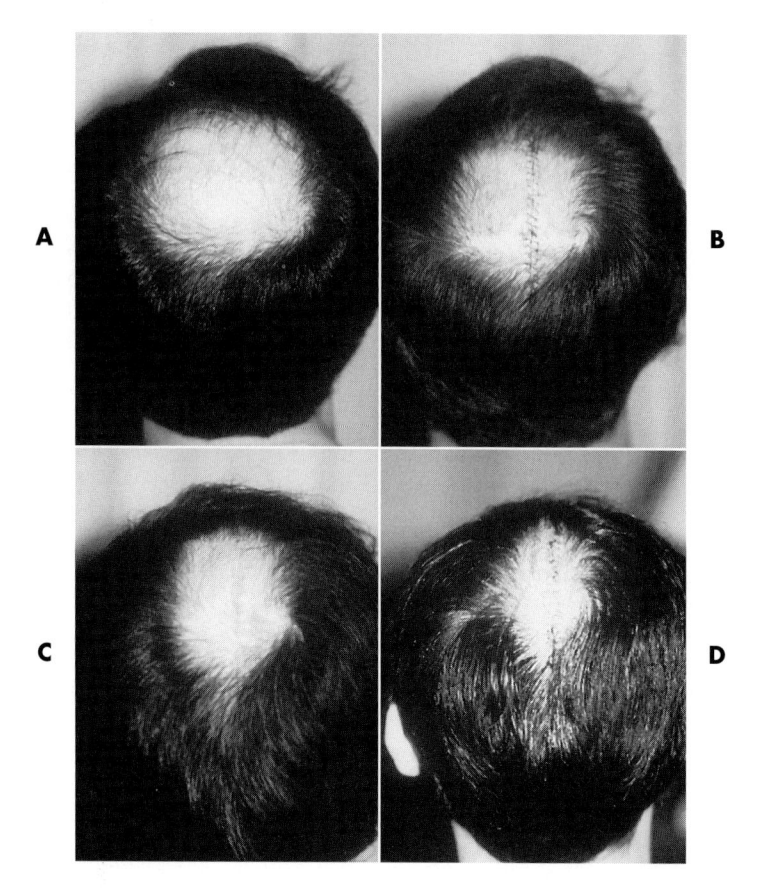

FIG. 9-31 **A,** Preoperative view. Vertex alopecia measures 12 cm. **B,** Postoperative view after first scalp reduction with an extender in place. Vertex alopecia measures 9 cm. **C,** View after first scalp reduction with extender still in place. The vertex alopecia has decreased from 9 cm to 6 cm. This decrease has taken place before extender removal. **D,** Postoperative view after second scalp reduction. Vertex alopecia measures 3 cm. A total of 9 cm has been removed after 30 days of extender use.

mated and closed. Slot formation is prevented with a triple hair-bearing transposition scalp flap procedure or Frechet flap.[3] Scalp extension followed by the Frechet flap is an integral part of the strategy in the surgical treatment of extensive baldness.

TIGHT SCALP

A few patients with extremely tight scalps and poor results with standard scalp reductions have undergone scalp extensions. They have uniformly experienced good results with scalp extenders placed in the vertex and/or the temporal area. The results were similar to those obtained with scalps of normal laxity. This subset of individuals were previously considered poor candidates for scalp reduction surgery.

LONG-TERM RESULTS

One patient has been followed up for over 4 years. No significant reduction of density, stretchback, or scar widening has occurred. Further studies of the long-term results are necessary.

TIME INTERVAL BETWEEN PROCEDURES

It is recommended that the scalp extender remain in place for 1 month before removal. The width of the scalp extender is limited to 5 cm to allow for easy placement and removal of the device. Two extenders (one behind the other) work best in cases of extensive baldness. The use of two extenders increases pain, and the patient should be so informed.

The number of reductions with scalp extenders depends on the strategy of the hair transplant surgeon. Some prefer to leave a bald area between the hair-bearing scalp, whereas others prefer to eliminate all of the top and posterior baldness. I use the latter approach and perform as many scalp extensions as are necessary to bring the hair-bearing lateral scalp together.

The only side effect induced by scalp extension is the decreased density of the lateral hair-bearing scalp. I have observed the same number and quality of grafts for transplanting after scalp extension.

CONCLUSION

The final aesthetic result appears to be far superior to that achieved with previous methods when scalp extension and slot correction surgery are used. A larger degree of alopecia can be corrected with this approach. The time interval to completion has been greatly reduced.

REFERENCES

1. Frechet P: Scalp extension, *J Dermatol Surg Oncol* 19:616-622, 1993.
2. Bosley L, Hope C, Montroy RE: MPR for surgical reduction of male-pattern baldness, *Curr Ther Res* 25:281-287, 1978.
3. Frechet P: A new method for correction of the vertical scar observed following scalp reduction for extensive baldness, *J Dermatol Surg Oncol* 16:640-644, 1990.

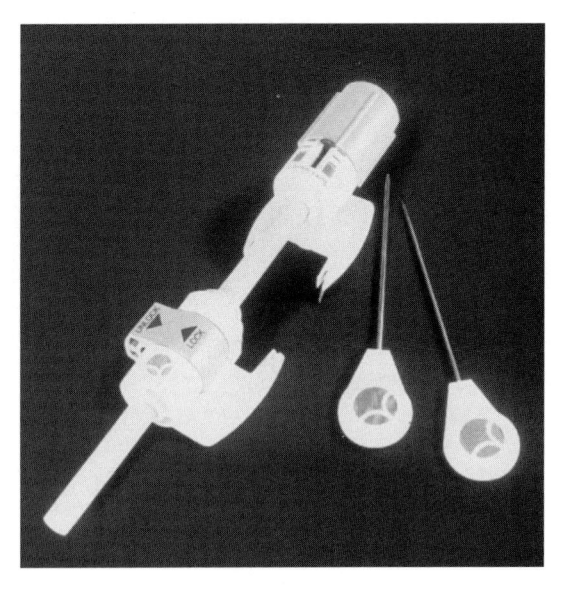

FIG. 9-32 Sure-Closure device. (Courtesy Life Medical Sciences, Inc.).

E. Intraoperative Scalp Extension

David M. Spencer and Dow B. Stough

There currently exist three possible modalities to accomplish expansion of the hair-bearing regions of the scalp. A complete understanding of each modality can be accomplished only by the correct usage of terminology[1] (see Chapter 9, Part C). Intraoperative scalp extension uses a nonvolumetric unidimensional skin-stretching device that creates a continuous inward movement during the intraoperative period. The incremental traction harnesses the viscoelastic property of the skin to produce skin stretching during the operative period.

Intraoperative scalp extension was pioneered by Cohen[2] with the suture tension adjustment reel device known as the Miami STAR. A second-generation product known as the Sure-Closure (Life Medical Sciences, Inc., Princeton, N.J.), a skin-stretching device, was developed by Hirschowitz and received Food and Drug Administration (FDA) approval October 1993 (Fig. 9-32). These devices, when applied to either side of a scalp reduction defect and tightened over 30 to 60 minutes, cause temporoparietal hair-bearing scalp to be advanced toward the midline over the scalp defect. The surgeon can then close the defect under minimal tension and can increase the amount of alopecic scalp excised by 20% to 30%.

NOTE: The authors have no proprietary interest in the Sure-Closure device or the Miami STAR.

INTRAOPERATIVE SCALP EXTENSION PROCEDURE WITH THE SURE-CLOSURE DEVICE

After prepping, draping, and anesthetizing the scalp in the usual manner for scalp surgery, the surgeon excises the previously marked reduction design. The surgeon then undermines in the avascular subgaleal plane and places the stretching device pins parallel to each other on both sides of the defect in the galea underlying the hair-bearing scalp (Fig. 9-33, A). The stretching device hooks abut the pins from the outside and are advanced toward the midline as the surgeon tightens the tension knob to the "lock-out" position (Fig. 9-33, B). The device maintains an extending force of 3 kg/cm^2 throughout the entire scalp between the pins for several minutes and then gradually loses this level of tension as a result of the progressive inward stretch of the galea and by the process of mechanical creep. The surgeon retightens the tension knob and/or repositions the pins and device to include a wider area of hair-bearing scalp over the next 30 to 60 minutes. Patients have reported a sensation of scalp tightening, but no pain attributable to the intraoperative extender has been described. In fact, many report scalp numbness for 6 to 12 hours immediately postoperatively, possibly secondary to stretch neuropraxia of neurovascular bundles in the galea. On removing the device and pins, the surgeon can elect to excise more of the extended alopecic scalp and reapproximate the wound edges with deep sutures and superficial staples or simply to reapproximate the wound margins without reexcising the ex-

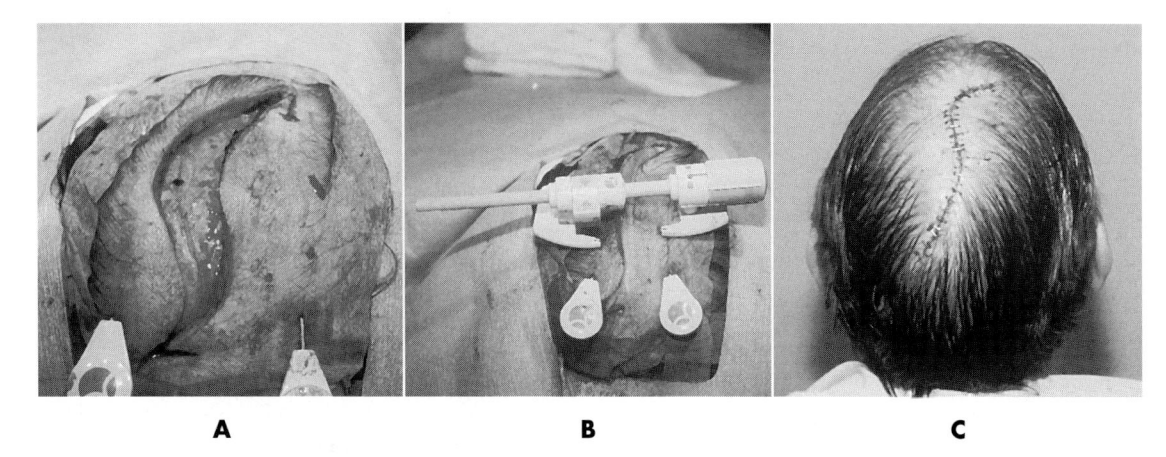

FIG. 9-33 A, After undermining, the Sure-Closure pins are placed parallel to each other on both sides of the defect. **B,** The stretching device hooks abut the pins from the outside and are advanced toward the midline. This advancement is accomplished by the surgeon tightening the tension knob. **C,** Postoperative view after closure.

tended scalp (Fig. 9-33, C). The latter choice minimizes undue tension, wound necrosis, and stretchback tendencies.

No scalp infections have been reported to date. We have not noted hematoma or sterile serosanguinous drainage from the approximated wound margins. We have observed a thickening of the scalp immediately surrounding the reduced area.

The Miami STAR works on the same principle as the Sure-Closure device but employs sutures under tension to produce incremental increases in traction.[2]

INTRAOPERATIVE SCALP EXTENSION

Advantages
1. Increases the amount of bald scalp removed by 20% to 30%.
2. Reduces the total number of reduction procedures by as much as 25% to 30%.
3. Associated with less stretchback tendency and less atrophic scarring.
4. Causes no appreciable postoperative hair loss to date.
5. Causes less postoperative discomfort to date.

Disadvantages
1. Causes intraoperative sensation of scalp tightness.
2. Lengthens reduction procedures by 30 to 60 minutes.
3. Requires increased cost.

ADVANTAGES

The advantages of using intraoperative scalp extension include decreased stretchback in many of the patients with excessive stretchback tendencies following previous scalp reductions and the obvious increase in the amount of alopecic scalp excised when compared with standard scalp reduction (see box).

DISADVANTAGES

Limitations or disadvantages of intraoperative scalp extension include (1) occasional arm hook penetration into the periosteum and subsequent blocking of the extension force during the operation, (2) increased amount of time to perform each scalp reduction, and (3) limited patient selection because the procedure is limited to patients with mild to moderate vertex baldness widths (bald scalp widths of 5 to 9 cm) because of the small size of the skin-stretching device (see box).

• • •

In the future, the Sure-Closure device will be modified to include hooks more adaptable to the galea.

REFERENCES
1. Cohen BH: Navigating through tissue expansion terminology, *J Dermatol Surg Oncol* 19:614-615, 1993.
2. Cohen BH, Cosmetto AJ: The suture tension adjustment reel, *J Dermatol Surg Oncol* 18:112-123, 1992.

F. The Biology of Skin Stretch and Tissue Expansion in Hair Restoration Surgery

James E. Vogel

As Vistnes[1] has pointed out, tissue expansion and acute skin stretch have made their way into the operating room without first passing through the research laboratory. Although this is a valid way of trying out reasonable ideas and techniques, the appropriate corollary now is to prove why and how they work. Surgeons performing hair replacement surgery using the techniques of tissue expansion and scalp advancement should now critically review the scientific data available on these techniques and review their anatomical basis. Such review is necessary so that traditional modalities and new advances in tissue expansion can be used with maximum safety and effectiveness.

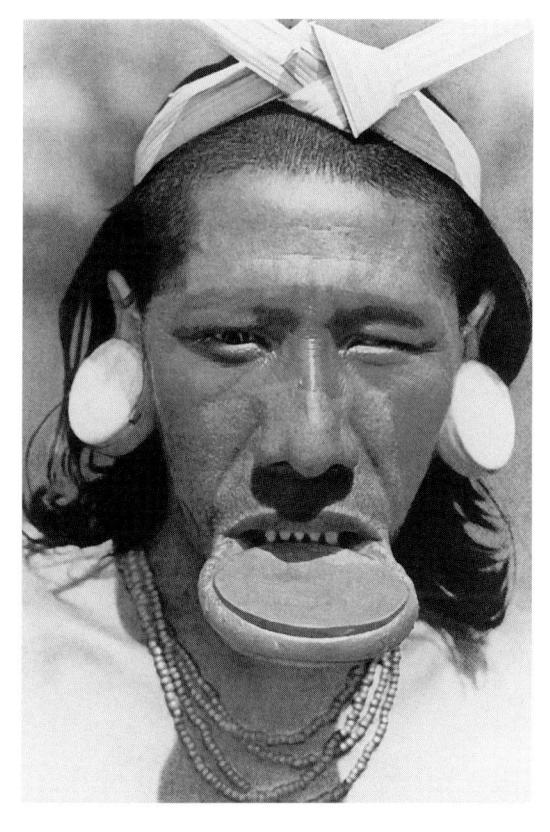

FIG. 9-34 Ubangi tribesman circa 1930. His stretched lower lip measures approximately 7½ inches in circumference. This tradition of self-mutilation was most likely begun centuries ago to make Ubangi tribespeople unattractive to slave traders. (From Rees TD, Wood-Smith D: *Cosmetic facial surgery,* Philadelphia, 1973, WB Saunders.)

The expansion of facial structures based on the elastic property of skin has been practiced for centuries in Eastern and African cultures (Fig. 9-34). This concept was used for the first time in medicine by Neumann,[2] who in 1957 reported tissue expansion for ear reconstruction. Despite this early report, little attention was focused on the applications of tissue expansion until Radovan[3,4] in 1976 reintroduced the concept and began using it successfully in breast reconstruction. Austad, Cherry, and associates[5-8] and Sasaki[9] in the 1980s pioneered applications of conventional tissue expanders and described the histology of expanded tissue. Until 1984, most tissue expansion applications used two operative procedures and an inflation time ranging from 4 to 10 weeks.[10,11] In 1987, Sasaki[9] and others[12,13] demonstrated that for limited tissue requirements, intraoperative tissue expansion was a viable alternative to conventional expansion techniques. Recently a variety of skin-stretching devices and clinical applications have been developed to immediately harness the viscoelastic properties of skin.[14-18] Other new techniques have been developed to reduce dramatically the time needed for skin expansion and to monitor the effects of expansion.[19-22]

ANATOMY AND PATHOPHYSIOLOGY OF STRETCHED SKIN

Fundamental to an understanding of what is accomplished in the operating room with tissue stretch and expansion techniques is an appreciation for the anatomy and histology of stretched skin. These anatomical details have practical and critical everyday implications for clinical practice. As

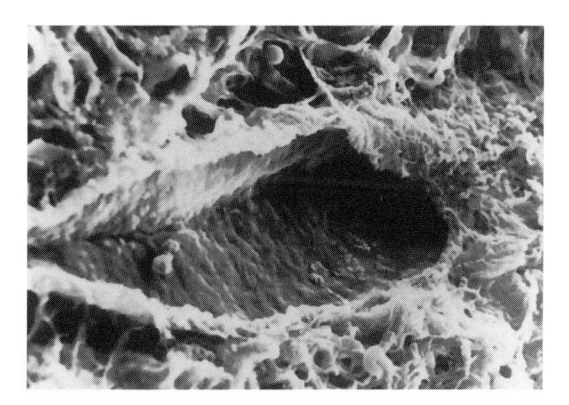

FIG. 9-35 Electron micrograph of an arteriole in the dermis. When the surrounding collagen fiber network is deformed, the lumen may become obliterated, producing ischemia, skin blanching, and possibly necrosis. (From McCarthy JG, editor: *Plastic surgery,* Philadelphia, 1990, WB Saunders.)

seen in Fig. 9-35, a small arteriole is coursing through the dermis. When the fibrous network is deformed through stretch or excessive tension, the lumen may become compressed and lead to telogen in the local area. If the lumen is obliterated, there will be blanching and ultimately necrosis. Similarly, nerve constriction, transection, or scar entrapment may cause pain or anesthesia. Interruption of lymphatics or obliteration results in edema. In addition, the fibrous networks of the scalp are transfixed by hair shafts (Fig. 9-36). This structure explains in part the relative immobility of scalp dermis compared with other areas of the body. Hair shafts are surrounded by follicles and sebaceous glands, which are attached to the main collagen network by fine fibrils. The elastin fibers and collagen network are the principal elements responsible for skin stretch.

Effect of Chronic (Traditional) Tissue Expansion on Tissue

EPIDERMIS

Statistical analysis of multiple skin sites over an expander reveals no significant variation in epidermal thickness during tissue expansion.[23-25] One week after placement of the prosthesis, some thickening may occur in the epidermis, but this thickening also occurs in sham-operated controls. The increased thickness probably represents postoperative and localized edema. By 4 weeks after placement of the prosthesis, epidermal thickness decreases to its normal baseline and essentially remains unchanged throughout expansion (Fig. 9-37). Accessory skin structures such as hair follicles show some degree of compression in the posteroanterior plane. The interfollicular distance increases as the tissue is ex-

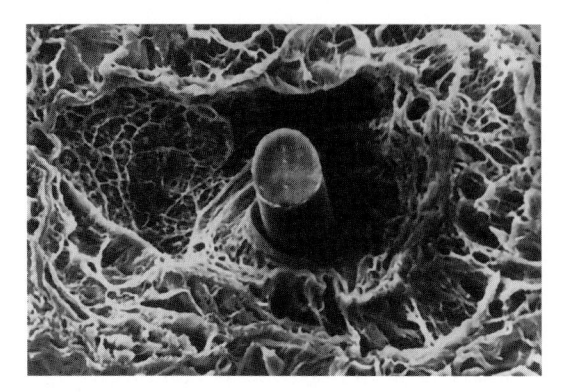

FIG. 9-36 Electron micrograph of a hair shaft surrounded by its follicle and sebaceous gland. They are shown attached to the main collagen network by fine fibrils. (From McCarthy JG, editor: *Plastic surgery*, Philadelphia, 1990, WB Saunders.)

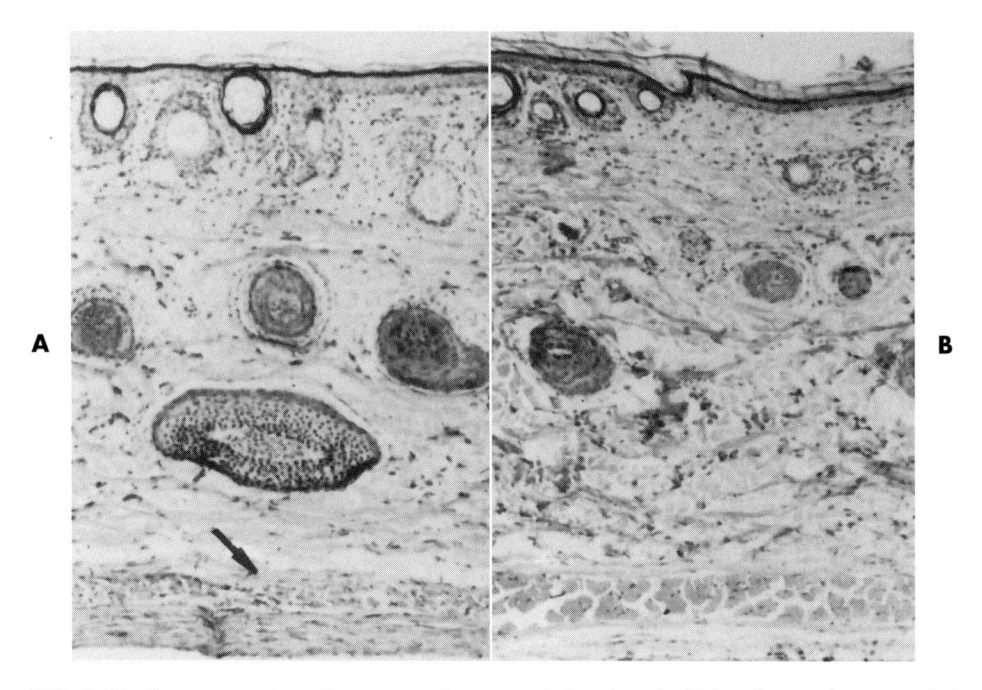

FIG. 9-37 Low-power view of guinea pig skin expanded at 4 weeks **(A)** and normal unexpanded implant site **(B)**. Note the following features in the expanded skin: (1) intact normal-appearing stratified squamous epithelium, (2) slight compression of hair follicle, (3) moderate atrophy of the panniculus carnosus muscle *(arrow)* and (4) well-formed fibrous connective tissue "capsule" surrounding the implant. (From Austad ED and others: *Plast Reconstr Surg* 70(6):704-710, 1982.)

panded progressively. It has been estimated that a twofold expansion in an average hair-bearing scalp can be performed before a noticeable increase in thinning of the hair occurs.

DERMIS

In contrast to the epidermis, there is rapid decrease in dermal thickness over the entire implant during the expansion process.[23-25] This effect is most pronounced during the first few weeks after implant placement and persists throughout the entire period of tissue expansion. Restoration of preexpansion dermal thickness occurs after the implant is removed. This return of dermal thickness can take up to 2 years.

MUSCLE/FAT

Considerable compression and some obliteration of fat occurs with tissue expansion. This fat is quickly restored on removal of the expander and subsequent weight gain. Significant atrophy of muscles occurs during the process of tissue expansion (Fig. 9-37). This effect is evident whether the tissue expander is placed above or below the muscle. Muscle function, however, remains active, and after removal of the tissue expander, muscle mass is diminished but maintains the ability to hypertrophy with use.

CAPSULE

A distinct capsule forms around the expander (see Fig. 9-37). Increased vasculature forms in the area adjacent to the capsule. The augmented blood supply around the periprosthetic capsule is a physiological and anatomical change in the tissue induced by the expander and expansion process. The presence of a foreign body, increased tissue tension, and ischemia are thought to bring about this physiological increase in blood supply. The increased blood supply in the capsule supports the surgical dogma of including this layer with the scalp flaps. An x-ray film of barium-injected blood vessels in expanded and nonexpanded flaps reveals the dramatic increase in vascularity of the tissue-expanded flaps (Fig. 9-38).

Electron Microscopic Studies

In 1982, Pasyk and associates[25] performed electron microscopic studies of expanded tissue in the guinea pig. Their work has elucidated the pathophysiology of skin expansion at the electron microscopic level. Active fibroblasts with prominent rough endoplasmic reticulum and mitochondria are identified in the expanded dermis and new immature collagen fibers of differing size are seen as well (Figs. 9-39 and 9-40). The presence of active fi-

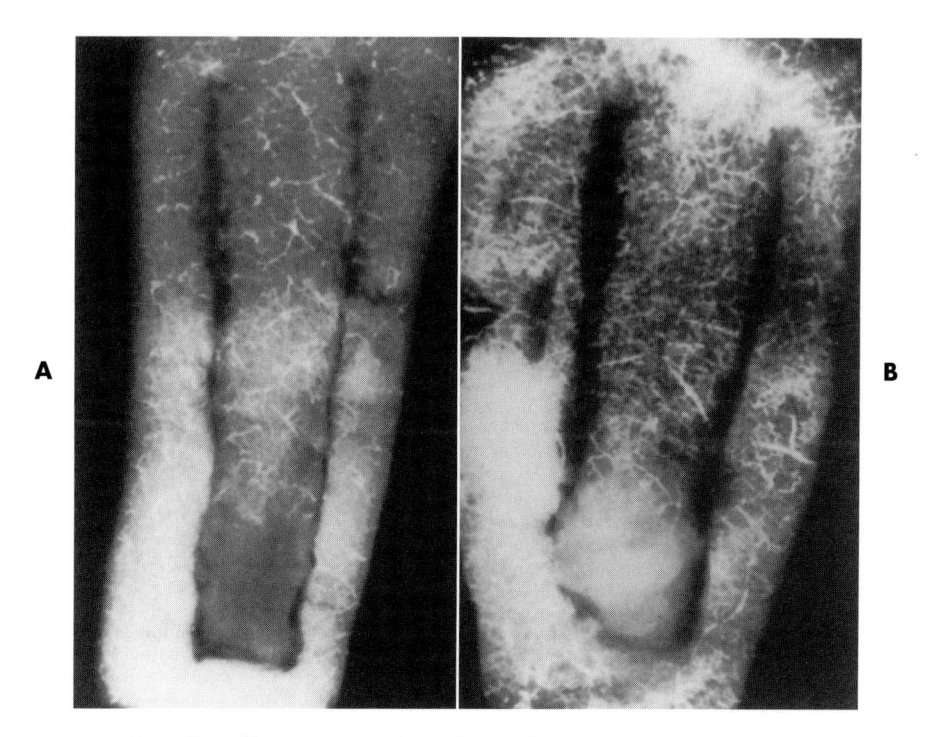

FIG. 9-38 X-ray film of barium-injected vessels of **(A)** a nonexpanded random pattern pig skin flap and **(B)** a matched skin flap that underwent tissue expansion. Note the dramatic increase in vascularity of the expanded flap. (From McCarthy JG, editor: *Plastic surgery*, Philadelphia, 1990, WB Saunders.)

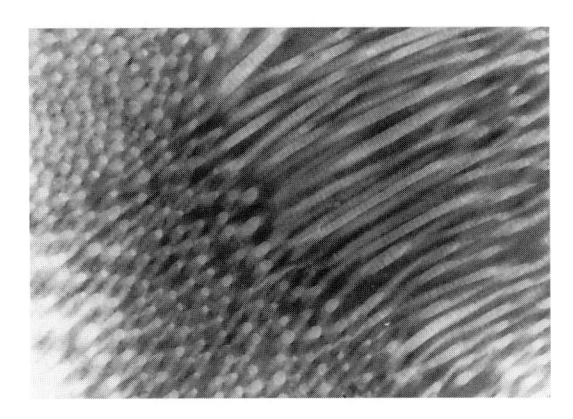

FIG. 9-39 Electron micrograph of expanded skin in 7-month-old guinea pig showing new and immature collagen fibers of differing size. (From Pasyk K and others: *Plast Reconstr Surg* 70(1):37-45, 1982.)

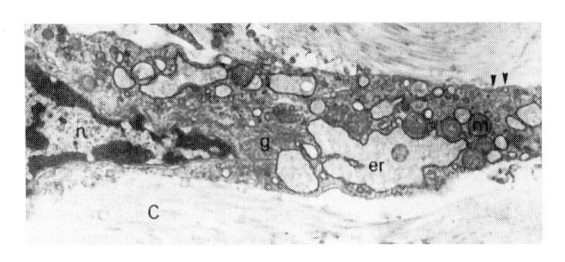

FIG. 9-40 Electron micrograph of expanded skin in 8-month-old guinea pig. Note the following: (1) part of a fibroblast with prominent rough endoplasmic reticulum *(er)*, (2) numerous mitochondria *(m)*, (3) golgi, *(g)*, (4) pinocytotic vesicles *(arrows)*, (5) nucleus *(n)*, and (6) collagen fibers *(C)*. (From Pasyk K and others: *Plast Reconstr Surg* 70(1):37-45, 1982.)

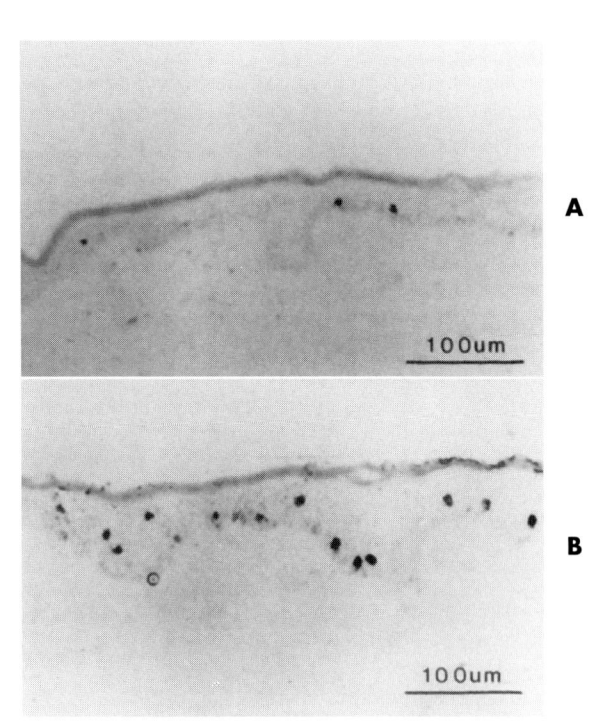

FIG. 9-41 First documented human response to tissue expansion reveals increased numbers of cells incorporating titrated thymidine **(A)** compared with nonexpanded skin **(B)**. (From Olenius M and others: *Plast Reconstr Surg* 91(2):213-216, 1993.)

broblasts in the expanded dermis is believed to be directly related to the origin of the immature collagen fibers that are present.

Origin of Expanded Skin

BIOLOGICAL ORIGIN
The presence of active fibroblasts and other histological clues were noted during the early 1980s and suggested the origin of expanded skin. However, the evidence remained circumstantial until 1986, when Austad, Thomas, and Pasyk[7] published their classic work entitled "Tissue Expansion: Dividend or Loan?" Research was performed using guinea pigs in which tissue expanders were inflated on a daily basis for 4 weeks. Using light microscopy and autoradiography with titrated thymidine, Austad, Thomas, and Pasyk were able to show a threefold increase in mitotic activity within 24 hours after tissue expansion compared with unoperated controls. These data provided the first conclusive evidence to document the biological origin of expanded tissue. This origin was from a net increase in cellular proliferation, a true tissue dividend.

Although tissue expansion was extensively used in human surgical procedures for over 30 years, the first conclusive evidence that this phenomenon existed in humans was only recently demonstrated. In 1993, researchers from Sweden substantiated the occurrence of increased DNA synthesis in expanded human epidermal cells as well.[26] The light micrographs in Fig. 9-41 reveal a significant milestone in our ability to define the human response to tissue expansion—namely, increased mitosis to create new tissue production. Although this analysis has never been performed on a human scalp, there is no reason to believe that the pathophysiology of expanded scalp would be different.

RECRUITMENT
The tissue dividend as a result of expansion over time explains only one component of the added availability of chronically stretched skin. The other component is tissue recruitment. The contribution

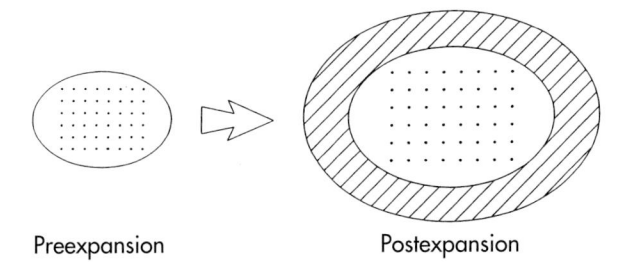

FIG. 9-42 Contribution of tissue recruitment to the overall process of tissue expansion. The dotted area represents the region in which the expander exerts its influence through cellular proliferation. The hatched area represents the phenomenon of the enlarging expander itself contributing to the recruitment process. (From Schmidt SC and others: *Plast Reconstr Surg* 87(1):10-15, 1991.)

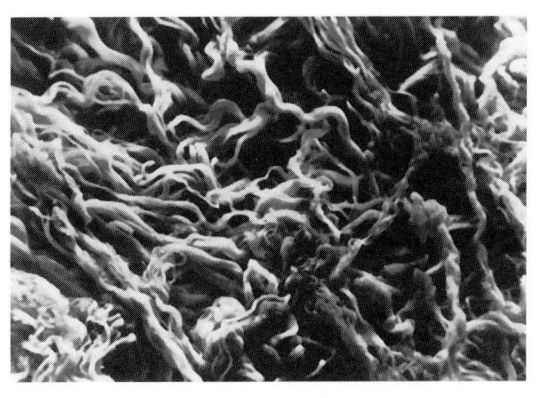

FIG. 9-43 Electron micrograph of collagen fibers in human dermis. Note the fiber length compared to the diameter and the random orientation. (From Montagna W, Bentley JP, Dobson RL, editors: *The dermis*, Norwalk, Conn., 1970, Appleton & Lange.)

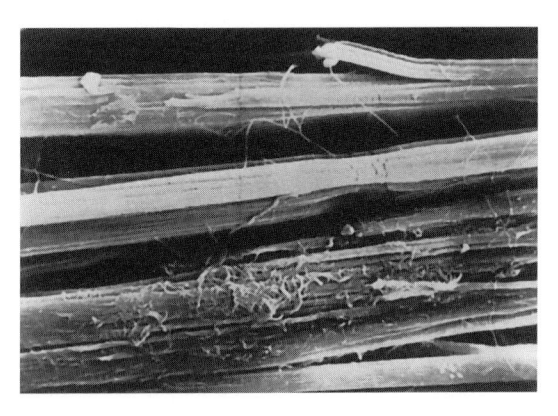

FIG. 9-44 Electron micrograph of collagen fibers in stretched skin. Note their straight alignment in the direction of stretch. This orientation places a limit on the skin extensibility in the direction of pull. (From McCarthy JG, editor: *Plastic surgery*, Philadelphia, 1990, WB Saunders.)

of tissue recruitment to the overall expansion process is best understood diagrammatically (Fig. 9-42). Surrounding loose skin is recruited by two processes: the undermining needed to place the implant and the dissection of the advancing expander itself as the implant volume increases.

• • •

Thus recruitment and increased mitosis are the two primary mechanisms to provide increased availability of tissue with expansion of tissue over time. Mechanical creep also contributes to the recruitment of available tissue with traditional methods of tissue expansion.

INTRAOPERATIVE TISSUE EXPANSION
Viscoelastic and Other Biomechanical Properties of Skin

In the past several years a popular method for obtaining additional transferable hair-bearing scalp has been to apply intraoperative stretch of the tissues for immediate tissue expansion. The acute gain in tissue availability through these maneuvers is possible as a result of the physical properties of skin. The viscoelastic properties of skin are the biomechanical elements primarily responsible for intraoperative expansion and acute stretch of skin. These dynamic and physical properties of skin have direct clinical applicability to every flap or advancement procedure that has been performed or designed on the scalp. Anatomically the ability of skin to stretch acutely primarily depends on the fibrous networks and architecture of collagen and elastin. The scanning electron micrograph (Fig. 9-43) clearly defines the structure of collagen fibers in the dermis. The fibers are long compared with their diameter and appear to be randomly oriented.

When skin is stretched in any direction, an increasing number of collagen fibers become aligned in the direction of the stretching force. When stretch is increased, the collagen fibers align in a parallel fashion (Fig. 9-44). Once the collagen fibers have fully realigned themselves parallel to the forces of pull, the skin is said to have reached its maximum degree of elastic stretch. At this point, the skin is highly resistant to further extension. If the stretched tissue is not pulled to the degree seen in the electron micrograph, the skin is said to have been stretched within the range of its elasticity and stretchback or recoil of the collagen can occur. Returning the deformed collagen to its relaxed position after acute stretch is the job of the much finer elastin fibers. If the skin is stretched far-

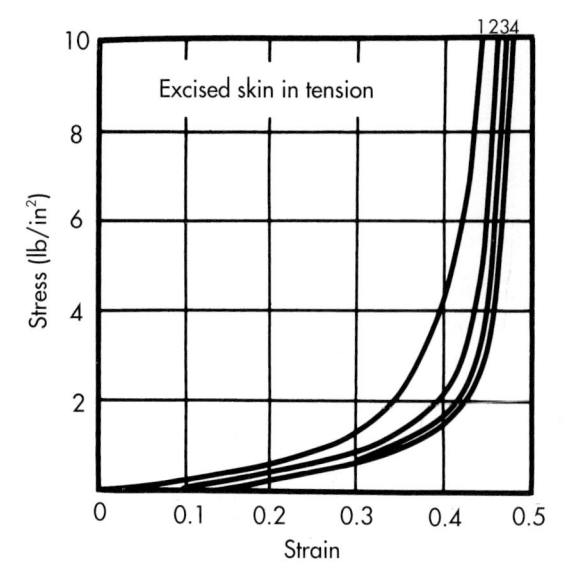

FIG. 9-45 Tissue creep occurs when a piece of skin is stretched and the stretching force is held constant. This results in a progressive increase in skin extension. The scientific basis of tissue creep (see text) explains the rationale for the technique of "load cycling," which is diagrammatically illustrated here. As skin pull (stress) is cyclically applied to the same or greater degree, additional length (strain or creep) is obtained. (From Montagna W, Bentley JP, Dobson RL, editors: *The dermis*, Norwalk, Conn., 1970, Appleton & Lange.)

ther than its maximum degree of elastic stretch, the collagen ruptures and, clinically, striae will result. It is well known from clinical and daily observation that the existence of striae is an irreversible phenomenon.

Creep and Stress Relaxation

Creep and stress relaxation were first described by Gibson[27] in 1967 (Fig. 9-45). Creep occurs when a piece of skin is stretched and the stretching force is held constant. Stress relaxation is the biomechanical reaction to creep. When skin is stretched for a given distance and that distance is held constant, the force required to keep it stretched gradually decreases. The decrease in force needed to maintain the increased length of stretched tissue is the definition of stress relaxation.

The mobile microarchitecture of skin and scalp that favors the phenomenon of creep requires an internal lubricant. This lubricant is provided by the mucopolysaccharide ground substance and the tissue fluid lying between the collagen fibers. As the tissues are stretched, the tissue fluid and ground substance are progressively displaced from the fibrous collagen network. This dehydration process is another mechanism responsible for increasing skin length with acute (i.e., immediate) stretch.

Creep and stress relaxation have traditionally been important in the operating room while closing donor scalp defects and advancing wound edges when a surgeon is faced with a wound that will not close easily. The usual technique for taking advantage of these viscoelastic properties of skin is familiar to most surgeons and is referred to as *load cycling*. The procedure of load cycling involves placing the sharp hook of a retractor under the dermis of each flap to be advanced and then pulling these flaps in opposite directions with as much force as the surgeon or an assistant can muster short of tearing the tissues. The pull usually lasts for at least a minute and is frequently cycled several times. On a microscopic level, the technique aligns the dermal collagen fibers. The tissue fluid and ground substance lying between the collagen fibers are progressively displaced from the fibrous network. This tissue dehydration process is maximized by performing the procedure several times. The scientific rationale for this technique of load cycling has been substantiated in the laboratory and is based on the principles of creep and stress relaxation. As seen in the strain (creep) vs. stress graft (see Fig. 9-45), by the third or fourth stress application (i.e., pull) more tissue length (i.e., creep) is obtained given a constant stress.

Stretchback

Although the acute stretch of scalp can produce dramatic intraoperative reduction in alopecia, the long-term gain can be reversed if stretchback of advanced flaps occurs. A seemingly endless clinical debate over the existence of stretchback has occurred during the past 10 to 15 years. Studies by Nordstrom[28] and others have addressed this issue and report significant loss of gained tissue advancement with acute skin stretch. However, reports by Unger have sharply refuted the finding of major stretchback after flap advancement with scalp reduction[29] (Unger MG: Personal communication). Stretchback is a clinical term and no one scientific element defines this phenomenon or measures it. Clearly the degree of collagen fiber realignment, degree of skin stretch within its range of elasticity, extent of tissue dehydration, local scar widening, and final wound tension all contribute to the tendency toward stretchback of advanced flaps. At this time, the most important component in determining the extent of predicted stretchback has not been scientifically scrutinized. However, clinically reduced intraoperative wound-closing tension seems to be a crucial factor.

To minimize stretchback of extensively advanced scalp flaps, one surgeon has used a retaining strip of alloplast to connet the two leading edges of the flaps.[14]

However, it remains to be proved whether higher wound-closing tensions that occur with extensive flap advancement supported with alloplast can counter the unrelenting forces of recoil over time.

The concept of stretchback in chronically expanded skin has been studied recently in laboratory experiments.[30] As pointed out earlier in this discussion, the presence of fibroblasts and their contribution to collagen synthesis in expanded skin are significant. This observation led Chang and others to ask whether tissue expansion alters dermal fibroblast function and whether the duration of tissue expansion alters the degree of fibroblast contractility and anticipated stretchback. Their findings in a rat model demonstrated what clinical surgeons have observed for years: that tissue expansion inhibits the in vitro contractile function of dermal fibroblasts in a time-related fashion. This scientific study is the first to provide support on a cellular level for the clinical impression that a longer duration of skin expansion may result in less stretchback.

• • •

Thus far, the scientific principles of chronic and acute tissue stretch have been reviewed. The controversial aspects of the various clinically reported techniques of scalp expansion, scalp stretch, and flap undermining can now be evaluated.

ANALYSIS OF SKIN STRETCH AND EXPANSION TECHNIQUES

Techniques for stretch in skin or scalp are most logically analyzed based on the length of time needed to accomplish the procedure.

Chronic (Traditional) Tissue Expansion

In clinical practice the greatest deterrent to the use of traditional methods of tissue expansion is patient acceptance. However, from a purely reconstructive standpoint, traditional methods of scalp expansion over time offer unparalleled flap mobility, improved vascularity, and decreased donor site complications when compared with the techniques of immediate tissue stretch. However, given the realities of what most patients are willing to go through, researchers have investigated the following questions: (1) How long does tissue need to be expanded and still develop additional new skin? (2) What techniques improve the efficiency of expansion? and (3) What is more important, wide undermining or intraoperative expansion?

Experimentally it appears that the peak of cell multiplication following expansion occurs between 12 and 24 hours after the expansion process is initiated.[6,7,23,31,32] This laboratory finding is important in helping to determine clinically how fast tissue expansion can be performed and still obtain a true increased cellular proliferative response to expansion. In 1986, Pietila and associates[33] demonstrated clinically that a 59% increase in the filling volume per filling session was achieved by a temporary overinflation of the expander in each session to a pressure at which the overlying tissues were blanching or the patient was not able to tolerate any higher pressure because of pain. This finding resulted in a corresponding increase in the speed of total expansion. Following this study, Schmidt, Mustoe, and associates[34] published experimental, histological, and laboratory data to substantiate what many clinicians (including Nordstrom) had observed in their practice for years. They noted that rapid expansion over 2 weeks could duplicate the accomplishment of traditional expansion over 6 weeks. This research was significant because it scientifically documented for the first time the ability to gain new tissue using a shorter expansion time. In a later study, this same group used a new concept of tissue expansion that is still experimental but may find clinical applicability (Fig. 9-46). They used an implantable, continuous tissue expander pump to demonstrate expansion in 3 days equal to that obtained in their earlier experiments over 2 weeks. This new concept of tissue expansion requires a microprocessor controller using a feedback loop to adjust the pressure in the expander on a continuous basis to maintain expander pressure just below capillary filling pressure. Most intriguing was the fact that collagen synthesis (and cellular proliferation) and other biological characteristics of the skin were equal over a 3-day expansion period to that over the more traditional 6-week period of expansion. In theory, this technique might allow hair restoration surgeons to harness the benefits of traditional expansion in only 3 days and thus gain greater patient acceptance. Other methods for improving the efficiency of tissue expansion have been attempted experimentally or in clinical practice, including using a texturized expander or locally injecting pharmacological agents.

One of the fundamental issues regarding tissue expansion continues to be the relative contribution of the various mechanisms to the overall expansion process. It will be recalled that two primary mechanisms are involved with traditional tissue expansion techniques: cellular proliferation and tissue recruitment. With traditional expansion techniques, it has been estimated that new tissue proliferation contributes 40% to expanded skin, whereas recruitment (undermining and mechanical tissue creep) comprises 60%.

The increasingly important role of undermining and tissue recruitment with traditional expansion was emphasized in 1993 by Fukuta, Jackson, and as-

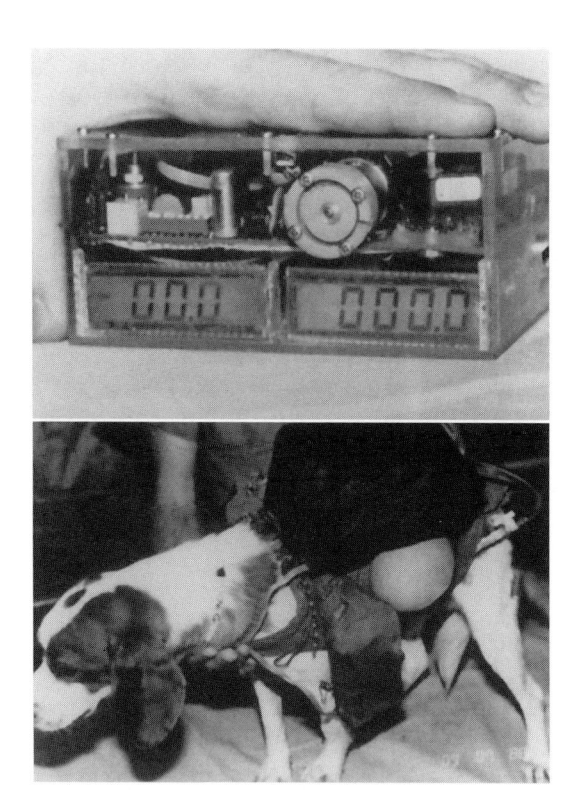

FIG. 9-46 An experimental continuous tissue expander pump that has been shown to dramatically shorten the time needed for tissue expansion. This technique requires a microprocessor controller to maintain a constant infusion pressure over a period of days. (From Schmidt SC and others: *Plast Reconstr Surg* 87(1):10-15, 1991.)

sociates.[35] Jackson and his coworkers used a canine model to demonstrate a more efficient and rapid expansion of available tissue over time but found that no increase in tissue proliferation occurred in the hyperexpanded animals. All additional surface area that was gained by rapid and massive hyperexpansion was provided by tissue recruitment from the mechanical dissection and acute tissue stretch of the expander. It is not known whether this increase in obtainable surface area by massive hyperexpansion is a reversible (i.e., temporary) phenomenon (a loan) or whether this increase is in fact a durable gain in tissue. Another relevant issue for the physician is whether massive and rapid tissue expansion would be tolerated by the patient.

Immediate Expansion

With regard to expansion techniques to provide acute stretch of the scalp, it has been shown experimentally by Sasaki[9] that intraoperative expansion provides a more efficient acute gain in tissue length than load cycling or stretching techniques. This finding does not negate the validity of load cycling as a technique but merely elucidates the improved three-dimensional efficiency of intraoperative tissue expansion compared with unidirectional techniques. Investigators in Israel have developed a skin-stretching device that can be used preoperatively or intraoperatively to harness the viscoelastic properties of skin.[14] The clinical application of this technique in alopecia reduction is being investigated. Frechet[36] has used another device to harness the biological properties of skin to internally advance scalp flaps. The exact mechanism of this device in achieving a surplus of scalp for advancement is currently under investigation (Vogel JE: Unpublished data). The prime advantage of internal, unidirectional scalp stretch over time is the absence of the cosmetic deformity of tissue expanders. At this time, the principal appeal of this technique rests in high patient acceptance, early reports of substantial tissue stretch, and low morbidity. Long-term clinical results of Frechet's exciting work will be required to validate this new technique.

A controversy exists regarding the relative importance of undermining vs. the direct benefit of the intraoperative expansion process. Studies in St. Louis and Hershey, Pennsylvania have independently evaluated this question and suggest that extensive undermining of tissue equals the benefit of reducing wound tension as a result of intraoperative expansion.[37,38] These scientific findings support the clinical experience that extensive undermining of the scalp has significant value in gaining flap advancement.[39] These reports do not necessarily mean that intraoperative expansion has limited value. Undermining advancement flaps or stretching them with an expander are two techniques that can be used by the hair restoration surgeon according to the clinical situation and location of the tissue to be advanced. The surgeon's experience, nature of the alopecia reduction, and patient's desires should be the guide to the preferred method of tissue advancement and stretch.

CONCLUSION

"Natural tissue expansion and skin stretch have been with us in the form of pregnancy for as long as mankind has existed. It takes keen observation, imagination, and a fertile mind to translate an observed phenomenon into an application for clinical surgery."[1] There is a definite but limited role for traditional tissue expansion in the treatment of male pattern baldness. Most likely there is a larger role for scalp advancement, reduction, and scalp-stretching techniques since they are more expedient and less deforming. Clearly clinical reports and techniques on tissue expansion and scalp stretch have far outstripped the number of scientific reports on this topic.

Hair replacement surgeons using techniques of tissue expansion and other forms of scalp stretch must fully understand the rationale and proven scientific basis for the techniques. This knowledge allows the safe use of the technology and development of a scientific basis for future advances and improved patient care.

REFERENCES

1. Vistnes LM: Discussion of "Tissue expansion in soft-tissue reconstruction" by CR Radovan, *Plast Reconstr Surg* 74:491-492, 1994.
2. Neumann CG: The expansion of an area of skin by progressive distension of subcutaneous balloon, *Plast Reconstr Surg* 19:124, 1957.
3. Radovan C: Breast reconstruction after mastectomy using the temporary expander, *Plast Reconstr Surg* 69:195-208, 1982.
4. Radovan C: Tissue expansion in soft tissue reconstruction, *Plast Reconstr Surg* 74:482-492, 1984.
5. Austad E: Complications of tissue expansion, *Clin Plast Surg* 3:549-550, 1987.
6. Austad E and others: Histomorphologic evaluation of guinea pig skin and soft tissue after controlled tissue expansion, *Plast Reconstr Surg* 70:704-710, 1982.
7. Austad E, Thomas S, Pasyk K: Tissue expansion: dividend or loan? *Plast Reconstr Surg* 78:63-67, 1986.
8. Cherry G and others: Increased survival and vascularity of random-pattern skin flaps elevated in controlled, expanded flaps, *Plast Reconstr Surg* 72:680-685, 1983.
9. Sasaki GH: Intraoperative sustained limited expansion (ISLE) as an immediate reconstructive technique, *Clin Plast Surg* 14:563, 1987.
10. Cohen M, Dolezal R, Schultz R: Tissue expansion in reconstructive surgery, *Contemp Surg* 30:21-31, 1987.
11. Vander Kolk C and others: Some further characteristics of expanded tissue, *Clin Plast Surg* 14:447-453, 1987.
12. McCauley R, Oliphant J, Robson M: Tissue expansion in the correction of burn alopecia: classification and methods of correction, *Ann Plast Surg* 25:103-115, 1990.
13. Nordstrom R, Devine J: Scalp stretching with a tissue expander for closure of scalp defects, *Plast Reconstr Surg* 75:587-591, 1985.
14. Hirschowitz B, Lindenbaum E, Har-Shai Y: A skin stretching device for the harnessing of the viscoelastic properties of skin, *Plast Reconstr Surg* 92:260-270, 1993.
15. Man D: Stretching and tissue expansion for rhytidectomy: an improved approach, *Plast Reconstr Surg* 84:561-569, 1989.
16. Baker S, Swanson N: Rapid intraoperative tissue expansion in reconstruction of the head and neck, *Arch Otolaryngol Head Neck Surg* 116:1031-1049, 1990.
17. Ehlert T, Thomas J: Rapid intraoperative tissue expansion for closure of facial defects, *Arch Otolaryngol Head Neck Surg* 117:1043-1049, 1991.
18. Machina B and others: Immediate versus chronic tissue expansion, *Ann Plast Surg* 26:227-232, 1991.
19. Barone F and others: The biomechanical and histopathologic effects of surface texturing with silicone and polyurethane in tissue implantation and expansion, *Plast Reconstr Surg* 90:77-86, 1992.
20. Brobmann G, Huber J: Effects of different shaped tissue expanders on transluminal pressure, oxygen tension, histopathologic changes, and skin expansion in pigs, *Plast Reconstr Surg* 74:731-735, 1985.
21. Hallock G, Rice D: Increased sensitivity in objective monitoring of tissue expansion, *Plast Reconstr Surg* 84:561-569, 1993.
22. Netscher D, Spira M, Peterson R: Adjunctive agents to facilitate rapid tissue expansion, *Ann Plast Surg* 23:412-416, 1989.
23. Argenta L, Austad E: Principles and techniques of tissue expansion. In McCarthy J, editor: *Plastic surgery*, Philadelphia, 1990, WB Saunders.
24. Bartell T, Mustoe T: Animal models of human tissue expansion, *Plast Reconstr Surg* 83:681-686, 1989.
25. Pasyk K and others: Electron microscopic evaluation of guinea pig skin and soft tissues "expanded" with a self-inflating silicone implant, *Plast Reconstr Surg* 70:37-45, 1982.
26. Olenius M, Dalsgaard C, Wickman M: Mitotic activity in expanded human skin, *Plast Reconstr Surg* 91:213-216, 1993.
27. Gibson T: Physical properties of skin. In McCarthy J, editor: *Plastic surgery*, Philadelphia, 1990, WB Saunders.
28. Nordstrom R: "Stretch-back" in scalp reductions for male pattern baldness, *Plast Reconstr Surg* 73:422-426, 1984.
29. Unger MG, Unger WP: Alopecia reduction. In Unger WP, editor: *Hair transplantation*, New York, 1979, Marcel Dekker.
30. Chang B and others: The effect of tissue expansion on dermal fibroblast contraction, *Ann Plast Surg* 28:315-319, 1992.
31. Argenta L: Controlled tissue expansion, *Surg Rounds* 65-86, Feb, 1986.
32. Mustoe T, Bartell, Garner W: Physical, biomechanical, histologic and biochemical effects of rapid versus conventional tissue expansion, *Plast Reconstr Surg* 83:687-691, 1989.
33. Pietila J and others: Accelerated tissue expansion with the "overfilling" technique, *Plast Reconstr Surg* 81:204-207, 1986.
34. Schmidt S and others: Continuous versus conventional tissue expansion: experimental verification of a new technique, *Plast Reconstr Surg* 87:10-15, 1991.
35. Fukuta K and others: Efficacy of cycled hyperinflation for rapid tissue expansion, *Plast Reconst Surg* 91:846-852, 1993.
36. Frechet P: Scalp extension, *J Dermatol Surg Oncol* 19:616-622, 1993.
37. Hochman M, Branham G, Thomas R: Relative effects of intraoperative tissue expansion and undermining on wound closing tensions, *Arch Otolaryngol Head Neck Surg* 118:1185-1187, 1992.
38. Mackay D and others: Stretching skin: undermining is more important than intraoperative expansion, *Plast Reconstr Surg* 86:722-730, 1990.
39. Brandy DA: New various approaches for the treatment of extensive baldness, *Am J Cosmet Surg* 7:129-139, 1990.

G. Rapid Intraoperative Tissue Expansion Created by Tension Clamps

James Arnold

Scalp surgeons have long recognized that the scalp is particularly responsive to tissue expansion techniques. Since the galea is loosely attached to the periosteum, large areas of the scalp can be undermined and mobilized and thereby allowed to participate in the expansion process. As a result of the intrinsic elasticity of the scalp, stretching (or expansion) occurs with particular ease. In addition, from the surgeon's point of view, the scalp is remarkably resilient. Despite repeated manipulations and invasive procedures, the scalp invariably heals well with few complications.

Even though the scalp responds favorably to tissue expansion, few surgeons presently are using tissue expansion techniques in scalp reduction procedures. Many surgeons are discouraged by the need for multiple procedures and expensive expansion devices. When complicated maneuvers are required, the surgeon may feel unprepared or hesitant to make a first attempt. Also, there is genuine concern that the surgical time involved may be unpredictably long.

Over a period of several years, I have developed a tissue expansion technique that is simple, effective, and easily adopted by any surgeon who performs scalp reductions. This technique involves the application of direct, forceful tension to the parietal scalp for a brief period as a means of inducing rapid intraoperative tissue expansion. The tension is created by using a modified version of a towel clamp, which is called a *tension clamp*. These clamps are convenient to use since they are applied to only the external surface of the scalp. Tension clamps are of simple design, inexpensive, reusable, and easily fashioned in the office. The skills required to use this technique can be self-taught with minimal investment in time and equipment. A 25% larger area of alopecia can be excised compared with that possible with a standard scalp reduction in less than 10 minutes of additional surgical time. This method has been used in over 500 scalp reductions with consistently good results and few complications.

INSTRUMENTS

A tension clamp is an innovative variation of a towel clamp. A standard 3½-inch towel clamp is modified by altering the curvature of the two prongs and bending the tips roughly parallel to each other (Fig. 9-47). A small amount of the original curvature is retained to help to prevent the clamp from slipping under tension. Since the modified clamp no longer functions as a towel clamp but is used exclusively to apply tension to the scalp, the term *tension clamp* has been adopted.

Anyone can make the simple changes needed to transform a towel clamp to a tension clamp. Roundnose pliers, designed for bending wire, greatly simplifed the bending of the prongs. Likewise, several of the surgical supply companies that sell towel clamps will make the necessary modifications if requested.

Tension clamps are applied to the scalp as demonstrated in Fig. 9-48. The prongs of the clamp span the incision and are inserted through the full thickness of the scalp. Closing the clamp draws the incision edges together, producing tension. Moving

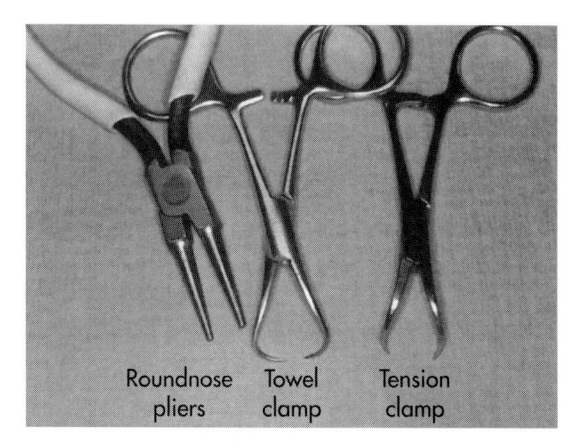

FIG. 9-47 Roundnose pliers are used to partially straighten the prongs of a standard 3½-inch towel clamp. The modified clamp functions in a new way and is called a *tension clamp*.

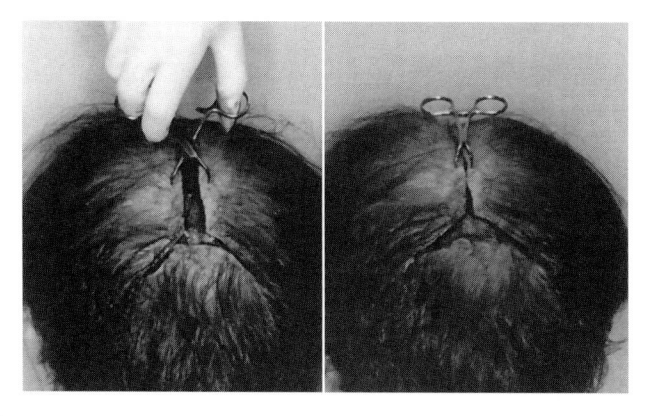

FIG. 9-48 The tips of the tension clamp are pressed through the full thickness of the scalp on both sides of the incision. When the clamp is closed, sufficient tension is created to stretch the scalp.

the clamp tips farther apart or closer together controls the amount of tension applied to the scalp when the clamp is closed. If too much or too little tension is present, the clamp may be quickly repositioned. The locking mechanism on each clamp allows the tension to be maintained.

SPECIAL CONSIDERATIONS

In the process of working with tension clamps on the scalp for several years, three observations have influenced the development of this procedure.

1. Different regions of the scalp vary in their response to tension. The greatest stretching occurs in the parietal regions, whereas meager stretching occurs in the occipital region. Consequently, tension clamps are placed across the midline to focus tension on the parietal areas. Performing a midline reduction with a posterior Y-plasty takes maximal advantage of parietal stretching.
2. Tension must be applied for a sufficient time period to adequately stretch the parietal scalp. If tension is released prematurely, the scalp will quickly rebound toward its prestretched position. Approximately 10 minutes of continuous, forceful tension is required in this procedure. If the scalp is under constant tension, it gradually relaxes and serial adjustments to tighten the clamps may be needed to maintain constant tension on the scalp.
3. This expansion technique allows for the resection of a larger area of alopecia than is obtainable with standard scalp reduction. The amount of excess scalp tissue that is safe to remove can be calculated in advance. The extra portion of resectable scalp tissue is equal to 25% of the redundant tissue produced by undermining the scalp. In each case, the amount of redundant scalp produced by undermining may vary greatly. A scalp that is "tight" and resistant to stretching may yield only 1 cm following extensive undermining, whereas a "loose" scalp may yield over 3 cm.

METHOD

A midline scalp reduction with a posterior Y-plasty advances three large flaps: the midline incision produces two parietal flaps, and the posterior Y creates an independent posterior flap. The sequence of steps used to perform a scalp reduction of this design, incorporating tissue expansion with tension clamps, is as follows.

STEP 1. Outline the principal midline area to be excised by drawing guidelines on the surface of the scalp (Fig. 9-49, A). The addition of two short lateroposterior lines defines the posterior flap (Fig. 9-49, B). Anesthesia is administered.

STEP 2. The first incision makes an angled turn as it follows the right parietal posterior guidelines (Fig. 9-50, A). Ideally the incision is made in one sweeping movement, but in reality the surgeon is often forced to pause along the way to maintain hemostasis. This incision separates the first of the three flaps, namely the right parietal flap.

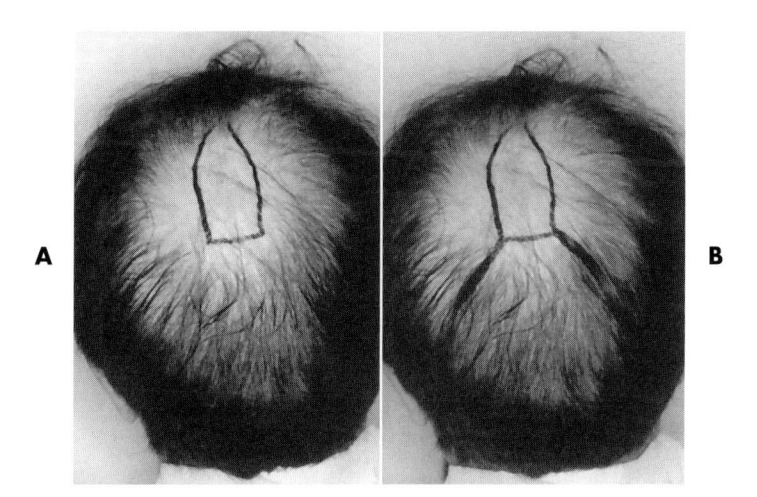

FIG. 9-49 A simple diagram drawn on the scalp creates a guideline for the surgeon's incisions. **A,** The diagram outlines the principal midline portion the surgeon hopes to remove. **B,** Two lateroposterior lines are added to define the shape of the posterior flap.

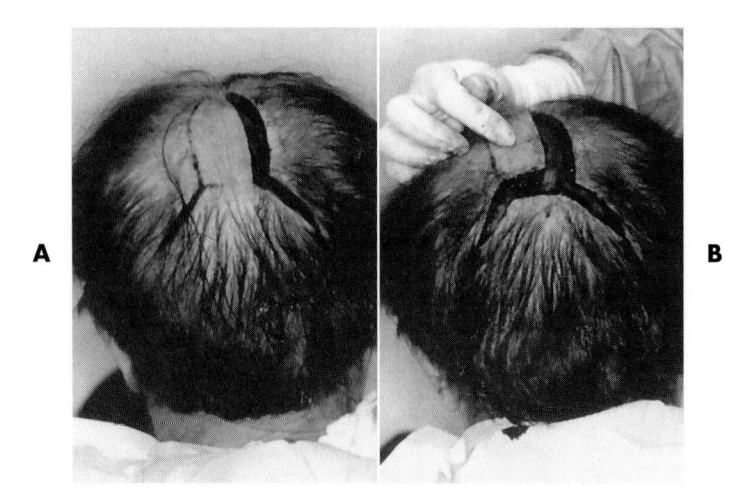

FIG. 9-50 Two incisions are used to separate the three flaps. **A,** The first angled incision separates the right parietal flap. **B,** The second angled incision completes the separation of the posterior flap.

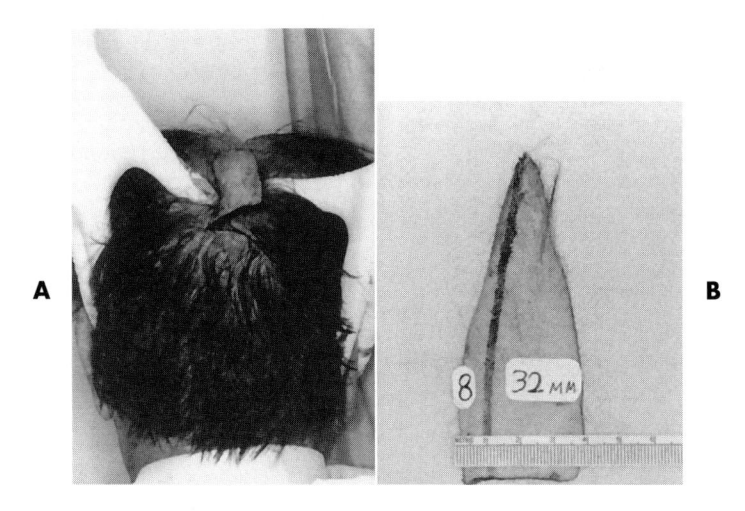

FIG. 9-51 A, After the scalp is undermined, the parietal flaps are advanced over the midline. The left flap overrides the right, allowing the surgeon to measure the width of the redundant scalp. **B,** The redundant portion plus an extra 25% is excised in one piece. In this case 32 mm of redundant scalp plus an additional 8 mm was excised.

STEP 3. The second incision makes an angled turn as it follows the remaining posterior guidelines, separating the posterior flap from the left parietal flap (Fig. 9-50, B). Just two incisions, each slightly angled, separate the three flaps: the posterior flap, right parietal flap, and left parietal flap.

STEP 4. The parietal scalp is undermined to the level of the ears while the posterior flap is undermined down to the nuchal ridge. The anterior 2 cm of the midline incision is *not* undermined. When undermining is not performed in the anterior area, scalp adhesion to the underlying periosteum is maintained. In this way the dog ear deformity that typically occurs in the anterior region is minimized or prevented.

STEP 5. After the scalp is undermined, the parietal flaps are advanced over the midline by applying hand pressure. The width of redundant scalp is measured by overlapping the right and left flaps (Fig. 9-51, A).

STEP 6. The measured redundant scalp plus an additional 25% is excised in one piece from the left parietal flap (Fig. 9-51, B).

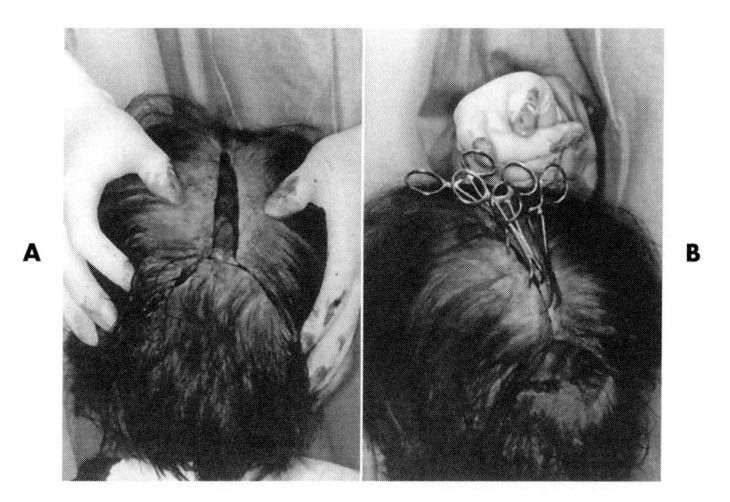

FIG. 9-52 **A,** After the excess scalp tissue is excised, hand pressure alone cannot approximate the parietal flaps. **B,** Several tension clamps are applied to stretch the scalp.

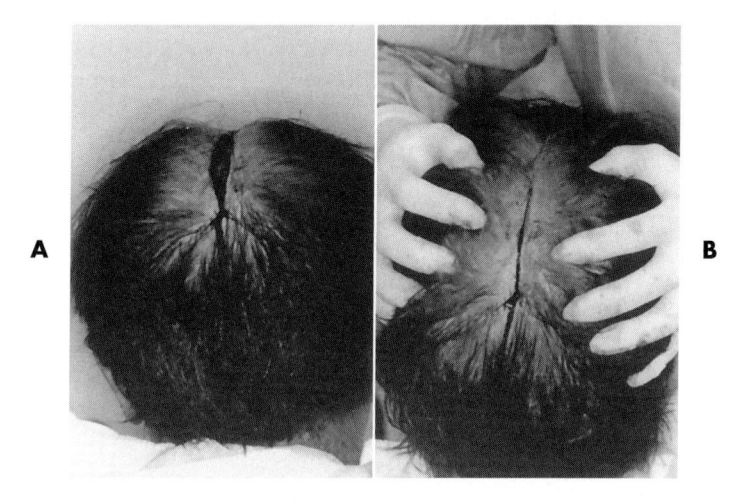

FIG. 9-53 **A,** The tension clamps are removed after the posterior flap is advanced and repaired. **B,** The stretched scalp enables approximation of the parietal flaps.

STEP 7. Because hand pressure alone cannot approximate the parietal flaps (Fig. 9-52, A), three or four tension clamps are placed along the midline incision to stretch the edges of the wound together. The tension clamp handles are positioned anteriorly to give the surgeon clear access to the posterior flap (Fig. 9-52, B).

STEP 8. During the 10 minutes required for the parietal scalp to stretch sufficiently, the posterior flap is advanced, trimmed of redundant tissue, and sutured into place (Fig. 9-53, A).

STEP 9. The tension clamps are removed. Hand pressure is applied by compressing the two parietal flaps towards the midline to determine if the parietal scalp edges will approximate easily (Fig. 9-53, B). If insufficient stretching has occurred, the tension clamps are reapplied with renewed force for a few additional minutes.

STEP 10. The midline incision is closed with interrupted sutures through the galea and a continuous running suture through the upper dermis.

DISCUSSION

Most surgeons agree that all the surgical steps described above are routine except Step 6. Note that the routine scalp reduction restricts removal of tissue to only that portion of redundant scalp that has been mobilized by undermining, whereas Step 6 of this method recommends excision of the redundant scalp plus an additional 25%. The routine scalp reduction follows the time-honored surgical principle of leaving adequate skin for wound closure. In contrast, this approach recommends removing more than the redundant tissue and thereby hints at a potential risk of a very difficult if not impossible closure. However, personal experience dictates that complete closure of the wound is possible. Review of the historical development of this method provides reassurance that the scalp can always be stretched and closed.

Initial attempts at performing this enhanced scalp reduction were very conservative. The redundant scalp was typically removed in three stages: first, the undermined redundant tissue was excised; second, tension clamps were applied to the scalp for 5 to 10 minutes; and third, the new portion of excess scalp created by tissue expansion was excised. The approach was to "cut, stretch, then cut again." Subsequently, numerous attempts were made to test the upper limits of this tissue expansion technique by increasing the length of time the tension was applied to the scalp. In some instances, tension clamps were left on the scalp as long as 30 minutes. Typically, the scalp would stretch an additional 30% to 50%. One extreme case allowed for the removal of an additional 2.7 cm, which was 76%. The more times the procedure was performed, the more confidence was gained in its safety and reproducibility. As time evolved, the three-stage procedure was condensed to a two-stage procedure of "cut first, then stretch." The main point is that the scalp is amazingly elastic. Removing an extra 25% of scalp tissue is a moderate measure considering that most scalps will tolerate the excision of an additional 30% to 50%.

When a surgeon first attempts to incorporate this tissue expansion technique into a scalp reduction procedure, he/she may prefer to take a cautious approach. Several options are available: the surgeon may initially elect to excise the redundant tissue in three stages (i.e., "cut, stretch, then cut again") or may decide to do a two-stage procedure but limit the amount of excess tissue removed in advance to 10% to 15% (i.e., "cut first, but only a little, and then stretch"). Even if the additional portion removed is only a few millimeters in width, the surgeon will benefit from the opportunity to see how the tension clamps function and how they can best be used.

A second use for tension clamps is to facilitate wound closure under tension. After stretching of the parietal scalp is completed and the wound edges are approximated by hand pressure, the scalp may have a tendency to slowly recoil. This development requires the surgeon to close the wound under moderate tension. Under these conditions, a tension clamp facilitates wound closure in the following way: (1) an interrupted suture is placed through the galea on both sides of the wound; (2) a tension clamp is then applied to reapproximate the edges; and (3) once the edges are approximated, the suture is tied with ease (Fig. 9-54). Sutures are removed on the seventh postoperative day. I have observed no differences in healing between wounds closed under moderate tension vs. wounds closed when no tension exists. My observations indicate

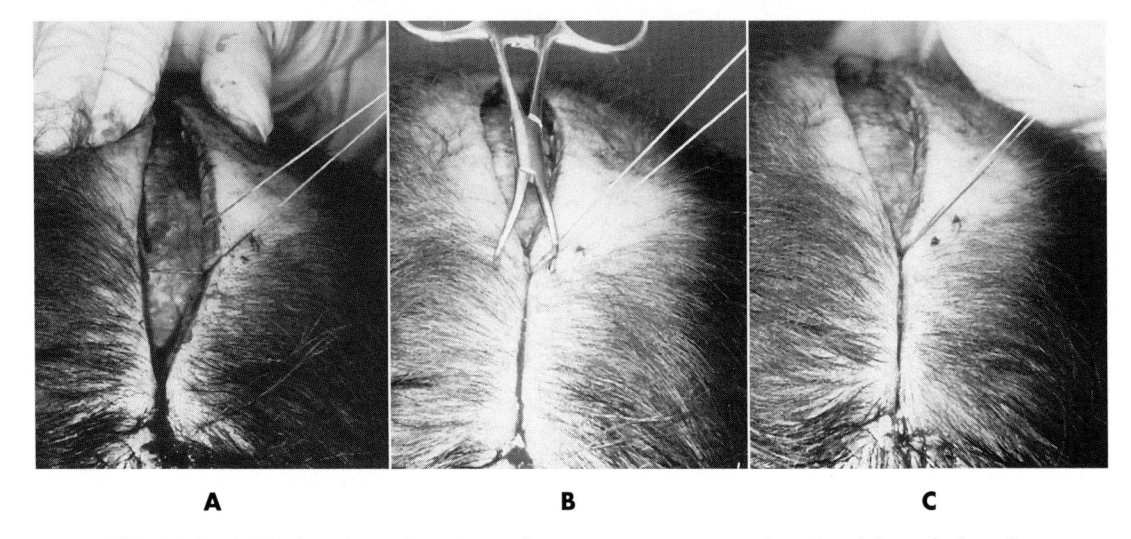

FIG. 9-54 A, To close the scalp under moderate tension, a suture is first placed through the galea on both sides of the wound. **B,** A tension clamp is applied to approximate the edges, allowing the suture to be securely fastened. **C,** When the clamp is removed, the edges remain approximated.

that a scalp closed under moderate tension will continue to relax and stretch for some time following surgery. Within 24 hours new mobility of the scalp develops and tension in the wound is no longer evident.

A third use for tension clamps is to hold them in reserve for emergency situations that may arise during traditional scalp reductions. Occasionally too much tissue is inadvertently excised, making wound closure difficult or impossible. In this situation, tension clamps can be applied briefly to stretch the scalp and thereby make closure possible.

COMPLICATIONS

This proposed method of scalp reduction, which incorporates a tissue expansion technique, is well tolerated by patients as long as the amount of tissue expansion applied is limited. With the limitation of the tissue excised to the redundant skin plus 25%, there is essentially no greater incidence of problems than is seen with a standard scalp reduction. Problems arise, however, when more than 25% of excess tissue is excised. Although the additional stretching required to remove more than 25% is easily accomplished, it correlates with a marked increase in postoperative pain and nausea for the patient.

CONCLUSION

In view of the tremendous benefits afforded by using tension clamps for tissue expansion (see box). I have routinely performed all scalp reduction procedures in this manner for the past several years. Although a 10-minute time period is needed to allow

---

TISSUE EXPANSION CREATED BY TENSION CLAMPS

Advantages
1. A 25% larger area of alopecia is resectable compared with that possible with standard scalp reduction.
2. Rapid tissue expansion is obtainable within 10 minutes.
3. Simple instruments are applied to the external surface of the scalp.
4. Skills are self-taught and easily acquired.
5. Tension clamps are inexpensive and reusable.
6. Results are consistent.
7. Complications are few.

Disadvantages
1. Overly aggressive use of the procedure may produce excessive postoperative pain.
2. Wound may require closure under moderate tension.
3. Expansion is limited to moderate amounts.

---

for adequate expansion to occur in the parietal regions, the surgeon may make good use of this time by repairing the posterior flap concurrently. Consequently, the time needed to add this technique to the procedure increases the total surgical time by only 1 to 2 minutes. The cosmetic improvements that result from this brief time investment are remarkable and are greatly appreciated by patients (Fig. 9-55).

Over the last decade, the field of scalp surgery has developed a burgeoning interest in the area of tissue expansion. There is little doubt that the demand

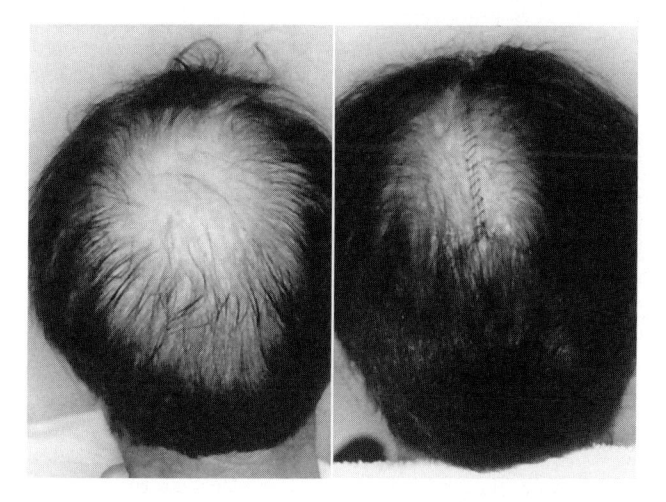

FIG. 9-55 These preoperative and postoperative views demonstrate the excellent results obtained by using tension clamps.

for tissue expansion will continue to grow. Surgeons who presently perform scalp reductions can easily incorporate the use of tension clamps into their existing procedures. Tension clamps provide an opportunity for the average scalp surgeon to add a simple form of tissue expansion to his/her present repertoire of skills.

H. The Integration of Scalp-Lifting with Small-Graft Hair Restoration Surgery

Dominic A. Brandy

HISTORY OF SCALP-LIFTING

Scalp-lifting is a procedure that is fairly representative of the rapid advancements that have recently occurred in the treatment of extensive baldness. In early years of hair restoration surgery, physicians would usually attempt to treat extensive baldness by covering the whole balding scalp with 4 to 5 mm punch grafts spread out over many sessions. This method was acceptable in most cases of frontal baldness; however, when coverage of the total head was attempted, a "baby doll" effect with poor density often resulted.

Progress was made in treating the posterior alopecic scalp when Blanchard and Blanchard[1] introduced the concept of midline scalp reduction in 1977. This procedure involved the fusiform excision of bald skin at the central bald scalp, undermining down to the superior ear, and subsequent closure of the defect with deep galeal and cutaneous sutures. The operation was then repeated every 2 to 3 months until the area of posterior alopecia was reduced in size.

Although this approach was a major advancement for treating the crown, successive procedures unfortunately were found to cause slot formation at the inferior crown because the length of the bald area increased by approximately 10% of its former length with each reduction.[2] In addition, the bald skin that was undermined and subsequently placed on tension during suturing was found to stretch back by 34% to 52%[3] depending on the amount of alopecic skin removed. Both of these problems were further exacerbated when the surgeon attempted to totally eliminate the baldness posteriorly.

Variations of this basic procedure (e.g., Y-shaped pattern,[4] paramedian[5]) have evolved over the years; however, many of the same problems previously mentioned for midline scalp reduction remain. These deficiencies exist primarily because bald skin is undermined and subsequently placed on tension, invoking stretchback.

When these problems were recognized, some surgeons turned to the method of slow tissue expansion,[6] which did eliminate extensive baldness in most patients. This technique, however, never really gained wide acceptance, primarily because of the gross cosmetic deformity that occurs during the instillation phase. This realization in combination with other complications[7] has caused midline scalp reduction to fall out of favor with most surgeons performing cosmetic hair restoration surgery for extensively bald patients.

In my view, it was not until the early 1980s that marked progress was made in scalp reduction surgery and the treatment of extensive baldness. It was at this time, that Marzola[8] introduced the concept of the lateral scalp-lift. His approach greatly reduced the problems of stretchback and slot formation while accomplishing the anterior and medial advancement of expanded flaps. It also became the rudiment of the other scalp-lifting flaps that I later developed.

SCALP-LIFTING PROCEDURES
Marzola Lateral Lift

The lateral lift is the groundwork for all of the scalp-lifting procedures. What Marzola did to create his procedure was to take the basic paramedian design and extend the anterior incision of this scalp reduction down to the mid-sideburn. This small but significant maneuver allowed him to visualize the occipital artery, sever it, and then undermine all the way to the hairline of the nape of the neck. Because the scalp below the nuchal ridge has no restrictive galea, he was able to remove approximately two times more bald skin than that possible with paramedian scalp reduction and he was able to do this without undermining bald skin, thereby eliminating stretchback. This approach also markedly elevated the posterior donor scalp, which helped to prevent slot formation (Fig. 9-56, A).

Recently, I demonstrated statistically that 60% more advancement is achieved with Marzola's procedure and all scalp-lifting procedures than with conventional scalp reduction (Fig. 9-57). I believe that this extra scalp mobility results from three primary factors:

1. There is no galea below the nuchal ridge to restrict the kinetics of the nape tissue.
2. The occipitalis and periauricular muscles are severed, which releases the inhibitory contractile forces of those structures.
3. There is a mild tenting effect below the occipital protuberance.

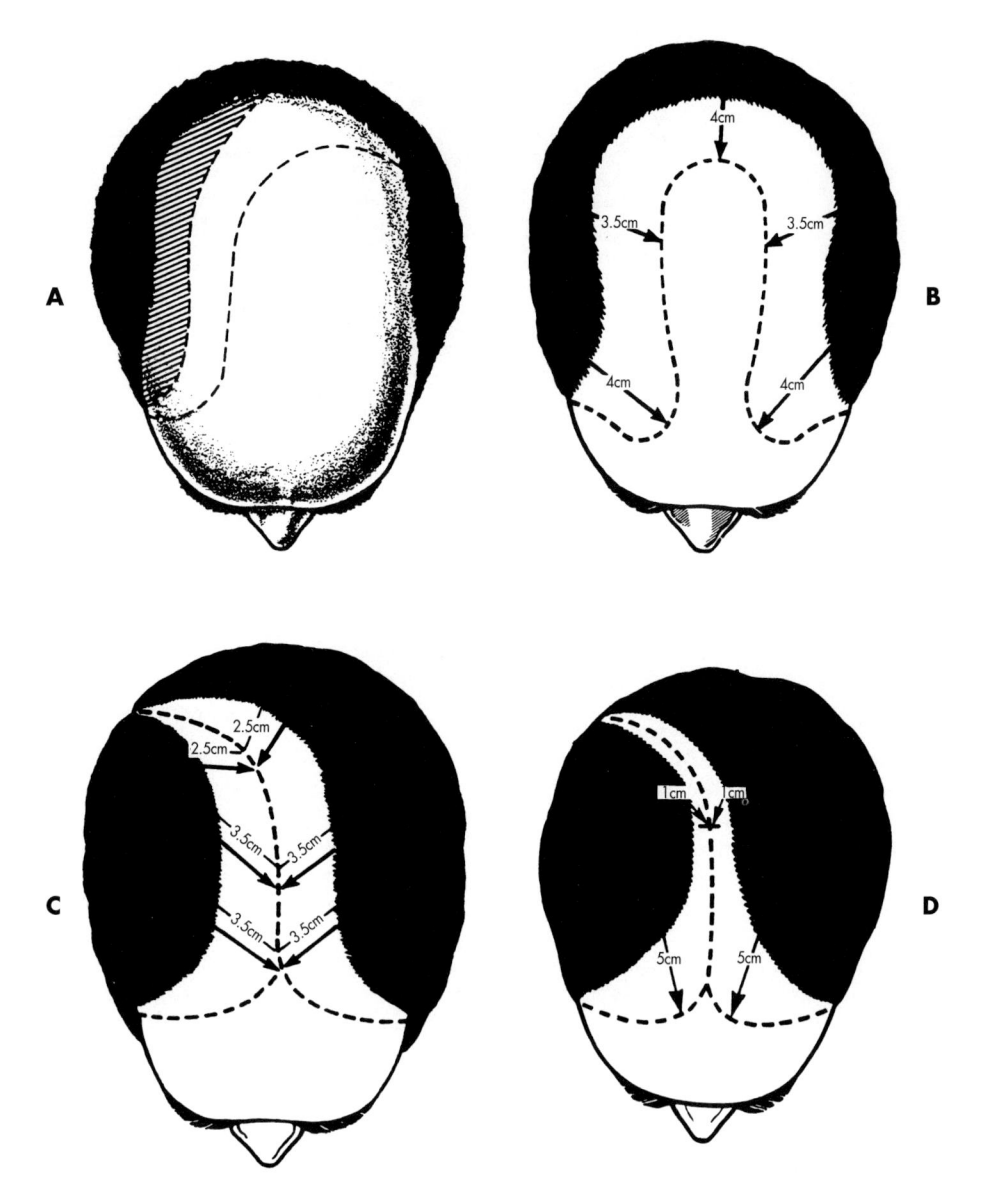

FIG. 9-56 A, Difference in alopecia removal between a paramedian scalp reduction and a Marzola lateral lift. Note the greater anterior and medial advancement of the Marzola lateral lift. This improvement is accomplished without undermining contralateral bald skin, which virtually eliminates the possibility of postoperative stretchback. **B,** Vectors and average advancements of a bilateral occipitoparietal flap. **C,** Vectors and average advancements of a Brandy bitemporal flap. **D,** Vectors of a bitemporal flap can be exchanged (medial for anterior). This greater anterior advancement works exceptionally well for patients with only bitemporal recessions and is called a modified Brandy bitemporal flap. (**A** and **B** from Unger WP: *Hair transplantation*, ed 3, New York, 1995, Marcel Dekker.)

Moreover, this extra movement is accomplished with minimal to no stretchback because the alopecic skin opposite the lift is not undermined as it is with conventional scalp reduction. Even more important, the probability of developing slot formation is dramatically decreased because the neck tissues are undermined down to the hairline of the nape, which allows a marked elevation into the vertex area. This anterior vector also significantly improves the temporal recessions.

Bilateral Occipitoparietal Flap

In 1985, I visited Marzola and learned his lateral technique. I also visited Bradshaw and found that

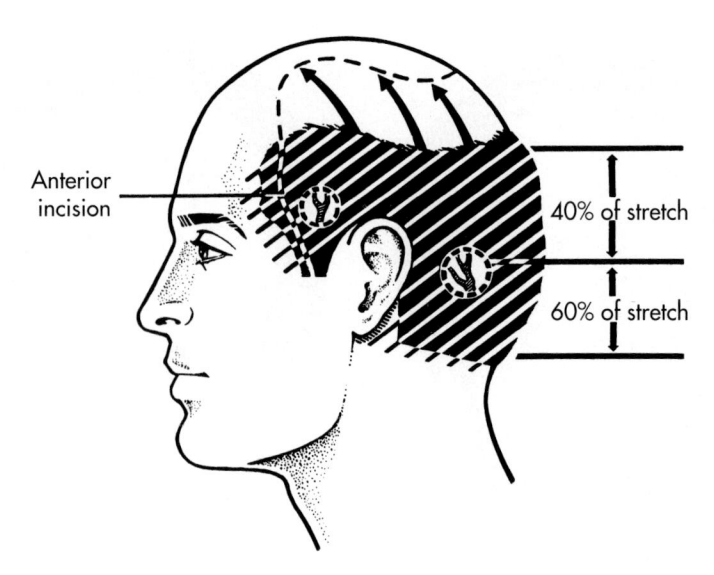

FIG. 9-57 The primary reason that scalp-lifting accomplishes a prodigious removal of alopecic scalp is because no galea exists below the nuchal ridge. Research has demonstrated that approximately 60% of the stretch of scalp-lifting comes from this galea-free area below the occipital protuberance. (From Unger WP: *Hair transplantation*, ed 3, New York, 1995, Marcel Dekker.)

he had just begun extending the Marzola incision from one mid-sideburn around the donor fringe to the opposite mid-sideburn. He was dividing both occipital arteries at the same time, undermining the entire scalp to the hairline of the nape, and then advancing the undermined area in an upward and inward fashion. This procedure resulted in an amazing removal of alopecic skin; however, Bradshaw's approach resulted in a 28.6% incidence of necrosis at the nuchal ridge,[9] and these necroses were sometimes of a serious magnitude.

Intrigued by the bilateral approach, I immediately changed several aspects of Bradshaw's method. The initial changes were:

1. I used a deeper plane of undermining. Instead of dissecting into the subcutaneous tissues of the neck, I divided the fascia of the trapezius and sternocleidomastoid muscles. This adjustment prevented major disruption of the random vasculature that exists below the nuchal ridge.
2. The patient was moved from a sitting position to a prone one. This positioning significantly improved visibility and enabled the assistants to get better retraction and thus enhanced the accuracy of the dissection.
3. A Prōn Pillō was used to keep the patient's head in a neutral position, thus preventing the head from extending during the advancement phase. This simple change ensured that excessive tension would not be applied to the skin overlying the occipital protuberance.
4. POR8 (vasoconstrictor available in Australia) was eliminated, and epinephrine was substituted.

With these early changes, I was able to decrease the necrosis rate from 28.6% to 3.5%. When the dramatic improvements of bilateral scalp-lifting were occurring on a consistent basis with minimal complications, I discussed the procedure with Dr. H. Pierce who suggested the name *bilateral occipitoparietal flap*.[10,11] To Pierce this procedure represented a major advancement in the treatment of extensive alopecia because of the amazing amount of bald skin that could be removed with just one procedure (Fig. 9-56, *B*). Moreover, this operation offered better visibility intraoperatively and, like the Marzola lift, significantly improved slot formation and the temporal recessions while essentially eliminating the stretchback problem.

Brandy Bitemporal Flap

The Brandy bitemporal flap[12] was the first procedure to evolve from the primary bilateral occipitoparietal flap. Geometrically this flap is a **C**-shaped flap that fits into a complementary **S**-shaped flap (Fig. 9-56, *C*) and can be used as a closure after a bilateral occipitoparietal flap or as a one-stage procedure for a patient with Norwood type IV baldness that is not likely to progress. When patients with type IV baldness are being treated, one bitemporal scalp-lift can replace the need for six or seven conventional operations (i.e., four hair grafting procedures to the recessions and two or three midline scalp reductions for midline alopecia).

The undermining for the bitemporal flap is similar to that for a bilateral occipitoparietal flap when it is performed as a primary, one-stage procedure for Norwood type IV baldness. On the other hand, when it is used as a secondary procedure after a bilateral occipitoparietal flap, undermining is frequently not required at the central 5 cm below the nuchal ridge because a more medial and less anterior vector is needed to accomplish closure after a bilateral occipitoparietal flap. In fact, more times than not, the undermining needs to proceed only to the nuchal ridge, a procedure I refer to as a bitemporal scalp reduction.[13]

Aesthetically, one of the most pertinent features of both the bitemporal flap and scalp reduction is the veer into the donor-dominant scalp, which helps to create a whorl-like configuration at the vertex. It accomplishes this pattern by transforming the hair direction from a divergent one to a more circular form. This configuration also significantly reduces the probability of developing slot formation inferiorly.

Modified Bitemporal Flap

After performing bitemporal flap procedures for approximately 1 year, I noticed that the advancement vectors could be exchanged—medial for anterior and vice versa. Because patients with bitemporal recessions and no future sign of posterior baldness desire more anterior movement into the recessions and no improvement at the crown, I exchanged the vectors (anterior for medial and medial for anterior) to create what is now called the *modified bitemporal flap*[14] (Fig. 9-56, *D*). This operation quickly gained popularity because the temporal recessions can be treated splendidly with just one procedure instead of three or four as is the case with hair grafting.

Frontoparietal Advancement Flap

The final procedure that evolved from the other procedures was the frontoparietal flap.[15,16] This flap was developed as a means to create a hairline for those patients who wanted nothing to do with hair grafting.

To achieve the anterior advancement that is necessary for hairline development, it is essential to make a back-cut at the temporal region, which in turn severs the posterior branch of the superficial temporal artery. Because this artery must be divided, the flap should be incised, the distal 8 cm elevated, and the flap laid back down so that revascularization can occur. This is essentially a delay. Two weeks later, the actual operation is performed with the undermining being similar to that for a Marzola lateral lift. In almost all cases, two frontoparietal flaps are required to accomplish a symmetrical hairline with good hair direction.

LIGATION PROCEDURES
Occipital Artery Ligation

In my early experience, the occipital arteries were divided at the time of the actual scalp-lifting procedure, which resulted in a 6.5% rate of necrosis on virgin scalps[17]—approximately 3.5% when secondary procedures were included in the statistics. I believed that a sudden curtailment of circulation at the nuchal ridge combined with stretch on the occipital skin was causing this complication. In an attempt to eliminate this complication, I began performing ligation of both occipital arteries 4 to 8 weeks prior to the first scalp-lift on a percentage of patients. I theorized that if the arteries were ligated before the surgery, the occipital scalp would acclimatize, which would prevent a sudden jolt of circulatory deprivation.

Horizontal Incision Ligation

Initially these occipital artery ligations were performed through horizontal incisions because of the excellent accessibility to the blood vessels that they offered. Although they reduced the average degree of the necroses by 47%, they did not have a positive effect on the incidence. In fact, the incidence was slightly higher at 7.5%. Because the necroses were *always* found directly below the horizontal scars from the ligation, it seemed that the necroses were occurring because the transverse scars from the ligation were blocking the crucial axial circulation from the temporal vessels.

Vertical Incision Ligation

In an attempt to eliminate the problem of necrosis, I switched exclusively to vertical incision ligation of the occipital arteries in March 1989. Since then, I have experienced only one case of a small necrosis, which is 0.31% of 324 virgin cases.

HISTORY OF MINIGRAFTING

As previously stated, the early days of hair transplantation surgery consisted of using rather large "plugs," which left the scalp looking more like a cornfield than a natural-appearing head of hair. This all changed in 1981 when Nordstrom[18] introduced the concept of a "micrograft." In his 1981 publication, Nordstrom described the use of three- to six-hair grafts at the anterior hairline to give this area a more aesthetically pleasing appearance.

Nordstrom's paper went relatively unnoticed until the 1984 International Congress of Hair Replacement Surgery in New York City where Bradshaw introduced the idea of quartering 4.5 mm punch grafts and placing these "quarter grafts" into small No. 15 blade incisions. Bradshaw, having had the procedure performed on himself, stunned the conference attendees by the natural appearance that resulted from the exclusive use of "minigrafts." The history of how this technique came about is covered more thoroughly by Orentreich in Chapter 2, Part A.

Since that time there has proliferated a multitude of ways to create these minigrafts. Some surgeons bisect 4 mm grafts (Lewis L: Personal communication), others trisect 3 mm grafts,[19] and the list goes on and on. I introduced the concept of using a multibladed knife for the development of minigrafts.[9] These knives create two or three 3 mm strips (depending on whether a triple- or quadruple-bladed instrument is used), which are then transected into 3 × 1.5 mm rectangular minigrafts[20] (Fig. 9-58). This idea was derived from the instrumentation by Coiffmann[21] and Bisaccia,[22] both of which consisted of 4 mm wide multibladed knives to make 4 × 4 mm square grafts. Others have since developed additional knives to meet the specific needs of their approaches.

In regard to the recipient area, the first approach, which was described by Bradshaw, was to make No. 15 blade incisions 2 mm apart and to arrange these rows circumferentially with each row being separated by 5 mm.[23] In a subsequent procedure, the same approach was used between the original rows of minigrafts. Although effective, this approach was found to be extremely cumbersome because the incisions were so close together.

The most common approach to the recipient area is simply to use random incisions or holes and then place the appropriate grafts into these openings. In essentially all of the articles published to date[19,24-26] this method seems to be the most prevalent.

As with Bradshaw's approach, this method can be effective, but it is too disorderly for my liking. This is especially true for patients with early baldness whose thinning hair creates a problem with detecting previously transplanted hair grafts. To bring more order and predictability to the minigrafting procedure, I developed the systematic, three-step approach.[27]

THREE-STEP MINIGRAFTING APPROACH

The systematic, three-step approach to minigrafting consists of a fully staggered pattern of No. 15 blade incisions, which is based on horizontal references lines with each incision being separated by 6 mm from the adjacent one regardless of whether it is the first, second, or third session (Fig. 9-59). The incisions for the second session are placed 2 mm to the right of those from the first growing session, and those for the third session are placed directly between and *slightly posterior* to the incisions for the first and second growing sessions. Anterior to these incisions, the surgeon makes random NoKor needle wounds. Into each No. 15 blade incision is placed a six- to eight-hair minigraft, and into each NoKor needle wound a single- or two-hair micrograft is placed.

INTEGRATION OF SCALP-LIFTING WITH THE THREE-STEP APPROACH

For most patients desiring alopecia reduction who have type VI extensive alopecia, a five-step protocol is used. This protocol entails a bilateral occipitoparietal scalp-lift followed by a Brandy bitemporal scalp-lift or scalp reduction and then three

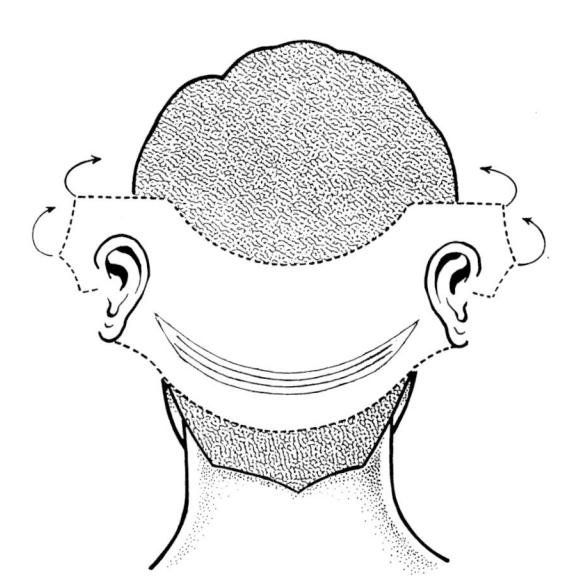

FIG. 9-58 The donor technique is a multistrip technique facilitated by a triple- or quadruple-bladed knife.

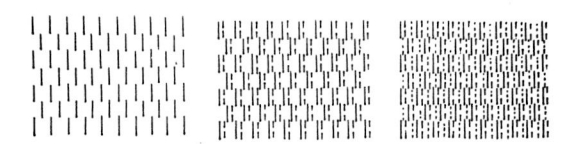

| 1st session of minigrafts
¦ 2nd session of minigrafts
⋮ 3rd session of minigrafts

FIG. 9-59 The three-step minigrafting approach consists of No. 15 blade incisions, separated by 6 mm and organized in a fully staggered pattern. These incisions are based on horizontal reference lines. The incisions from the second session are 2 mm to the right of those from the first session, and those from the third session are between and *slightly posterior* to the incisions from the first and second sessions.

The Integration of Scalp-Lifting with Small-Graft Hair Restoration Surgery 271

Key to grafting symbols

| 1st session of minigrafts
¦ 2nd session of minigrafts
┆ 3rd session of minigrafts
· Single-hair micrograft
• Three-hair micrograft

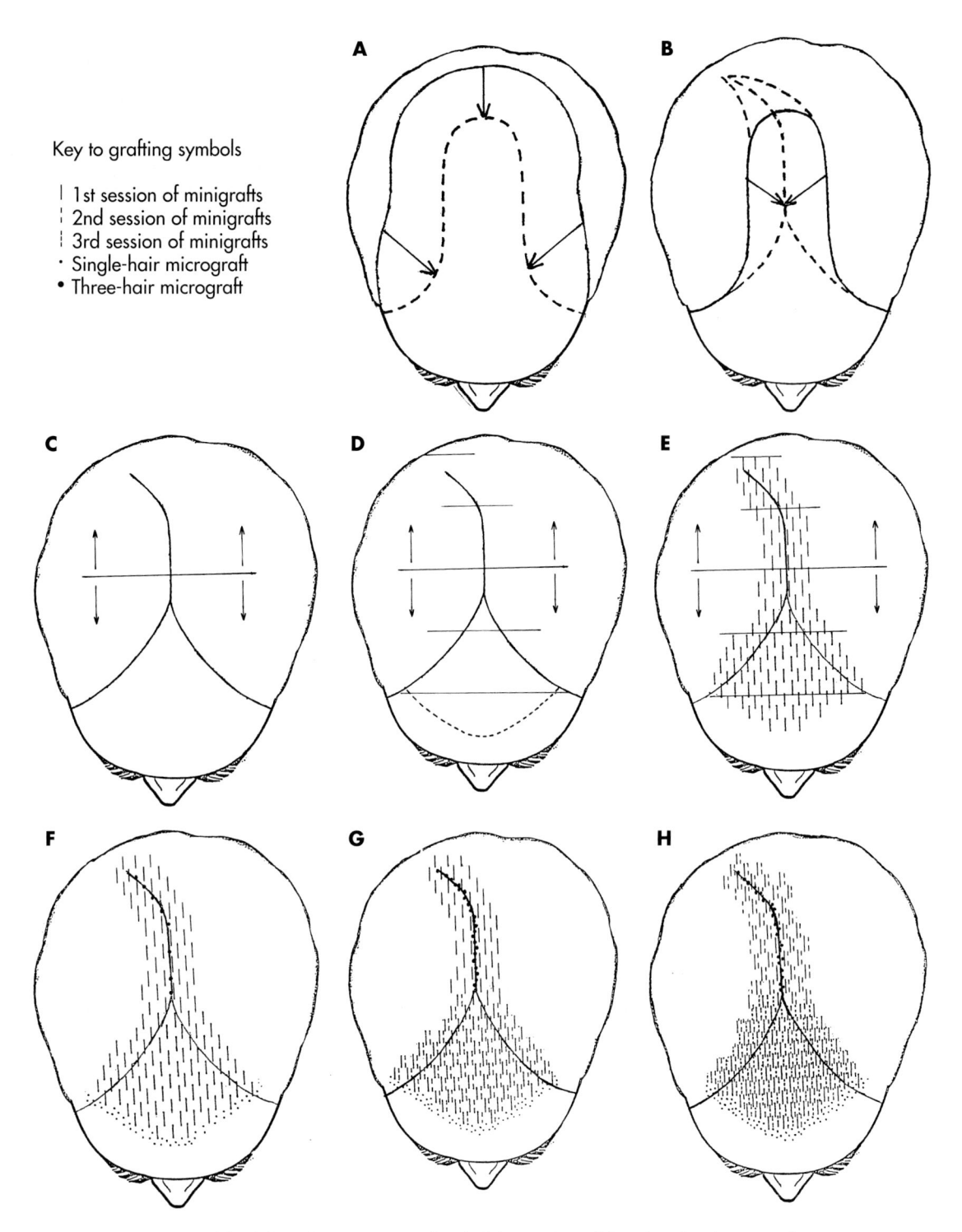

FIG. 9-60 **A,** The bilateral occipitoparietal scalp-lift is performed 2 to 6 weeks after vertical incision ligation of the occipital arteries. **B,** The Brandy bitemporal scalp-lift or scalp reduction is performed 3 months after the bilateral occipitoparietal scalp-lift. **C,** A large horizontal reference line is first drawn at the vertex (the highest point of the head). **D,** Smaller horizontal reference lines are then drawn to guide the three-step minigrafting approach. **E,** A stencil is used to mark all of the proposed No. 15 blade incisions. **F,** The first session of mini-micrografts is performed 3 months after bitemporal scalp-lift or scalp reduction. **G,** In the second session of mini-micrografts, the grafts are placed 2 mm to the right of those transplanted in the first frontal session. **H,** In the third session of mini-micrografts, the grafts are placed directly between and slightly posterior to those transplanted in the first and second sessions.

sessions of minigrafts and micrografts to the frontal and posterior areas.

Step One: Bilateral Occipitoparietal Scalp-Lift

Initially, ligation of both occipital arteries is performed through vertical incisions. The occipital vessels are first located with Doppler ultrasonography and then are ligated or cauterized through a vertical incision that is easily retracted with a Weitlaner retractor. The most crucial point in occipital artery ligation is that the main trunk must be disrupted. Three cauterized or ligated vascular stumps must be remaining at the end of the procedure (i.e., the main, ascending, and descending branches). The vertical incisions are closed with 4-0 degradable suture. Two to 6 weeks later the patient returns to the surgical suite, at which time the bilateral occipitoparietal scalp-lift is performed (Fig. 9-60, A). During the occipitoparietal scalp-lift, it is critical to follow the strict precautionary measures, which are discussed later. This scalp-lift is closed with 0 degradable suture galeally and 5-0 degradable suture cutaneously. One month after surgery the patient is advised to start stretching the scalp by hand and/or with a special scalp stretcher.[28] This early stretching prevents excessive fibrosis between the skin and undersurface and also significantly improves scalp laxity.

Step Two: Brandy Bitemporal Scalp-lift or Scalp Reduction

Three months are allowed to elapse, at which time the Brandy bitemporal scalp-lift or scalp reduction is performed. In the majority of cases undermining needs to proceed only to the nuchal line. Therefore a bitemporal scalp reduction is usually the procedure performed at this time (Fig. 9-60, B). As with the bilateral occipitoparietal scalp-lift, scalp stretching is begun 1 month after this surgery.

Step Three: First Mini-Micrograft Session

Again 3 months are allowed to pass, at which time the first mini-micrograft session is performed. This first grafting session is crucial and sets the tone for the final result. Therefore careful planning is essential.

First I place the patient in the Frankfort position and place a comb on the head parallel to the floor (Fig. 9-61). A large horizontal reference line, perpendicular to the scar, is then drawn at the point at which the head begins to descend posteriorly (Fig. 9-60, C). This extremely important line dictates where the hair grafts will change from an anterior to a posterior angle. Once this step is completed, the hairline is drawn, and the horizontal reference lines for the three-step minigrafting approach are scribed (Fig. 9-60, D). These lines are drawn at the frontal region and continue all the way back to the inferior end of the scar.

After the horizontal reference lines are completed (Fig. 9-62, A), a specially developed stencil[20] with 20 slits per square inch is aligned over them. An Acculine marker is then pushed up and down through the openings of the stencil (Fig. 9-62, B). When the marks are completed, the surgeon uses a Pilot marker to make the Acculine marks more indelible (Fig. 9-62, C). This pattern begins at the hairline (Fig. 9-62, D) and continues all the way to the inferior end of the scar. This pattern should be blended into the donor-dominant scalp 2 to 3 cm adjacent to the scar (Fig. 9-62, E), and slit grafting should be the only method used in this area. Blending with slit-minigrafts adjacent to the scar accomplishes two goals:

1. It builds in a degree of insurance in case the surgeon misjudges the future extent of the alopecia.
2. It softens the divergence that usually occurs when extensive baldness is completely eliminated with alopecia-reducing procedures.

Once all of the markings are finished (see Fig. 9-60, E), the surgery is begun. Strip donor harvesting is usually performed with a quadruple-bladed knife with the patient's head resting in a Prōn Pillō. I usually start at the most inferior aspect of good donor hair and take the harvest from ear to ear. The three 3 mm strips that are harvested can usually be transected into 240 to 260

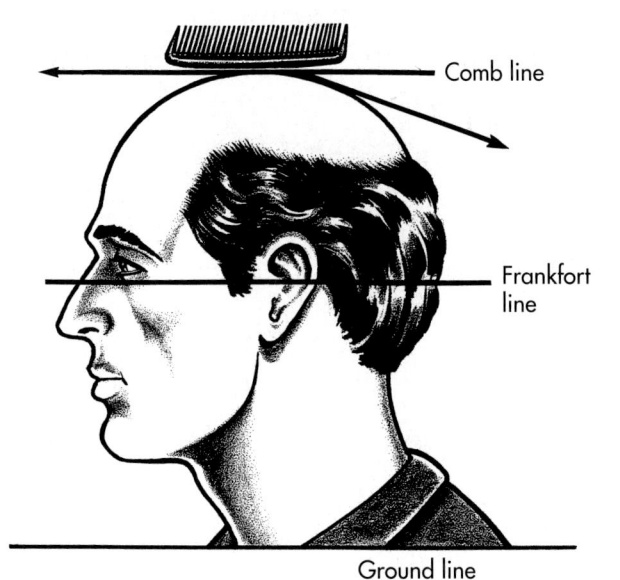

FIG. 9-61 To determine the vertex, the patient is placed in the Frankfort position and a comb is placed on the head parallel to the floor. All grafts posterior to the point where the head begins to descend posteriorly are angled posteriorly. All grafts anterior to this point are angled anteriorly.

six- to eight-hair (3 × 1.5 mm) minigrafts. One hundred micrografts are also dissected from the distal ends of the harvested scalp.

After the remaining defect is sutured with 0 degradable suture galeally and 3-0 monofilament suture cutaneously, incisions are begun at the posterior aspect of the scalp. The first No. 15 blade incisions are begun at the large horizontal reference line that was previously drawn to indicate where the scalp begins to descend. All incisions posterior to this line are made directly into the lines previously marked and are angled approximately 45 degrees posteriorly in relation to the skin surface. Likewise, all incisions anterior to this line will be pointed 45 degrees anteriorly. The incisions at the line are angled a little less acutely to soften the transition. In addition, 16-gauge NoKor needle incisions are made directly into the scar in areas

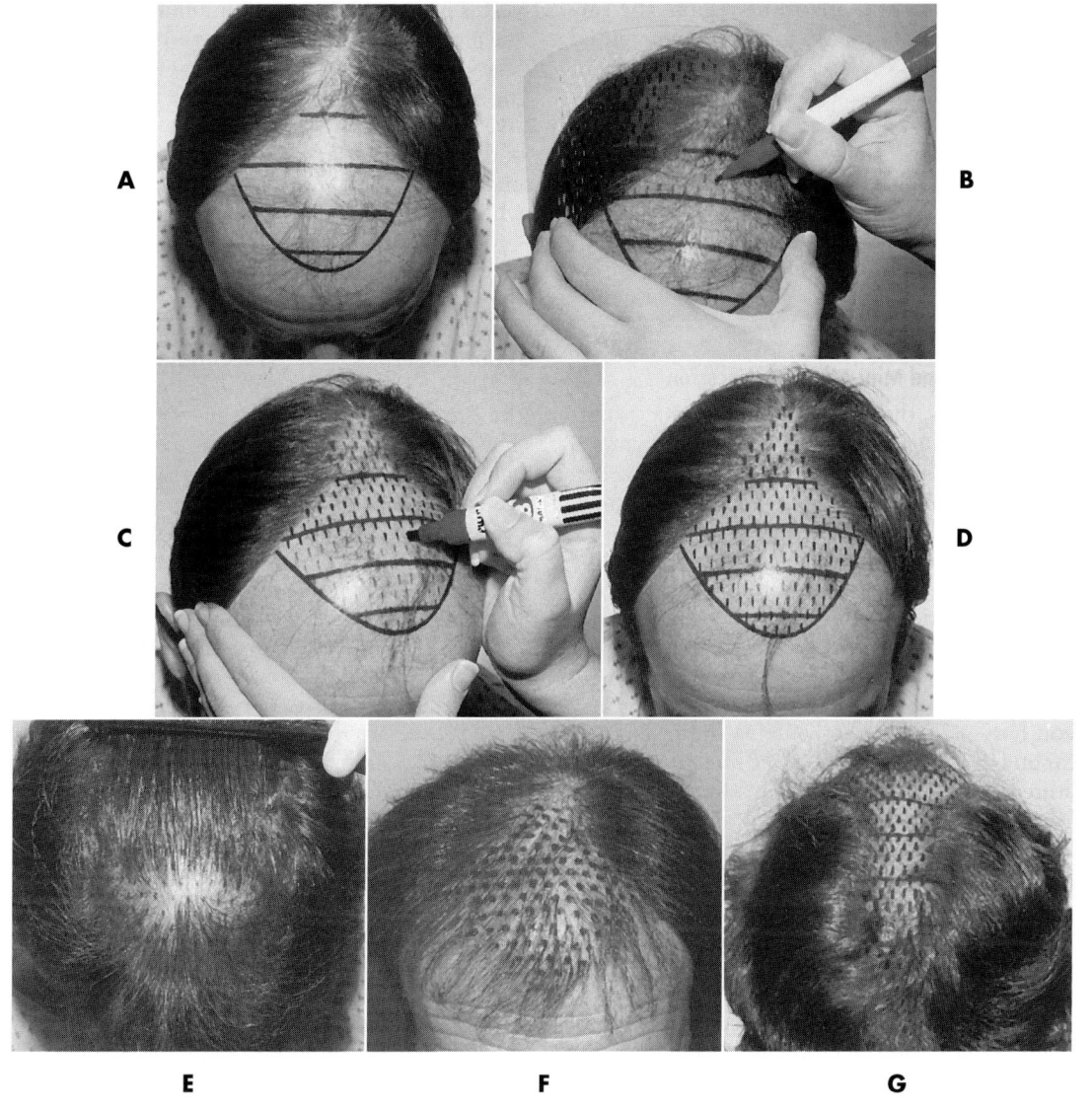

FIG. 9-62 **A,** The horizontal reference lines are first scribed with a Pilot marker. **B,** A stencil with 20 slits per square inch for six- to eight-hair minigrafts is placed over the area to be grafted, and an Acculine marker is pushed up and down through the openings of the stencil. **C,** A Pilot marker is then used to make the marks more indelible. **D,** The stenciled marks are completed and the first mini-micrografting session can commence. **E,** Stenciled marks are also made adjacent to the midline scar. **F,** Immediately before the second session, small dots are scribed over the growing grafts from the first session. The incisions are made 2 mm to the right of the growing grafts. **G,** Immediately before the third session, large dots are made over the growing grafts from both the first and second sessions. The incisions are made directly between and slightly posterior to these large dots.

Discussion

Scalp-lifting is probably the most efficient way (along with slow tissue expansion) for treating patients with extensive male pattern baldness and scalp defects.[11,30] The primary reason for this fact is that every single donor hair on the patient's head is being used to accomplish the final result. Having used this technique frequently, I have accomplished consistently good outcomes on properly selected patients with type VI extensive baldness (Figs. 9-63 and 9-64). With adherence to sound surgical principles and constant review of ways to improve results and lessen the complications, the procedure can be one that is virtually complication free.

The most critical manipulation added to the operative protocol is the vertical incision ligation of the occipital arteries performed 2 to 6 weeks before the actual bilateral scalp-lift. Because of the recent findings by Taylor and associates[31,32] that the choke vessel acclimatization effect lasts for 6 weeks after major perforators are ligated, I changed the interval between ligation and actual scalp-lift from the

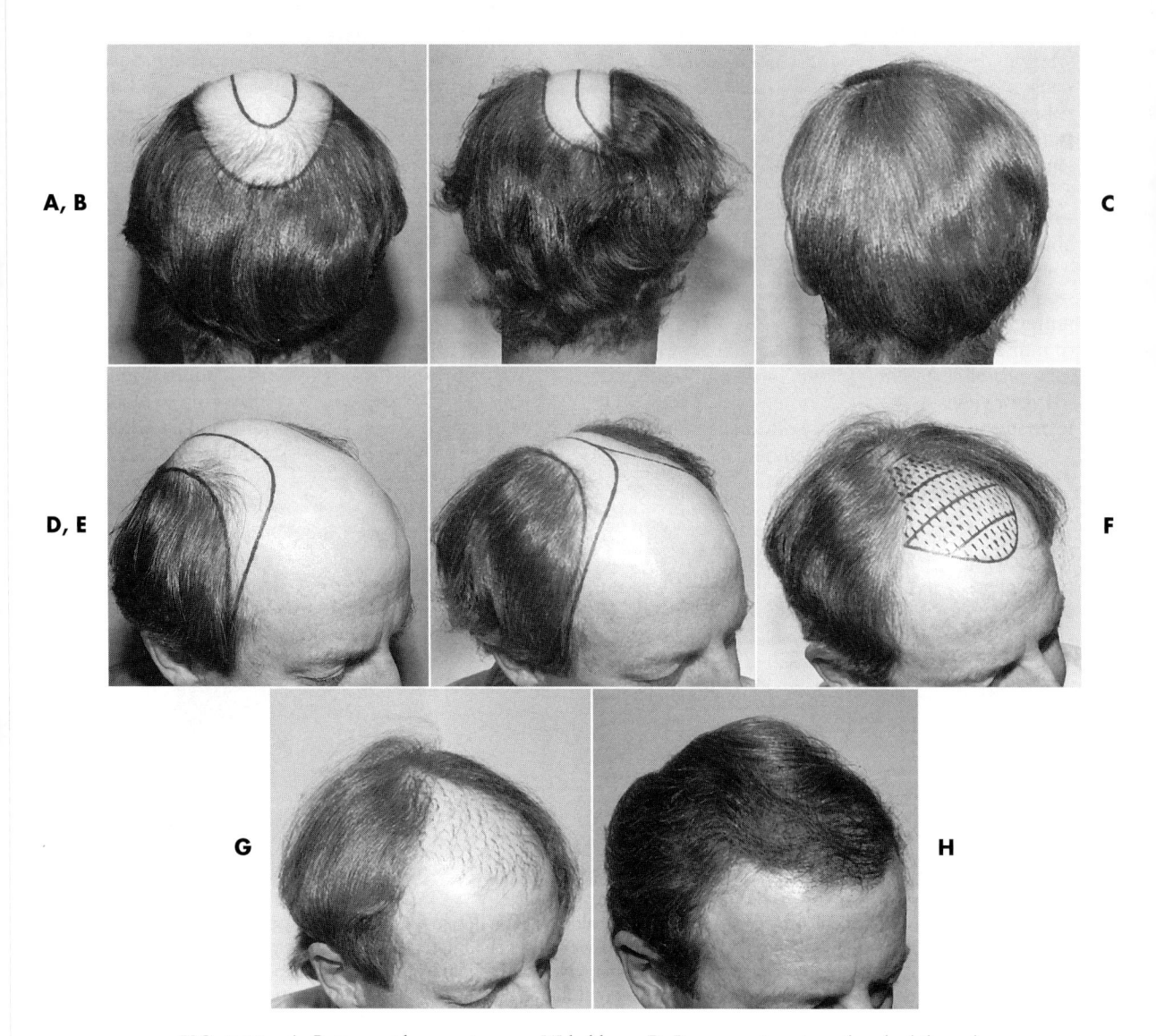

FIG. 9-64 **A,** Patient with extensive type VI baldness. **B,** Postoperative view after the bilateral occipitoparietal scalp-lift and immediately before the Brandy bitemporal flap. **C,** Postoperative view after the Brandy bitemporal flap. **D,** Preoperative oblique view. **E,** Postoperative oblique view after the bilateral occipitoparietal scalp-lift and immediately before the Brandy bitemporal flap. **F,** Postoperative oblique view after the Brandy bitemporal flap. The hairline is stenciled in immediately before first grafting session. **G,** Result after the first growing graft session. **H,** Final result after two scalp-lifts and three mini-micrograft sessions. *Continued.*

original 4 to 8 weeks to 2 to 6 weeks. Taylor's angiographic findings, in combination with my statistical evidence,[17] dictate that vertical incision ligations should be considered a standard procedure before the actual lifting surgery.

Almost as important as occipital artery ligations is the proper plane of undermining below the nuchal ridge. To ensure that this proper plane is achieved, the surgeon should attempt to divide the fascia of the trapezius and sternocleidomastoid muscles, which lie in this region. This task can be dramatically facilitated by using two assistants and by using a specially designed suction retractor[33] that I developed (Robbins Instruments, Chatham, N.J.). The proper plane is ensured by making certain that a glistening surface is evident on the underside of the flap. If fat or hair follicles are visible, the plane is much too superficial, and the chances of developing necrosis postoperatively increase significantly. Conversely, if the scissors fall into an inferior hole, the plane is too deep and the scissors should be turned upward.

To guarantee proper tension on the flap, the patient's intraoperative head position should be neutral and the surgeon's tactile sense acute. To ensure this neutral head position, the patient should be placed prone with the head on a Prōn Pillō, which automatically will keep the head relatively neutral. As mentioned previously, this was one of the earliest changes made from Bradshaw's original technique and probably had more to do with dramatically reducing the necrosis rate than any other early adaptation.

Equally important is the surgeon's tactile sense during the advancement. Obviously this "feel" will not be exquisitely sensitive during the early stages of the learning curve. The surgeon should therefore lean toward the conservative side until this sense becomes more developed through experience.

Another critical precept to follow with these procedures is that only Marzola scalp-lifting should be performed on patients who have undergone prior hair grafting. During the early phases of the development of this technique, I experienced a 12.5% necrosis rate in patients who had bilateral procedures after having undergone punch hair grafting. Because of this high necrosis rate,[34] I began performing only Marzola lateral lifts (without prior ligation) on individuals who had previous hair grafting. The necrosis rate with this adaptation was dramatically reduced to 1.6% *with the necrosis always occurring after the second lateral lift.* Since collating this information, I now perform the first lateral lift, dividing the occipital neurovascular bundle

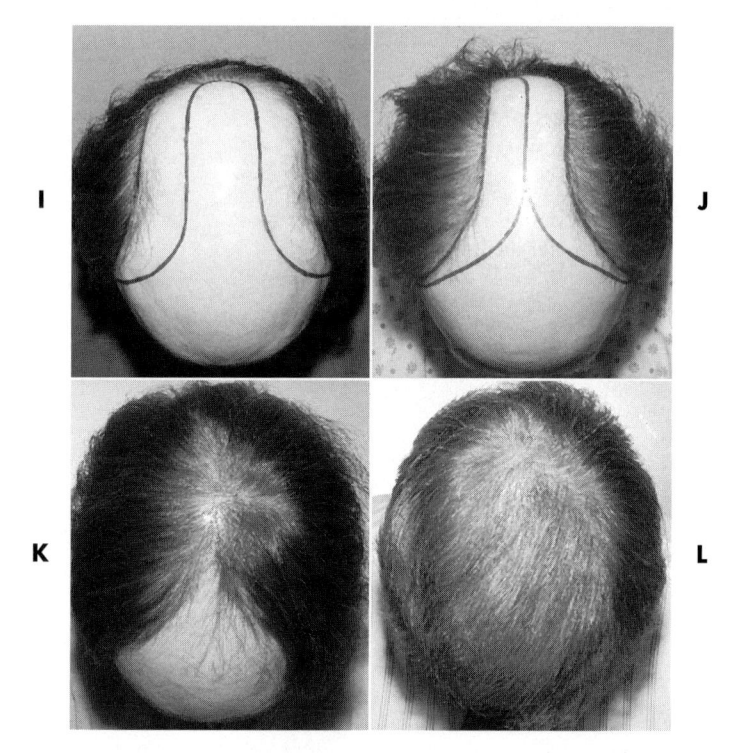

FIG. 9-64, cont'd. **I,** Preoperative top view before bilateral occipitoparietal scalp-lift. **J,** Postoperative view after the bilateral occipitoparietal scalp-lift and before the Brandy bitemporal flap. **K,** Postoperative view after the Brandy bitemporal flap. **L,** Final result after two scalp-lifts and three mini-micrograft sessions.

on that side, and simultaneously perform an occipital artery ligation percutaneously on the opposite occipital artery. The second lateral lift is then performed 4 to 6 weeks after the first lateral lift. This maneuver allows the choke vessels to expand on the contralateral side and has thus far prevented necrosis from occurring after the second lateral lift (the only lateral procedure ever to experience necrosis).

Finally, it is critical to use Doppler ultrasonography to locate and scribe the temporal arteries preoperatively to avoid cutting the superficial temporal artery.

In regard to the grafting that is combined with these scalp-lifting procedures, it is my strong belief that the hair transplanting ability of the surgeon "makes or breaks" the final result. It is also my strong opinion that if the surgeon cannot perform good hair grafting or does not have access to a physician who performs good hair transplantation, scalp-lifting, or for that matter any alopecia-reducing procedure, should not be undertaken. This dogmatism is expressed because the scarring that develops from all alopecia-reducing procedures can at times be cosmetically bothersome to the patient, and the surgeon *must* be able to effectively deal with this issue. It is for this reason that the surgeon should also be able to perform Frechet-type transposition flaps for the correction of the occasional deep-lying scar at the occiput.

The three-step micro-minigrafting approach is one of the most predictable, organized, and yet simple methods to date. The four primary reasons for this are:

1. Even, uniform coverage is accomplished with each procedure. The stencil significantly enhances the surgeon's ability to achieve this uniformity.
2. Each graft receives even nutritive circulation, thereby increasing the survival rate of each graft.
3. The speed of placing the grafts is significantly improved because each graft is an equal distance from the adjacent graft. This equal distancing allows for an easy system of placement to be developed while decreasing the amount of graft "popping."
4. The speed of making the appropriate incisions is tremendously improved, especially during the second and third sessions in patients with early thinning when random patterns make it extremely difficult to visualize growing grafts from a previous session.
5. The straight, forward, and backward direction of the incisions ensures that previously growing grafts will not be destroyed from misdirection of subsequent incisions.

As stated previously, scar management is very important in alopecia reduction, and I believe that the aforementioned approach gives the surgeon a "no-nonsense" protocol to tackle the task. The

FIG. 9-65 A more refined stencil with 40 small holes per square inch for three- to four-hair minigrafts is used for black-haired patients and for those who desire undetectability from the beginning of the surgical transplantation.

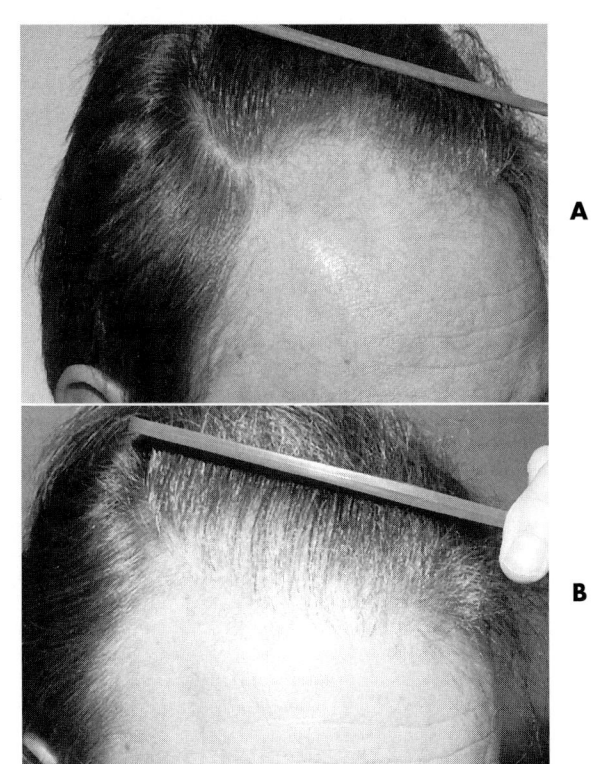

FIG. 9-66 **A,** Preoperative view. **B,** Postoperative view after only one session using the more refined stencil system.

shingling effect that is put to use at the posterior aspect of the scalp helps to create a fuller look than would be accomplished if the grafts were pointed in a forward direction in the area below the highest point of the head. The slit-grafting that is used beside the scar lines effectively softens the divergence that can sometimes occur after alopecia reduction while causing minimal damage to the existing hair in those regions. And finally, the straight, forward, or backward direction gives excellent versatility for hairstyling and prevents destruction of previous transplants.

If a more intense refinement is desired for the patient early in hair transplantation, I use a more refined stencil that consists of 40 holes per square inch for the organization of three- to four-hair micrografts into holes or slits. This is a change from the formerly described stencil that had 20 slits per square inch for six- to eight-hair grafts (Fig. 9-65). This more refined stencil is used for patients who request undetectability even from the first session (Fig. 9-66), those with black hair on white skin, or those with tight scalps who need holes so that compression does not become a cosmetic hinderance.

CIRCUMFERENTIAL SCALP REDUCTION

For the surgeon with less skill or without an intricate surgical setup or who has fear of complications, the same geometrical designs of scalp-lifting can be used, but the undermining can be limited to the nuchal ridge—a procedure I call *circumferential scalp reduction*.[35] This limited undermining, however, increases the number of procedures required for closure to three to five because of the reality that 60% of the stretch with scalp-lifting comes from the area below the nuchal ridge (Fig. 9-67). If additional scalp mobility is desired, the occipitalis and postauricular muscles can be severed bilaterally, and more aggressive undermining can be performed lateral to the occipital neurovascular bundles and inferior to the nuchal ridge (Fig. 9-68). Undermining can also be performed deep to the nuchal ridge, medial to the occipital bundles, so that more donor scalp can be advanced into the crown, thus reducing slot formation.

Scalp Extension

If the patient wants to shorten the interval between procedures, the surgeon has the surgical accessibil-

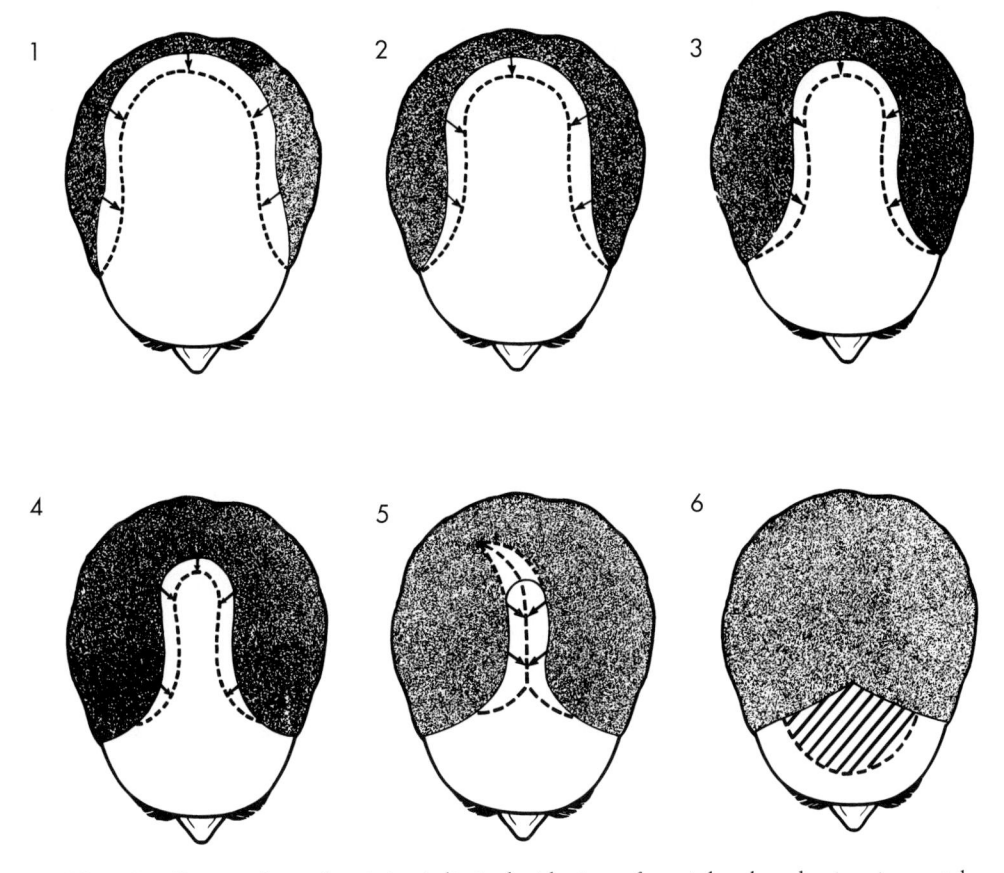

FIG. 9-67 Because the undermining is limited with circumferential scalp reduction, it may take from three to five procedures to achieve closure in extensively bald patients. (From Unger WP: *Hair transplantation*, ed 3, New York, 1995, Marcel Dekker.)

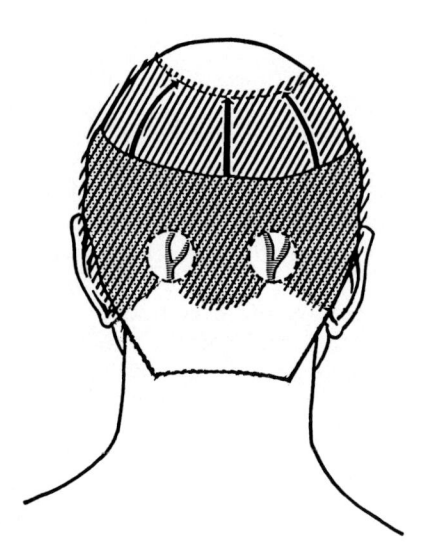

FIG. 9-68 More aggressive undermining laterally and medially can significantly improve the amount of scalp mobility of the circumferential scalp reduction.

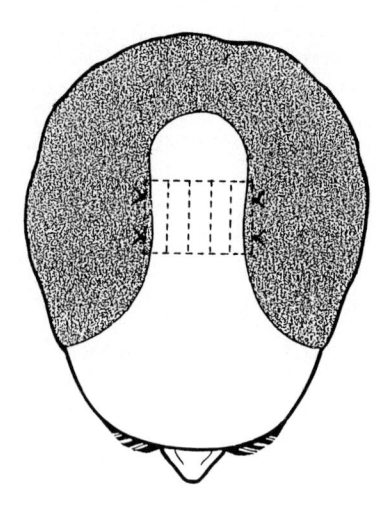

FIG. 9-69 With circumferential scalp reduction, the surgeon sutures a bioelastic silicone sheet under tension under a tunnel formed at the midline. This adjunct will allow the surgeries to be separated by 1 month. (From Unger WP: *Hair transplantation,* ed 3, New York, 1995, Marcel Dekker.)

ity with this circumferential approach to suture a 4 to 5 cm wide, 0.01-inch strip of bioelastic silicone sheeting (Duralastic; Applied Biomaterial Technology) to one edge of the galea, pass it under a 5 cm wide tunnel, stretch the strip to maximum tension, hold tension with needle holders, and then suture the strip to the opposite galeal edge (Fig. 9-69). This strip should be stretched as far as possible and sutured under as much tension as possible to accomplish the best result.[36] Normally with this technique the interval between surgeries can be decreased to 1 month (Fig. 9-70).

With regard to the prospect of the Duralastic strip sutured under tension increasing the amount of alopecia excision, it would be necessary for the strip to be stretched further than the amount that would normally be excised. For instance, if a subsequent circumferential reduction would normally have required excision of 3 cm of bald skin, it would be necessary to stretch the Duralastic sheeting 4 cm to accomplish 1 cm of extra movement. Because of this fact, I believe that the primary advantage of scalp extension with a "suture-in-place" Duralastic extender is to decrease the time interval between surgeries.

Alternatively, a silicone hook device developed by Frechet[37,38] can be used. However, this device is costly compared with a hand-cut Duralastic strip (approximately $500 vs. $10). The other advantage of the Duralastic strip is that it can be custom-cut for the individual operation. Hook devices, on the other hand, cannot be custom-cut for variable distances. They are, however, the only physically possible way to attach a silicone sheet under tension while using midline scalp reduction because of the lack of surgical accessibility for suturing afforded by midline scalp reduction.

LONG-TERM RESULTS

I believe that if the extensively bald patient is selected properly, those who have had alopecia reduction (i.e., scalp-lifting, circumferential scalp reduction) fair much better over the long term than those who undergo hair grafting alone. The primary reason for this opinion is that if the patient's hair loss progresses past the point that was predicted, it will usually look much better when the thinning occurs on top of the head (a natural position for thinning) than when an unnatural halo of baldness develops all the way around a central area of hair grafts. In addition, this thinning on top of the head can be more easily camouflaged than that around the balding area.

I also believe that if very thorough hair wetting is done at the time of consultation, a fairly accurate assessment of future baldness can be given. Most hair surgeons do not perform this maneuver routinely and therefore get into trouble 10 to 15 years down the road. All and all, if hair density, hair quantity, hair texture, and hair color are acceptable after hair wetting, the patient will be offered the best cosmesis long term with scalp-lifting and/or circumferential scalp reduction.

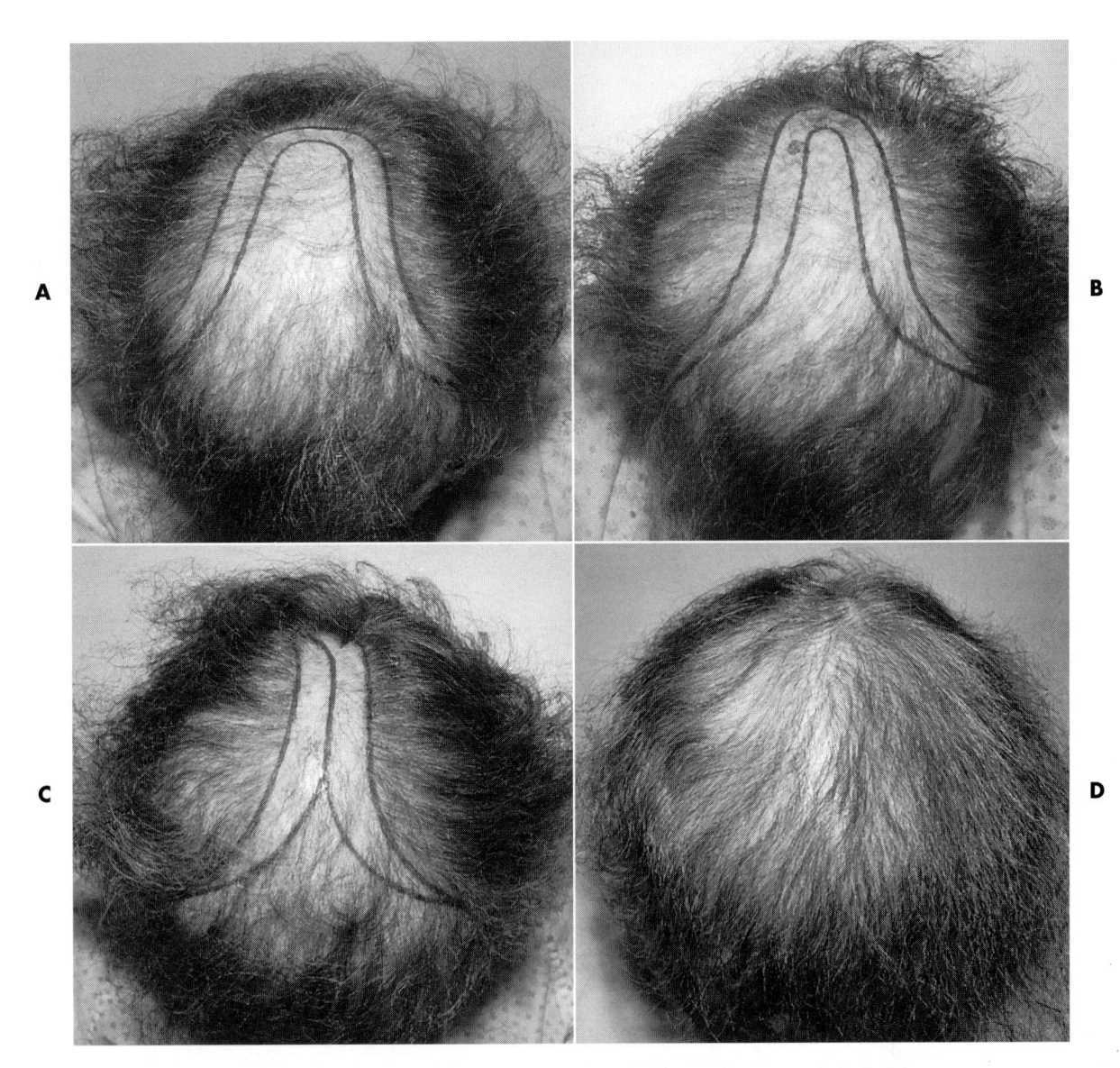

FIG. 9-70 A, Preoperative view of patient with extensive baldness who previously had undergone two lazy-S scalp reductions that had since stretched back. **B,** Postoperative view 1 month after the first circumferential scalp reduction with extender and immediately before second circumferential scalp reduction with extender. **C,** Postoperative view 1 month after the second circumferential scalp reduction and immediately before the bitemporal scalp reduction with extender. **D,** Postoperative result 1 month after the bitemporal scalp reduction with extender.

CONCLUSION

Scalp-lifting is an extremely effective and expedient method for treating extensive and moderate types of alopecia. The keys to keeping the complication rate to an almost nonexistent level and cosmesis to the highest level are:

1. Use vertical incision occipital artery ligations 2 to 6 weeks before the first scalp-lifting procedure.
2. Perform precise undermining and advancement.
3. Perform a delay procedure before frontoparietal advancement flaps.
4. Do not use frontoparietal advancement flaps on patients with prior punch hair grafting.
5. Use only Marzola lateral lifts on patients who have had prior hair transplantation.
6. During the first Marzola lateral lift, perform an occipital artery ligation on the contralat-

eral side percutaneously immediately after the completion of the first side lift. The contralateral side should be lifted within a 4- to 6-week window.

7. Locate and then draw in the temporal arteries with Doppler ultrasonography preoperatively.
8. Always try to perform lifts first and grafts subsequently for the following five reasons:
   - Any necrosis can be corrected at the time of the donor harvest.
   - The scar can be adequately corrected with proper grafting techniques while the frontal hairline is being developed.
   - Frechet transpositional flaps, in combination with grafting, can be performed only after lifts are completed.
   - More artistry can be applied to the development of the hairline shape.
   - Bilateral scalp-lifting procedures can be used. If grafting begins before scalp-lifting, only lateral procedures can be performed, which prolongs treatment.

REFERENCES

1. Blanchard G, Blanchard B: Obliteration of alopecia by hairlifting: a new concept and technique, *J Natl Med Assoc* 69:639-641, 1977.
2. Nordstrom REA: Scalp kinetics in multiple excisions for correction of male pattern baldness, *J Dermatol Surg Oncol* 10:991-995, 1984.
3. Nordstrom REA: "Stretch-back" in scalp reductions for male pattern baldness, *Plast Reconstr Surg* 73:422-426, 1984.
4. Unger MG: The Y-shaped pattern of alopecia reduction and its variation, *J Dermatol Surg Oncol* 10:297-303, 1984.
5. Alt TH: History of scalp reductions and paramedian method. In Norwood OT, editor: *Hair transplant surgery*, ed 2, Springfield, Ill, 1984, Charles C Thomas, pp 221-244.
6. Manders EK, Schenden MJ, Furrey J: Skin expansion to eliminate large scalp defects, *Ann Plast Surg* 12:305, 1984.
7. Austad ED: Complications of tissue expansion, *Clin Plast Surg* 14:549-550, 1987.
8. Marzola M: An alternative hair replacement method. In Norwood OT, editor: *Hair transplant surgery*, ed 2, Springfield, Ill, 1984, Charles C Thomas, pp 21-44.
9. Brandy DA: A new instrument for the expedient production of minigrafts, *J Dermatol Surg Oncol* 18:487-492, 1992.
10. Brandy DA: The bilateral occipitoparietal flap, *J Dermatol Surg Oncol* 10:1062, 1986.
11. Brandy DA: Extensive scalp-lifting as a reconstructive tool for a large scalp defect, *J Dermatol Surg Oncol* 18:806-811, 1992.
12. Brandy DA: The Brandy bitemporal flap, *Am J Cosmet Surg* 3:11-15, 1986.
13. Brandy DA: The bitemporal scalp reduction, *Am J Cosmet Surg* 8:33-39, 1991.
14. Brandy DA: The modified bitemporal flap for the treatment of bitemporal recessions, *Aesthetic Plast Surg* 13:203-207, 1989.
15. Brandy DA: New various approaches for the treatment of extensive baldness, *Am J Cosmet Surg* 7:129-189, 1990.
16. Brandy DA: A new surgical approach for the treatment of extensive baldness, *Am J Cosmet Surg* 3:19-25, 1986.
17. Brandy DA: The effectiveness of occipital artery ligations as a priming procedure for extensive scalp-lifting, *J Dermatol Surg Oncol* 17:946-949, 1991.
18. Nordstrom REA: "Micrografts" for the improvement of the frontal hairline after hair transplantation, *Aesthetic Plast Surg* 5:97, 1981.
19. Lucas MWG: The use of minigrafts in hair transplantation surgery, *J Dermatol Surg Oncol* 14:1389-1392, 1988.
20. Brandy DA: Use of a stencil for the improved accuracy, speed and aesthetics in mini-micrografting, *J Dermatol Surg Oncol* (In press).
21. Coiffmann F: Use of square scalp grafts for male pattern baldness, *Plast Reconstr Surg* 60:228-232, 1977.
22. Bisaccia E, Scarborough D: A technique for square plug hair transplantation. Presented at the 17th Annual Scientific and Clinical Meeting of ASDS. Maui: February 13-17, 1990.
23. Bradshaw W: Quarter grafts: a technique for minigrafts. In Unger WP, editor: *Hair transplantation*, ed 2, New York, 1988, Marcel Dekker, pp 333-350.
24. Norwood OT: Hair transplant surgery: innovative designs, *J Dermatol Surg Oncol* 16:50-54, 1990.
25. Nelson BR and others: Hair transplantation in advanced male pattern alopecia, *J Dermatol Surg Oncol* 17:243-253, 1991.
26. Swinehart JM, Griffin EI: Slit-grafting: the use of serrated island grafts in male and female pattern alopecia, *J Dermatol Surg Oncol* 17:567-573, 1991.
27. Brandy DA: A three-step systematic incisional-slit minigrafting approach, *J Dermatol Surg Oncol* 19:421-426, 1993.
28. Brandy DA: A special scalp garment for prestretching prior to alopecia-reducing procedures, *J Dermatol Surg Oncol* (In press).
29. Brandy DA, Meshkin M: Utilization of NoKor vented needles for the improvement of slit-micrografting, *J Dermatol Surg Oncol* (In press).
30. Brandy DA: Combining extensive scalp-lifting and coronal brow-lifting for the treatment of cicatricial alopecia, *Am J Cosmet Surg* 7:45-50, 1990.
31. Callegari PR and others: An anatomic review of the delay phenomenon: I. Experimental studies, *Plast Reconstr Surg* 89:397-407, 1992.
32. Taylor GI and others: An anatomic review of the delay phenomenon: II. Clinical applications, *Plast Reconstr Surg* 89:408-418, 1992.
33. Brandy DA: Two new retractors for hair replacement surgery, *J Dermatol Surg Oncol* 19:881-883, 1993.
34. Unger MG: Postoperative necrosis following bilateral lateral scalp reduction, *J Dermatol Surg Oncol* 14:541-544, 1988.
35. Brandy DA: Circumferential scalp reduction: the application of the principles of extensive scalp-lifting for the improvement of conventional scalp reduction, *J Dermatol Surg Oncol* (In press).
36. Brandy DA: The use of retention sutures and tensed Silastic-Dacron strips for the prevention of stretchback after alopecia reducing procedures, *J Dermatol Surg Oncol* (In press).
37. Frechet P: Scalp extension, *J Dermatol Surg Oncol* 19:616-622, 1993.
38. Frechet P: The extender—a new tool for scalp reduction. Presented at the First Annual Meeting of the International Society of Hair Restoration Surgery. Dallas: April 30-May 2, 1993.

I. Scalp-Lifting

James M. Swinehart

The development of extensive scalp-lifting has presented a significant advance in hair restoration surgery. Properly performed, this procedure can remove large amounts of bald scalp in a safe manner, generally in two operations.

The concept of scalp-lifting was initiated by Marzola and has been extensively analyzed, developed, and perfected by Brandy. Modifications of the procedure have considerably lessened the associated side effects and complications.[1-3]

Careful attention to the "Ten Commandments of Scalp-Lifting" will maximize the probability of a successful outcome (see box). Ignoring one or more of these guidelines, on the other hand, may lead to increased risk of complications or lack of effective scalp-lifting.

> **"TEN COMMANDMENTS" OF SCALP-LIFTING**
>
> 1. Establish a master plan and understand the goals.
> 2. Perform proper patient preparation (preoperative expansion).
> 3. Obtain effective anesthesia and analgesia.
> 4. Plan the incision line.
> 5. Obtain optimal visualization with help from surgical assistants.
> 6. Understand the anatomy and surgical planes of dissection.
> 7. Obtain effective hemostasis.
> 8. Use proper instrumentation.
> 9. To advance the scalp correctly, understand the relationship of the extent of undermining to the amount of lift obtained.
> 10. Perform correct closure methods to prevent stretchback.

PROPER PLANNING: UNDERSTANDING THE GOALS

Given the complexity of scalp-lifting, why perform this operation instead of a simple midline or paramedian scalp reduction? The answer is that with scalp-lifting far more bald skin can be removed than with any other type of operation, saving valuable donor grafts for the frontal scalp and hairline.

The surgeon plans a scalp-lift operation to elevate all portions of the scalp vertically and anteriorly—especially the occipital scalp. Midline or paramedian scalp reductions, on the other hand, lift the scalp only from side to side. As the parietal scalp is advanced, the occipital scalp dog ear recedes, creating the unsightly slot deformity so common in these older procedures.[4-8]

The proper master plan enables the surgeon to remove *all* of the bald skin on the posterior and central crown, replacing it with natural scalp hair rather than grafts. Ideally, scalp-lift candidates should have Hamilton type IV, V, or VI (not VII) hair loss with a bald crown width of less than 12 or 13 cm and an occipital donor scalp height of at least 9 to 10 cm, without an unusually high initial posterior scalp hairline.

In most instances the bilateral occipitoparietal flap is first performed to lift the scalp in every di-

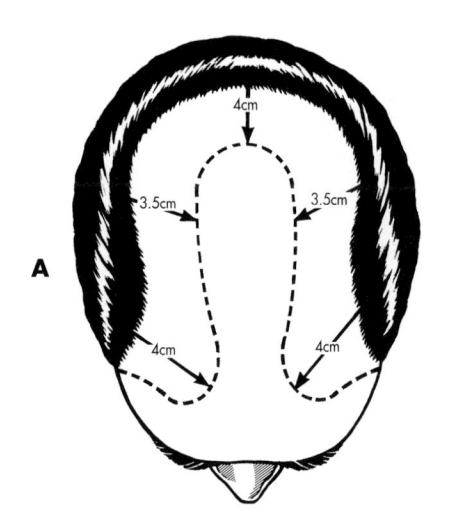

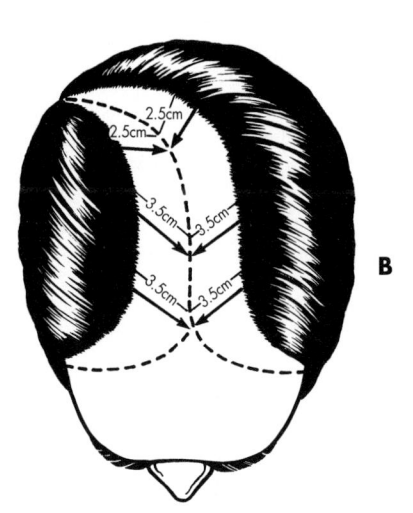

FIG. 9-71 A, Scalp movement in the bilateral occipitoparietal flap. **B,** Scalp movement in the bitemporal flap. (From Unger WP: *Hair transplantation,* ed 3, New York, 1995, Marcel Dekker.)

rection (especially upward from the occiput), removing a horseshoe-shaped section of bald skin from the vertex (Fig. 9-71, A). The second operation, a bitemporal flap, seeks to unite both sides of the parietal scalp in the midline, removing the remaining bald skin in the central crown (Fig. 9-71, B). The posterior curve of the bitemporal flap follows the patient's natural whorl and eliminates the possibility of slot formation posteriorly. Both flaps move anteriorly (the bilateral occipitoparietal flap more than the bitemporal flap), serving to eliminate the temporal recession (Fig. 9-72). Ideally, scalp-lifting should be performed before hair graft transplantation to ensure an adequate blood supply and to avoid distortion of graft placement areas. The advantages of scalp-lifting over

TABLE 9-1 Scalp-Lifting vs. Scalp Reduction

SURGICAL OUTCOME	SCALP-LIFTING	MIDLINE OR PARAMEDIAN SCALP REDUCTION
Number of operations needed to completely remove the bald crown	Usually 2	Often 4-7 (without scalp extension)
Number of future hair transplant grafts needed after reduction is completed	Smaller number	Larger number
Amount of bald skin removed	Maximum	Limited (without scalp extension)
Scalp stretch	Maximum (60% to 70% from areas beyond the galea)	Much less (galea is hard to stretch)
Lifting of occipital scalp	Excellent	Little or none
Slot formation	None	A potential problem
Stretchback	Less marked	Often significant
Surgical visibility	Excellent	Fair to poor
Correction of temporal recession	Yes	No
Extent of undermining	Maximum	Usually not beyond galea
Blood loss	Generally 100-200 ml	Generally <100 ml
Cost	Higher	Lower
Operative time involved	Approximately 1½-2 hr	Generally <1 hr
Combination with scalp extension	May facilitate correction of type VI alopecia	Decreased number of midline reductions with increased removal of bald skin

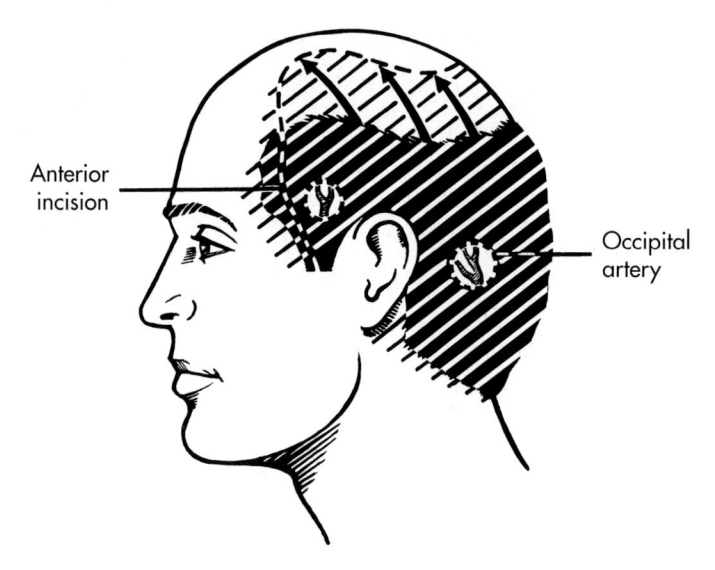

FIG. 9-72 Advancement of flap in relationship to the principal blood supply of the scalp. (Courtesy Dr. Dominic Brandy.)

traditional scalp-reduction methods are summarized in Table 9-1.

PATIENT PREPARATION (PREOPERATIVE EXPANSION)

In years past, hair restoration surgeons focused on operative methods to overcome the lack of ability of the galea aponeurotica to stretch. These methods included intraoperative expansion, preoperative expansion, galeotomies, presuturing, and surgical winches.[9-14] However, a valuable principle was overlooked; namely, the ability of tissue to stretch over a period of time as a result of prolonged tension, similar to that used in the past by African tribes for stretching lips or ears.

The "30-30-30-30" Scalp Massage

To accomplish the "30-30-30-30" scalp massage, the patient initiates scalp massage at least 30 (up to 60) days before the scalp-lift. The patient grasps the lateral or posterior scalp hair, presses upward with the heels of the hands, and lifts the scalp up as far as possible for 30 seconds at a time. These 30-second lifts are alternated with 30 seconds of relaxation for at least 30 minutes a day. Additional stretch can be obtained from a Velcro stretch device (Anthony Products, Indianapolis Ind.), whose tension is adjusted every 2 to 3 minutes. This device consists of circumferential and transverse straps around the entire scalp. We are continually surprised at the amount of laxity generated over a 2-month period in a previously "tight" scalp.

Prevention of Scalp Necrosis

In the past, necrosis of a portion of the posterior scalp was a risk because both occipital arteries were cut during a bilateral occipitoparietal scalp-lift, sometimes leaving the posterior scalp without sufficient circulation (Fig. 9-73). This risk can be virtually eliminated, however, by one of two operative methods: either transecting only one occipital artery at a time (during each of the two scalp-lifts)[15] or the performance of prior occipital artery ligation[5] (Fig. 9-74).

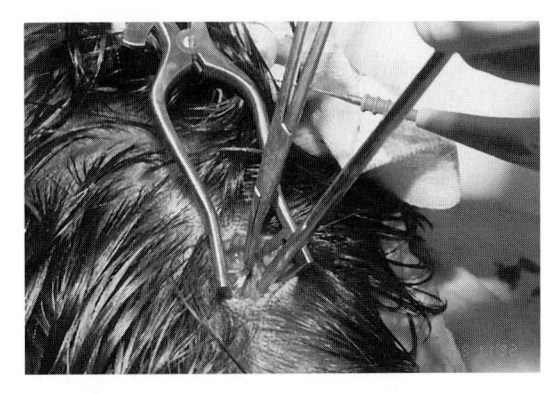

FIG. 9-73 Electrocoagulation of main occipital artery.

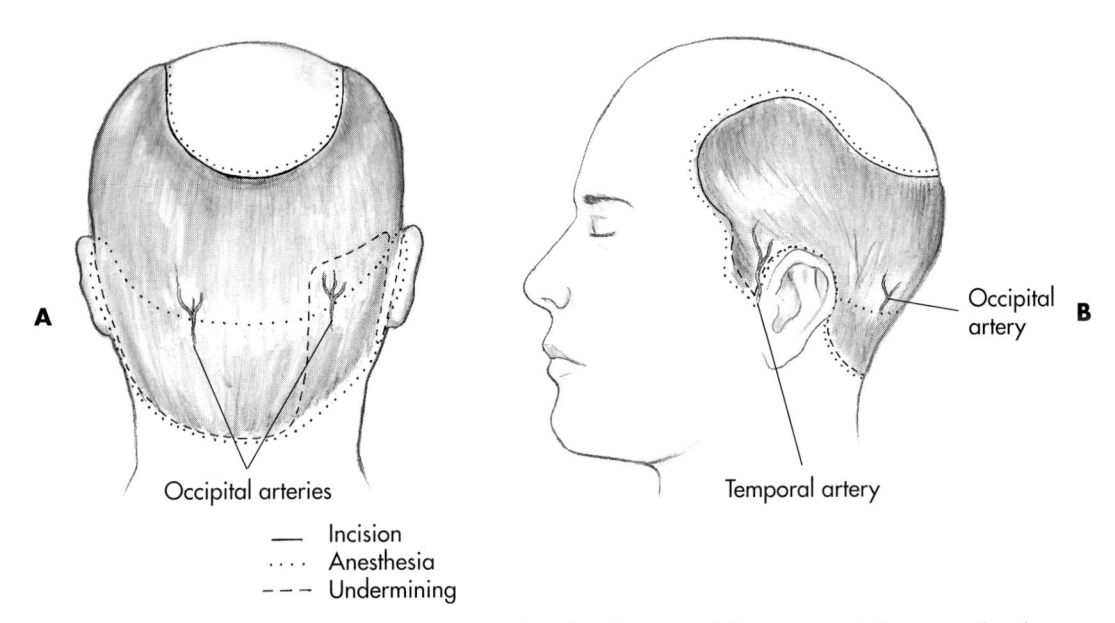

FIG. 9-74 Extensive scalp-lifting with unilateral undermining. The location of the occipital and temporal arteries and the extent of the anesthesia, incision line, and undermining are indicated. **A,** Posterior view. **B,** Lateral view.

Prior occipital artery ligation has been shown to be quite beneficial.[16] Performance of bilateral occipital artery ligation 4 to 6 weeks before the first scalp-lift has decreased the risk of scalp necrosis to less than 2%. Since the occipital arteries must be cut at some point during extensive scalp-lifting, collateral circulation is necessary to preserve the occipital scalp's blood supply. This prior ligation encourages the development of "choke vessels" from the superficial temporal arteries and postauricular arteries to supply in advance this occipital region of the scalp. Intraoperative bleeding is also noticeably diminished posteriorly by prior ligation.

To perform occipital artery ligation, each vessel is identified with Doppler ultrasonography and marked. With the patient under local anesthesia, a 3 cm vertical incision is made through the scalp to the fascia. Careful blunt and sharp dissection is used in identifying each main occipital artery and its two vertical branches. These two sets of three arteries are electrocoagulated and transected. Closure is then performed with 4-0 degradable suture.

ANESTHESIA AND ANALGESIA

Because of the length of the operation (approximately 1½ to 2 hours) and the use of the prone position, patient sedation and relaxation are essential. Although the procedure may be performed with the aid of oral or intramuscular analgesia and sedation, intravenous sedation producing "twilight sleep" provides ideal anesthesia for this operation. Medications may be administered effectively by a certified registered nurse anesthetist (CRNA), relieving the surgeon of this task. Commonly used drugs include propofol (Diprivan), midazolam (Versed), fentanyl citrate, as well as droperidol (Inapsine) for nausea. Near the end of the operation, the CRNA may administer dexamethasone (Decadron) for prevention of postoperative edema, dimenhydrinate (Dramamine) for prevention of nausea, and intramuscular ketorolac tromethamine (Toradol) for prevention of postoperative pain. (We have not noticed an increased bleeding tendency with the latter drug in patients with normal hematological and platelet functions.) Cephalosporin administration initiated preoperatively is continued for 5 days postoperatively.

Local Anesthesia

Once sedation has been obtained, local anesthesia is commenced. A ring block of the scalp is performed with approximately 20 ml of 2% lidocaine (Xylocaine) with 1:100,000 epinephrine. Another 10 ml of this mixture is injected along the proposed incision line (see Fig. 9-74). Approximately 30 ml of 0.25% lidocaine with 1:400,000 epinephrine or 100 ml of tumescent solution (0.1% lidocaine with 1:1,000,000 epinephrine) is then used to "connect" these areas and to thoroughly infiltrate the entire area below the nuchal ridge from ear to ear.[17] Intraoperatively, during a more extensive procedure, this vascular area below the nuchal ridge can be reinfiltrated with a 50/50 combination of 1% lidocaine with 1:100,000 epinephrine mixed with 0.5% bupivacaine (Marcaine) (approximately 15 to 20 ml) with or without hyaluronidase (Wydase), 1 ml per 10 ml of local anesthetic, affording long-lasting postoperative pain relief and increased intraoperative hemostasis.

PLANNING THE INCISION LINE

In contrast to the midline or paramedian incision line, which provides limited visibility and allows undermining in only one direction, the bilateral circumferential incision of extensive scalp-lifting allows the surgeon to remove at least twice as much bald skin since the undermining is carried down to and beyond each postauricular region down to the nape of the neck posteriorly.[18,19] This incision also generates excellent visibility since the scalp is "rolled back" or lifted during the operation.

Immediately before surgery, both superficial temporal arteries (which provide the primary blood supply to the scalp) are carefully identified with a handheld Doppler device (Huntleigh Technologies, Bedfordshire, Great Britain) and marked.[15] Anteriorly, the incision lies 1 cm posterior to the temporal hairline but well in front of the just-marked temporal artery (Fig. 9-75). The incision begins at a level even with or close to the superior pole of the helix bilaterally. The bilateral occipitoparietal flap incision line then extends superiorly, following the outline of the bald crown in a posterior direction in a generally bilaterally symmetrical fashion[20] (see Fig. 9-74). When the bitemporal flap is subsequently executed 3 months later, the temporal scar from the bilateral occipitoparietal flap is excised as the incision traces the same course.[21] Posteriorly, however, both parietal incisions meet at a point that veers approximately 45 degrees in the direction of the whorl on the crown, eliminating any possibility of a slot deformity or dog ear. Thus with two procedures the right and left parietal scalp and occipital scalp all meet at the central crown, covering this region with the patient's natural hair. The anterior crown is subsequently covered in three or four sessions with minigrafts and micrografts.[22,23]

ROLE OF SURGICAL ASSISTANTS IN OBTAINING VISUALIZATION

During extensive scalp-lifting, five staff members should always be present: the CRNA, circulating nurse, surgeon, and two surgical assistants. The lat-

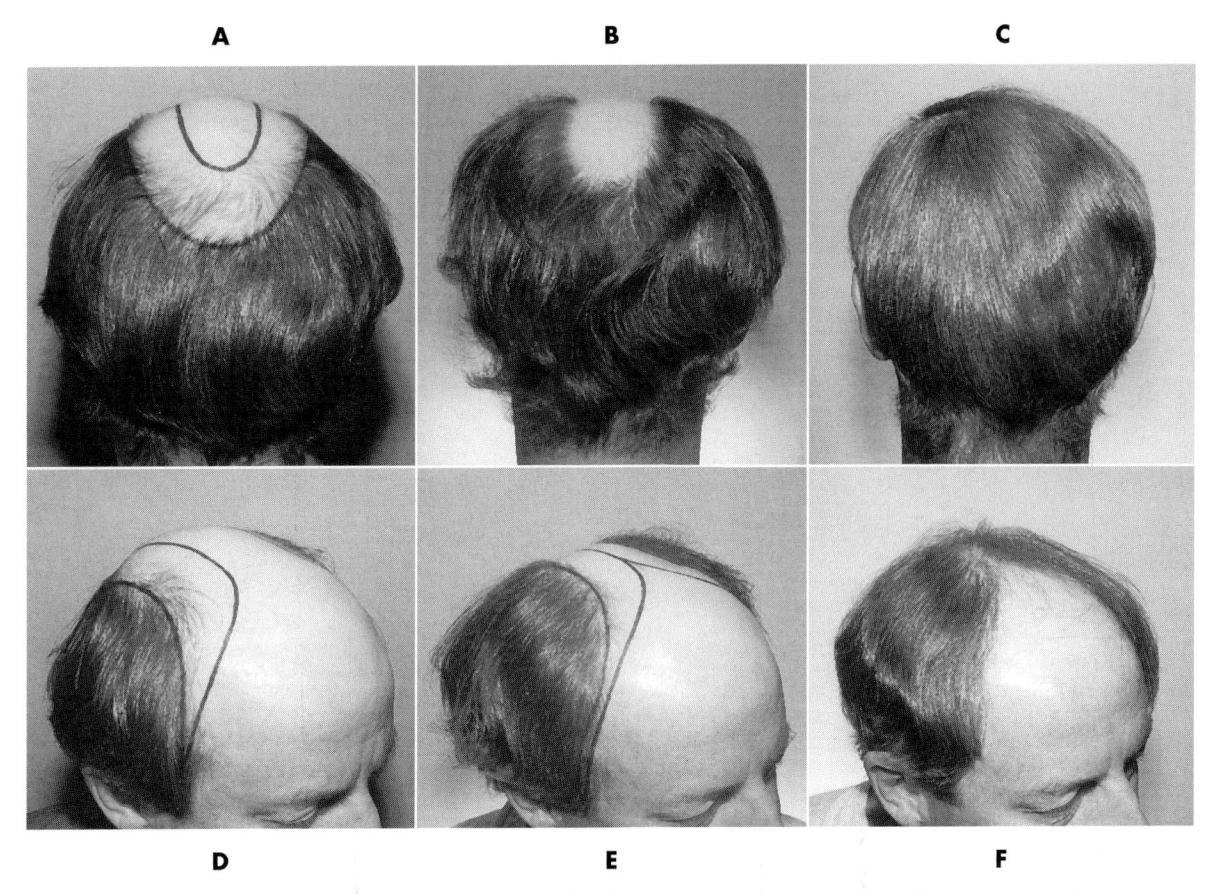

FIG. 9-75 **A,** Preoperative posterior view. **B,** Postoperative view after bilateral occipitoparietal scalp-lift before bitemporal lift. **C,** Postoperative posterior view after bitemporal lift. **D,** Preoperative oblique view. **E,** Postoperative view after bilateral occipitoparietal scalp-lift before bitemporal lift. **F,** Postoperative oblique view after bitemporal lift. (From Unger WP: *Hair transplantation*, ed 3, New York, 1995, Marcel Dekker.)

ter three are gowned, gloved, and masked in sterile operating room fashion. As the surgeon strives to maintain hemostasis and to dissect in the proper surgical planes, visibility is critical. During the initial phase of the operation (subgaleal undermining to the ears and to the nuchal ridge), the assistants roll back the scalp, providing easy access for the surgeon.

As the surgeon proceeds deeper inferiorly, past the level of the occipitalis muscles, the assistants must vigorously elevate the scalp as much as possible from the underlying structures. One assistant continually lifts the occipital hair with one hand, forcing the frontal scalp down with the other (Fig. 9-76). The second assistant also elevates the scalp with one hand, using the other hand for handling surgical instruments. The surgeon also elevates the scalp with a suction retractor in one hand, undermining with a scissors or scalpel in the other. Thus, for patients undergoing scalp-lifting, the longer the hair, the better!

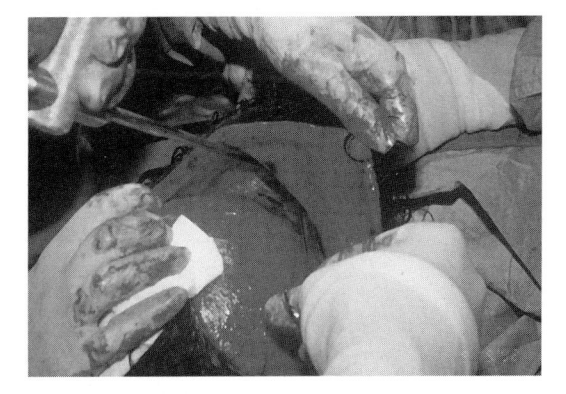

FIG. 9-76 Obtaining proper visualization. The assistant pushes down on anterior scalp with the right hand and lifts the hair with the left hand. The surgeon elevates the flap with a suction retractor.

UNDERSTANDING THE ANATOMY AND SURGICAL PLANES OF DISSECTION

One side at a time, the surgeon commences the incision at the inferior temporal aspect (mid-sideburn) and carries it superiorly and posteriorly to the midline. The initial undermining is carried out in the avascular plane underneath the galea but above the temporalis muscle fascia (Fig. 9-77, A). Care is taken to remain deep to the superficial temporal arteries anteriorly (Fig. 9-77, B). This undermining is carried out inferiorly until the area just above the level of the ear is reached (Fig. 9-77, C). During all phases of the operation, the surgeon creates three or four tunnels by a spreading motion of the scissors

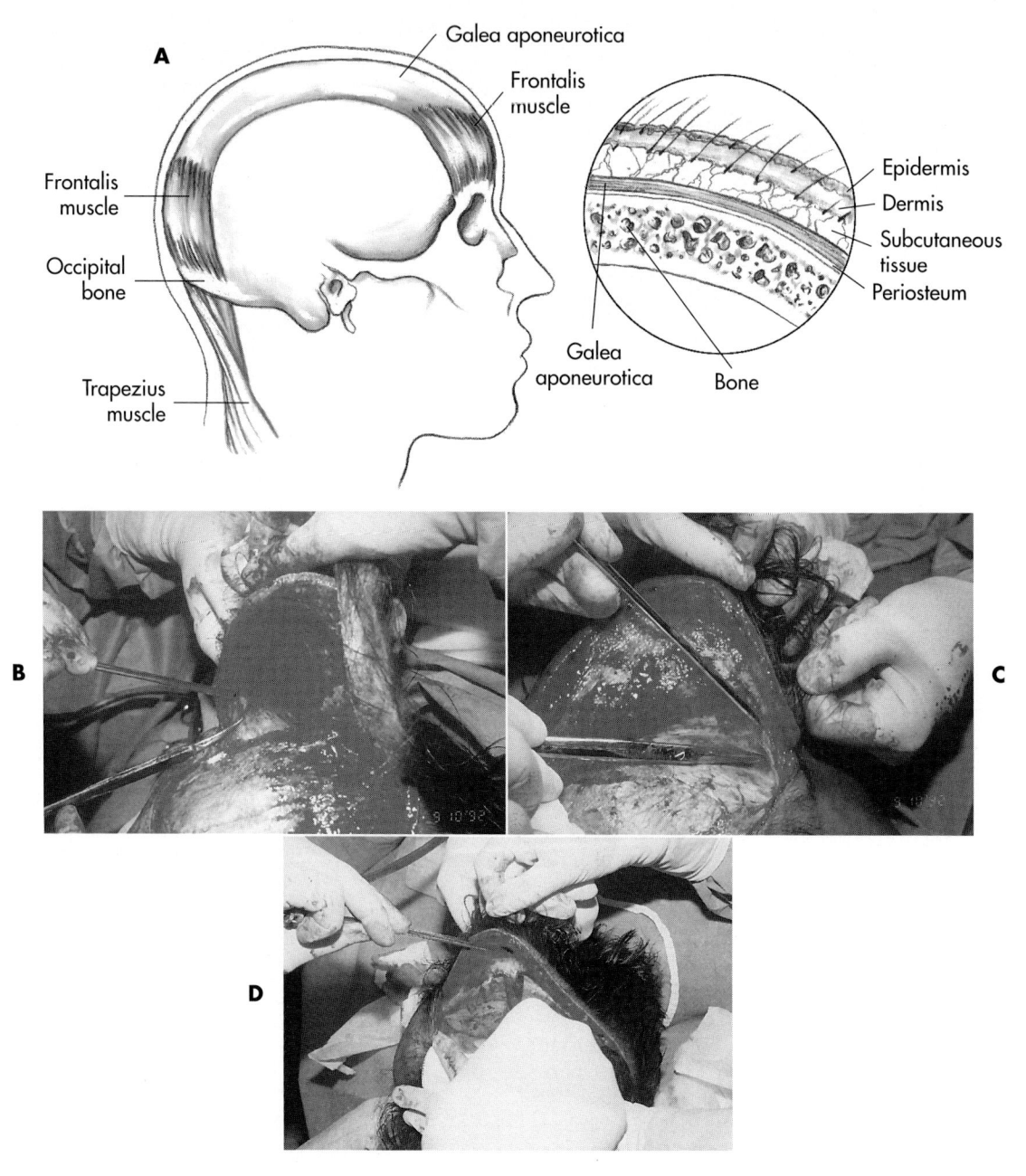

FIG. 9-77 A, Lateral view of planes of dissection in extensive scalp-lifting. **B,** Temporal artery is visualized 2 cm posteriorly to anterior incision line. **C,** Subgaleal undermining in temporal area. **D,** Sharp dissection through tunnels, which were created by blunt dissection. (**A** redrawn from *Gray's Atlas of Anatomy.*)

and then the tunnels are connected through sharp dissection (Fig. 9-77, D).

In this conservative fashion, major structures can be approached cautiously. Posteriorly the undermining is then executed subgaleally as well, proceeding inferiorly until the nuchal ridge is approached. At this point, both occipitalis muscles come into view. These thin muscles, each approximately 3 to 4 cm long and 5 to 6 cm in width, originate from the fascia overlying the bony nuchal ridge and insert into the galea of the posterior crown of the scalp (Fig. 9-78, A).

The dissection is then carried inferiorly in the avascular subcutaneous postauricular "face-lift" plane by a spreading motion of the dissection scissors (Fig. 9-78, B). This dissection is carried down to the perichondrium of the ear (Griffin E: Personal communication). Cutting the small postauricular muscles bilaterally may add another 0.5 to 1 cm of stretch and elevation bilaterally.

To proceed further inferiorly the surgeon comes to the most difficult part of the operation: connecting both postauricular dissections by undermining the posterior scalp down to or close to a line drawn horizontally from the inferior aspect of each earlobe along the nape of the neck. To reach the proper fascial plane, the occipitalis muscles must be transected. Although the neurovascular bundle containing the occipital artery has previously been ligated in many cases, residual perforators or stumps may still bleed briskly. Therefore the use of the cutting current on the electrosurgical machine allows this incision to be made with relatively little bleeding (Fig. 9-79, A).

The undermining now proceeds in a plane deep to the subcutaneous fat (and hair follicles) of the inferior occipital scalp but above the sternocleidomastoid and trapezius muscles (Fig. 9-79, B and C). The surgeon literally attempts to split the fascia of these muscles, remaining in a relatively avascular plane (Fig. 9-79, D). In this phase, the lifting maneuver of the surgical assistants is of paramount importance. If the surgeon sees subcutaneous fat or hair follicles, he/she should proceed more deeply; if muscle is visualized through the fascia, he/she must dissect more superficially (Fig. 9-79, E and F).

After careful, persistent undermining, the hairline of the nape of the neck is reached (Fig. 9-79, G). The surgeon next creates a drain stab wound behind one or both ears, placing a drain in one or both locations. Last, meticulous hemostasis is performed; the surgeon may spray topical thrombin (2500 U) under the flap before advancement.

EFFECTIVE HEMOSTASIS

Fig. 9-80, which depicts the anatomy of the scalp, reveals a generous blood supply. Four main arteries supply the scalp in paired fashion: the occipital artery to the posterior scalp, the postauricular artery to the posterior parietal scalp and posterior crown, the supraorbital artery to the frontal scalp, and the superficial temporal artery to the bulk of the temporal and parietal scalp and the crown. This latter arterial supply must be preserved at all costs during the operation because it eventually replaces the supply from the occipital artery.[24]

Generous amounts of lidocaine with epinephrine used preoperatively and intraoperatively greatly aid hemostasis, as mentioned earlier. An excellent suction machine and a fiberoptic headlamp for optimal visualization are essential. The use of a cutting current for dissection in vascular areas, when possible, can considerably decrease bleeding. The electrosurgery machine must be relatively powerful to afford effective coagulation (examples include those manufactured by Valleylab Inc., Boulder, Colo.; CR Bard, Inc., El Monte, Calif.; or the Bovie specialist unit, Cincinnati, Ohio). In most instances, the use of long tonsil hemostats combined with a monopolar current (patient grounded) provided optimal results, although some surgeons prefer a one-piece fingertip suction coagulation device such as that

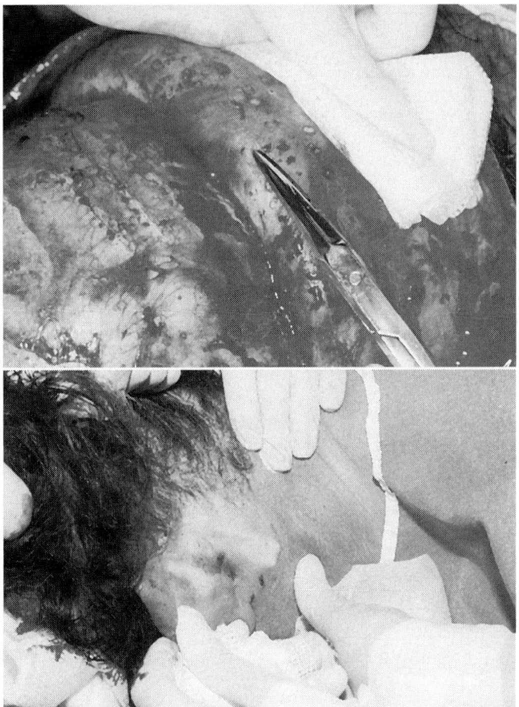

FIG. 9-78 **A,** Superior insertion of the occipitalis muscle into the galea aponeurotica. **B,** Subcutaneous undermining by blunt dissection in the postauricular region.

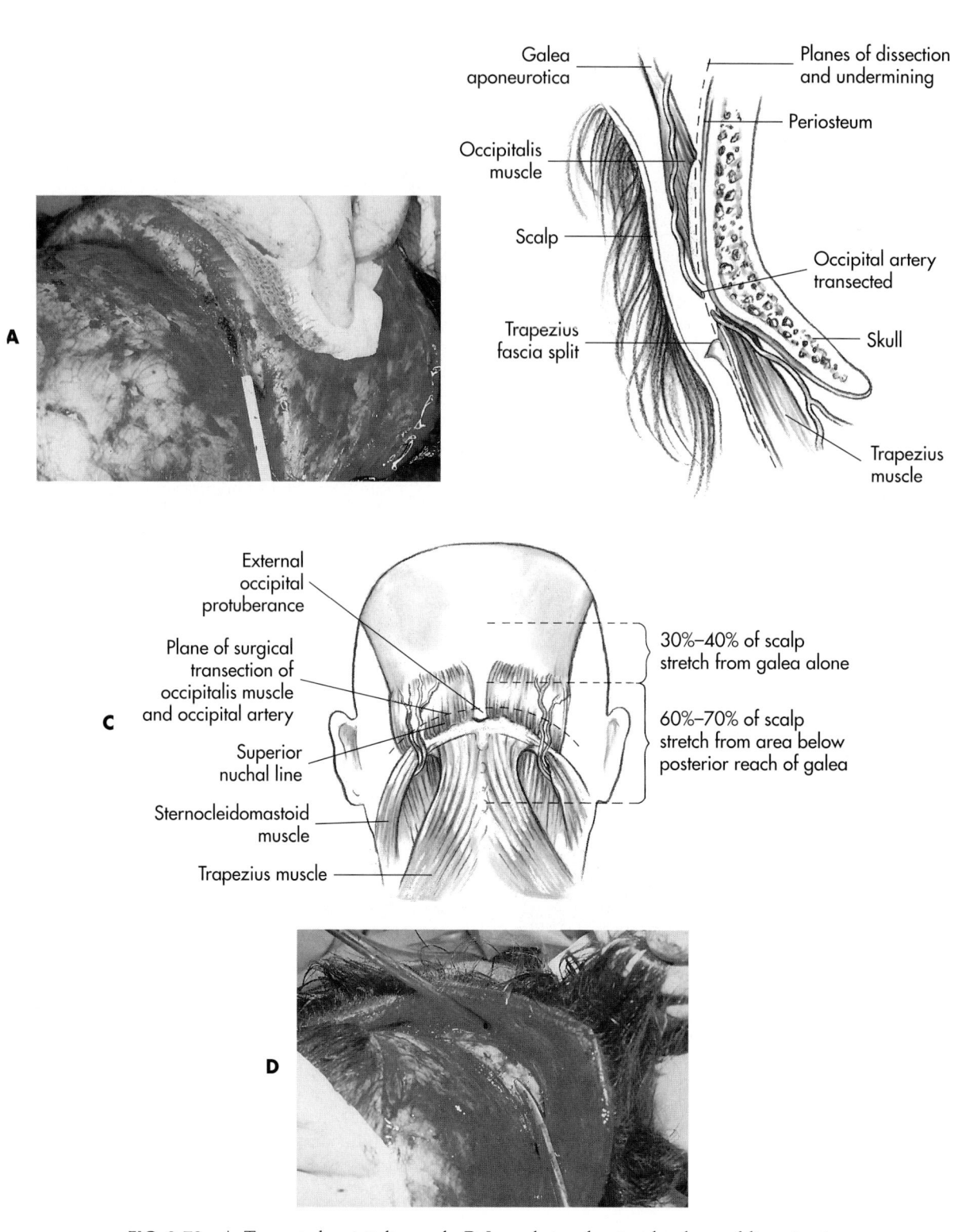

FIG. 9-79 **A,** Transected occipitalis muscle. **B,** Lateral view showing the planes of dissection in extensive scalp-lifting. **C,** Posterior view showing the planes of dissection with scalp stretch obtained from each dissection. **D,** Undermining continues in the posterior subcutaneous plane after transection of the occipitalis muscle.

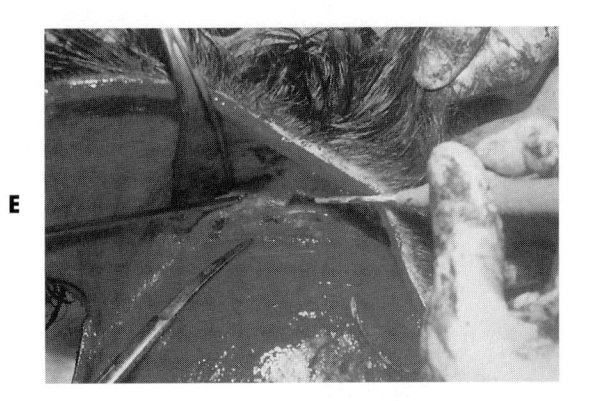

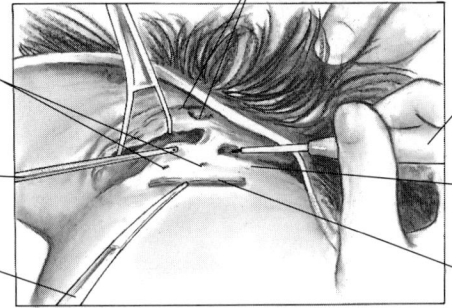

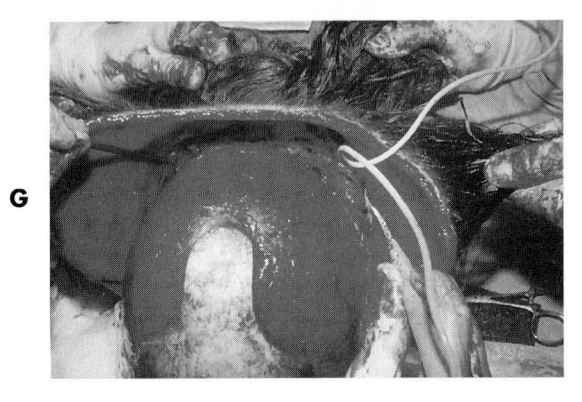

FIG. 9-79, cont'd. **E,** Splitting of the trapezius and sternocleidomastoid fascia near the nape of the neck with an intraoperative view of the cut occipitalis muscle and ligated occipital arteries. **F,** View of dissection below the nuchal ridge. **G,** Scalp flap completely elevated after full dissection to the nape of the neck bilaterally.

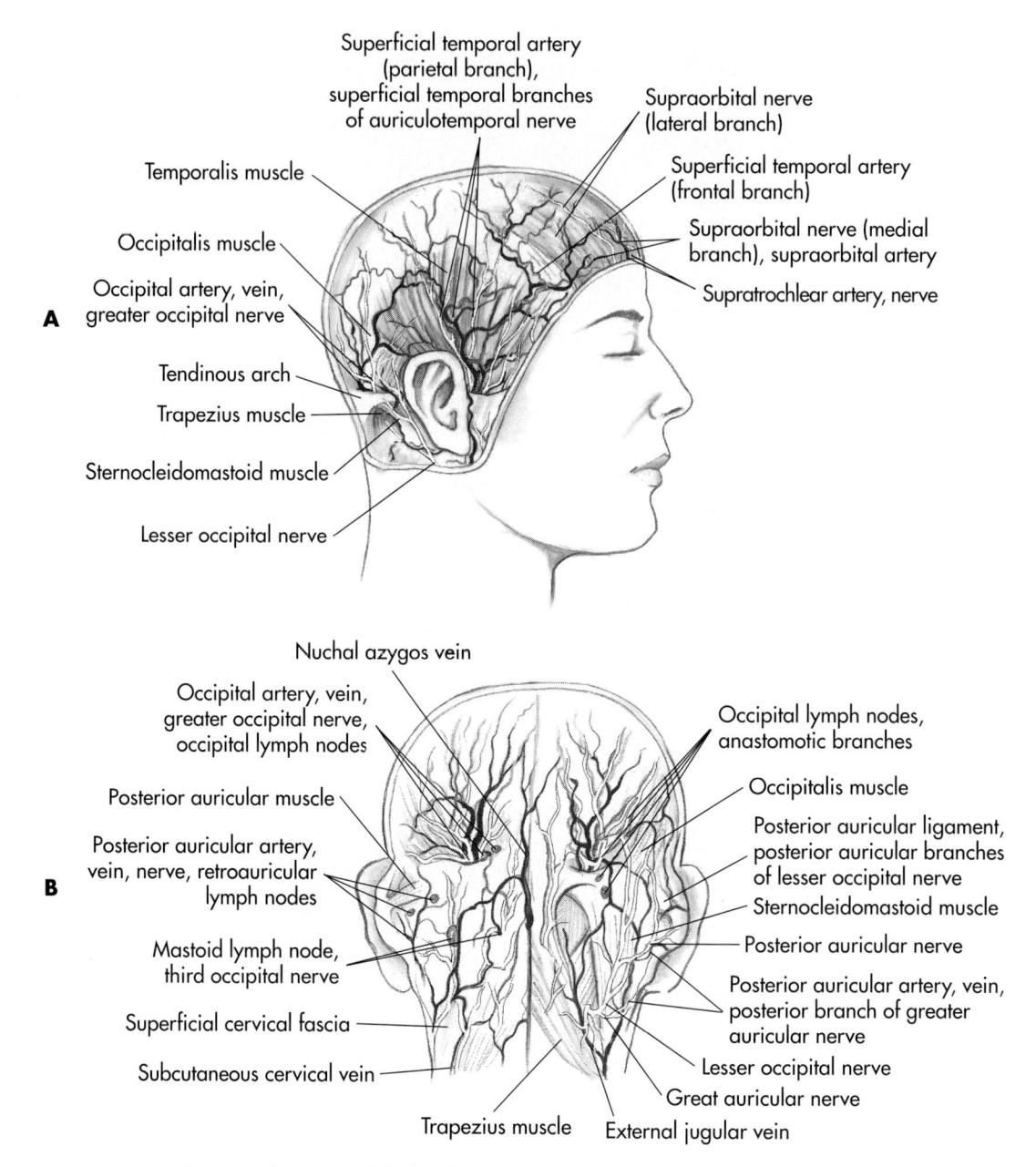

FIG. 9-80 Anatomy of the head and neck. **A,** Lateral view. **B,** Posterior view.

produced by Valleylab. More recently, I have used a monopolar finger-switch bayonet coagulating forceps with teeth (Olson, Concord, Calif.) with excellent and swift hemostatic results. In addition, an argon beam photocoagulator (Birtcher, El Monte, Calif.) has proved to be quite effective.

Finally as vascular structures such as both occipitalis muscles and arteries and the nuchal azygos vein are approached, the assistants can clamp both ends of these structures as the surgeon first transects them with the cutting current and then touches each hemostat with a coagulation current. Bone wax proved invaluable in one instance in which an anomalous perforator originating from the bony skull was encountered. With these methods, the average blood loss during extensive scalp-lifting should be no more than 100 to 200 ml.

PROPER INSTRUMENTATION

The use of specially designed surgical instruments can enhance the surgeon's skills and considerably diminish operative time. A combination suction retractor (Robbins Instruments, Inc., Chatham, N.J.) enables a surgeon to elevate the scalp flap, simultaneously identifying and removing the source of bleeding before electrocoagulation. A long-handled hooked "skeleton" retractor (Robbins Instruments, Inc., Chatham, N.J.) can facilitate hemostasis by isolation of various bleeding points. Long-bladed "supercut" scissors are a valuable aid in undermining. A Weitlaner retractor (Miltex, Lake Success, N.Y.) is of particular importance during occipital artery ligation 4 to 8 weeks before the scalp-lift. D'Assumpcao retractors (Padgett Instruments, Kansas City, Mo.), originally designed for face- and brow-lifting, are invaluable for determining the exact amount of overlap during the actual elevation of the flaps (see Fig. 9-82). The importance of a handheld Doppler device, fiberoptic headlamp, electrosurgery machine with finger-switch cautery, and powerful suction have been discussed previously.

ADVANCING THE SCALP: RELATIONSHIP OF UNDERMINING TO AMOUNT OF LIFT

Because of the inability of the galea to stretch, scalp reductions in which only the galea is undermined (e.g., the midline or paramedian reduction) are doomed to removal of relatively little scalp. The secret to success in extensive scalp-lifting lies with the fact that most of the stretch comes from areas that do not possess an underlying galeal layer. These regions include the supraauricular and postauricular areas as well as the lower occipital scalp inferior to the nuchal ridge beyond the level of the occipitalis muscles. Indeed, intraoperative studies in the occipital scalp and on the parietal scalp have revealed that only 30% to 40% of the stretch, or advancement, comes from the area between the posterior incision line and nuchal ridge (with underlying galea), whereas 60% to 70% of the advancement is provided by undermining the more elastic lower occipital or lower parietal scalp mentioned earlier (with no underlying galea) (see Fig. 9-81).

Once undermining has been completed in a bilateral occipitoparietal scalp-lift, the occipital scalp is advanced superiorly with D'Assumpcao retractors (Fig. 9-82). A "blood print" on the bald scalp of the crown delineates the area to be excised, which is generally 3 to 4 cm (Fig. 9-83). Galeal 0 PDS II or 0 Monocryl (Ethicon) sutures or staples hold this area in place.

Next (or initially in a bitemporal flap), the parietal scalp is advanced medially and anteriorly. Again blood prints determine the exact amount of the temporal recession to be excised (Fig. 9-84). The incision line is gradually joined with the initial inferior incision in the temples. In this fashion, a horseshoe-shaped crescent of bald scalp is removed in the bilateral occipitoparietal scalp-lift (see Fig. 9-71, A); an inverse V-shaped segment with a posterior veer is excised in the bitemporal lift (see Fig. 9-71, B).

CLOSURE METHODS: PREVENTION OF STRETCHBACK

Once the bald scalp has been overlapped and excised, subcutaneous closure is effected with approximately 10 to 12 "figure-of-eight" 0 PDS II sutures. Deep bites into the galea, especially posteriorly, help to ensure a narrow suture line. Stretchback is avoided by the fact that the remaining bald scalp is not undermined and by the fact that stretch vectors range in several different directions. One or more retention sutures of 2-0 Ethibond (Ethicon) or tensed Silastic-Dacron strips can be tunneled under the remaining bald crown in the initial bilateral occipitoparietal flap operation to further deter stretchback (Fig. 9-85). The wound edges have long since healed by the time the PDS sutures dissolve (generally 2 to 3 months). In addition, the use of a contractile implant similar to the Sure-Closure, as described in Chapter 9, Part E can be used. Alternatively, a scalp extender, as described by Frechet, can be placed under the central bald area to enhance the stretch of the hair-bearing scalp before the bitemporal lift.[25]

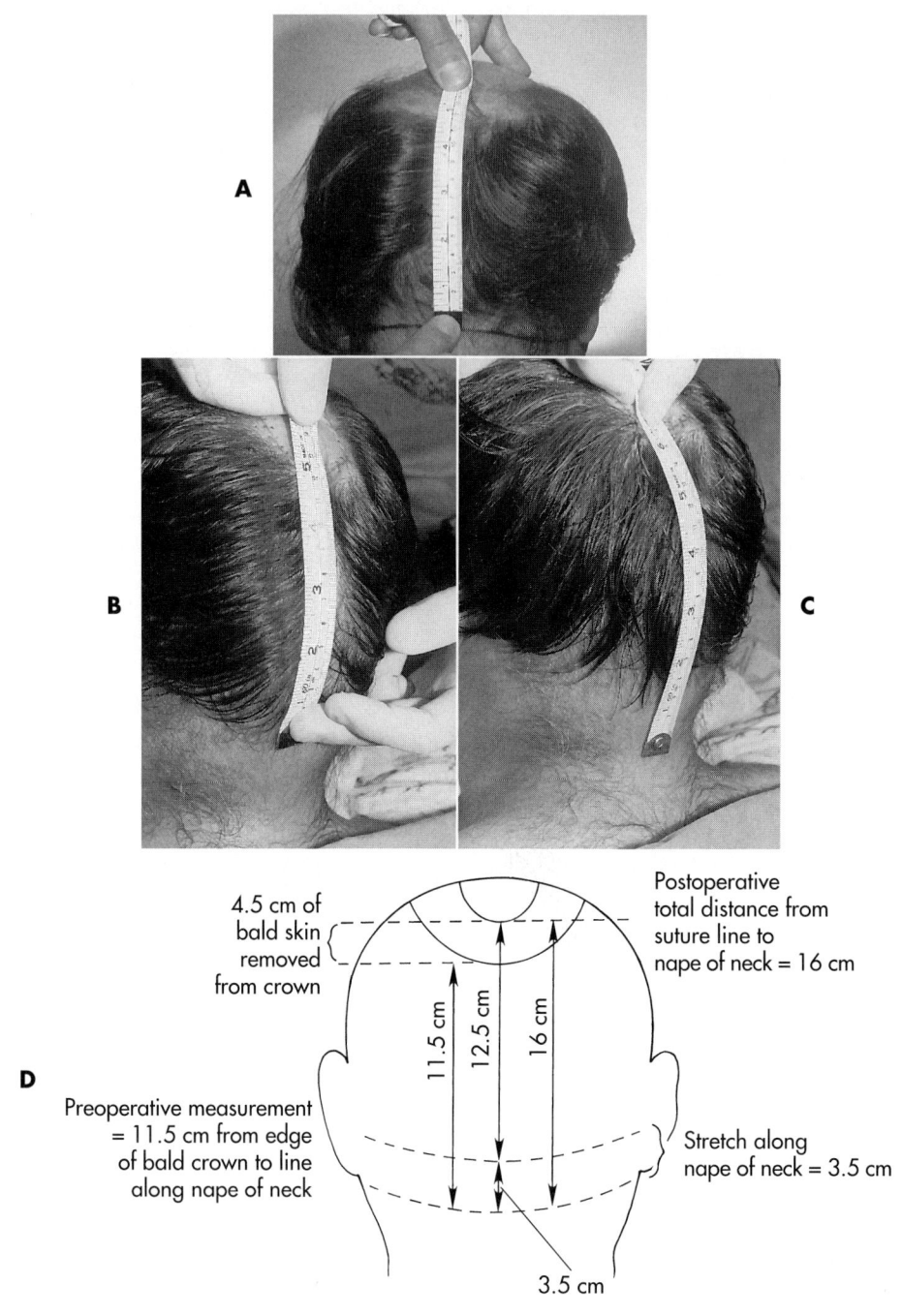

FIG. 9-81 **A,** Preoperative measurement of 11.5 cm from the posterior aspect of the bald crown to the horizontal line along the nape of the neck drawn from earlobe to earlobe. **B,** Same measurement postoperatively equals 12.5 cm. **C,** Measurement from the posterior incision line to the new line drawn from earlobe to earlobe equals 16 cm. **D,** Preoperative and postoperative measurements from a bilateral occipitoparietal scalp-lift.

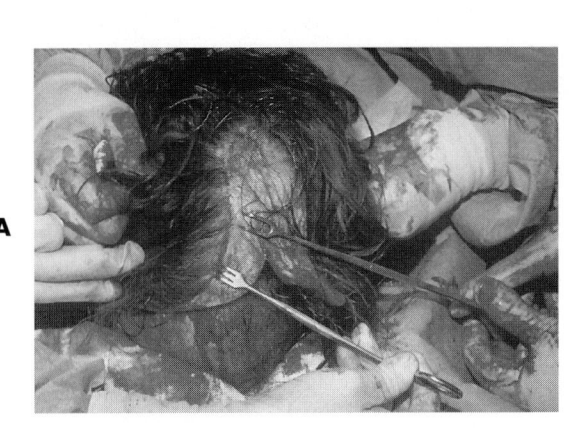

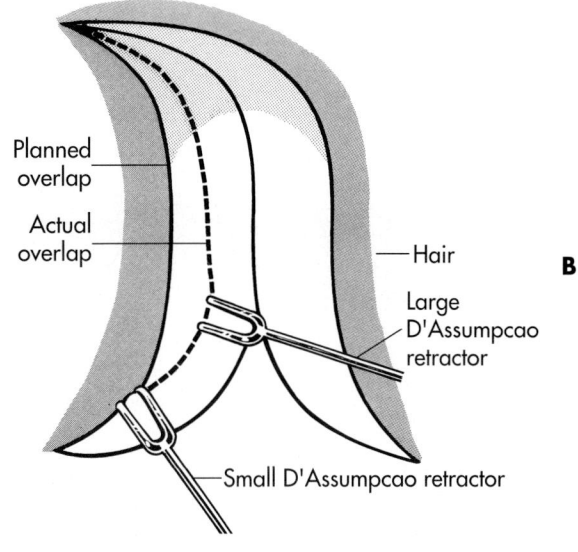

FIG. 9-82 **A,** Advancement of the bitemporal flap before excision of the bald scalp. **B,** Advancement of the bitemporal flap before excision of the bald scalp showing use of D'Assumpcao retractors. (Courtesy Dr. Dominic Brandy.)

Some surgeons close the skin with staples or nonabsorbable synthetic sutures. However, we use running colorless 4-0 PDS II because of its properties of high-tensile strength, lack of conspicuous visibility, and gradual dissolution (Fig. 9-86).

COMPLICATIONS

Should the "Ten Commandments" described herein be followed carefully, complications from extensive scalp-lifting can be minimized. Scalp necrosis from compromise of the vascular supply was described before. However, with the use of either unilateral intraoperative occipital artery ligation or prior bilateral occipital artery ligation, only one case of minor necrosis was encountered by one author (DAB) in over 200 recent cases (Brandy DA: Personal communication, 1993). One case of localized telogen effluvium on the occipital scalp with regrowth within 3 months was noted. The deep PDS sutures may occasionally extrude from the surface 1 to 2 months postoperatively. Paresthesia or anesthesia of the posterior crown secondary to cutting of the occipital nerves may last for months and may even be permanent. Spreading of the coronal scar can occur if suture tension is too tight. In some instances, micrografting will be required to cover the scalp-lift scar once both lifts have been executed.

The prophylactic administration of preoperative antibiotics and the generous scalp blood supply have prevented the development of infection. Other surgical complications, including postoperative nausea and vomiting, pain and bleeding, and hematomas, are minimal if the proper techniques as described in this discussion are used.

THE FUTURE: AREAS FOR POSSIBLE IMPROVEMENT

Improved methods for increasing the stretch of the scalp and decreasing bleeding would considerably facilitate the performance of scalp-lifting. Improved preoperative scalp massage techniques, as well as the use of inconspicuous expanders after the initial lift, could provide this advantage. Alternatively, the use of a contractile implant, hooked to the undersurface of both sides of the lateral and posterior hair-bearing scalp at the conclusion of the initial reduction would gradually stretch the hair-bearing scalp before the second, and final, reduction.

Improved hemostasis may be afforded in the future by the use of argon laser photocoagulators or by use of hemostatic laser beams during the undermining of vascular areas.

Finally, educational residency training programs, didactic courses, and "round-the-operating-table"

296 Scalp Reductions and Scalp-Lifting

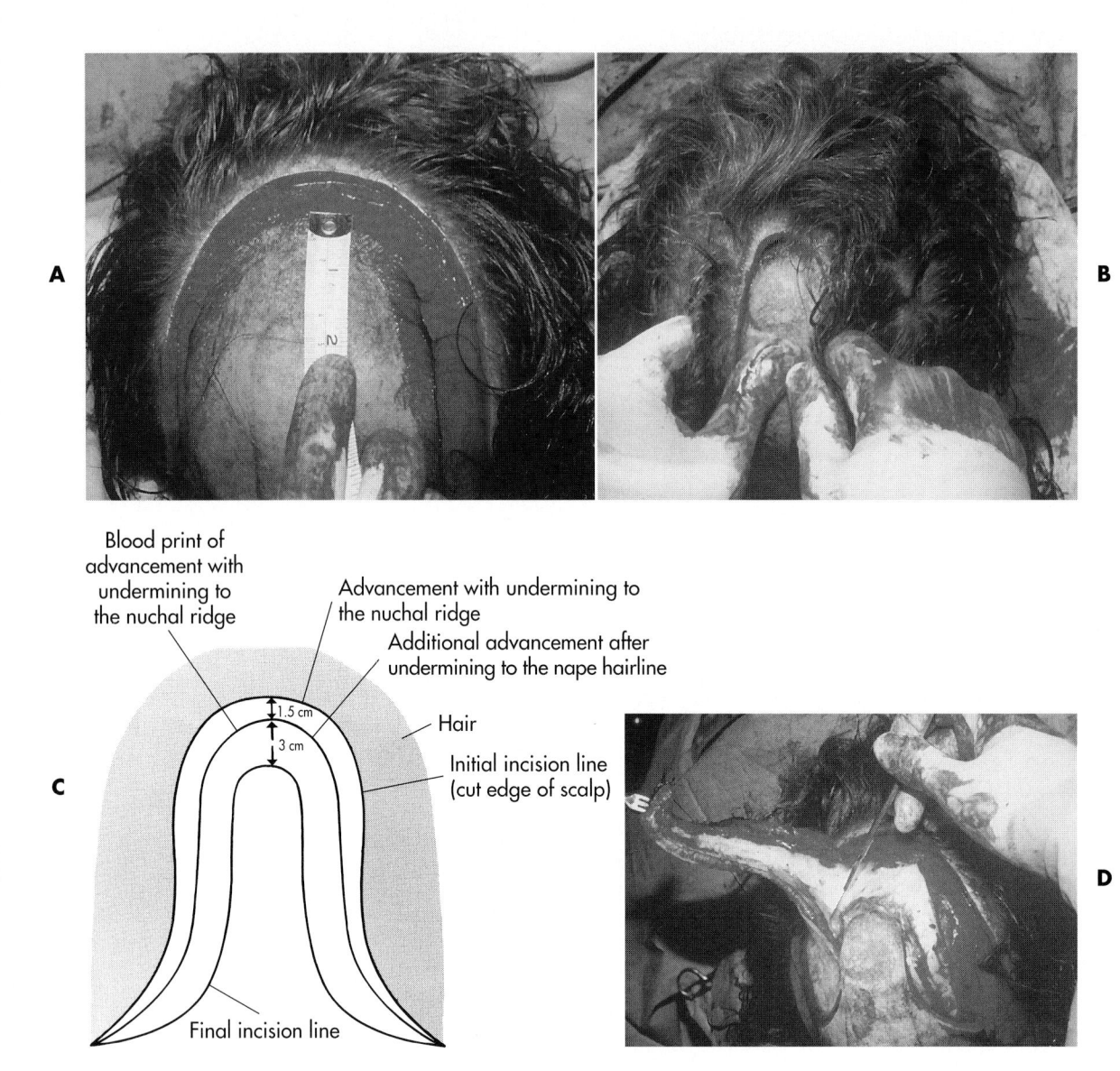

FIG. 9-83 **A,** Subgaleal undermining only to nuchal ridge without transection of occipitalis muscle produces overlap of only 1.5 cm (blood print). **B,** Full undermining to the nape of the neck produces overlap (lift) of 4.5 cm. **C,** Overlap before and after undermining past the level of the occipitalis muscle (nuchal ridge). **D,** Excision of bald skin on the posterior crown. (**C** from Unger WP: *Hair transplantation*, ed 3, New York, 1995, Marcel Dekker.)

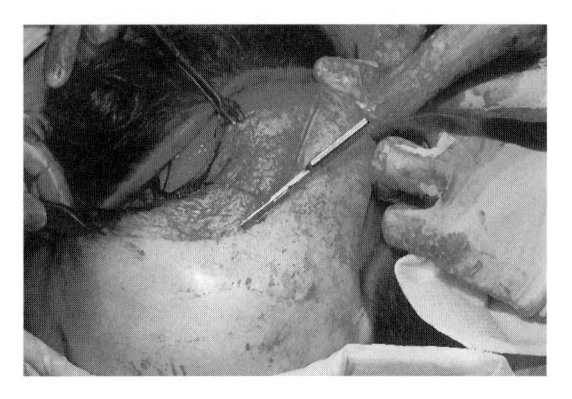

FIG. 9-84 Excision of bald skin at the temple along a line produced by a blood print.

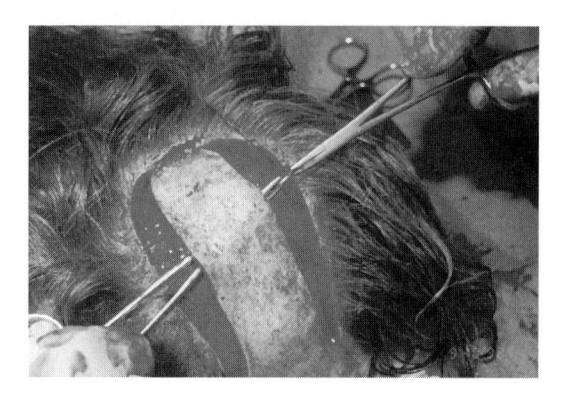

FIG. 9-85 Retention suture under the bald crown following bilateral occipitoparietal scalp-lift to prevent stretchback.

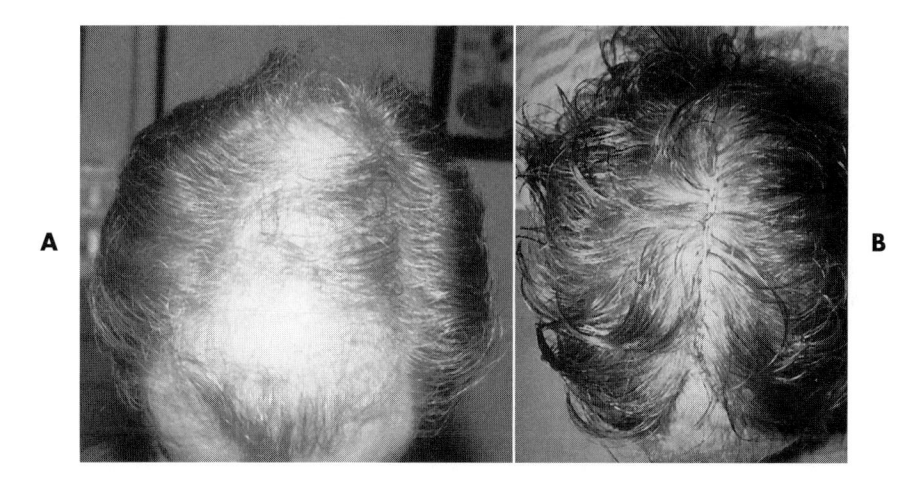

FIG. 9-86 A, Preoperative view before bitemporal lift. **B,** Postoperative view after excision of 6 cm of bald skin, uniting both parietal scalps in the midline. The area to be grafted anteriorly is now minimal.

surgical seminars would enable hair restoration surgeons to better understand the anatomical and technical considerations involved in this operation.

In summary, extensive scalp-lifting represents the state of the art in scalp reduction surgery. Careful attention to the 10 critical points described will enable the surgeon to remove maximal amounts of bald scalp with minimal adverse effects. It is hoped that this detailed description will further advance the armamentarium of the surgeon in the treatment of male pattern alopecia.

REFERENCES

1. Brandy DA: Point: extensive scalp-lifting, *J Dermatol Surg Oncol* 14(4):352, 1988.
2. Unger MG: Counterpoint: the risks of the bilateral lateral scalp reduction, *J Dermatol Surg Oncol* 14:353-354, 1988.
3. Unger MG: Postoperative necrosis following bilateral lateral scalp reduction, *J Dermatol Surg Oncol* 14:541-543, 1988.
4. Unger MG, Unger WP: Management of alopecia of the scalp by a combination of excisions and transplantation, *J Dermatol Surg Oncol* 4:670-672, 1978.
5. Bosley LL and others: Male pattern reduction (MPR) for surgical reduction of male pattern baldness, *Curr Ther Res* 25:281-287, 1979.
6. Bosley LL and others: Reduction of male pattern baldness in multiple stages: a retrospective study, *J Dermatol Surg Oncol* 6:498-503, 1980.
7. Unger MG: The modified major scalp reduction, *J Dermatol Surg Oncol* 14(1):80-84, 1988.
8. Blanchard G, Blanchard B: Obliteration of alopecia by hairlifting: a new concept and technique, *J Natl Med Assoc* 69:639-641, 1977.
9. Alt TH: Scalp reduction as an adjunct to hair transplantation: review of relevant literature, presentation of an improved technique, *J Dermatol Surg Oncol* 6:1011-1018, 1980.
10. Alt TH: Scalp reduction, *Cosmet Surg* 1:1-19, 1981.
11. Alt TH: Aids to scalp reduction surgery, *J Dermatol Surg Oncol* 14:309-315, 1992.
12. Cohen BH, Cosmetto AJ: The suture tension adjustment reel: a new device for the management of skin closure, *J Dermatol Surg Oncol* 18:112-114, 1992.
13. Sasaki GH: Intraoperative sustained limited expansion (ISLE) as an immediate reconstructive technique, *Clin Plast Surg* 14:563-573, 1987.
14. Norwood OT, Shiell RC: *Hair transplant surgery*, ed 2, Springfield, Ill, 1984, Charles C Thomas, p 207.
15. Swinehart JM, Griffin EI: Extensive scalp lifting, *J Dermatol Surg Oncol* 18:796-804, 1992.
16. Brandy DA: The effectiveness of occipital artery ligations as a priming procedure for extensive scalp lifting, *J Dermatol Surg Oncol* 17:946-949, 1991.
17. Klein J: Tumescent technique, *Am J Cosmet Surg* 4:263-267, 1987.
18. Marzola M: The Marzola scalp reduction. Presented at the Fifth National Symposium on Hair Replacement Surgery. Miami, Fla.: 1983.
19. Marzola M: An alternative hair replacement model. In Norwood OT, editor: *Hair transplant surgery*, ed 2, Springfield, Ill, 1984, Charles C Thomas, pp 315-324.
20. Brandy DA: The bilateral occipito-parietal flap, *J Dermatol Surg Oncol* 10:1062-1066, 1986.
21. Brandy DA: The Brandy bitemporal flap, *Am J Cosmet Surg* 3:11-15, 1986.
22. Brandy DA: A new surgical approach for the treatment of extensive baldness, *Am J Cosmet Surg* 3:19-25, 1986.
23. Brandy DA: A six-step approach for the treatment of extensive baldness, *J Dermatol Surg Oncol* 13:519-525, 1987.
24. Brandy DA: Pitfalls and pearls of extensive scalp-lifting, *Am J Cosmet Surg* 4:217-223, 1987.
25. Frechet P: The extender—a new tool for scalp reduction. Presented at International Society of Hair and Scalp Surgery. Dallas: April 30-May 2, 1993.

10
Complications

A. The Overwhelming Responsibility*

Emanuel Marritt

The longer I perform hair transplants, the more I realize how complicated and intricate a procedure it truly is. Sixteen years ago, when I didn't know what I didn't know, growing hair in blissful ignorance seemed so easy. In retrospect, growing hair is still easy; it's trying to make it look natural and undetectable that's so damn difficult!

Now, whenever I begin to draw the hairline on a 30-year-old grade V patient with dark, straight hair and light skin, I am aware of an anxiety that never afflicted me 15 nostalgic years earlier. It is the anxiety of awareness, the apprehension of experience.

At that moment I must be aware of the variables of hair color, curl, texture, density, present balding pattern, future balding pattern, present styling preferences, future styling preferences, facial features, forehead contour, temporary graft concealment, and, of course, the fact that hair transplantation is the only cosmetic procedure that deliberately and intentionally plans to disfigure its patients for an entire NBA season, including the playoffs!

As I step back and look at the hairline I have just drawn, I further remind myself that this hairline and the graft dispersement must look natural, not only when he is 35 but also when he is 45, 55... and 65.

That "simple office procedure" has, in reality, just handed me a life sentence of follicular responsibility. The weight of this awareness is not only humbling, it can be, at times, simply overwhelming.

---

*Reprinted from *Hair Transplant Forum International*, Special Edition, 1993, p 4.

B. Adverse Consequences in Hair Restoration Surgery

Dow B. Stough and Francisco Jimenez

Despite the surgeon obtaining a thorough history and using meticulous technique, complications will develop in a small percentage of all surgical cases involving hair restoration. This chapter addresses only those patients with poor results that can be minimized by careful preoperative planning. Correction of these problems and others is addressed by Leavitt in Chapter 10, Part C.

Complications such as unexpected drug reactions, hematoma formation, severe edema, neuralgia, keloid formation, wide scarring, arteriovenous malformations, posttransplant epidermal cysts, and infection are unforeseeable events that are beyond the surgeon's control.

POOR CANDIDATE SELECTION

Patients with dark, coarse hair and pale skin are generally less than optimal candidates for hair transplantation. Although it is possible to obtain good results in those patients with a high degree of contrast between their skin color and hair color, traditional punch autografts (≥ 3 mm) should be avoided in this subset of patients (Figs. 10-1 and 10-2).

IMPROPER HAIRLINE PLACEMENT

The most common mistakes made by both novice and experienced hair transplant surgeons involve hairline placement. Physicians often err by placing the hairline too low in accordance with the patient's wishes. Hairlines placed at a level below a point 6 cm from the glabella almost always fall short of both patient and physician expectations (Figs. 10-3 and 10-4). In general, the higher the hairline, the more pleasing the cosmetic result.

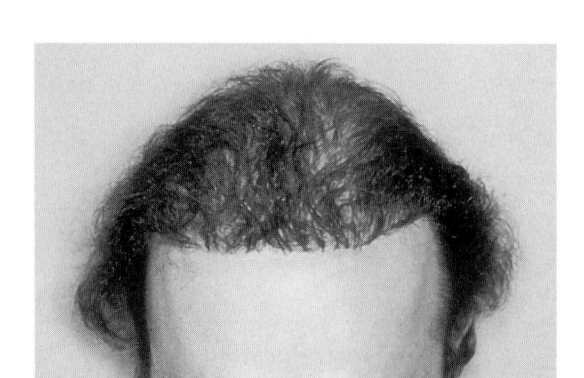

FIG. 10-1 Patient with black hair and pale skin. In addition to using large 4 mm autografts in the frontal hairline, the surgeon compounded the problem by creating a wide, flat hairline, which draws attention to the forehead. The creation of temporal recessions would have resulted in a much more natural appearance, despite the patient being a marginal candidate.

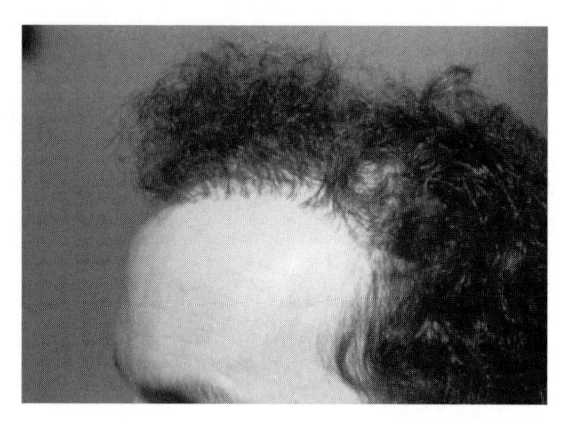

FIG. 10-2 Patient with dark hair and light skin. The patient's hair displays curl, which is beneficial. The hairline in this patient was transplanted with large grafts approximately 3.5 mm in size. Similar to the patient in Fig. 10-1, this patient's hairline is poorly drawn. The surgeon attempted to bridge the area between the temporal and parietal zones. An upward triangular recession should always be created. In this case the temporal recession has been blunted with punch autografts.

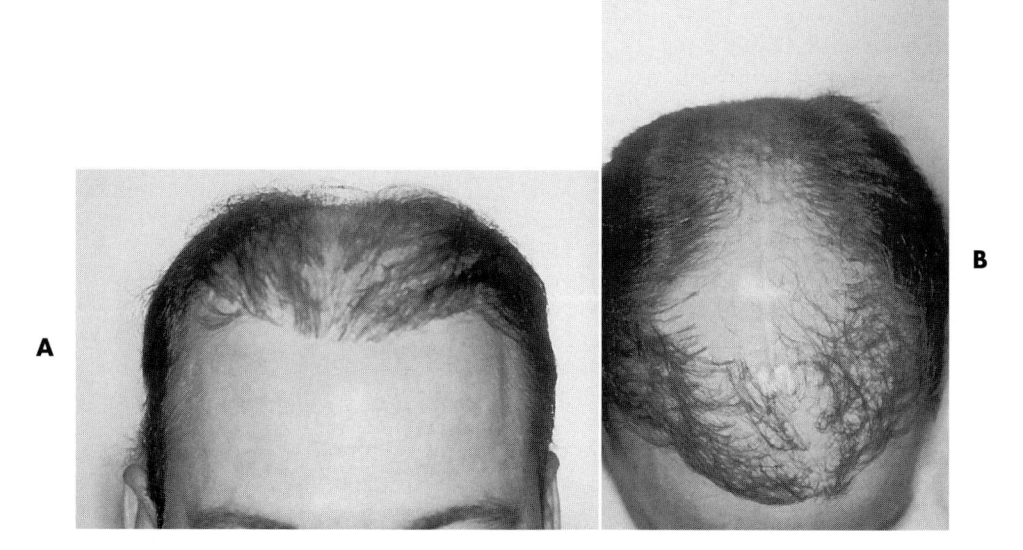

FIG. 10-3 A, The hairline on this patient was placed too low. The problem was compounded by a poor hair-skin color contrast and the lack of irregularity within the hairline. **B,** Result after multiple midsagittal reductions. Such reduction patterns will push the anterior hairline lower, making the overall appearance worse.

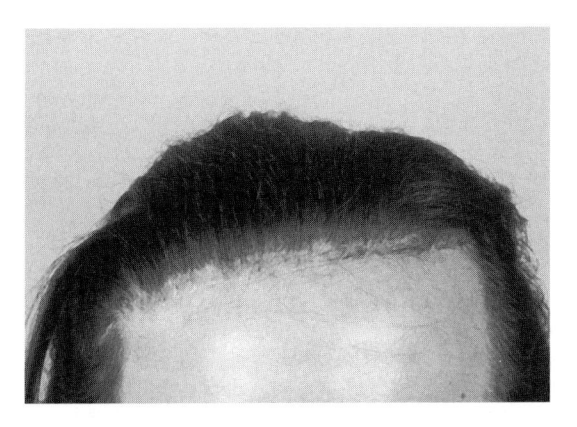

FIG. 10-4 This patient underwent a temporoparietooccipital flap. The resulting hairline is abnormal in that it is lower in the area of attachment of the flap to the base and higher in the region of the distal tip of the flap. The use of micrografts will achieve a marginal improvement.

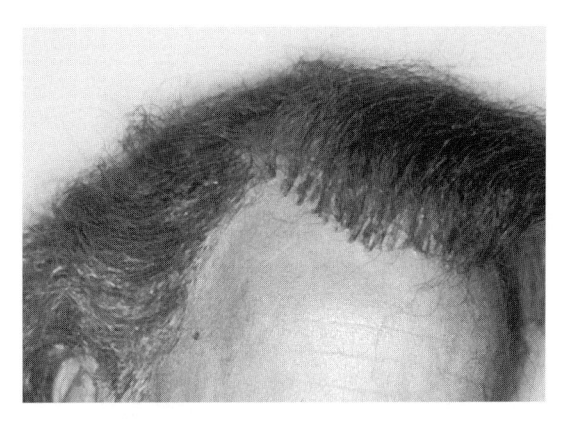

FIG. 10-5 This patient has a mixture of dark and gray hair and is a wonderful candidate for transplantation. However, the surgeon erred by placing extremely large (4.5 mm) grafts along the frontal hairline, resulting in a cornrow appearance. A partial correction could be performed using single- and two-hair grafts along the frontal zone.

PATIENTS WITH DENSE, COARSE HAIR

Surgeons generally prefer to perform hair transplant surgery on patients who have a high density of hair in the donor area. However, those with excessive density are also at risk for an unnatural result consisting of a "clumpy" or "cornrow" appearance (Fig. 10-5). This result can be minimized by a properly placed hairline and by the use of single-hair grafts in the anterior 2 cm of the hairline. In patients with high hair density (trichoscope counts of >25), caution is urged in placing any grafts that contain four or more hairs (Fig. 10-6).

BUILDING A WALL

When grafts of any size are placed in a horizontal line along the forehead, an abrupt transition appears between the non–hair-bearing area of the forehead and the scalp. In an attempt to create as dense a hairline as possible, surgeons often create a "wall" of hair. This "wall effect" can appear abnormal, even when the hairline has been properly drawn, small grafts have been used, and the patient does not have a high degree of hair-skin color contrast (Fig. 10-7). This unnatural appearance is prevented by building a soft zone of single-hair grafts in the anterior 2 cm. We refer to this technique as a feathering zone approach.

DIFFUSE VELLUS THINNING

Some patients display no frank alopecia but only widespread diffuse thinning. When the thinning hair regions consist mainly of vellus hairs, it is often

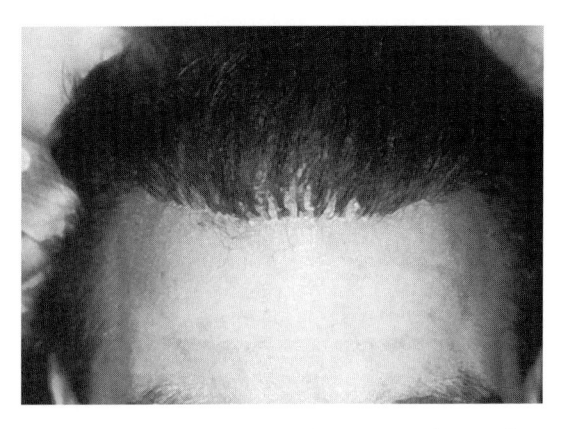

FIG. 10-6 This patient has dense, coarse hair and an abnormally low hairline. A high degree of coarseness in association with high hair density should be a preoperative warning that a poor result is likely if "traditional" grafts are used.

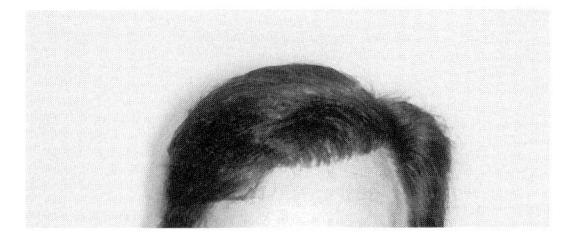

FIG. 10-7 This patient underwent hair transplantation performed by an experienced hair transplant surgeon who did not use the feathering zone technique. Despite an adequate hairline and excellent graft growth, the wall effect is readily apparent. This defect can be prevented by using the feathering zone approach.

302 Complications

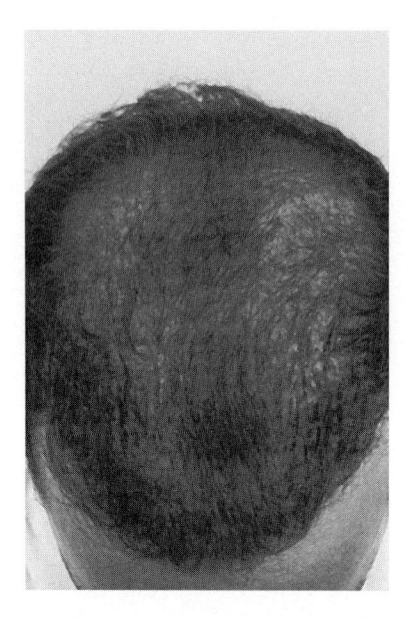

FIG. 10-8 This patient underwent successful hair transplantation in the frontal region. However, he complained that the transplant in the midfrontal area of the scalp was unsuccessful. Close inspection revealed a high graft yield of the 1.25 mm grafts. However, in the area posterior to the hairline, these grafts were not substantial enough in numbers or in density to overcome the high rate of loss and to achieve a "fuller look." Further transplanting should not be performed until more extensive alopecia develops.

difficult to achieve a significant increase in density with smaller grafts (Fig. 10-8). If a 1 mm punch cannot be used in the recipient area without transecting a hair follicle, the patient is not considered a good candidate for surgery (Fig. 10-9). Some surgeons choose slit grafting for this subset of patients.

THE VERTEX

The vertex should be approached cautiously. This region is of marginal importance to one's appearance and hair in this area does little in achieving facial framing, but it has the capacity to consume an almost endless quantity of grafts. The vertex is positioned as a transition point between hairs directed posterior to anterior and superior to inferior. The concealment of grafts of any size is much more easily accomplished in the frontal region than in the vertex area. No traditional 3 mm or larger grafts should be used in this area (Fig. 10-10). We use only grafts of up to 1.25 mm in size in the vertex area (Fig. 10-11). Most patients do not receive extensive vertex grafting (Figs. 10-12 and 10-13).

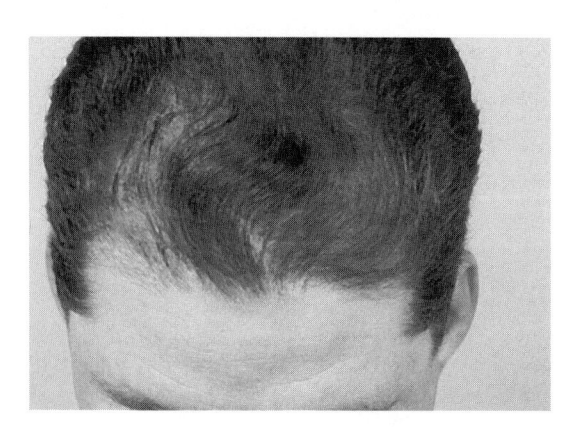

FIG. 10-9 This 30-year-old patient presented for hair transplantation with a goal of achieving a "thicker look." The patient was temporarily rejected because of the inability to produce a significant increase in density with current techniques. Furthermore, the natural hair growth is directed posteriorly and would be poorly mimicked by hair restoration surgery. The patient may become a candidate for surgery as the alopecia progresses.

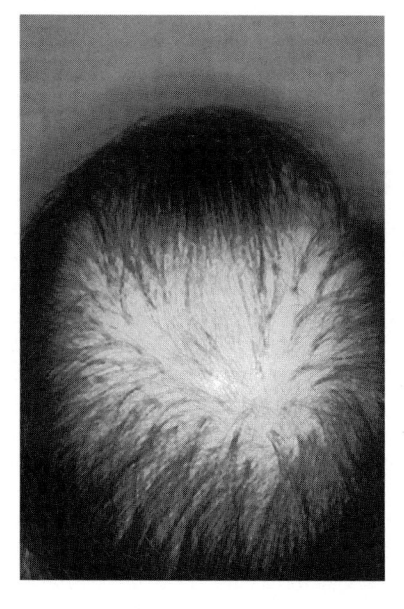

FIG. 10-10 Typical patient with vertex alopecia after attempted grafting with 4 mm round grafts. In the rare event the grafted area is concealed with transplants, the beneficial cosmetic result will be short-lived because alopecia will progress. There is no role for traditional grafts in the vertex.

LINEAR STRIP GRAFTING

From time to time, various hair transplant surgeons have advocated strip grafting. There are numerous theoretical advantages to strip grafting: increased hair density, full-appearing hairline, decreased requirement for multiple micrografting sessions, and ability to predetermine hair direction for styling. However, despite these theoretical advantages, clinical experiences with strip grafting have been uniformly disappointing.

The first author (DS) has seen numerous cases in which strip grafting failed to produce significant hair growth. The consistency of hair growth, even within an individual strip, is quite variable and often poor compared with other modalities (Fig. 10-14). Fortunately, strip graft transplantation is seldom practiced by hair restoration surgeons.

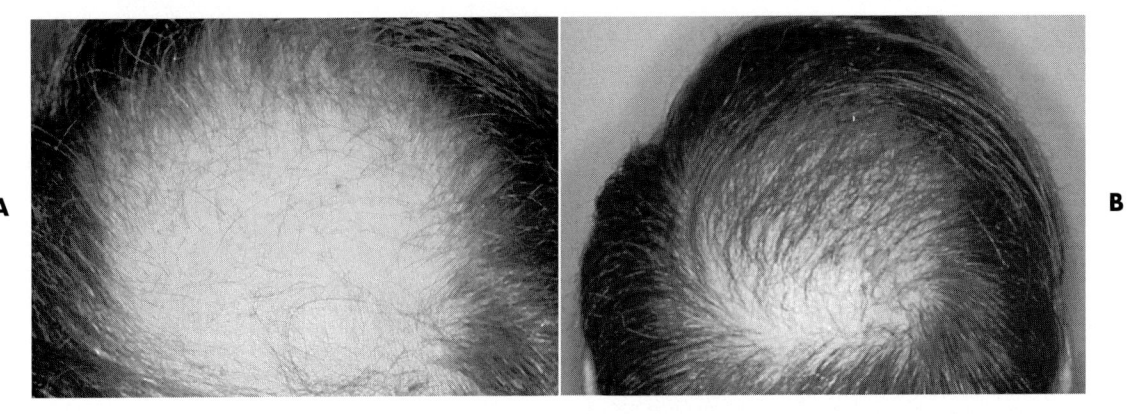

FIG. 10-11 **A,** Preoperative view of 61-year-old patient. The patient displayed a dense frontal hairline and alopecia limited to the vertex region. He was classified as having Norwood type III baldness. He had excellent donor hair density. **B,** Result 4 months after a single session of 100 single-hair grafts, 100 1 mm grafts, and 100 1.25 mm grafts. No attempt will be made to completely correct this vertex alopecia because we anticipate further extension of the alopecia. To attempt a complete restoration of this area with small grafts would be fruitless.

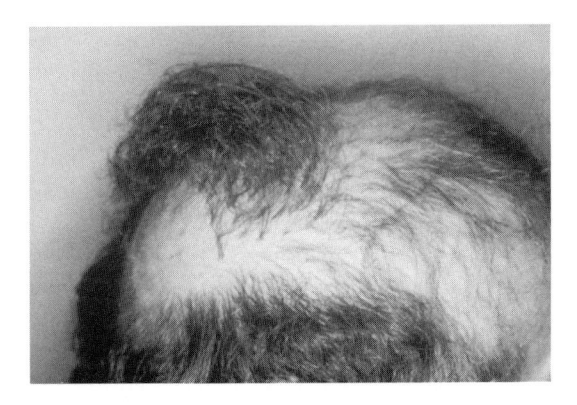

FIG. 10-12 Result 15 years after 154 grafts were placed at vertex. (Courtesy Dr. Henry Clamp.)

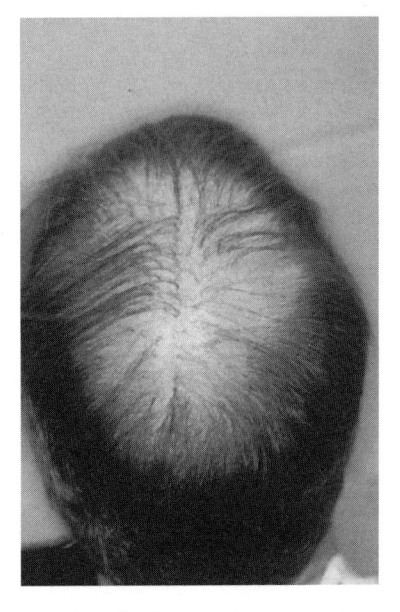

FIG. 10-13 Result 10 years after two scalp reductions and approximately 400 4 mm grafts. A linear line of grafts or "zipper effect" is responsible for the unnatural result. (Courtesy Dr. Henry Clamp.)

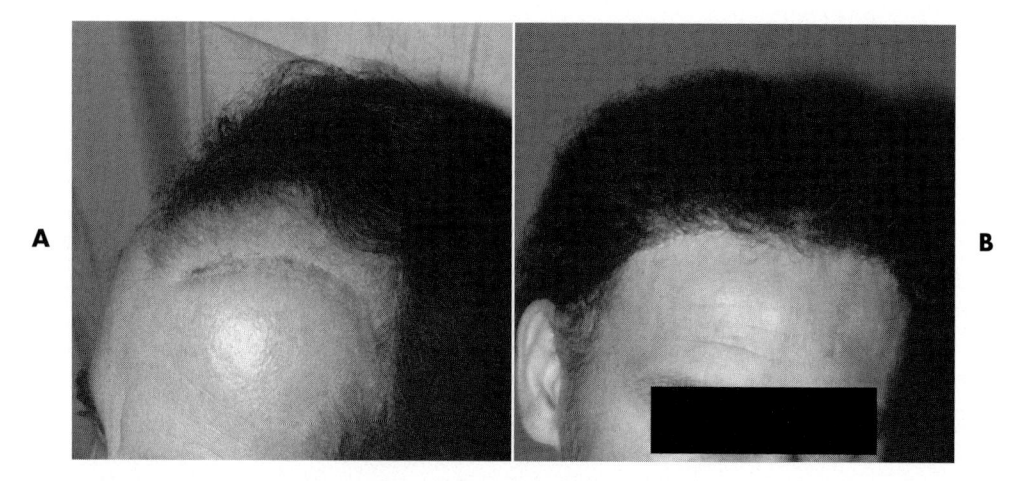

FIG. 10-14 **A,** Postoperative view 2 years after an attempt to re-create the frontal hairline using a strip graft. There was marginal hair growth. **B,** Result 8 months after repair with punch grafts. (Courtesy Dr. Marcelo Gandelman.)

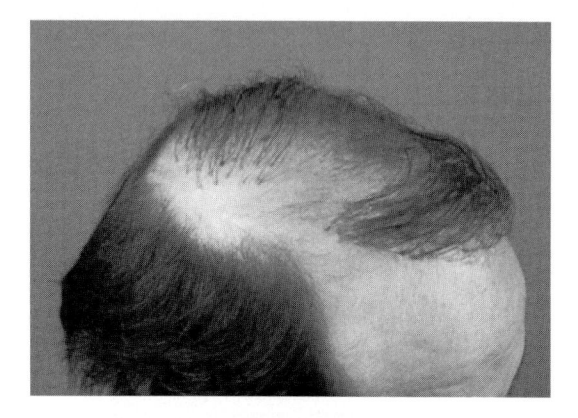

FIG. 10-15 This patient presented for consultation with the history that he had undergone hair transplantation 7 years earlier at the age of 21 years. The patient, now 28 years old, has experienced further alopecia progression, creating an unnatural result.

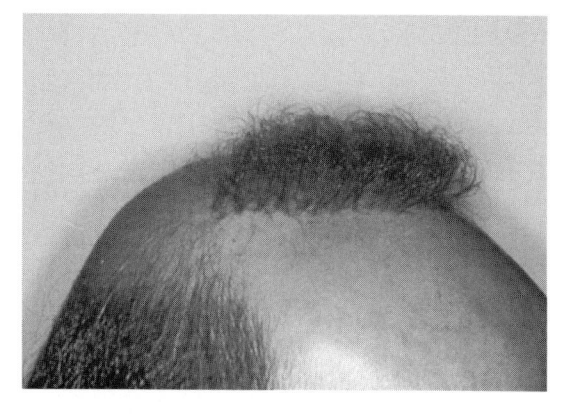

FIG. 10-16 This 32-year-old man of Malaysian descent underwent hair transplantation 10 years earlier. The temporal fringe has recessed, creating gap areas. The dense frontal hairline has now become a detriment to his cosmetic appearance. A soft, thin look produced initially would have been more advisable.

ALOPECIA PROGRESSION

Hair transplantation is a calculated risk. In the vast majority of cases, the surgeon can minimize these risks by proper candidate selection. We generally accept no patients for hair transplantation who are younger than 25 years of age. The progressive nature of alopecia is more unpredictable in the younger patient (Figs. 10-15 and 10-16). However, despite optimal candidate selection, some long-term risks exist. Patients may undergo successful hair transplants with an excellent cosmetic appearance for 10, 15, and even 20 years' duration only to eventually realize an unnatural result because of the progression of alopecia (Figs. 10-17 to 10-19). Fortunately, these severe long-term consequences do not materialize in the vast majority of cases (Fig. 10-20).

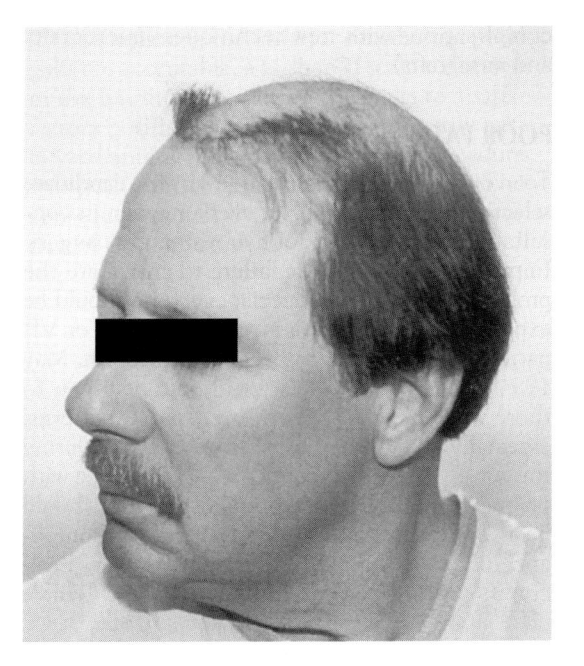

Adverse Consequences in Hair Restoration Surgery **305**

FIG. 10-17 This patient demonstrates the long-term consequences of transplanting only in the regions of the frontal recessions. The patient underwent hair transplantation approximately 12 years ago. Fortunately, he has donor hair available for approximately three more sessions.

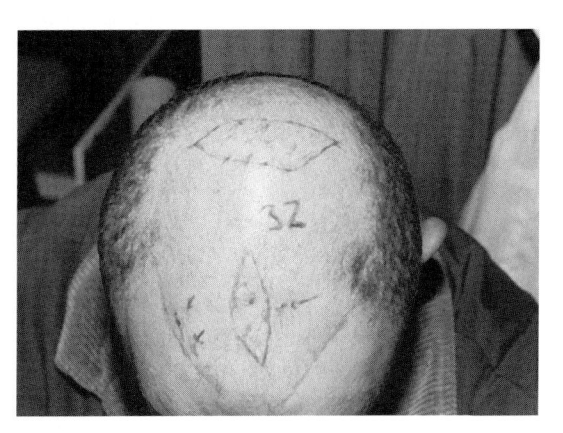

FIG. 10-18 In this patient scattered grafts had been placed at the hairline and vertex 20 years earlier. Hairline grafts have been excised, and the markings indicate lines of excision of remaining grafts. (Courtesy Dr. Henry Clamp.)

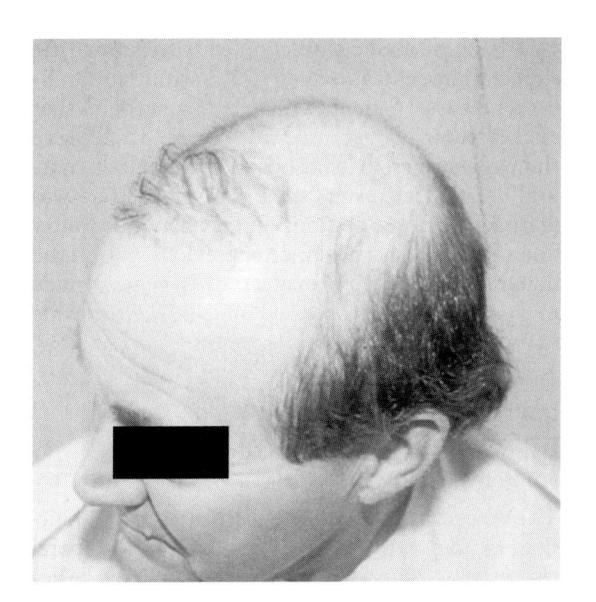

FIG. 10-19 This patient underwent hair transplantation 15 years before presenting for consultation. The patient has the appearance of a frontal forelock. From a forward angle, the transplant is quite presentable. The natural result is aided by the thin appearance and lack of creation of a "wall" of hair.

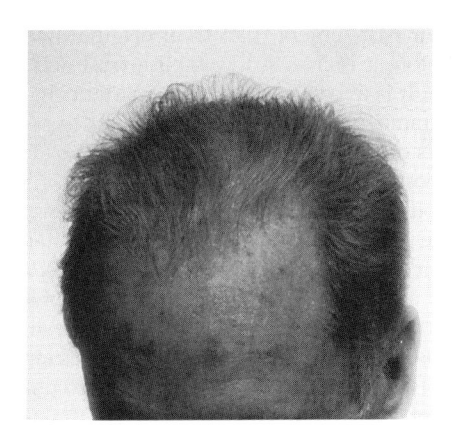

FIG. 10-20 A happy ending. This patient received hair transplants more than 25 years ago with excellent results and no long-term sequelae. Parietal hair remained and the patient has minimal contrast between hair color and skin color.

3. A low hairline can be corrected with a coronal-incision forehead lift.
4. Wedge excisions can be used to remove grafts in the temporal gulf or in locations that are inappropriately low. Micrografting is suggested over the incision lines (Figs. 10-21 and 10-22).
5. Punching out grafts and suturing the sites individually or as a group is another alternative. We routinely retransplant the hair that has been removed.
6. Non–hair-bearing grafts can also be used to replace the tissue that is removed.
7. Electrolysis with subsequent dermabrasion is sometimes used but has met with variable results. It is unsuccessful in cases in which severe scarring is present. Any excisional techniques can result in hypopigmentation and/or scar tissue. In almost all cases an aesthetic result is produced with appropriate micrografting or minigrafting or following dermabrasion. The micrografts should be taken from areas where the hair is soft and fine. Proper forward angulation and correct direction are essential, particularly in frontal hairline transplantation.

Unanticipated Recession of Temporal Area

One of the most common complaints from patients with several years between hair transplants is the large area of baldness between the lateral aspects of the parietal hairline and the temporal peaks. Recession of the temporal area should always be considered. In these patients the natural progression of alopecia was not fully anticipated. The patient's only recourse was an unnatural hairstyle to hide this defect. Historically, traditional transplants—punch grafts placed into areas of frontal recessions—were problematic in re-creating a natural temporoparietal fringe. Transplanting micrografts (one or two hairs) or minigrafts (three to five hairs) into the superior temporal region and fringe posteriorly anchors the hairline permanently and naturally (Fig. 10-23).

It is essential to transplant, even if conservatively, into areas of vellus hair. An exception should be made when a frontal forelock is planned since no transplantation will be needed in the temporal area.[2]

Close examination of these hairlines should reveal temporal angles that are blunted or barely perceptible because of randomly distributed fine, soft hair.

Hairline Inappropriately Placed Too High

Lowering a cosmetically undesirable hairline is best achieved with the use of several rows of micrografts (Fig. 10-24). If it is to be lowered more than 3 mm, minigrafts should be placed into small holes (0.5 to 1.75 mm) immediately anterior to the existing hairline. This technique produces an excellent result. Small holes are preferred to slits in the hairline for two reasons. First, the area is usually devoid of hair, and the holes remove bald tissue. Second, the holes allow for a more natural distribution of hair. Slits may result in compression of hair and create unnatural tufts. The ultimate goal is to create a natural zone of soft, fine, acutely angled hair.

Hair Transplantation in the Vertex and Crown

Hair transplantation in the vertex and crown should be performed only after determining that sufficient donor area is available to completely transplant the anterior frontal scalp. I agree with Marritt's assertion that with the passage of time, most men become more psychologically concerned about the effects of frontal baldness and less concerned about the back of the head (vertex, crown).[2] Since future hair loss is virtually impossible to pre-

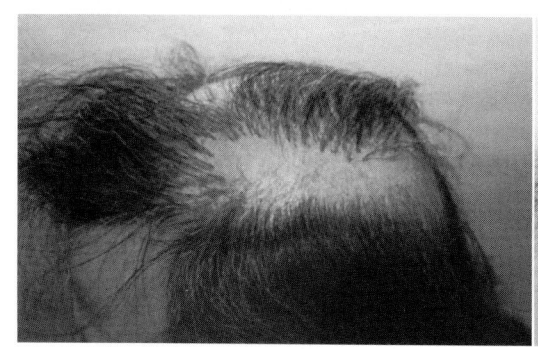

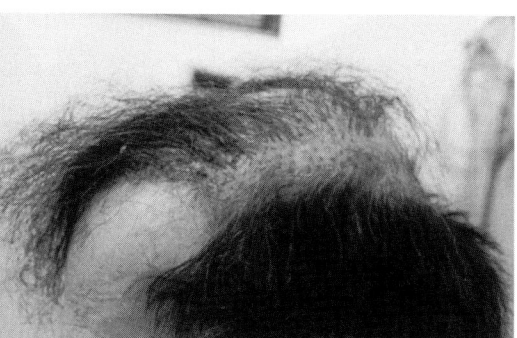

FIG. 10-23 **A,** This patient presented with recession in the temporal area many years after initial transplantation with traditional 4 mm grafts. **B,** Correction was achieved with micrografts and minigrafts. It is important to realize that some grafts will be directed almost completely inferiorly in raising the temporal zone and others will be directed anteriorly in the frontal region.

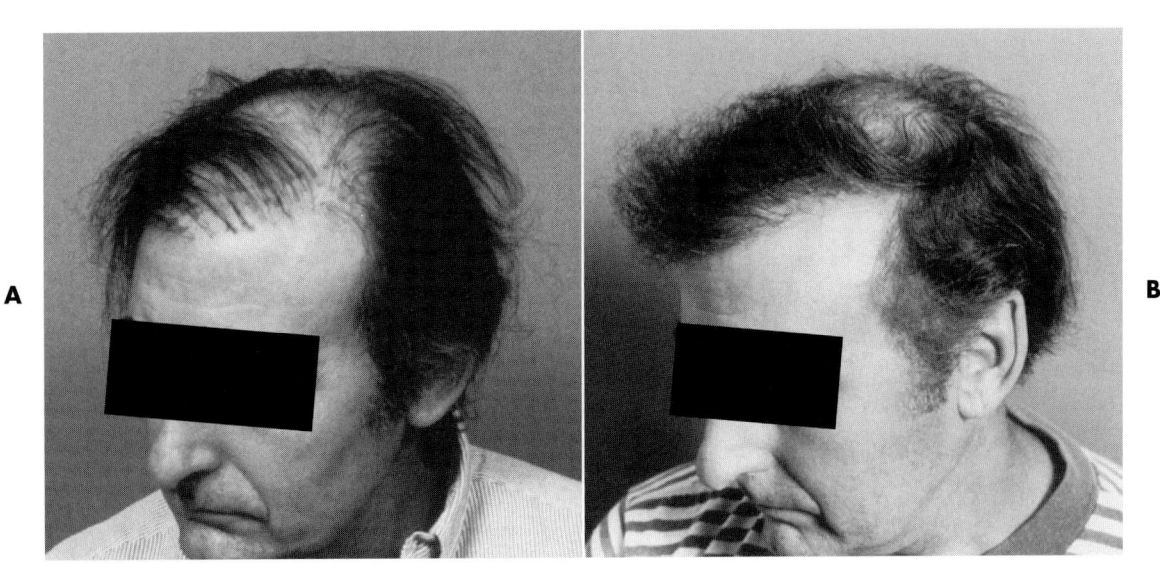

FIG. 10-24 A, This patient presented with large circular grafts in the front hairline. There was also receding in the temporal area. **B,** Correction was achieved with 120 minigrafts placed into 1.5 to 2 mm holes and 130 micrografts.

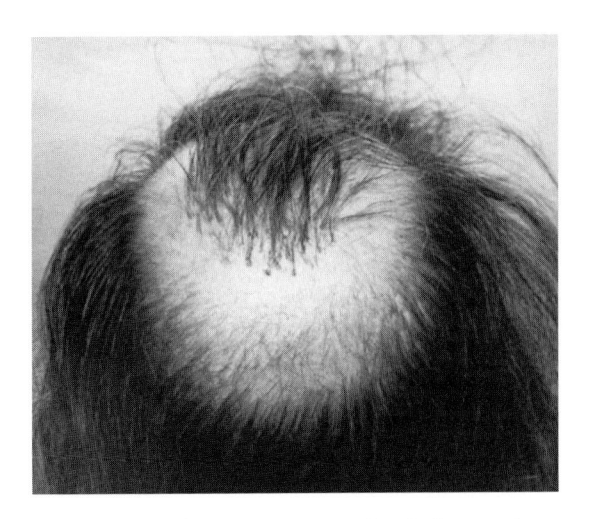

FIG. 10-25 This patient presented with the complaint of large visible grafts in the crown and vertex after hair loss in the area surrounding the grafts. A U-shaped scalp reduction was performed followed by micrografts and minigrafts to temporarily correct the problem.

dict, transplantation of the crown and vertex often results in a decreased availability of donor hair for later thinning problems, and patients should be counseled appropriately (Fig. 10-25).

A partially transplanted vertex/crown without sufficient donor hair to complete the surgery presents an embarassing problem that is difficult to hide. In rare cases corrective surgery may be performed by customizing scalp reduction incisions to remove as many grafts and as much bald tissue as possible or by punching out the grafts (Fig. 10-26). Scalp reductions can result in disfiguring scars that may magnify the problem. Removal of grafts is frequently most prudent. As noted earlier, grafts should not be wasted and should be retransplanted into an appropriate area after they are trimmed to the desired size. Punching out grafts may produce some scarring and possible hypopigmentation; this potential drawback must be weighed against the fact that the existing grafts look unnatural.

INAPPROPRIATE DONOR HARVEST TECHNIQUES

Strip harvesting can be performed in areas where round grafts were previously obtained for transplanting and where bands of scars separate patches of hair. Adjusting the blades of the knife to excise two scars and one strip of hair is most efficient[3] (Fig. 10-27). This technique results in large strips of hair suitable for micrografts and minigrafts and eliminates scar tissue, thus giving the perception of more hair. Closure of this donor site can be more difficult than with unharvested zones. Undermining and subcutaneous sutures are often required. Close examination of the density and caliber of the hair determines which donor hair is most appropriate for the area to be grafted. When the number of grafts from a scarred area is being calculated, it should be remembered that fewer grafts are obtained compared with a strip taken from virgin scalp.

310 Complications

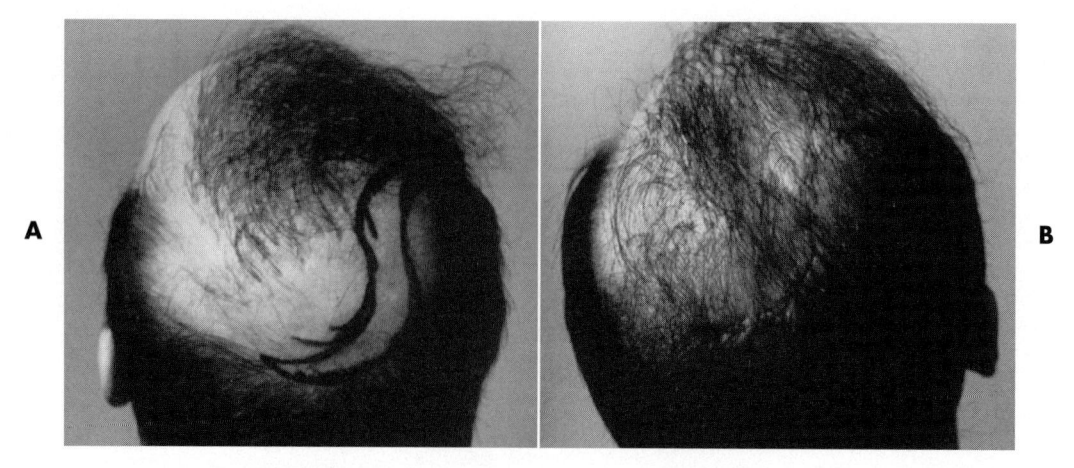

FIG. 10-26 A, This patient presented with recession in the temporal area several years after the initial transplant. Minimal donor hair existed for future surgery. **B,** Result after one modified-S reduction. The temporal recession has been almost completely diminished and there is improved coverage in the crown. Next, grafts will be transplanted over the incision and in the front hairline.

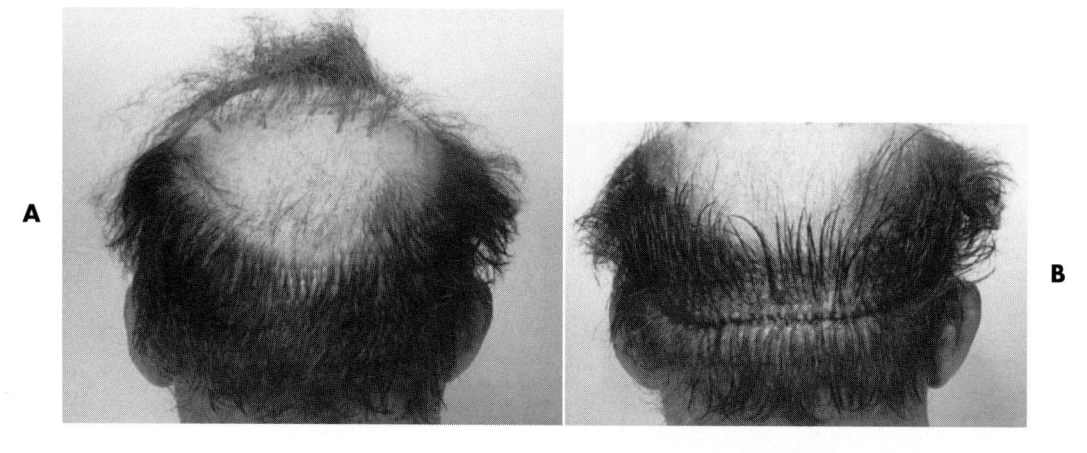

FIG. 10-27 A, In this patient, round grafts had been previously harvested from the occipital area. **B,** A large strip was excised with a triple-bladed scalpel (with the center blade removed) and the defect was then sutured closed. This technique resulted in not only a decrease of visible scar tissue but also the production of 180 minigrafts of four to six hairs and 80 single- and two-hair micrografts.

Two potential donor sites that are often untouched and may be available are the temporal and inferior occipital areas. Caution should be used in these areas because visible scars, recession in the temporal area, or raising of the hairline in the neck can occur. These regions should not be overharvested. Patients who are subjected to shotgun harvesting techniques may have excessively thin areas. The patient's hair can be wetted and then loosely combed to identify these spots. One should avoid harvesting from places genetically susceptible to androgenic alopecia. If virtually no donor hair remains, use of tissue from areas vulnerable to androgenic alopecia may need to be considered for patients in desperate need of grafts. Patients must be informed that these grafts may be lost.

USE OF OLD TECHNIQUES
Poor Growth/Hair Yield

Poor havesting techniques, such as the use of dull punches, overzealous trimming of fat from the base of the graft, improper instrument usage, and compromised circulation can all be reasons for limited hair growth and reduced yield.[4]

Patients frequently express dissatisfaction with insufficient hair density and ask for larger, thicker grafts. This is inappropriate (Fig. 10-28). The best solution for poor hair growth is micrografting and minigrafting. Patients should be informed that micrografts and minigrafts have superior viability and cover more surface area while using the same amount of donor hair. Patients who are accustomed to large grafts should be informed that a greater number of micrografts and minigrafts will be necessary to achieve desirable density. Small grafts also create a more natural distribution of hair.

Cosmetically significant areas such as the part side of the hairline and the part side ledge in the crown should be transplanted first. A session with fewer grafts should be considered if poor circulation is suspected or when transplantation into an area of cicatrix is performed. In patients who display minimal bleeding, the use of epinephrine is optional.

Poor Distribution of Hair

When donor hair is limited, it can be removed from areas that are relatively unimportant cosmetically and then trimmed appropriately and retransplanted into a priority area (i.e., non–part side transplanted into part side) (Fig. 10-29).

Ridging, Hyperfibrotic Transplants, and Peripheral Scarring

Ridging is thickening and elevation in a transplanted zone; it is most likely a result of fibrosis at and above the galeal levels.[5] Peripheral scarring refers to a ring or partial ring of scar tissue in a graft, resulting in absence of hair.

Peripheral scarring and ridging are treated by punching and inserting the appropriately sized minigrafts (0.5 to 2 mm) in the scarred region. Micrografts may be used in front of peripherally scarred grafts in the first row of the hairline.

Cobblestoning

Cobblestoning refers to elevation of a graft and involves scar tissue. It occurs if grafts are improperly cut or if the recipient site is at an incorrect depth. At the point of insertion, the graft is raised or bumpy, resembling a cobblestone road (Fig. 10-30). Conservative treatment includes:

1. Topical steroid lotions (may be beneficial if treated very early)
2. Intralesional triamcinolone (Kenalog, 10 mg/ml to 40 mg/ml)
3. Light electrocautery with careful curetement may be performed as soon as 4 weeks postoperatively or at the time of next surgery after initial anesthesia is instituted.
4. Tangential shave excision performed with razor blades (Personna Plus blades work well) at the edges of the graft; thus hairs are not injured sufficiently to damage future growth.

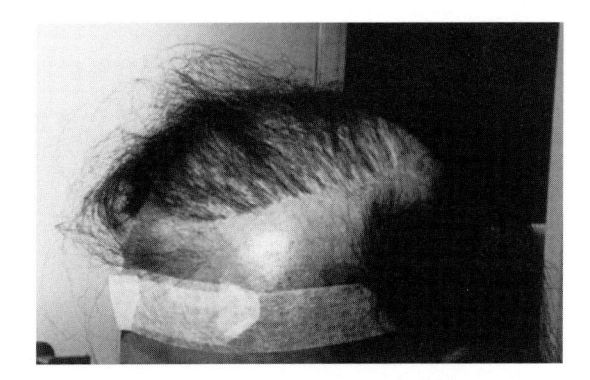

FIG. 10-28 Result of transplantation with large 4 to 6 mm traditional grafts. Hypopigmented scarring is visible in the anterior region.

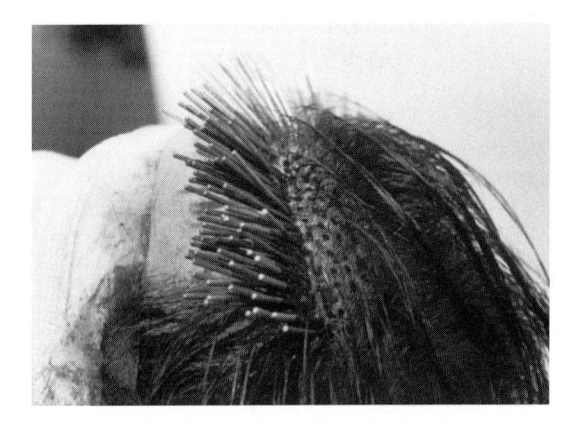

FIG. 10-29 Intraoperative view demonstrating high-density micrografts using Merritt microdilators and four- to seven-hair round grafts placed into 1.5 to 2 mm holes.

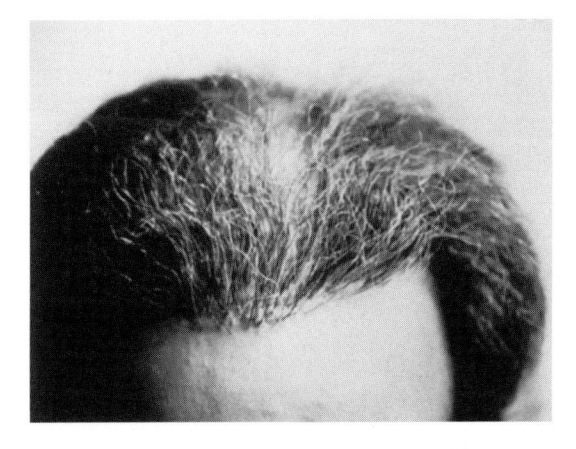

FIG. 10-30 This patient presented with cobblestoning. The cobblestoning has made it difficult for the patient to achieve a natural result.

If cobblestoning is severe, the appropriately sized punch should be selected and the graft removed, making sure that the same angle of insertion is used. The hole can be sutured or transplanted with a smaller graft. The base of the hole must be free of scar tissue.

Color and Texture (Caliber) Mismatch

Color mismatch is usually noted in persons with graying hair. Graying frequently occurs in the temporal and parietal scalp region before it occurs in the occipital area. Hair in the temporal and parietal scalp may be used as donor hair if a color discrepancy exists and the patient does not wish to color the hair.

Hairlines that are transplanted with coarse hair, particularly in dark-haired persons, are somewhat conspicuous even if the technique used is flawless. Micrografts should be transplanted using soft hair for the hairline. Single-hair micrografts are the preferred size for dark-haired persons.

Improper Direction and Angulation

Treatment of misdirected hair depends on the location and severity of the problem. In cosmetically insignificant areas, only extremely misdirected or misangled grafts should be treated. Cosmetically significant areas should be treated as follows.

ISOLATED GRAFTS. Isolated grafts that are misdirected or inappropriately angled should be punched out. Care must be given to correctly align or angle the punch to avoid dissection of hairs. If the angle is completely unsuitable, the hole may then be sutured (3-0 or 4-0 nylon should be used). In a subsequent session the area should be transplanted with the grafts inserted at an appropriate angle. If the direction is wrong, a new graft should be properly directed into the hole.

GROUP OF GRAFTS. If a group of grafts is improperly directed or angled, complete correction is difficult. Disregarding this misdirection makes styling the hair almost impossible. It is usually not feasible to cut out an entire area of grafts if the front few rows of grafts are angled at 90 degrees instead of a more acute angle. If grafts in the front row are misdirected randomly without knowledge of correct direction, the hair will form unnatural patterns.

If less than 20% to 30% of the hair transplant has been completed, the treatment of choice is to graft the remaining areas appropriately. These correctly positioned grafts will somewhat "overpower" the other grafts and allow reasonable styling options.

If 30% or more of any cosmetically significant area is transplanted with incorrect or randomly angled or misdirected grafts, a realistic goal is to blend the area. This partial correction of direction will allow easier and more appropriate styling.

CHANGING THE HAIRSTYLE. If a part side cannot be styled well and the non–part side has been transplanted to a lesser extent, the remaining non–part side should be transplanted with grafts at the appropriate direction and angulation to become the new part side. If both sides are equally lacking, the hairline should be moved down if cosmetically favorable and if sufficient donor hair exists. If neither of these treatment options is feasible, the severely misdirected and angled grafts should be removed and the area transplanted with micrografts and minigrafts.

The grafts should be directed and angled to "split the difference"; if existing grafts are angled at 90 degrees and 45 degrees is the desired angle, then future grafts should be angled at about 70 degrees. This technique creates a feathered zone and allows for easier and more appropriate styling. Micrografts are especially useful in blending areas because they can be transplanted adjacent to the incorrect grafts in large numbers without using significant donor hair.

NEW TECHNIQUES

Micrografts and minigrafts are not a panacea. Although patient complaints with micrografts and minigrafts are far fewer than those associated with larger circular grafts, problems nevertheless exist.[6]

Inadequate Density

If a patient complains about a lack of density, providing treatment and achieving satisfaction are not difficult provided the patient has been educated appropriately and has realistic expectations. Patients must be told in their preoperative consultations, and it must be reinforced thereafter, that hair transplantation is a multistep process. Although each patient determines his own desired degree of density, the natural progression of alopecia coupled with telogen defluvium may necessitate the addition of grafts in any given area. The patient must be cognizant of this fact and reminded of it repeatedly. Obviously, lack of density is corrected by adding more grafts. If the results look natural, one should not fall into the trap of trying to obtain maximum density with grafts that are too large in diameter.

Unnatural Appearance

Problems with poor growth are rare. Small grafts tend to grow better than standard grafts, but they are easier to damage.[5] It is important to remember that unnatural results may occur in good candidates even when the proper surgical technique is used. Realistically, the natural progression of baldness may overtake hair transplantation.

Telogen Defluvium Secondary to Transplantation

Telogen defluvium describes the acceleration of hair loss in the recipient region during the early postoperative months. This occurs in the final telogen stage of the hair cycle. The precise reason for this phenomenon is unknown. It may be a result of mechanical trauma, decreased microcirculation, or injected fluids and drugs.[7] It is essential to anticipate some telogen defluvium and graft accordingly. Failure to plan for this phenomenon may lead to an unacceptable result. Schiell's suggestion[7] of high-density micrografting and minigrafting to obtain a hair "credit balance" in light of the expected loss works best. This technique allows for a fuller, denser, and more aesthetically pleasing hair transplant.

"Plug" or "Toothbrush" Look

The "plug" or "toothbrush" look is less common with the use of micrografts and minigrafts. This look is best corrected by the creation of an irregular zone (feathering zone) of scattered micrografts. The surgeon must use more micrografts and fine hair in patients with coarse, dark brown, or black hair. If a patient has this problem, I recommend increasing the number of micrografts and using very soft, fine hair transplanted anterior to the hairline. In the first row, single-hair micrografts are preferred, with two- or three-hair micrografts used in rows two and three. If the hairline is already too low, the problem grafts should be punched out (they can be used in the crown or other, less cosmetically significant area) and micrografts using only the softest, finest hair should be transplanted. In this case, the more micrografts, the better.

Compression

Compression is the term used to describe the appearance of hair that has an unnatural, increased density because the grafts were placed into recipient sites that were too small. Compression most often occurs when large grafts (≥ 4 mm) are cut in half and placed into slits. It has been my experience that smaller grafts and fine, light-colored, and salt-and-pepper hair appear more natural in slits. Grafts that contain dense, dark-colored, coarse hair should be placed in small holes (0.5 to 2 mm) and contain fewer hairs (three or four) if inserted near the hairline. Correction is most important in the first few rows of the hairline. Correction is achieved by punching out a portion or even all of the grafts and replacing them with softer, finer, less dense hair. In addition, single-, two-, or three-hair micrografts should be transplanted anteriorly.

If compressed grafts are near the frontal hairline, they should be removed and replaced with grafts the appropriate color and texture. Again, micrografts should be transplanted anteriorly.

Pitting or Pinched Appearance

Pitting or *pinched* describes a graft that lays inferior to the skin, thus creating shadows and an unnatural appearance. This problem can occur with any type of graft but is associated most often with slit grafts. One should check carefully to ensure that the grafts are flush with the skin.

Popping

It is more difficult to perform hair transplantation in patients who have undergone multiple scalp reductions because they are more susceptible to graft popping. With patients whose grafts have a tendency to "pop," the reason should be immediately determined and the cause eliminated in subsequent surgeries. To help to correct the problem, the use of a compression bandage for the first 48 hours should be considered. After the bandage is removed, the patient should apply firm, even pressure with 4×4 gauze pads dampened with saline solution at 5-minute intervals several times a day. If a patient has a history of graft elevation, fewer grafts should be transplanted in each session and the grafts should be spaced farther apart. Treatment for popping and resultant cobblestoning is the same as that described for circular grafts (see p. 311).

A FINAL THOUGHT

Performing corrective surgery and doing it well are important to all of us. To quote Dr. O'Tar Norwood: "Good results go unnoticed, but bad results are obvious. One bad result can damage the entire hair transplant community."[8]

REFERENCES

1. Unger W: *Hair transplantation*, New York, 1988, Marcel Dekker, p 416.
2. Marritt E: Yes Virginia, you can remove all the baldness, *Hair Transplant Forum* 3(6):5, 1993.
3. *Hair Transplant Forum* 5(5):7, 1993.
4. Fleming R: *Aesthetic and reconstructive surgery of the scalp*, St Louis, 1992, Mosby, p 85.
5. Kabaker S: Ridging at a graft hairline, *Hair Transplant Forum* 3(4):9, 1993.
6. Schiell R: Trouble in paradise, *Hair Transplant Forum* 3(4):3, 1993.

7. Straub P: The knife, *Hair Transplant Forum* 2(4):1, 1992.
8. Norwood O: New publication aims at idea, *Hair Transplant Forum* 1(1):1, 1990.

D. Poor Hair Growth after Hair Transplantation: The X Factor

Richard C. Shiell

It must first be clearly defined what is meant by the term *poor hair growth*. Who is to be the arbitrator: the surgeon, the patient, or some third party, such as the patient's ex-wife? A patient may present with beautiful hair growth and yet have a glum countenance, claiming dissatisfaction with the results. Further questioning may reveal a marital separation in which the wife cited "your stupid hair transplant" as one of the precipitating factors in the disharmony leading to separation. Another patient may complain 8 weeks postoperatively about a lack of hair growth because he has forgotten that new hair growth can take 12 to 24 weeks to appear.

Poor hair growth is best defined as growth that is less than that normally expected by the surgeon when the time after surgery and the quality of donor hair are taken into consideration.

SORTING OUT PATIENT COMPLAINTS

Fortunately, patient's complaints are few, but when they occur, they may concern lack of hair density, donor or recipient scars, tender lumps or pimples, noticeable hair tufts, painful donor or recipient sites, lack of naturalness or "crinkle" in the newly growing hair, "picket fence" appearance of the hairline, difference in color of the new hair, and increase in hair loss since the operation. All of these situations are a source of concern to the patient, but only the first needs to be examined more closely to see if it constitutes poor hair growth.

In the past when the 4 mm graft was the standard in hair transplant surgery, hair content varied from about 8 to 28 hairs per donor plug, with an average of about 20. If there was a significant decrease in hair yield 12 months postoperatively from the growth that was noted before graft insertion, "poor growth" was easily identified. With minigrafts, however, there may be no clear indication of the size of graft used by the surgeon.

When surgeons keep careful operative records, it may be possible to assess the results objectively. For instance, if 500 grafts that each contain approximately three hairs have been inserted, a 6-month yield of approximately 1500 hairs should be expected. From my experience, such a yield is not always found for a number of possible reasons.

POOR-QUALITY DONOR SITES

With the advent of shorter hairstyles for men, it is becoming increasingly difficult to identify "whisker hair" preoperatively. This hair type is notorious for its incapacity to achieve good density or length postoperatively. Some surgeons favor the lower hair margins at the back and sides of the scalp as donor sites in an attempt to obtain hair of finer quality for the future hairline region. They not only risk obtaining whisker hair but also may be using hair that has a much shorter life span. The lower hair-bearing zones frequently become bald in later life, and the fine hair may represent hair already in transition to the vellus state and subsequent baldness. Stough and Haber refer to these "danger zones" in their chapter on donor harvesting.

PHYSICAL FACTORS

The follicles may sustain damage during preparation of the plugs as a result of drying or excision of growth centers. Damage may also occur during insertion of the grafts because of compression caused by rough handling. Postoperative damage may result from failure to establish a good blood supply or because of acute infection.

FOLLICULITIS

A severe acute staphylococcal or fungal infection may cause follicular damage, but in my experience this event is unusual. Chronic low-grade bacterial folliculitus, on the other hand, may continue over months or years and is a more common cause of follicular damage and hair loss. Although chronic folliculitis is occasionally seen by most hair transplant surgeons, its exact cause has not been completely investigated. A rarer cause of folliculitis appears to be coloring sprays used to thicken the hair of balding men. This possibility has an allergic basis and resolves rapidly once the coloring agents are removed from the scalp.

CENTRAL NECROSIS OR "DONUTTING"

Central necrosis was a common phenomenon in large grafts in the past, and its occurrence with minigrafting has been argued. It is difficult to identify central necrosis in small units, but an overall assessment of the number of hairs present 12 months postoperatively sometimes shows significantly fewer hairs than expected. Whether this reduction is the result of follicular destruction, poor vascularity, or some other factor such as graft trauma has never been established.

GRAFTS TOO LARGE

The optimal size of grafts to achieve full vascularization has been disputed for decades and probably varies from patient to patient. If significant "donutting" occurred (loss of hair in center of graft with ring of viable hair remaining), it was accepted that the graft was too large, and smaller grafts were used in subsequent operations. The size differential between the graft and the recipient site is obviously important as well because compression of the graft tissue as a result of an overtight fit could prevent adequate oxygenation of the graft.

GRAFTS TOO CLOSE TOGETHER

In the past it was considered important to allow adequate spacing of about 4 mm between grafts to ensure that blood vessels penetrated to the central regions of the scalp. With the advent of minigrafts and the increasing density with which these tiny units are being inserted, these old principles are being ignored or abandoned. It is not known what the density limit is, but it surely varies between patients and may certainly be exceeded in many patients.

COBBLESTONING

Grafts that are slightly raised in the early postoperative period generally flatten over subsequent months. The patient who has persistent "cobblestoned" grafts generally has wide and lumpy donor sites as well (Fig. 10-31). This result may be due to an inherited trait in which there is a propensity to form hypertrophic scars. Hair growth in cobblestoned grafts is not as good as that expected after assessment of the donor hair density (Fig. 10-32).

POOR HAIR GROWTH ASSOCIATED WITH HAIRPIECE USE

Many surgeons have noticed that when a wig or hairpiece is worn too soon after hair transplantation, there is an increased rate of infection in the grafts. Sometimes wig wearing is associated with later poor hair growth in hair transplants, but a direct correlation between these two factors has not been studied to date. In my experience many patients have reported increased hair growth once they stopped wearing a hairpiece. No study has been undertaken to ascertain if these observations are valid and objective or purely anecdotal. If the poor growth is validated, possible causes could be low-grade infection, mechanical trauma, or increased humidity beneath the hairpiece.

USE OF SALINE PRESERVATIVES

It has been reported that some preparations of normal saline solution contain an alcohol preservative that may interfere with hair growth. With the increasing volumes of saline solution and epinephrine being used to minimize bleeding, the potential toxic effects of this solution may become significant. It is advisable to make sure that the isotonic saline solution is free of alcohol.[1]

MISADVENTURE

Improperly trained staff can inadvertently be the cause of poor growth at times. I remember well an

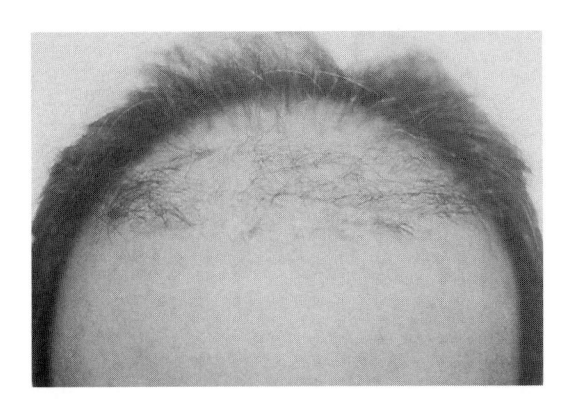

FIG. 10-31 This patient's hair was transplanted by another physician. The patient presented to Dr. Dow Stough with complaints of poor hair growth. Examination displayed prominent "donutting." The hairline was revised and reconstructed with smaller grafts.

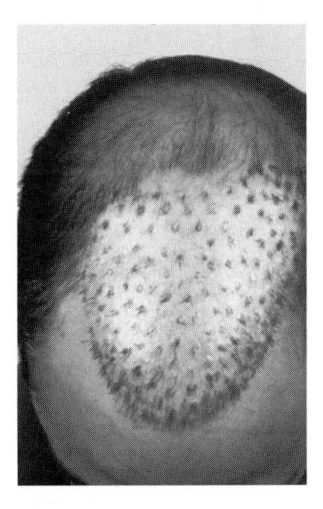

FIG. 10-32 Graft elevation and cobblestoning in a patient with traditional 4 mm grafts.

occasion when a new assistant neatly cut off "all the little black things" from the base of the first dozen 4 mm plugs passed to her for trimming and debridement. On another occasion, 50 plugs were passed to a new nurse with instructions to immerse them in normal saline solution. Twenty minutes later the surgeon was horrified to find that they had been immersed in formalin solution like all the other biopsy specimens she had handled that day.

X FACTOR

In 1984, I postulated that in addition to the known causes of follicular destruction, there was an unknown cause or "X factor" that was responsible for the loss of follicles in a small percentage of my patients (approximately 0.5% to 1%).[2]

I still believe that in a small percentage of patients the hair growth is regularly worse than can be explained by known factors such as those previously outlined. This poor growth persists after subsequent transplantation sessions and despite attempts by the surgeon to vary the operative techniques used.

Surgeons who deny the existence of this X factor have frequently not thought about it or searched for its effects because no one likes to find problems or identify failure.

Other surgeons, such as Quinlan, Stough, and Norwood, have experienced cases with poor hair growth of unknown cause. Until the cause of this poor growth is elucidated, we must continue our search for the cause of the X factor.

REFERENCES

1. Straub P: The cause of poor hair growth? *Hair Transplant Forum* 3(5):17, 1993.
2. Shiell RC, Norwood OT: *Hair transplant surgery*, Springfield, Ill., 1984, Charles C Thomas.

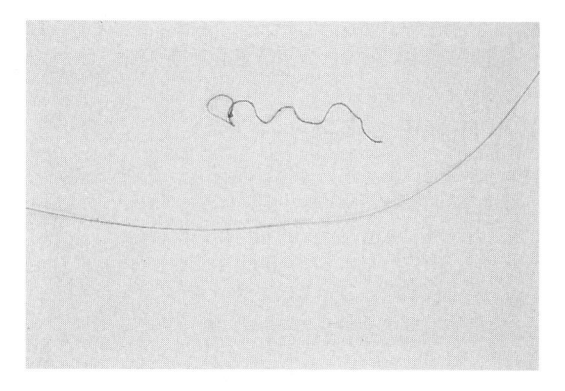

FIG. 10-33 Pretransplantation straight hair *(bottom)* vs. posttransplantation kinky, lusterless hair *(top)*.

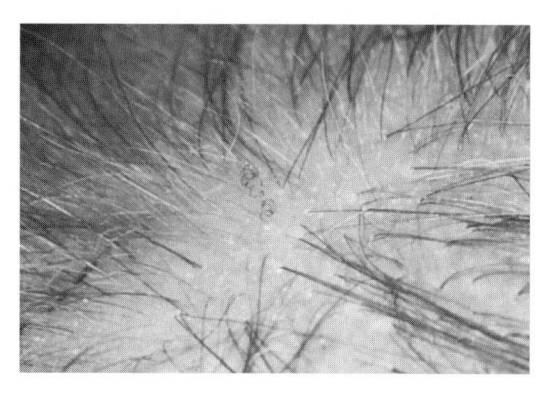

FIG. 10-34 Kinky posttransplantation hair shows lusterless sheen and difficult-to-control manageability.

E. Anatomical Hair Shaft Sequelae of Hair Transplantation

Neil S. Sadick and Ken N. Hashimoto

It is a well-known fact that after hair transplantation, a significant subset of patients with androgenic alopecia develop hair that is often significantly more kinked or wavy compared with their original nontransplanted hair (Fig. 10-33). In addition, the hair may appear to be somewhat without luster and with decreased sheen (Fig. 10-34). These characteristics often lead to pronounced difficulty in hair grooming. The lack of luster or sheen often improves somewhat over the years with continued use of conditioners or hair straighteners. This phenomenon may be referred to as acquired posttransplantation hair kinking (APTHK).

HISTOPATHOLOGICAL FINDINGS

The anatomical rationale for these changes has been studied by several investigators by means of scanning electron microscopy and routine light microscopy. These results are summarized in the accompanying box. Light microscopic evaluation has revealed that the transplanted hair has a "wavy" pattern compared with the straight donor hairs.[3] Scanning electron microscopy has revealed alterations largely confined to the cuticular layer of transplanted hairs. Whereas donor hairs have shown a normal pattern of imbrication (i.e., overlapping of the cuticular scales with characteristic spiral edges), hair shafts of posttransplanted hair have revealed a number of pathological changes. In the series of Nelson and associates,[3] hair shafts of

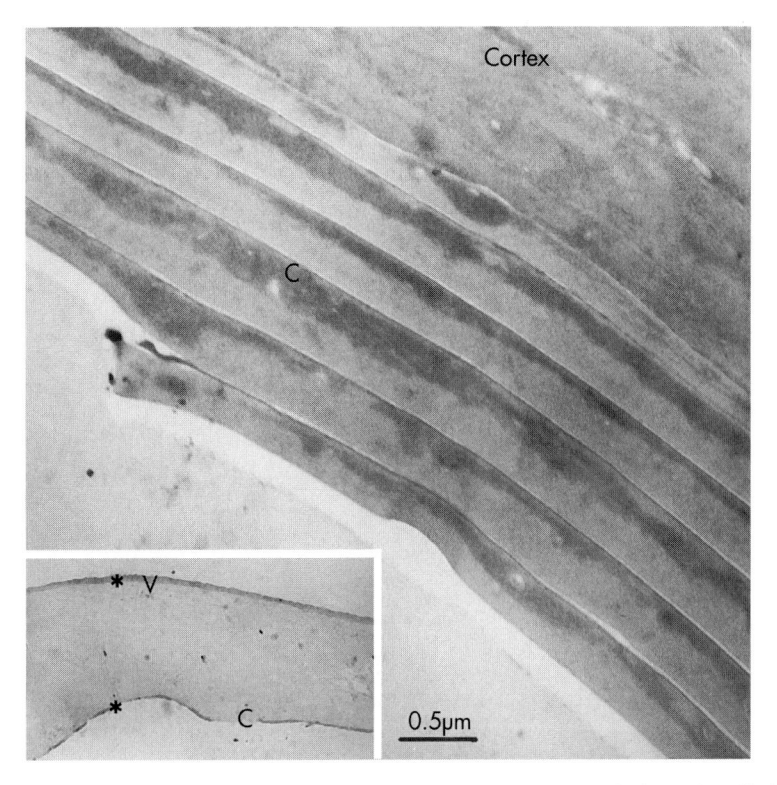

FIG. 10-35 On the concave side of a curled hair, the thickness of individual cuticle cells (C) is approximately 365 nm and the number of cuticle cells is six (original magnification × 30,000). **Inset,** Curled hair has a thicker cuticle (*) on the convex surface (V) than on the concave (C) surface. Araldite-embedded hair is stained with 0.1% azure B.

LIGHT/SCANNING ELECTRON MICROSCOPIC CHANGES NOTED IN ACQUIRED POSTTRANSPLANTATION HAIR KINKING

Light Microscopic Findings
1. Wavy pattern

Scanning Electron Microscopic Findings
1. Partially to completely denuded cuticular scales[1]
2. Loss of spiral edge of cuticle[1]
3. Loss of overlapping "shingle effect" of cuticle[1]
4. Nonuniformity of the thinned cuticle[2]
5. Decreased diameter of the concave side of the cuticles; 365 nm vs. 485 nm on the convex side[2]
6. Desquamation of cuticular scales on the concave side[2]
7. Exposure of cortical fibers[2]

---

posttransplanted hair revealed completely to partially denuded cuticular scales with a loss of the characteristic spiral wavy edges.

In the recently completed studies of Sadick, Hashimoto, and Teiscberg,[2] the curly transplanted hair had a similar number of cuticular cells vs. nonkinked donor hairs. However, there was a significant difference in the uniformity of the cuticle of the kinked transplanted hair. This resulted in a thinned, nonuniform appearance. Thick sections cut at 1 μm and stained with 0.1% azure B showed a difference in the thickness of cuticles between the concave side and the convex side, the former being significantly thinner than the latter (Fig. 10-35 [inset]). This difference in cuticular thickness was not the result of the number of cuticle cells but rather the diameter or width of each individual cell (Figs. 10-35 and 10-36). The average diameter of each cuticular cell on the concave side was only 365 nm vs. 485 nm on the convex side. Normal hairs from the same person demonstrated an average diameter of 546 nm (Fig. 10-37), slightly wider than the cuticle cells on the convex side. The cuticular cells of normal hair seemed to be more uniform in width

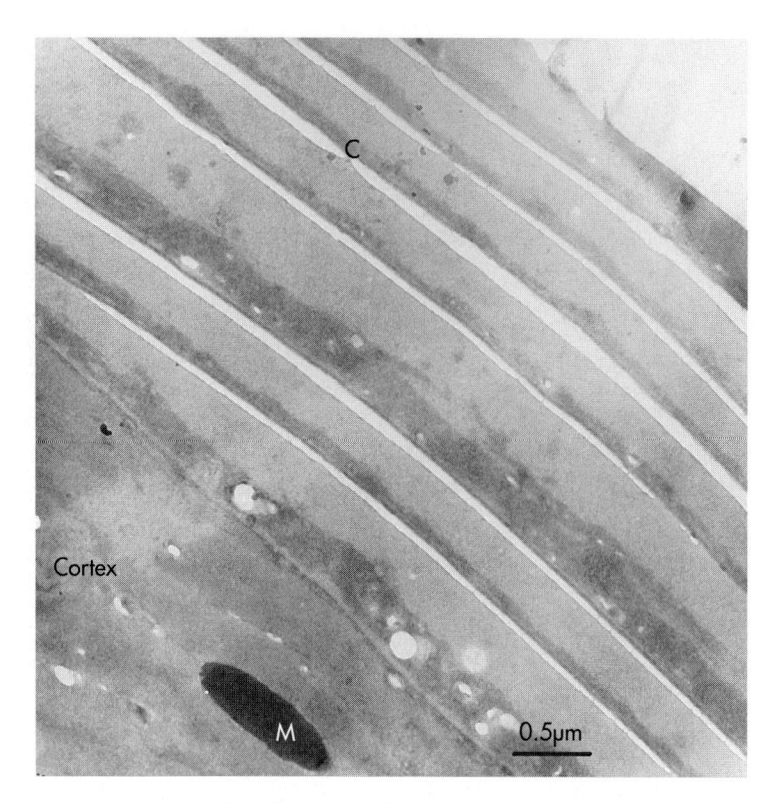

FIG. 10-36 On the convex side of the same curled hair as shown in Fig. 10-35, *inset*, the thickness of the cuticle cells (C) is on average 485 nm and the number of cuticle cells is seven. Melanosome (M) is present in the fiber cortex (original magnification × 30,000).

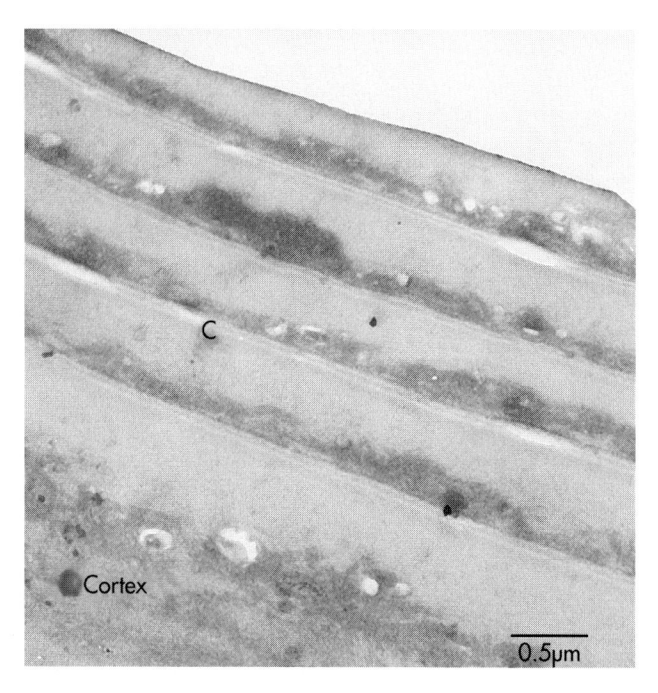

FIG. 10-37 Normal hair from the same patient. The thickness of the cuticle cells (C) is 546 nm, comparable with that of the cuticle cells on the convex side. The number of cuticle cells is five. The thickness of individual cuticle cells is more uniform than that of curled hair (original magnification × 30,000).

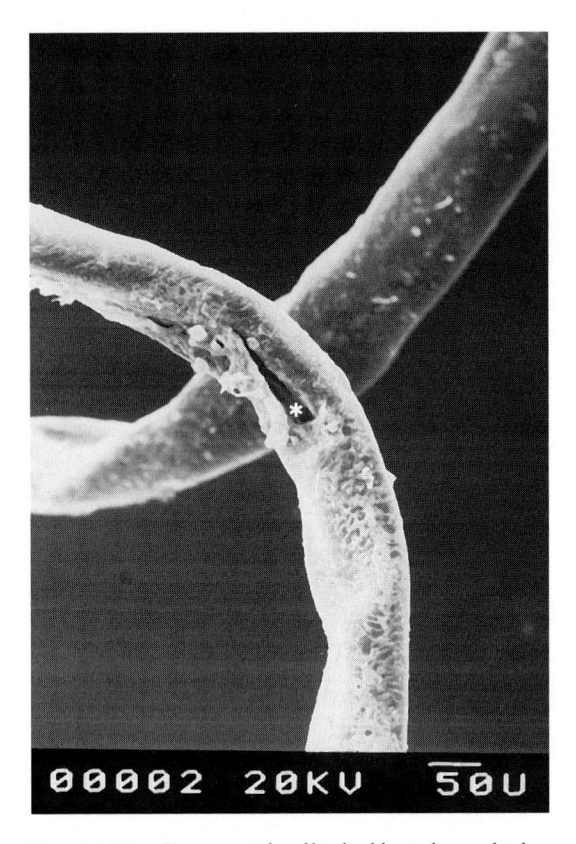

FIG. 10-38 Concave side of kinked hair shows the loss of cuticles and a breakage resulting in an exposure of fiber cortex (*).

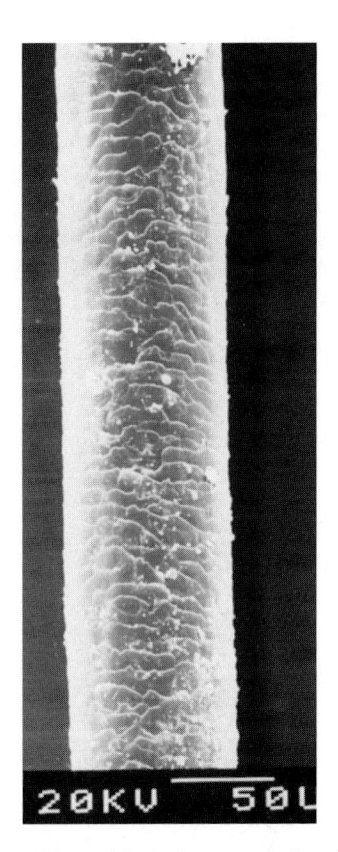

FIG. 10-39 Normal hair shows a regular, shinglelike scale pattern of the cuticle.

than the affected hairs on both the concave and convex sides. Scanning electron microscopy revealed desquamation of cuticular scales on the concave side and exposure of cortex fibers (Fig. 10-38). Normal hairs from the same patient showed a regular, shinglelike scale pattern (Fig. 10-39).

DISCUSSION

The cause of the aforementioned clinical and pathophysiological changes noted after hair transplantation in a subset of patients remains an enigma. The changes are most similar to those described under the eponym of acquired progressive kinking of the hair (APKH), a rare disorder.[4] Its onset is usually in young adulthood, and a strong male predominance has been noted. The condition is characterized by extreme curliness of the hair, mainly on the frontoparietal region of the scalp and vertex, often in association with an increasingly coarse texture, diminished luster, and striking unruliness. The hair may darken or remain unaltered in color. Likewise, the rate of growth may decrease or may be unchanged.[5-7] Light microscopic alterations have included changes in hair shaft diameter, partial twisting of the hair on its longitudinal axis, and "beading" of the hair subsequent to the previously described changes.[1,5-7] Investigators have hypothesized an androgen-dependent mechanism because of the onset of this disorder after puberty, its associated color changes, and the increased tendency for these patients to develop common male pattern alopecia. Finally, several of the patients have had spontaneous regression of the condition. The cause of this unusual trichomalady remains unknown to date.[1,5]

Although clinically similar to the findings noted after transplantation, none of the associated histopathological change noted in APKH have been noted in the patient group previously studied, which suggests an alternative pathophysiological mechanism of APTHK.

The cause of APTHK remains unknown. Although a mechanical destruction of the hair bulb or hair bulge regions during hair transplantation could be hypothesized to be the cause, only a proportion of all patients who undergo hair transplanation experience this condition. When it is observed, all transplanted hairs are involved. We hypothesize that certain persons may undergo a change in transducer signal-mediated growth characteristics, which leads to an alteration. This change could take place at the matrix level or in the bulge of the hair follicle, so that the newly emerging posttransplantation hair fibers containing the cortex and its associated cuticular structure may manifest the clinical changes herewith described as APTHK.[8] Alternatively it is possible that matrix cells of the cuticle are more susceptible to trauma or nutritional deprivation and that in certain patients or selected hair follicles the weakness is accentuated.

The lack of luster and its clinical improvement over time with the use of conditioners may be related to the filling in of altered cuticular defects by these agents.[1]

CONCLUSION

After the hair transplantation grafting technique, APTHK develops in a percentage of patients. APTHK is manifested by kinky, unruly, lusterless hair that is difficult to manage. This phenomenon is clinically similar to the previously described APKH,[1,5-7] although the ultrastructural findings in APTHK differ from those of APKH. The major structural alterations noted in APTHK, as proved by scanning electron microscopy, are confined to the hair cuticle, where irregular cuticular thickness occurs because of alterations in the diameter and width of cuticular cells. This leads to a loss of the characteristic spiral edge and overlapping "shingle" effect with subsequent exposure of cortical fibers through the breakage of the cuticles in involved hairs.[2,3]

The exact cause of APTHK remains unknown. Further studies are necessary to further elucidate the mechanisms leading to the altered histological and ultrastructural findings.

Although conditioners may somewhat improve the lusterless effect associated with APTHK and make the hair somewhat more manageable by filling in and coating the various cuticular defects noted,[3] there remains no effective treatment for this clinical phenomenon, which is often bothersome to the patient after successful hair transplantation surgery. Studies testing the effect of systemic retinoids in APTHK are presently under way in the hope that they may prove effective in reversing the trichopathological alterations noted in this clinical setting.

REFERENCES

1. Cullen SI, Fulghum DD: Acquired progressive kinking of the hair, *Arch Dermatol* 125:252-255, 1989.
2. Sadick NS, Hashimoto KN, Teiscberg SL: Acquired post hair transplantation kinking syndrome (APTHK) (in press).
3. Nelson BR and others: Curly lusterless hair: anatomic surface changes on transplanted hair shafts, *J Derm Surg Oncol* 19:1129-1133, 1993.
4. Wise F, Sulzberger MD: Acquired progressive kinking of the hair accompanied by changes in its pigmentation correlation of an unidentified group of cases presenting circumscribed areas of kinky hair, *Arch Dermatol* 25:95-110, 1932.
5. Esterly NB, Lavin MP, Garancis JC: Acquired progressive kinking of the hair, *Arch Dermatol* 125:813-815, 1989.
6. Mortimer PS and others: Acquired progressive kinking of hair: report of six cases and review of literature, *Arch Dermatol* 121:1031-1033, 1985.
7. Rebora A, Guarrera M: Acquired progressive kinking of the hair, *J Am Acad Dermatol* 12:933-936, 1985.
8. Furslind B: The growing anagen hair. In Orfanos CE, Napple R, editors: *Hair and hair disorders*, Berlin, 1990, Springer-Verlag.

F. Posttransplant Epidermoid Cysts Secondary to Small-Graft Hair Transplantation

David A. Whiting and Dow B. Stough

The insertion of a micrograft or minigraft sometimes leads to the formation of an epidermoid cyst at the graft site. The percentage of small grafts that form cysts is unknown, but this phenomenon is not uncommon. The cyst usually remains small but may become secondarily infected. We have coined the term *posttransplant epidermoid cyst* to denote that these cysts, although similar to epidermal inclusion cysts, derive their origin from the hair transplant procedure.

ETIOLOGY

The cyst is caused by the implantation of a small hair-bearing graft. Cyst formation is presumably dependent on the displacement of an epidermal fragment from its normal site, with subsequent proliferation of the ectopic epidermal cells deep in the dermis or in the subcutaneous tissue. The epidermal fragment may be detached from the overlying epidermis and implanted by the hypodermic needle used for making the recipient track for a micrograft. In cases in which a small 1 to 2 mm trephine is used to make the recipient hole for a round minigraft, skin fragments may be pushed down into the subcutaneous tissue rather than up into the trephine. This is more likely to occur when the trephine is blunt. The displaced cutaneous tissue is easily lost and remains buried under the scalp skin, where its epidermal cells can give rise to a cyst. The transplanted small graft itself may be the source of the buried epidermal cells that cause the cyst, whether the graft was implanted correctly, upside down, or just too deeply into the recipient needle track, trephine hole, or slit-graft incision. Regardless of the mechanism of implantation, the buried epidermal cells are derived from the host. They are therefore not liable to immediate rejection.

Experiments with deep reimplantation of human skin biopsy specimens into the host have shown that although some autografts are necrosed and resorbed, many others show epithelial proliferation.[1] In due course the buried epithelial cells form a loose mass of keratin, which acts as a nidus for cyst formation. More epithelial cells stream around this horny core and form stratified squamous epithelium that partially or completely encloses the keratinized center. It in turn produces more keratin and the cyst enlarges.[1] Presumably the process is similar to that which occurs in epidermal inclusion cysts that are the result of epithelial cells implanted in a finger pad, for example, by a splinter, thorn, or needle.[2-4]

CLINICAL DESCRIPTION

At a variable time after hair transplantation surgery, but usually within a few months, one or more small cystic swellings may develop at the sites of micrografts or minigrafts (Fig. 10-40). A hair may actually protrude from the cyst (Fig. 10-41). The cyst may reach a diameter of 1 to 8 mm and, more important, may become infected and painful (Fig. 10-42). The patient usually complains about the cyst for cosmetic reasons or because of discomfort.

HISTOPATHOLOGY AND PATHOGENESIS

The histopathology of a posttransplant cyst is illustrated in Fig. 10-43. In one section of the biopsy a portion of the epidermoid cyst is evident in the lower dermis, projecting into the subcutaneous tissue (Fig. 10-43, A). It contains laminated layers of keratin and is lined by a thick wall of stratified squamous epithelium (Fig. 10-43, B). The prominent granular layer indicates that this epithelium was derived from surface epidermis, follicular infundibulum, sebaceous duct, or acrosyringium. Further sections of the biopsy show a transplanted hair follicle positioned horizontally in the subcutaneous tissue (Fig. 10-43, C). The follicular infundibulum and its adjacent epidermis around one end of the transplanted hair are clearly visible (Fig. 10-43, D), and the cyst appears to have arisen from this portion of the follicle. The buried hair has provoked a foreign body reaction around it consisting of lymphocytes, histocytes, neutrophils, plasma cells, and foreign body giant cells (Fig. 10-43, D and E). This type of reaction is consistently seen when fragments

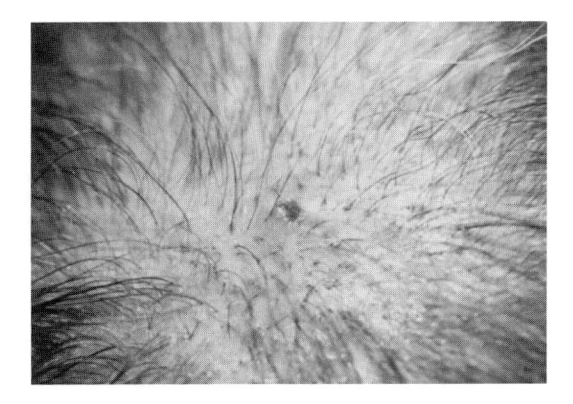

FIG. 10-40 Small domed cyst with overlying crust at the site of micrografts.

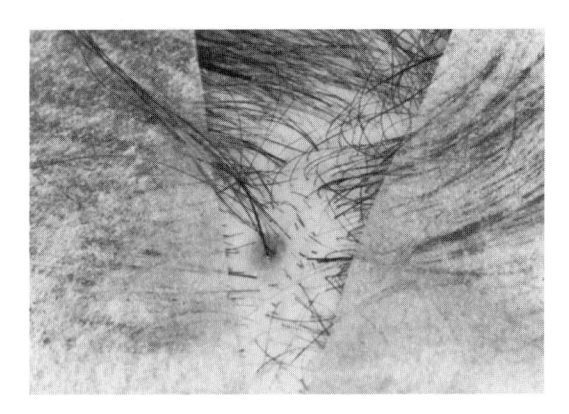

FIG. 10-41 A clump of hair from a small graft protrudes through a posttransplant cyst.

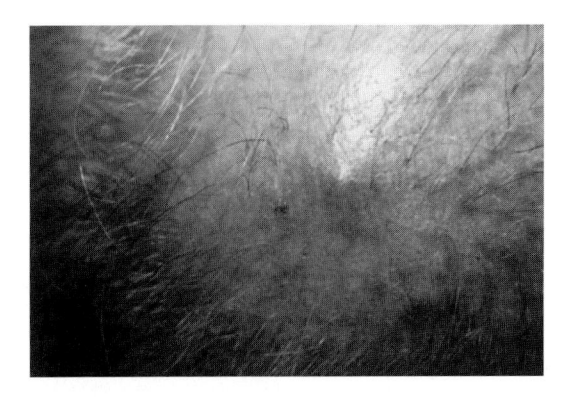

FIG. 10-42 Infected cyst secondary to micrografting shows erythema and swelling.

322 Complications

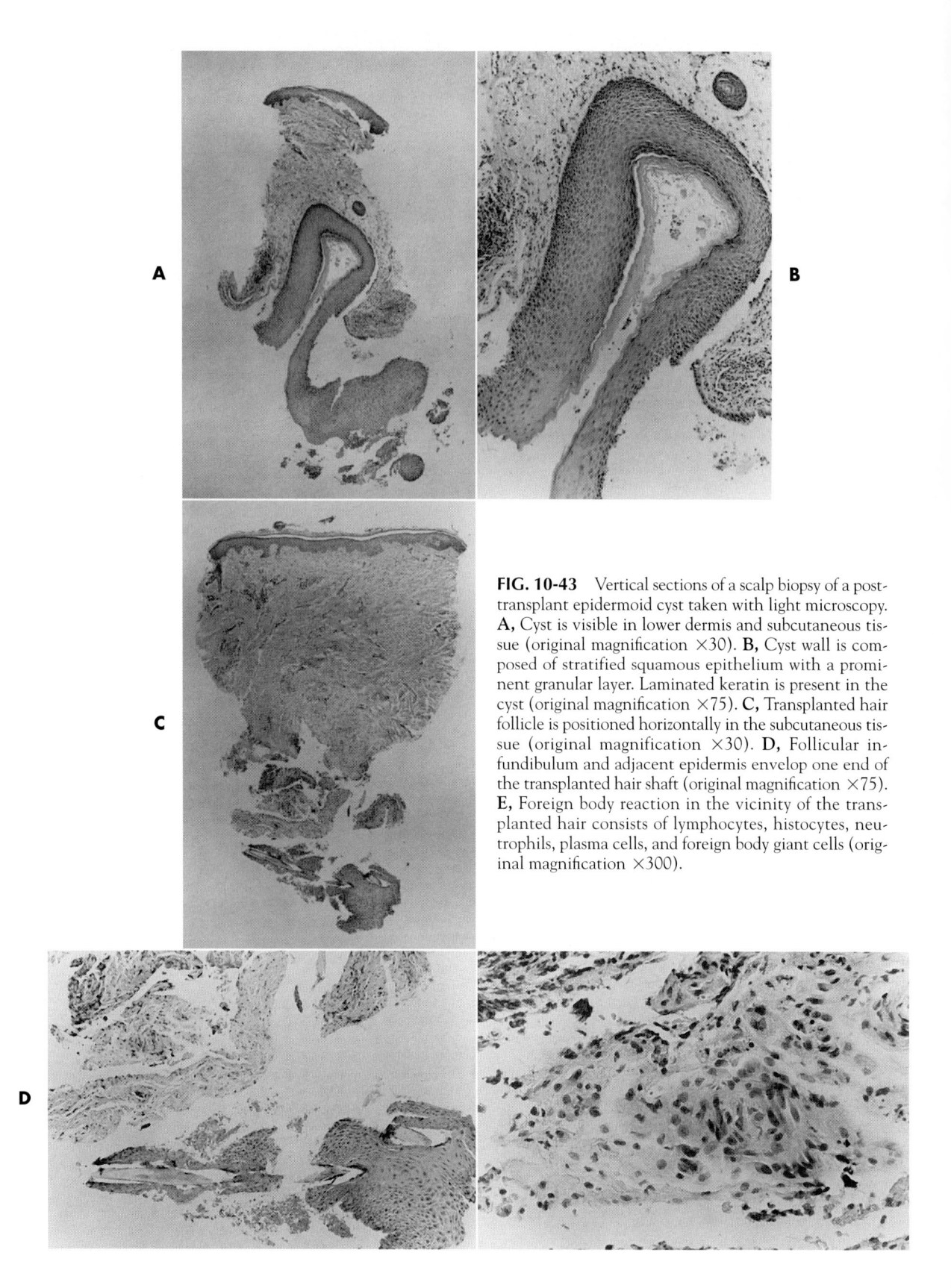

FIG. 10-43 Vertical sections of a scalp biopsy of a posttransplant epidermoid cyst taken with light microscopy. **A,** Cyst is visible in lower dermis and subcutaneous tissue (original magnification ×30). **B,** Cyst wall is composed of stratified squamous epithelium with a prominent granular layer. Laminated keratin is present in the cyst (original magnification ×75). **C,** Transplanted hair follicle is positioned horizontally in the subcutaneous tissue (original magnification ×30). **D,** Follicular infundibulum and adjacent epidermis envelop one end of the transplanted hair shaft (original magnification ×75). **E,** Foreign body reaction in the vicinity of the transplanted hair consists of lymphocytes, histocytes, neutrophils, plasma cells, and foreign body giant cells (original magnification ×300).

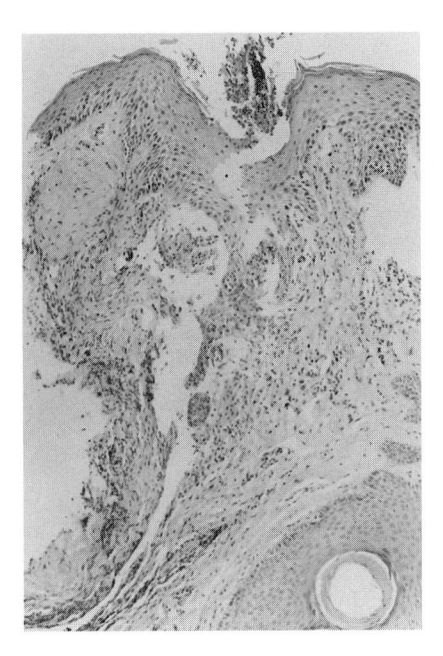

FIG. 10-44 Horizontal section of scalp biopsy of implant track after rejection of micrograft. A foreign body reaction surrounds the empty track, which is incorrectly placed at a right angle to the existing follicle seen in horizontal section (original magnification ×75).

of hard or soft keratin are released into the dermis after follicular rupture from any cause, so it seems likely that the hair transplant was damaged and follicular keratin was exposed. A similar foreign body reaction to a damaged graft with exposed follicular keratin may result in graft rejection. A section from a biopsy of the implant track after such a rejection shows the foreign body reaction involving the empty track (Fig. 10-44). Presumably secondary bacterial infection could also cause extrusion of the implanted hair. It should be noted that in some posttransplant cysts the associated hair is undamaged and growing well. In such a case the cyst could have arisen from surface epithelium implanted by the hollow needle used for making the recipient track or from fragments of skin punched out by the trephine from the recipient area and lost in the subcutaneous tissue.

It seems possible that posttransplant cysts could also result from the proliferation of epidermal cells from the outer root sheath, or trichilemma, of the implanted hair follicle. In that case the histological findings of a trichilemmal or pilar cyst,[5] or even of a hybrid cyst,[6] could be expected in some cases.

INVESTIGATION AND DIAGNOSIS

It is usually easy to diagnose epidermoid cysts caused by small grafts because they are of recent origin, are small in size, may be infected, and are associated with recent hair transplants. Preexisting epidermoid or pilar cysts, hidrocystomas, hemangiomas, and other skin tumors are usually easy to differentiate from posttransplant epidermoid cysts.

TREATMENT

If infection is present, incision, drainage, and administration of appropriate antibiotics are indicated. Uncomplicated cysts should be excised as conservatively as possible to preserve the surrounding hair transplants.

PREVENTION

With correct operative technique, most small grafts containing one or several hair follicles can be successfully transplanted. Consistently good results depend on the implantation of undamaged follicles into well-directed recipient sites. The implants must be inserted the right way up and should fit firmly but not be buried. To minimize the implantation of epidermal fragments by the needle used for making the recipient site, consideration should be given to using solid needles with perfectly ground points rather than hollow needles with jagged points. If a small trephine is used to remove a core of skin to make the recipient hole, it must be kept as sharp as possible to avoid implanting skin fragments into the subcutaneous tissue.

REFERENCES
1. Epstein WL, Kligman AM: Epithelial cysts in buried human skin, *Arch Dermatol* 76:437-455, 1957.
2. Greer KE: Epidermal inclusion cyst of the sole, *Arch Dermatol* 109:251-252, 1974.
3. Pinkus H: Epidermoid cysts or epidermal inclusion cysts? *Arch Dermatol* 111:130, 1975.
4. Wein MS, Caro MR: Traumatic epithelial cysts of the skin, *JAMA* 102:197-200, 1934.
5. Pinkus H: "Sebaceous cysts" are trichilemmal cysts, *Arch Dermatol* 99:544-555, 1969.
6. Brownstein MH: Hybrid cyst: a combined epidermoid and trichilemmal cyst, *J Am Acad Dermatol* 9:872-875, 1983.

G. Scarring and Keloid Development after Alopecia Correction Surgery

John Karl Randall and Dow B. Stough

Scarring associated with hair restoration can be seen in the donor area and less commonly in the recipient area. Scarring and slot defects can be quite noticeable in scalp reductions. Scalp-lifting can also lead to noticeable scarring. Distal tip

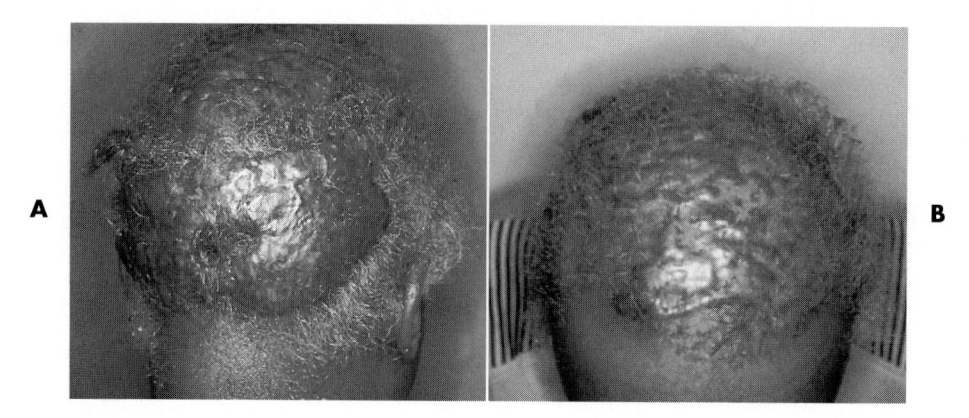

FIG. 10-45 **A,** Severe keloid formation in the donor area after hair transplantation. **B,** Keloid formation in recipient area after hair transplantation. (**A** Courtesy Dr. Marc D. Brown.)

necrosis and scarring associated with flaps are seen with some frequency.

Multiple factors contribute to noticeable scar formation including patient selection, genetic factors, and surgical technique. Scarring is the normal healing process below the epidermis. When scar biopsy goes awry, significant problems ensue.

KELOIDS AND HYPERTROPHIC SCARRING

Keloids display a genetic and familial predilection. Keloids occur more frequently in blacks than in whites.[1] Fig. 10-45 reveals severe keloid formation after hair transplantation. By definition, keloids are benign tumors that extend beyond the border of the original wound and do not regress. Hypertrophic scars show spontaneous remission and stay within the borders of the original scar.

Both types of abnormal scarring are best avoided by obtaining a thorough history, examining existing scars, and possibly performing a test graft area in high-risk patients.

Treatment

Treatment options for keloids and hypertrophic scarring are listed in the accompanying box. It should be emphasized that keloids can be notoriously difficult to treat and that surgical excision without pharmacological intervention will almost always fail. Because a complete discussion of the biology of keloids and treatment options is beyond the scope of this discussion, the reader is referred to more comprehensive resources.[2-4]

The prevention of unsightly scars associated with hair restoration is best accomplished by meticulous surgical technique and the reduction of risk factors such as smoking.

KELOID TREATMENT OPTIONS

1. Intralesional corticosteroids (i.e., triamcinolone acetonide at 40 mg/ml—multiple treatment sessions)
2. Surgery (scalpel or destructive laser) combined with pharmacological intervention
3. Pressure
4. Silicone sheeting (commercially available)
5. Excision followed by radiation therapy
6. β-aminopropionitrile (BAPN), which should be used only by those who have experience using this agent
7. D-Penicillamine, as with BAPN
8. Colchicine, as with BAPN
9. Flashlamp-pumped pulsed dye laser and intralesional steroids
10. Stanozolol (anabolic steroid), as with BAPN
11. Transcutaneous electrical stimulation of skin with TENS-like unit

---

DONOR SITE SCARRING

A problem that deserves special attention is donor site scarring. The occurrence of wide, cosmetically significant scarring in the donor area is relatively uncommon. However, some persons seem prone to developing wide scars regardless of the method of donor closure used. If such a person has dark hair and pale skin, the scarring can be clinically apparent and the patient may require longer occipital hair length to cover the scarring (Fig. 10-46, *A*).

Wide donor area scars are seen more often in the lower occiput along the nuchal ridge (Fig. 10-46, *B*). Scars also appear to be wider in the postauricular zones compared with areas more anterior (Fig.

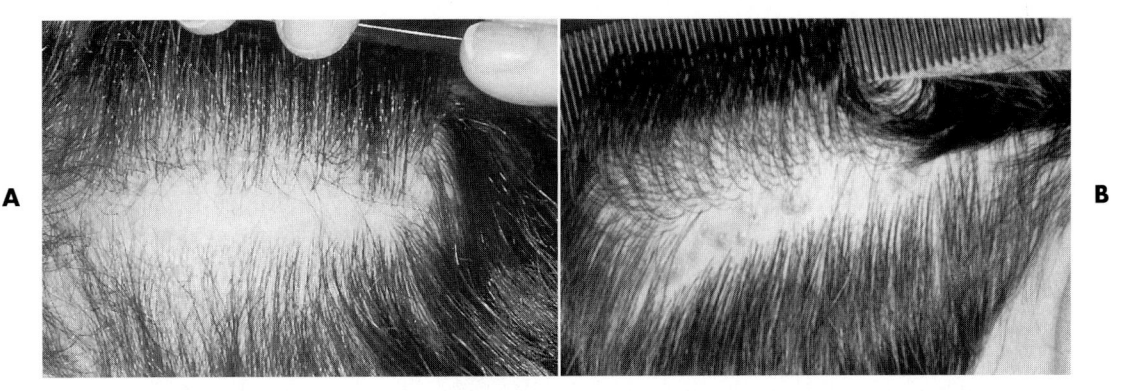

FIG. 10-46 A, Unusually wide scarring in the donor region. The scarring occurred despite meticulous wound closure with sutures and no subsequent dehiscence. Fortunately such cases are relatively rare. **B,** Wide donor area scarring along the nuchal ridge. The patient also displays a folliculitis reaction within the scar tissues. Since no deep sutures were used, this reaction may result from the regrowth of transected hair follicles.

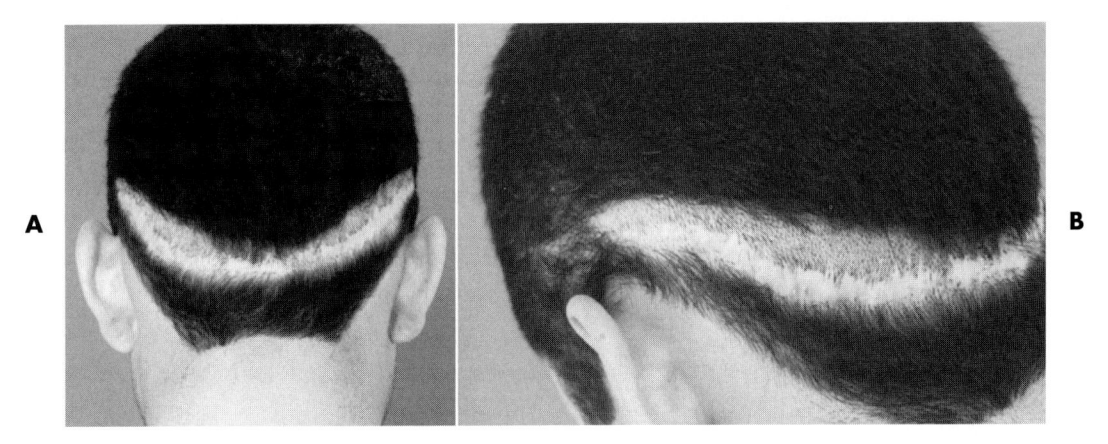

FIG. 10-47 A, Donor scarring is always more apparent in a person with dark hair and pale skin. **B,** Closeup view. (Courtesy Dr. Arturo Sandoval Camarena.)

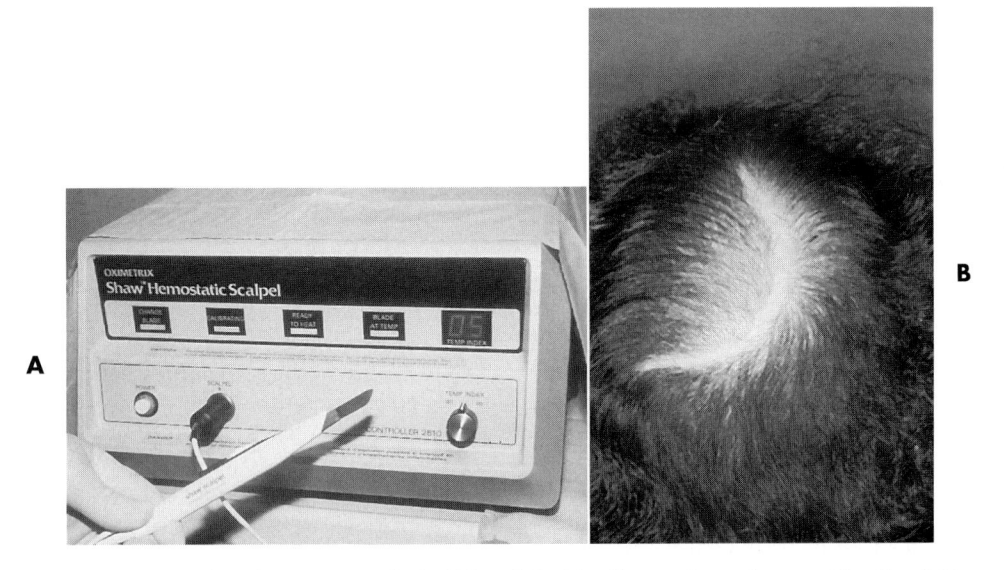

FIG. 10-48 A, Shaw hemostatic scalpel. Although highly effective for producing a bloodless field, this device may cause wide, cosmetically unacceptable scars. **B,** This patient underwent a modified-S scalp reduction in which the surgeons used a Shaw hemostatic scalpel.

10-47). We have seen numerous cases in which individuals had acceptable scars higher in the occiput and cosmetically significant scars in the lower occipital regions.

ELECTROCOAGULATION

The Shaw hemostatic scalpel has been used as an aid to accomplish scalp reduction surgery (Fig. 10-48, A). This cautery blade is highly effective in producing a bloodless field and greatly decreases operative time. We have used this device for approximately 4 years in hundreds of scalp reduction cases. Although the Shaw hemostatic scalpel is a useful adjunct to accomplishing scalp reduction surgery, it creates a cosmetically unacceptable scar in a significant percentage of patients. We no longer advocate the use of this device because of the high probability of scarring (Fig. 10-48, B).

• • •

Cosmetically acceptable scarring is best achieved by careful patient selection, reduction of risk factors, and meticulous surgical technique. Despite these precautions, a small percentage of patients will develop significant scarring.

REFERENCES

1. Brauner GJ: Cutaneous disease in the black races. In Moscella SL, Hurley HJ, editors: *Dermatology*, ed 2, Philadelphia, 1985, WB Saunders, pp 1924-1925.
2. Stucker FJ, Shaw GY: Keloids and hypertrophic scars. In Papel ID, Nachlas NE, editors: *Facial plastic and reconstructive surgery*, St Louis, 1992, Mosby, pp 53-55.
3. Cuono CB: Scars and keloids. In Jurkiewicz MJ and others, editors: *Plastic surgery principles and practice*, St Louis, 1990, Mosby, pp 1411-1428.
4. Klumpar DI, Murray JC, Anscher M: Keloids treated with excision followed by radiation therapy, *J Am Acad Dermatol*, 31(2):225-231, 1994.

H. Arteriovenous Malformation after Hair Transplantation

Jeffrey C. Weidig

Arteriovenous fistulas are relatively rare after hair transplantation surgery but can occur in both the recipient and donor areas.[1-3] Their occurrence was more common in the days of standard round grafting.[4,5] With the older techniques of shotgun harvesting, these fistulas generally developed in the donor area.

The clinical presentation of these fistulas is rather straightforward[6,7]: a pulsatile enlarging mass develops in the area in which surgery was performed.

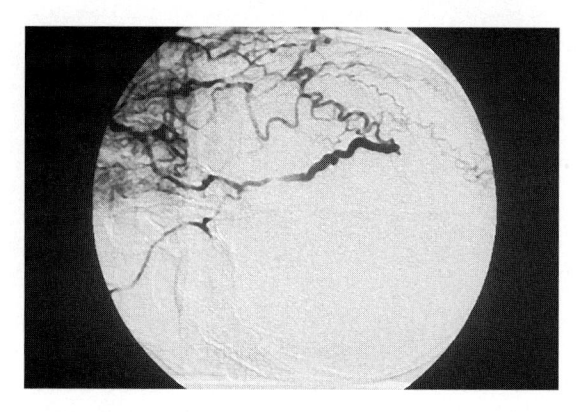

FIG. 10-49 Arteriogram of the right temporal artery, which illustrates the arteriovenous malformation.

The successful treatment of arteriovenous fistulas involves identification of the aneurysm by palpation and the placement of a large suture. Ligation may be successful and obviate the need for incision and dissection. The sutures should be left in place for at least 2 weeks.

For fistulas that do not respond to ligation, incision with complete dissection can be undertaken. Rarely arteriography may be indicated to define the extent of the arteriovenous fistula.[8] Doppler ultrasonography can be helpful in assisting operative correction.[8]

The following case is typical for its presentation but unusual in that this arteriovenous fistula developed after extensive micrografting.

CASE HISTORY

P.H. is a 41-year-old white man who initially presented for hair transplantation in the frontal area. The first two hair transplant sessions were performed without difficulty and there were no sequelae. However, after the transplant session along the hairline with micrografts, which took place 6 months after the second transplant procedure, a large swelling of the frontal vein developed. The patient noticed this problem approximately 2 weeks after the transplantation of the micrografts. The area became quite noticeable and on examination it was readily apparent that the frontal vein had now become pulsatile; auscultation revealed a bruit. The results of a repeat physical examination and blood work proved to be entirely within normal limits. The patient was referred to a vascular surgeon. The surgeon performed an arteriogram through the right temporal artery, which disclosed an arteriovenous malformation in the frontal projection (Fig. 10-49). Once the area was identified,

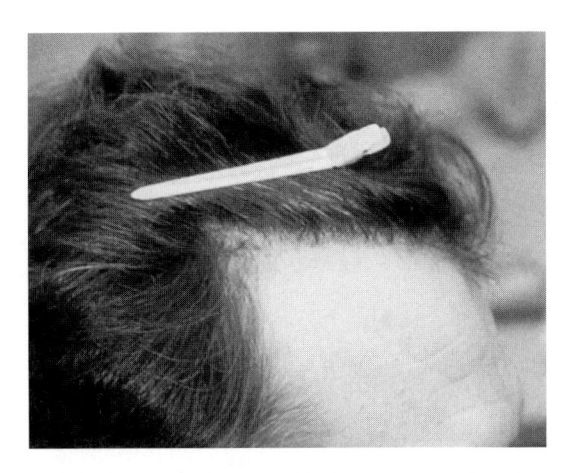

FIG. 10-50 This 41-year-old white man developed an arteriovenous fistula in the frontal hairline after extensive micrografting. Surgical excision was successfully undertaken. The patient is shown with no evidence of arteriovenous fistulas.

I. Long-Term Problems Associated with Hair-Bearing Flaps for Male Pattern Baldness

Sheldon S. Kabaker and Jeffrey S. Epstein

Hair-bearing flaps have been used effectively for many years to correct scalp baldness. Until the 1970s, most of these flaps were used to treat cicatricial alopecia secondary to burns, infections, and other trauma. During the past 20 years the emphasized application of these flaps has been on the treatment of male pattern baldness. The most popular of these flaps are those pedicled on the superficial temporal artery, conveniently located for rotation into the frontal hairline region. The temporoparietooccipital flap, which is a long flap based on the posterior (parietal) branch of the superficial temporal artery, was popularized by Juri[1,2] in 1975. This flap, which is sufficiently long enough to span the frontal hairline, is twice delayed to secure arterial and venous circulation. Numerous variations pertaining to shape, dimensions, and delay technique have been described, but the essence of the flap remains unchanged.[3-6] Nondelayed rotation of long temporoparietooccipital flaps has also been described.[7,8]

Temporoparietal flaps, which were introduced by Lamont[9] and Passot[10] and then refined by Elliott[11,12] in 1977, are short flaps that are also pedicled on the posterior branch of the superficial temporal artery. The shorter length allows for nondelayed transfer, but bilateral flaps are required to create a frontal hairline. I (SSK) have used the temporoparietal flap much less frequently than the temporoparietooccipital flap in my practice because, although the technical expertise required is equal, the potential tissue yield is much less with the temporoparietal flap. Other advantages of temporoparietooccipital flaps include the avoidance of notching in the frontal hairline where two temporoparietal flaps would meet, the more concealable sequela if necrosis of the flap tip should occur, and a single donor site that is easier to close than bilateral temporoparietal flap donor sites.

Although the temporoparietooccipital and temporoparietal flaps comprise the basic armamentarium for most surgeons who use hair-bearing flaps to treat male pattern baldness, other flaps have been described, a testament to the extensive blood supply to the scalp.[2,6,7,13-15] Microvascular free flaps, although rarely performed in the United States because of the technical expertise and extensive allocation of resources they require, are used with regularity in Japan.[16,17] The most recent advance-

the arteriovenous fistula was taken down surgically. Four months postoperatively there was no evidence of any further dilatation of the frontal vein. There was no obvious arteriovenous fistula, and a photograph of the area revealed complete resolution (Fig. 10-50). Subsequent hair transplantation in this same area with micrografts has produced no abnormality, and in fact the patient is satisfied with the result.

REFERENCES

1. Semashko D and others: Arteriovenous fistula following punch-graft hair transplantation, *Derm Surg Oncol* 15:754-755, 1989.
2. Barros AAJ, Heard GE: Arteriovenous fistula after hair transplantation, *Br Med J* 1:340-341, 1978.
3. Stough DB: Complications of hair transplantation, *Cutis* 6:645-651, 1970.
4. Orentreich N: Hair transplantation: the punch-graft technique, *Surg Clin North Am* 51:511-518, 1971.
5. Norwood OT: Arteriovenous fistulae resulting from hair transplant surgery, *Cutis* 8:263-264, 1971.
6. Lanzieri CF and others: Arteriovenous fistula after hair transplantation, *AJNR Am J Neuroradiol* 6:111-112, 1985.
7. Souder DE, Beauregard LB: Arteriovenous fistula secondary to hair transplantation, *N Engl J Med* 283:473-474, 1970.
8. Williams LR, Robinson JK, Yao JST: Hair transplantation producing arteriovenous fistulization, *Ann Vasc Surg* 1:241-243, 1986.

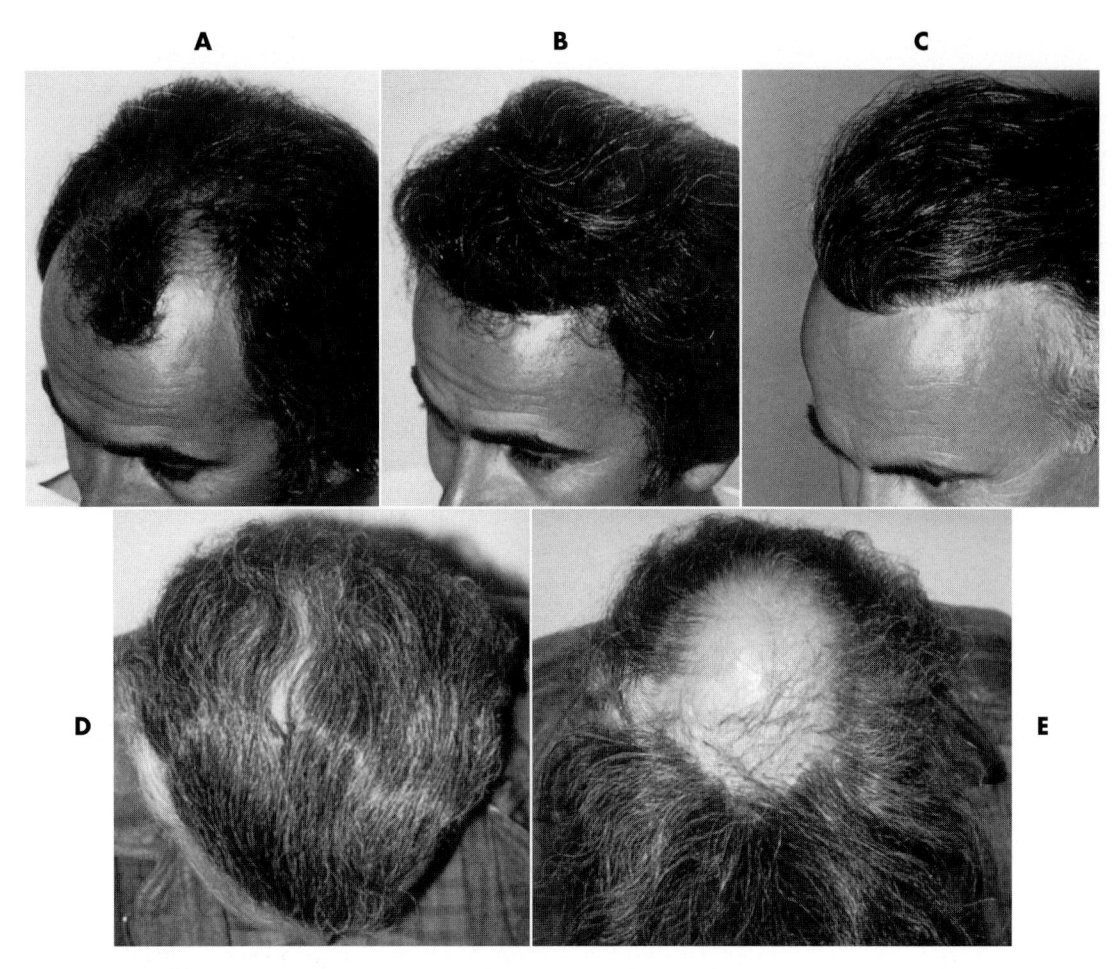

FIG. 10-51 **A,** Preoperative superior oblique view. **B,** Postoperative view 4 years after surgery (two Juri flaps). **C,** Postoperative view 13 years after surgery. **D,** Postoperative top view (with hair styled) 13 years after surgery. **E,** Postoperative top view 13 years after surgery with hair combed forward to show the bald area, the result of progressive male pattern baldness.

ANTICIPATED LONG-TERM PROBLEMS WITH SCALP FLAPS

Improperly positioned or asymmetrical frontal hairline
Detectable frontal hairline
Hair loss behind the flap because of progressive baldness
Hair loss in the flap resulting from male pattern baldness
Peninsula effect resulting from progressive temporal recession
Detectable donor site

ment in aesthetic scalp flap surgery is the expanded bilateral advancement transposition (BAT) flap procedure, which in two or three stages allows for the total resurfacing of the scalp with the flap hair growing in a normal anterior direction.[18]

Because most of these flaps are now used for purely cosmetic purposes, higher standards of results are expected. The potential long-term problems associated with scalp flaps are listed in the accompanying box. Most of these concerns relate to the progressive nature of baldness.

To assess the validity of these potential long-range problems, long-term follow-up was conducted on a randomly chosen series of 20 patients who had temporoparietal or, more commonly, temporoparietooccipital scalp flaps for the treatment of male pattern baldness. The follow-up period ranged from 10 to 18 years (Figs. 10-51 and 10-52).

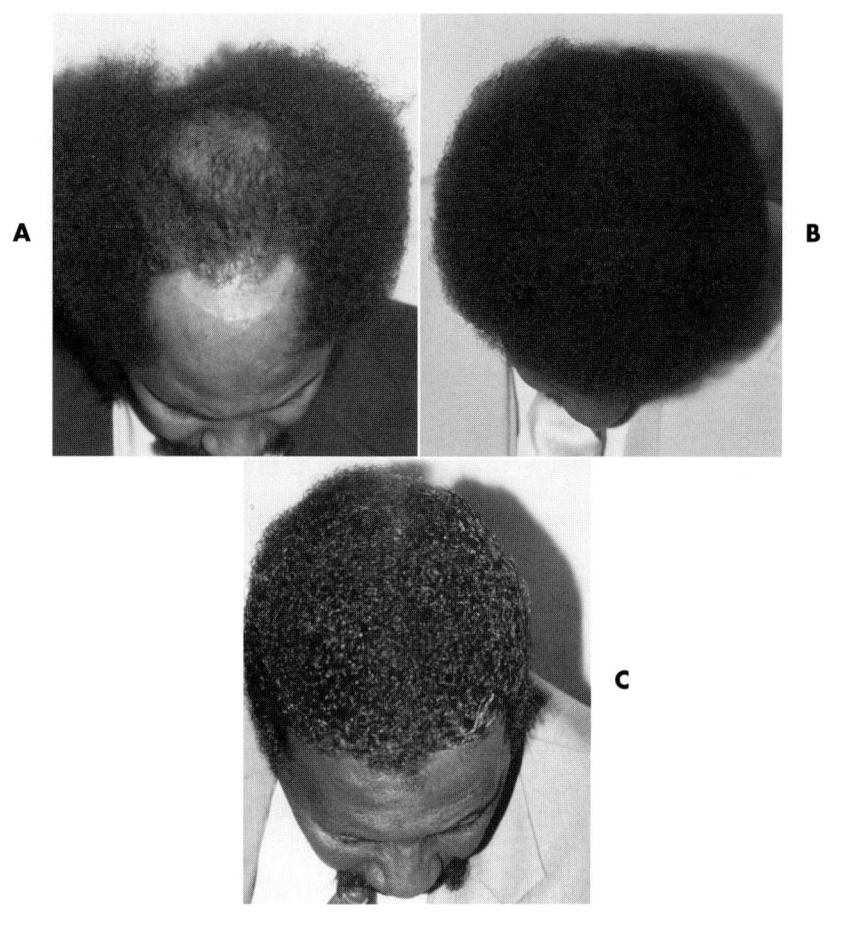

FIG. 10-52 A, Preoperative top view. **B,** Postoperative view 2 years after surgery (two Juri flaps). **C,** Postoperative view 18 years after surgery. The patient has maintained satisfactory cosmetic coverage even with a shorter hairstyle.

LONG-TERM OUTCOMES

Improperly Positioned Frontal Hairline

To achieve consistently good results with all types of hair replacement surgery, it is essential to properly position the frontal hairline. Two common mistakes are creating a simian appearance because of inadequate frontotemporal recession and placing the hairline too low, which is inappropriate for the patient as he ages and increases the amount of scalp that requires resurfacing from a limited donor supply. When a frontal hairline is created with flap(s), the recipient site is positioned where desired. The midline (trichion) is positioned approximately 8 to 10 cm superior to the nasal root (nasion), with the lateral aspects of the flap curving posteriorly to create frontotemporal recessions located along a line drawn superior from the lateral canthal region.

Three of the patients had asymmetry of the frontal hairline, which was repaired with a scalp reduction posterior to the lower flap side. Because of proper planning at the time of flap rotation, in no cases was the final hairline position too low.

Detectable Frontal Hairline

A detectable frontal hairline spans a spectrum of manifestations, the mildest of which is an abrupt hairline resulting from dense flap hair compared with the adjacent frontal skin. Compounding this problem is the often decreased pigmentation of the flap skin. The most extreme manifestation of a detectable frontal hairline is a visible scar, which can usually be prevented by beveling and deepithelializing the anterior edge of the flap so that hair grows through and thus conceals the scar. Notching along the frontal hairline can occur at the junction point when two temporoparietal flaps are used to create a hairline.

Micrografting of the hairline anterior to the flap, with the hairs inserted parallel to the posteriorly directed flap hairs, is the best way to create a natural-appearing, nonvisible frontal hairline. Micrografting was subsequently performed in several patients. Curly or kinky hair does not usually require micrografting.

Hair Loss behind the Flap

Progressive hair loss posterior to the flap is expected. It has been estimated that 60% of all men 60 years of age have significant baldness, which increases to 80% at 80 years.[19] The importance of anticipating future hair loss cannot be overemphasized. In most persons who are candidates for flap procedures, the temporoparietooccipital flap is preferable because a second flap is available for additional scalp coverage. Although the typical flap candidate is not as concerned about future hair loss as he is about his current receding hairline, future hair loss will almost surely take on increased importance in future years. Subsequent procedures performed on the patients who were studied for hair loss behind the frontal scalp flap(s) included scalp reductions, a second temporoparietooccipital flap, and hair grafting. The interval between flap placement and the first subsequent adjuvant procedure ranged from 2 to 12 years.

Hair Loss in the Flap

Since the earliest procedures were performed, the senior author (SSK) has always been concerned about the assumption that with progressive baldness the hair in the flap could eventually be lost because it came from some area of the fringe. Because of this assumption, the flap was always taken from as low as possible to prevent this phenomenon. Only one in more than 300 of our early cases eventually reported thinning of hair in the flap. This particular patient was operated on at age 21 years when he was significantly bald. He was warned of and understood the potential for this problem. He planned to wear and indeed wore a hairpiece behind the flap to cover the remaining baldness. Fifteen years after the surgery, he reported thinning in the flap. On examination it was found that the baldness had progressed to the level of the donor site scar and the front of the flap was thinning. He was advised that when the thinning created a cosmetic problem, minigrafts and micrografts would be performed. He has yet to require this additional surgery. Because of patient selection and proper flap design, hair loss in the flap is a rare problem.

One case of complete alopecia of the flap associated with total hair loss secondary to chemotherapy for Burkitt's lymphoma occurred 9 years after flap transposition. Complete hair regrowth occurred in the flap and the rest of the scalp.

Peninsula Effect

With progressive temporal and downward recession associated with the natural course of balding, there is a conceptual risk with temporoparietooccipital

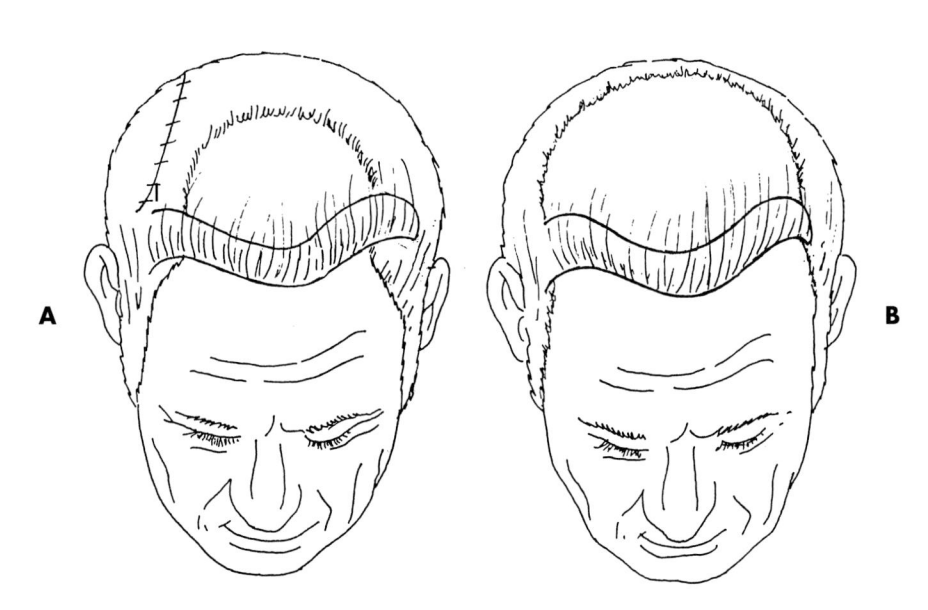

FIG. 10-53 **A,** Design of the temporoparietooccipital flap. The tail should be long enough to extend into the temporal hairline and should be harvested sufficiently distal from the fringe. **B,** Long-term result. With downward recession of the fringe, a peninsula effect is avoided because the tail of the flap extends into the temporal recession. The donor site scar remains covered by fringe hair.

flaps that an artificial-appearing frontal hair-bearing peninsula will be created. This situation could occur if the temporal hair were to recede from the tail end of the flap. This deformity is prevented by extending the tail end of the flap into the temporal hair region. The single base of a temporoparietooccipital flap and the two bases of bilateral temporoparietal flaps run through the temporal tuft and frontotemporal recession area, ensuring permanent hair unilaterally and bilaterally with a temporoparietooccipital and two temporoparietal flaps, respectively (Figs. 10-53 and 10-54).

Although progressive hair loss occurred in the patients who were studied, in no cases was a peninsula created.

Detectable Donor Site

A visible donor scar is usually the result of closure under tension. Most of these widened scars occurred when bilateral flaps were raised as a result of the increased closure tension. The anterior parietal portion of the second flap donor site is the most likely to visibly scar.

Patients with a history of keloid formation are at risk for hypertrophic scarring. Although hypertrophic scarring occurs rarely in the scalp, such a scar developed in one black patient. In addition, if the flap is taken from too high on the fringe, the scar will be exposed with progressive baldness. This problem was seen in one patient, as described earlier.

FINAL THOUGHTS

The subjects in this long-range follow-up study represent a small percentage of the senior author's (SSK) total experience with scalp flaps for baldness. More than 300 flaps (80% of them temporoparietooccipital flaps) have been performed in the past 20 years. Long-term patient follow-up is a valuable learning tool for the aesthetic surgeon. The long-term follow-up in these patients is unique but may not be typical because these patients had additional procedures, which allowed us to locate them and their records.

In our practice scalp flaps play a limited but important role in the armamentarium against baldness. Whereas some of the problems with flaps also occur with other surgical procedures for baldness, others are unique. Proper planning, a respect for the progressive nature of baldness, and meticulous surgical technique are keys to minimizing problems in flap surgery.

REFERENCES

1. Juri J: Use of parieto-occipital flaps in the surgical treatment of baldness, *Plast Reconstr Surg* 55:456-460, 1975.
2. Juri J, Juri C: Temporo-parieto-occipital flap for the treatment of baldness, *Clin Plast Surg* 9:255-261, 1982.
3. Kabaker SS: Experiences with parieto-occipital flaps in hair transplantation, *Laryngoscope* 538:73-84, 1978.
4. Kabaker SS: Juri flap procedure for the treatment of baldness: two-year experience, *Arch Otolaryngol* 105:509-514, 1979.

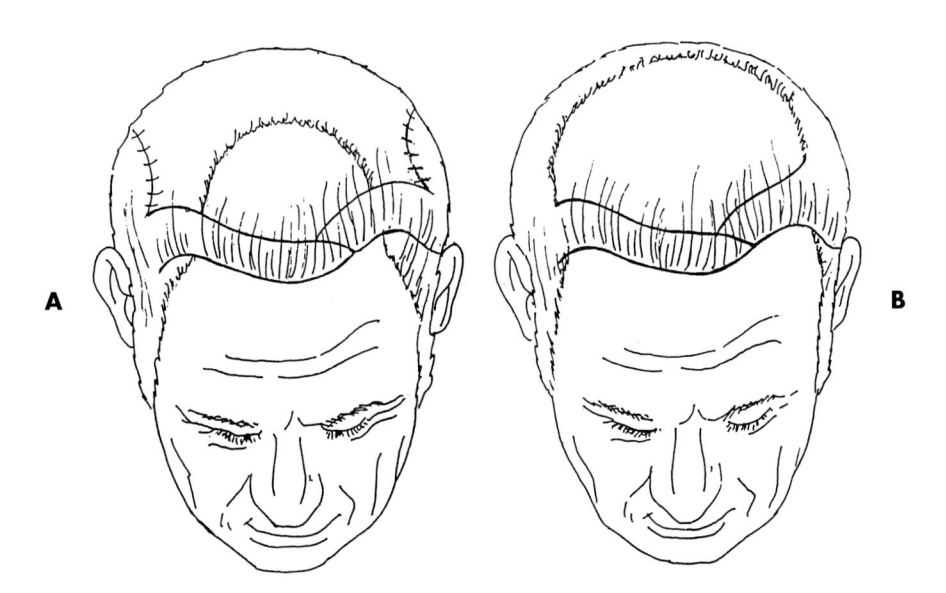

FIG. 10-54 A, Design of temporoparietal flaps. The flaps should be harvested sufficiently distal from the fringe and of different lengths to prevent notching at their junction. **B,** Long-term result. With recession of the fringe, the properly planned donor sites are not visible. Unlike with a single temporoparietooccipital flap, there is no risk of a peninsula effect because the flap bases fill in the temporal hairline tuft with permanent hair.

5. Mayer TG, Fleming RW: *Aesthetic and reconstructive surgery of the scalp*, St Louis, 1992, Mosby, pp 93-182.
6. Stough DB, Freilich IW: Hair-bearing flaps for baldness, *Facial Plast Surg* 2:283-286, 1985.
7. Nataf J: Surgical treatment for frontal baldness; the long temporal vertical flap, 74:628-635, 1984.
8. Nordstrom REA: One variety of a long, non-delayed temporo-parieto-occipital flap, *J Dermatol Surg Oncol* 14:755-761, 1988.
9. Lamont ES: A plastic surgical transformation: report of a case, *West J Surg* 65:164-165, 1957.
10. Passot R: *Chirurgie esthetique pure (technique et resultats)*, Paris, 1931, Doin et Cie.
11. Elliott RA: Lateral scalp flaps for instant results in male pattern baldness, *Plast Reconstr Surg* 60:699-703, 1977.
12. Elliott RA: The lateral scalp flap for anterior hairline reconstruction, *Clin Plast Surg* 9:241-253, 1982.
13. Bouhanna P: The post-auricular vertical hair-bearing transposition flap, *J Dermatol Surg Oncol* 10:551-554, 1984.
14. Chajchir A, Benjaquen J, Arellano A: A new scalp flap for baldness, *Aesthetic Plast Surg* 15:271-278, 1991.
15. Dardour JC: Treatment of male pattern baldness with a one-stage flap, *Aesthetic Plast Surg* 9:109-112, 1985.
16. Harii K, Ohmori K, Ohmori S: Hair transplantation with free scalp flaps, *Plast Reconstr Surg* 53:410-413, 1974.
17. Ohmori K: Microsurgical free temporoparietal flaps in surgery for male pattern baldness, *Clin Plast Surg* 18:791-796, 1991.
18. Anderson RD: The expanded "BAT" flap for treatment of male pattern baldness, *Ann Plast Surg* 31:385-391, 1993.
19. Hamilton JP: Pattern loss of hair in men: types and incidence, *Ann N Y Acad Sci* 53:708-728, 1951.

J. Hiccups Following Surgery of the Scalp

James Arnold

The word "hiccup" onomatopoetically describes the characteristic sound that results from the act of hiccupping. The peculiar noise is produced by a "diaphragmatic spasm causing a sudden inhalation that is interrupted by a spasmodic closure of the glottis."[1] The "he" sound mimics the sudden inbreathing, whereas the "kup" sound is produced by the sudden closure of the glottis. A variety of equally descriptive words are used in other languages to describe this phenomenon: "hipo" in Spanish, "hoquet" in French, "skihuk" in Hebrew, and "hikke" in Danish. An alternative spelling for the word in English is hiccough. Although the proper medical term for hiccups is *singultus*, the preferred word by conventional use is *hiccups*.

There are many curious facts about hiccups. No physiological benefit results from hiccupping. The hiccup phenomenon has been observed in many mammals besides man including dogs, cats, horses, and cows. Hiccupping often occurs in the fetus in utero and may be quite frequent during the third trimester. Men are affected more often than women with intractable hiccups. Whereas other reflex reactions such as a cough or sneeze evoke concern, hiccups are often viewed as amusing. Mundane situations, enlivened by the addition of hiccups, can provide an author with a rich source of humorous material.[2]

Whereas short spells of hiccups may be entertaining, longer episodes are troublesome. Occurrences that last anywhere from several minutes to 48 hours are referred to as *hiccup bouts* and may be associated with patient discomfort.[3] Spells that last more than 48 hours are considered *persistent* or *protracted hiccups* and may interfere with eating and sleeping. *Intractable hiccups* are episodes that last more than 1 month and may be life threatening.[4] In rare instances hiccups have been known to persist for decades.[5]

DISCUSSION

The fact the hiccups may occur after scalp surgery is not well known (see box). Most cosmetic surgeons acquire extensive surgical experience before attempting hair replacement procedures. As a result they become familiar with recognizing and treating common postoperative complications such as infections and hematomas. However, they are unaware that scalp surgery may be associated with the additional postoperative complication of hiccups. Somehow, manipulation of the scalp seems to be uniquely responsible for triggering hiccups. Cosmetic procedures performed on the skin elsewhere on the head and neck do not produce hiccups. When hiccups develop, the uninitiated surgeon may fail to recognize the cause-and-effect relationship between the surgery on the scalp and this postoperative complication. It is therefore important that surgeons undergoing training in hair replacement surgery be informed of the possible occurrence of this complication.

Similarly, patients do not usually associate hiccupping with their recent scalp surgery, especially because the hiccups occur several hours postoperatively. Patients often endure persistent hiccups for 24 hours or more before notifying their physician. When postoperative instructions are given after a

HICCUPS AFTER SCALP SURGERY	
Incidence:	≥5%
Onset:	Several hours after surgery
Duration:	Hours to days
Treatment:	Chlorpromazine, 25 mg po q 4 hr

scalp procedure, it is important that patients are made aware that hiccups may occur.

Norwood and Shiell[6] report that the incidence of hiccups after scalp surgery is approximately 2%. Although there are no other published studies in the literature, I have questioned several hundred patients 1 week postoperatively on the occurrence of hiccups. The true incidence of this complication appears to be 5% to 10%. In addition, it is my impression that the incidence of hiccups after scalp surgery varies with the type of scalp procedure performed; hiccups appear to occur more frequently after hair transplantation than after scalp reduction surgery. Furthermore, it seems that particular patients may have a predisposition toward this complication. Some persons experience hiccups repeatedly after scalp surgery regardless of the procedure performed.

A review of the literature reveals that many causes are known to precipitate hiccups.[3] The causes can be grouped into five general categories:

1. Diaphragmatic irritation (e.g., gastric distention after abdominal or thoracic surgery)
2. CNS lesions, particularly posterior fossa tumors
3. Toxic, metabolic, or drug-induced causes (e.g., alcohol intoxication)
4. Peripheral nerve stimulation of the vagus or phrenic nerves
5. Idiopathic causes

Careful review of these five general categories may help to identify the causal relationship between scalp surgery and hiccups. At the onset it is easy to eliminate the first three categories because diaphragmatic irritation, CNS lesions, and toxic-metabolic conditions are all causes that do not seem relevant to this situation. Although hiccups can develop as an adverse side effect of a medication, the drugs used for scalp procedures are also used with other surgical procedures in which hiccups do not occur. Idiopathic causes also seem unlikely because patients in whom hiccups develop postoperatively do not experience random bouts at other times. However, there does appear to be a direct correlation between the surgical manipulation of the scalp and the development of hiccups in these patients. This observation suggests that the cause of postoperative hiccups is located specifically in the scalp. In my opinion, peripheral nerve stimulation is the most plausible explanation for this hiccup phenomenon. Either the vagus or phrenic nerve receives stimulation as a result of the surgery performed on the scalp.

The vagus nerve, the longest of the cranial nerves, has a complex origin, numerous pathways, and great individual variation. The innervation pathways of the posterior scalp come into close approximation with the pathways of the vagus nerve in at least two locations. First, the spinal nerves C2 and C3 innervate most of the posterior scalp. Also originating from the C2 and C3 spinal nerves is the sensory branch of the vagus nerve, called the *auricular nerve*.[7] The auricular nerve provides sensation to the posterior auricle and the tympanic membrane. There are several reports of injury or irritation of the auricular nerve producing hiccups.[8] Surgery performed on the scalp may similarly irritate the auricular nerve, either in a direct or indirect manner, and thereby cause hiccups. Second, both the vagus nerve and the spinal nerves C2 and C3 communicate with the superior cervical sympathetic ganglion.[9] Scalp surgery that stimulates the C2 and C3 spinal nerves may indirectly stimulate the vagus nerve by way of this ganglion.

The phrenic nerve predominantly originates from the C4 spinal nerve but is augmented by fibers from the C3 spinal nerve. It is conceivable that stimulation of the C3 spinal nerve in the region of the scalp could also send signals to the phrenic nerve. Most authorities agree that stimulation of the phrenic nerve anywhere along its pathway can cause hiccups.

I recognize the speculative nature of the anatomical connections between the scalp and the vagus and phrenic nerves. However, direct or indirect stimulation of these nerves appears to be the most plausible explanation of postoperative hiccups.

TREATMENT

The treatment of choice for hiccups is the administration of chlorpromazine. It is very effective and is the only medication approved by the Food and Drug Administration (FDA) for this purpose. A standard regimen consists of chlorpromazine, 25 mg orally every 4 hours, until the hiccups ease. Patients should be cautioned about potential side effects, including drowsiness and postural hypotension in particular. There are anecdotal reports of chlorpromazine preventing hiccups in susceptible patients when the drug is given preoperatively. The literature recommends haloperidol, 2 mg three times per day, as an alternative regimen if chlorpromazine is ineffective.[3]

CONCLUSION

The hiccup phenomenon is an uncommon but not rare sequela after scalp surgery. Left untreated, hiccups may last several days and may interfere with the patient's ability to eat and sleep. Postoperative instructions given to patients after scalp surgery should include a directive to notify the physician should hiccups occur. Surgeons who are learning hair replacement techniques should be informed of the low but real incidence of this postoperative complication. Chlorpromazine is an effective treatment. This information should adequately prepare the surgeon for any postoperative call he/she may receive in which the patient says, "Hiccup."

REFERENCES

1. Taylor E: *Dorland's Illustrated Medical Dictionary*, Philadelphia, 1985, WB Saunders, p 547.
2. Fulghum R: *Uh-Oh*, New York, 1991, Villard Books, p 51.
3. Kolodzik PW, Eilers MA: Hiccups (singultus): review and approach to management, *Ann Emerg Med* 20:565, 1991.
4. Johnson L: Hiccups: causes and cures, *J Clin Gastroenterol* 7(6):539-552, 1985.
5. Boehm D: *Guiness 1994 Book of World Records*, ed 33, New York, 1994, Sterling, p 177.
6. Norwood OT, Shiell RC: *Hair transplant surgery*, ed 2, Springfield, Ill., 1984, Charles C Thomas, p 208.
7. Goss CM: *Gray's anatomy*, ed 27, Philadelphia, 1959, Lea & Febiger, p 1070.
8. Cardi E: Hiccups associated with hair in the external auditory canal: successful treatment by manipulation, *N Engl J Med* 265:286, 1961.
9. Goss CM: *Gray's anatomy*, ed 27, Philadelphia, 1959, Lea & Febiger, p 1010.

K. Emergency Situations in Hair Transplantation

William H. Beeson

Fortunately, emergency situations in hair restoration surgery are extremely rare. However, it is imperative that the surgeon be cognizant of their potential and adept in dealing with them (Table 10-1).

INTERACTIONS WITH MEDICATIONS

Although noting allergies to specific medications is critical, the surgeon must also be aware of potential interactions between medications commonly used by hair transplant patients.

Many surgeons use prophylactic antibiotics. Macrolides, especially erythromycin, are frequently prescribed for patients with an expressed allergy to penicillin (see box). Concomitant use of these medications with the commonly prescribed antihistamine terfenadine (Seldane) or astemizole (Hismanal) can result in lethal arrhythmias.[1] These antihistamines undergo metabolism in the liver by a specific cytochrome P450 isoenzyme. Macrolide antibiotics inhibit this isoenzyme and can lead to elevated terfenadine plasma levels associated with QT prolongation and increased risk of ventricular tachyarrhythmias.[2] For this reason concomitant use of macrolide antibiotics with terfenadine should be avoided.

MACROLIDES	
GENERIC NAMES	TRADE NAMES
Erythromycin	
Ethylsuccinate	E.E.S.
Estolate	Ilosone
Lactobionate	Lactobionate-IV
Gluceptate	Ilotycin
Azithromycin	Zithromax
Clarithromycin	Biaxin

Triazolam (Halcion) is frequently used as an amnestic in hair restoration surgery. It should be noted that erythromycin reduces clearance and results in increased plasma concentration of triazolam.

Ketorolac (Toradol) is a nonsteroidal antiinflammatory medication that has been advocated as an analgesic for hair restoration surgery because of its lack of psychomotor effects. Intramuscular doses of 30 to 60 mg are given 30 to 45 minutes before surgery. Time of onset is approximately 15 minutes, with peak activity noted in approximately 50 minutes. Ketorolac is a nonnarcotic agent that is equivalent to approximately 12 mg of morphine or 50 to 100 mg of meperidine.

Physicians who prescribe ketorolac should be aware of at least one reported case of hyperkalemia after a single 30 mg intramuscular injection of ketorolac. A potassium level of 6.9 mmol/L was noted 4 hours after administration. Consideration should be given to monitoring potassium in patients who receive this agent.[3]

Ketorolac is also noted for inhibiting platelet function. Bleeding time is prolonged because of the inhibition of platelet agglutination and thromboxane production[4] (Stough DB: Personal communication, February 1994).

β-Adrenergic blocking agents are commonly prescribed for a wide variety of cardiovascular disorders, including hypertension (see box, p. 337). Noncardiovascular uses include hyperthyroidism, migraine, potential tremors, glaucoma, and anxiety. A potentially life-threatening interaction can occur between these commonly prescribed agents and local anesthetics that contain epinephrine.[5,6] Gandelman and Barretto have five well-documented cases of β-blocker–epinephrine interaction in patients undergoing hair transplantation (Stough DB: Personal communication, February 1994).

Brummett[7] has pointed out the physiological mechanism for this interaction. β-Adrenergic re-

Emergency Situations in Hair Transplantation 335

TABLE 10-1 Emergency Situations in Hair Transplant Surgery and Treatment

PROBLEM	CAUSE	SYMPTOMS	SIGNS	TREATMENT
Allergic reaction	Allergy to medication	Pruritus	Urticaria, edema	1:1000 epinephrine subcutaneous 0.01 ml/kg (maximum 0.5 ml); repeat q 20-30 min as necessary Diphenhydramine 50-100 mg IM or IV
Anaphylaxis	Allergic reaction to medication	Vomiting, pruritus, respiratory distress	Diaphoresis, hypotension, nausea, bradycardia, edema, urticaria, respiratory stridor	1:1000 epinephrine subcutaneous 0.01 ml/kg (maximum 0.5 ml); repeat q 20-30 min as necessary Aminophylline IV 6 mg/kg loading dose over 20 min then 0.5-1 mg/kg/hr maintenance Oxygen Diphenhydramine IV 50-100 mg
Anaphylactoid reaction	Nonimmune reaction Possible reaction to contrast dyes or nonsteroidal antiinflammatory medications	Vomiting, pruritus, respiratory distress	Diaphoresis, hypotension, nausea, bradycardia, edema, urticaria, respiratory stridor	1:1000 epinephrine subcutaneous 0.01 ml/kg (maximum 0.5 ml); repeat q 20-30 min as necessary Aminophylline IV 6 mg/kg loading dose over 20 min then 0.5-1 mg/kg/hr maintenance Oxygen Diphenhydramine IV 50-100 mg
Anesthetic toxicity	Excessive volume, intravascular injection	Numbness in tongue and lips, "copper penny" taste in mouth	Agitation, tachycardia, increased talkativeness, nausea Progressive symptoms—drowsiness, tremors, seizures, respiratory depression, coma, hypotension, bradycardia	Oxygen supplementation Valium 5-10 mg IV Metaraminol (Aramine) 0.5-1 ml IV over 2-3 min for hypotension if needed Isoproterenol (Isuprel) 1-2 mg (5-10 ml) diluted in 250-500 ml D5W; infuse at rate to increase heart rate to 60 beats/min—used for decreased cardiac output as necessary; be alert for cardiac and respiratory arrest
Myocardial infarction	Coronary artery disease	Chest pain, nausea, shortness of breath	Chest pain radiating into arm and neck, hypotension, cardiac arrhythmia	Nitroglycerin sublingually if prescribed Monitor pulse, blood pressure, ECG Oxygen supplementation Establish IV Provide pain control—morphine 2 mg IV q 5 min as needed for pain relief Prepare to administer advanced cardiac life support measures
Cardiopulmonary arrest	Cardiac arrest or ventricular fibrillation	—	Loss of consciousness, without pulse or respiration	Initiate advanced cardiac life support protocol

Continued.

TABLE 10-1 Emergency Situations in Hair Transplant Surgery and Treatment—cont'd

PROBLEM	CAUSE	SYMPTOMS	SIGNS	TREATMENT
Hypoglycemia	Decreased blood sugar	Weakness, trembling, nausea	Diaphoresis, tachycardia, somnolence, normal blood pressure	Carbohydrate—½-1 amp D5W IV
Seizures	Seizure disorder, anesthetic toxicity	—	Loss of consciousness, muscular rigidity	Prevent injury with Valium, 5-10 mg IV Oxygen supplementation
Syncope (vasovagal)	Fright	Weakness, nausea	Pallor, diaphoresis, hypotension, bradycardia, loss of consciousness	Place patient in a reverse Trendelenberg position, apply cold compresses to head and neck; aromatic ammonia, atropine 0.5 mg IV or sublingually
Hereditary angioedema	Plasma regulator deficiency (C1 inhibitor), trauma	Abdominal pain, respiratory distress	Brawny nonpitting edema, urticaria, possible respiratory distress	1:1000 epinephrine 0.2-0.3 ml subcutaneous and repeated every 20-30 min ×3 Nebulized racemic epinephrine Diphenhydramine 50-100 mg IM or IV Stabilize airway; consider tracheotomy
Malignant hyperthermia	Triggering inhalation anesthetic agent and/or depolarizing muscle relaxant	—	Masseter muscle rigidity, high fever, tachycardia, arrhythmias, hypotension, tachypnea, elevated end-tidal CO_2, peripheral mottling	Terminate anesthesia immediately, oxygen supplementation, sodium bicarbonate 1-2 mEq/kg IV, cool body immediately with ice packs and ice gastric lavage Dantrolene sodium 2.5 mg/kg IV

β-ADRENERGIC BLOCKERS	
GENERIC NAME	TRADE NAME
Noncardioselective	
Alprenolol	Aptine
Zarteolol	Cartrol
Labetalol	Normodyne, Trandate
Nadolol	Corgard
Penbutolol	Levatol
Pindolol	Visken
Propranolol	Inderal
Sotalol	Betapace
Timolol	Blocadren, Timolate, Timoptic, Timoptol
Cardioselective	
Acebutolol	Sectral
Atenolol	Tenormin
Betaxolol	Kerlone
Bisoprolol	Zebeta
Esmolol	Brevibloc
Metoprolol	Lopressor

ceptors located in the myocardium increase rate and force of contraction when stimulated. β-Adrenergic and α-adrenergic receptors are found in most blood vessels. When epinephrine is administered, the normal physiological response of the blood pressure would be an increase in systolic pressure because of α-adrenergic receptor stimulation of blood vessel contraction and a β-adrenergic receptor elevation in cardiac output. Simultaneously, a decrease in diastolic blood pressure occurs because of β-adrenergic receptor stimulation of blood vessel relaxation.

Brummett[7] points out that in patients who are being treated with β-adrenergic receptor blockers, the only effect of epinephrine that can occur is an activation of the α-receptors in the blood vessels. The result is a profound increase in peripheral resistance with a resultant increase in blood pressure. The increase in blood pressure will act as a carotid baroreceptor that will activate the parasympathetic nervous system–mediated (vagus) slowing of the heart. Because the β-receptors in the heart are blocked, the sympathetic nervous system is unable to restore a normal heart rate; thus if the vagal response is strong enough, bradycardia can progress to complete cardiac arrest.[7,8]

Atropine sulfate given intramuscularly or intravenously before epinephrine is administered may inhibit the reflex vagal-induced brachycardia resulting from the elevated blood pressure. If possible, β-blockers should be discontinued approximately 2 weeks before surgery. Termination must be gradual and not abrupt.[1]

ANESTHETIC TOXICITY

Most adverse reactions to local anesthetics are really manifestations of epinephrine toxicity. Faintness, sweating, pallor, and tachycardia are usually caused by epinephrine.

The maximal effect of most local anesthetics injected into the skin occurs approximately 40 minutes after administration. Thus it is most likely that an anesthetic reaction will manifest itself within that time. It is important to be alert for the initial signs of toxicity such as nervousness, excessive talkativeness, slurred speech, complaints of a taste ("like a penny in my mouth"), and confusion (Table 10-2). When these signs are noted, oxygen should be administered immediately. Death from an anesthetic reaction is usually a result of hypoxia because oxygen demands on the brain are increased 300% during a seizure. Thus cerebral hypoxia ensues and inevitably results in death. One should also be prepared to administer diazepam in increments of 2.5 to 5 mg. The patient should then be watched closely for progression of the reaction and appropriate treatment steps should be initiated.[9]

Later signs of anesthetic reaction include somnolence, muscular twitching, convulsions, cardiovascular collapse, and respiratory and/or cardiac arrest. Oxygen should be administered at the slightest suggestion of a reaction.[10]

MALIGNANT HYPERTHERMIA

Malignant hyperthermia is an autosomal dominant hypermetabolic disorder of the skeletal muscle that can result in death. A malignant hyperthermic crisis can be precipitated in any susceptible person who receives volatile inhalational anesthetics and depolarizing muscle relaxants. The incidence of malignant hyperthermia is reported to be 1 in 250,000 persons who receive general anesthesia. If such agents are used in one's practice, it is imperative that patients be screened carefully preoperatively (see box, p. 338) and that appropriate precautions be taken with at-risk patients. The amide local anesthetics have proved safe for use in patients susceptible to malignant hyperthermia[11] (see box, p. 338).

Should clinical signs of malignant hyperthermia be detected (masseter muscle rigidity, high fever, tachycardia leading to arrhythmias, hypotension, tachypnea, elevated end-tidal CO_2, cutaneous erythematous flush, and peripheral mottling), appropriate treatment should be initiated immediately. The box on p. 339 presents the suggested emergency treatment of malignant hyperthermia as recom-

TABLE 10-2 Local Anesthetic Toxic Symptoms

STAGES	ORGANS AFFECTED	SYMPTOMS
1. Excitation of the central nervous system	Cerebral cortex	Excitement, disorientation, rambling speech, seizures
	Brainstem	Tachycardia, hypertension, vomiting, sweating
2. Depression of the central nervous system	Cerebral cortex	Coma
	Brainstem	Bradycardia, hypotension, apnea
3. Depression of the cardiovascular system	Heart	Bradycardia
	Circulatory system	Hypotension, shock
4. Cardiorespiratory arrest		
5. Death		

Modified from Lee KJ: *Essential otolaryngology,* ed 5, Norwalk, Conn., 1991, Appleton & Lange.

POSITIVE RISK FACTORS FOR MALIGNANT HYPERTHERMIA

Family history of malignant hyperthermia
History of complication or death arising from anesthesia
Personal history of malignant hyperthermia
History of significant anesthesia complication
High fevers of unknown etiology following anesthesia
Dark cola-colored urine following anesthesia
History of muscle disorder, weakness, or muscle cramps (may occur during sleep or at times of inactivity)
Muscle hypertrophy of bulky muscle groups

ANESTHETIC AGENTS CONSIDERED SAFE IN PATIENTS SUSCEPTIBLE TO MALIGNANT HYPERTHERMIA

Barbiturates
Thiopental
Methohexital

Intravenous Anesthetics
Propofol
Etomidate
Ketamine

Inhalation Anesthetics
Nitrous oxide

Benzodiazepines
Diazepam (Valium)
Midazolam (Versed)
Lorazepam (Ativan)

Opioids
Morphine
Meperidine (Demerol)
Hydromorphone (Dilaudid)
Fentanyl (Sublimaze)
Sufentanil (Sufenta)
Alfentanil (Alfenta)

Neuromuscular Blocking Agents
Pancuronium
Atracurium
Vecuronium
Doxacurium
Pipecuronium
Mivacurium

Local Infiltration Anesthetics
Lidocaine (Xylocaine)
Bupivacaine (Marcaine)
Mepivacaine (Carbocaine)
Tetracaine (Pontacaine)
Procaine (Novocain)
Chloroprocaine (Nesacaine)
Cocaine

mended by the Malignant Hyperthermia Association of the United States.[12-14]

ANAPHYLAXIS AND ANAPHYLACTOID REACTIONS

Anaphylaxis is an immune reaction that depends on the formation of IgE antibody, the immunoglobulin responsible for typical allergic reactions. An initial sensitization occurs and subsequent exposure to the offending agent, even in minute concentrations, is potentially fatal.[15]

Anaphylactoid reactions are defined as systemic reactions that have the same symptoms as anaphylaxis but are not caused by IgE and are usually not immune in nature. They occur as a result of substances that cause direct nonimmune release of mast cell products, which can cause urticaria, angioedema, chest pain, wheezing, and hypotension. Reactions to radiographic contrast dye and nonsteroidal antiinflammatory drugs such as acetylsali-

> **SUGGESTED EMERGENCY THERAPY FOR MALIGNANT HYPERTHERMIA (Revised 1993)***
>
> *Acute Phase Treatment*
> 1. Immediately discontinue all volatile inhalation anesthetics and succinylcholine. Hyperventilate with 100% oxygen at high gas flows, at least 10 L/min. The circle system and CO_2 absorbent need not be changed.
> 2. Rapidly administer dantrolene sodium in a 2 to 3 mg/kg initial bolus with increments up to 10 mg/kg total. Continue to administer dantrolene until signs of malignant hyperthermia (e.g., tachycardia, rigidity, increased end-tidal CO_2, and temperature elevation) are controlled. Occasionally a total dose greater than 10 mg/kg may be needed. Each vial of dantrolene contains 20 mg dantrolene and 3 gm mannitol. Each vial should be mixed with 60 ml of sterile water for injection USP without a bacteriostatic agent.
> 3. Administer sodium bicarbonate to correct metabolic acidosis as guided by blood gas analysis. In the absence of blood gas analysis, 1 to 2 mEq/kg should be administered.
> 4. Simultaneous with the first three steps, actively cool the hyperthermic patient. Use intravenous iced saline solution (not Ringer's lactate), 15 ml/kg every 15 minutes × 3.
>   a. Lavage stomach, bladder, rectum, and open cavities with iced saline solution as appropriate.
>   b. Surface cool with ice and hypothermia blanket.
>   c. Monitor closely because overvigorous treatment may lead to hypothermia.
> 5. Arrhythmias will usually respond to treatment of acidosis and hyperkalemia. If they persist or are life threatening, standard antiarrhythmic agents may be used, with the exception of calcium channel blockers, which may cause hyperkalemia and cardiovascular collapse.
> 6. Determine and monitor end-tidal CO_2; arterial, central, or femoral venous blood gases; serum potassium; calcium; clotting studies; and urine output.
> 7. Hyperkalemia is common and should be treated with hyperventilation, sodium bicarbonate, intravenous glucose, and insulin (10 U regular insulin in 50 ml 50% glucose titrated to potassium level). Life-threatening hyperkalemia may also be treated with calcium administration (e.g., 2 to 5 mg/kg of calcium chloride).
> 8. Ensure urine output >2 ml/kg per hr. Consider central venous or pulmonary artery monitoring because of fluid shifts and hemodynamic instability that may occur.
> 9. Boys <9 years of age who experience sudden cardiac arrest after receiving succinylcholine in the absence of hypoxemia should first be treated for acute hyperkalemia. In this situation calcium chloride should be administered along with other means to reduce serum potassium. These patients should be presumed to have subclinical muscular dystrophy.
>
> *Postacute Phase Treatment*
> 1. Observe the patient in an ICU setting for at least 24 hours because recrudescence of malignant hyperthermia may occur, particularly after a fulminant case resistant to treatment.
> 2. Administer dantrolene 1 mg/kg IV q 6 hours for 24 to 48 hours after the episode. After that, dantrolene 1 mg/kg PO q 6 hours may be used for 24 hours as necessary.
> 3. Arterial blood gases, creatine kinase, potassium, calcium, urine and serine myoglobin, clotting studies, and core body temperature (e.g., rectal, esophageal) should be continuously monitored until stable.
> 4. Counsel the patient and family regarding malignant hyperthermia and provide further precautions. Refer the patient to MHAUS. Fill out an Adverse Metabolic Reaction to Anesthesia (AMRA) report available through the North American Malignant Hyperthermia Registry, 717-531-6936.
>
> *As recommended by the Malignant Hyperthermia Association of the United States, Darien, Conn.

cylic acid, indomethacin, and ibuprofen would be examples of anaphylactoid reactions.

The diagnosis of systemic anaphylaxis may not be obvious. It may be difficult to exclude a vascular, cardiac, or neurological problem. The differential diagnostic possibilities to consider include acute myocardial infarction, pulmonary embolism, acute asthma, hereditary angioedema, seizure disorder, anaphylactoid reaction, or vasovagal reaction. Vasovagal reactions may occur after an injection (e.g., lidocaine [Xylocaine], penicillin) and include symptoms such as pallor, diaphoresis, bradycardia, nausea, and hypotension, which can be confused with anaphylaxis. Although anaphylactic reactions are rare, vasovagal reactions are not rare. Orentreich[16] has reported a 1:1000 incidence for syncope associated with hair transplantation. However, a high index of suspicion is prudent in such situations to avert a possible catastrophe.

In the event of an anaphylactic reaction, 1:1000 epinephrine 0.01 ml/kg up to a maximum of 0.5 ml is administered subcutaneously and repeated every

When proper protocol is followed, these patients can undergo hair transplantation with successful results.

REFERENCES

1. Lazarovich M: Urticaria and angioedema: a practical approach, *Resident Staff Physician* 2:9, 1992.
2. Donaldson VH, Rosen FS: A biochemical abnormality in hereditary angioedema, *Am J Med* 35:37, 1963.
3. Rosen FS and others: Genetic heterogeneity of the C1 esterase inhibitor in patients with hereditary angioedema, *J Clin Invest* 50:2143, 1971.
4. Middleton E and others: *Allergy principles and practice*, ed 4, St Louis, 1993, Mosby, p 1568.
5. Sheffer AL, Fearon DT, Austen KF: Clinical and biological effects of stanozolol therapy for hereditary angioedema, *J Allergy Clin Immunol* 68:181, 1981.
6. Stites D, Terra A: *Basic and clinical immunology*, ed 7, Norwalk, Conn., 1991, Appleton & Lange, p 365.
7. Frank MM and others: Epsilon aminocaproic acid therapy of hereditary angioedema: a double blind study, *N Engl J Med* 286:808, 1972.

M. Von Willebrand's Disease and Hair Restoration Surgery

Dow B. Stough and Marc R. Avram

Unexpected bleeding with delayed hemostasis is a rare event in hair restoration surgery. When encountered, it is prudent that the hair restoration surgeon seek a cause for the abnormal hemostasis.[1] A partial list of the causes of delayed hemostasis is found in the accompanying box. When it is evident that ingested medications, such as aspirin, vitamin E, or nonsteroidal antiinflammatory medications are not responsible, von Willebrand's disease should be considered.

Von Willebrand's is the name given to a wide family of bleeding disorders, all with a quantitative or qualitative abnormality of von Willebrand's factor.[2] Von Willebrand's disease is the most common hereditary bleeding disorder and may occur in up to 1% of the population.[1-3] In some patients factor VIII is also reduced. In patients with classic hemophilia, the primary problem is a decreased or absent factor VIII, whereas the von Willebrand's factor is normal.

The absence of a normal plasma level of von Willebrand's factor will result in a decreased platetet adherence to damaged blood vessels. The plasma von Willebrand's factor functions as a carrier protein for plasma factor VIII. These two proteins, that is, von Willebrand's factor and plasma factor, are termed the *factor VIII molecular complex*.

SYMPTOMS

Von Willebrand's disease may be discovered at any age. Bruising can be a sign of von Willebrand's disease rather than the muscle or joint bleeding that occurs with hemophilia. Oftentimes this disorder is initially discovered after prolonged bleeding at the time of a surgical procedure. Most patients with this disorder have very mild symptoms and many are undiagnosed unless a family member is identified with the disease or preoperative hemostasis testing is performed. Thus recognition of the condition is very important. Hair restoration surgeons should be aware of the disorder and order specific laboratory tests for von Willebrand's disease if necessary. The usual hemostasis screening test may be normal in mild forms of von Willebrand's disease.

INHERITANCE

Von Willebrand's disease affects both men and women and is inherited as an autosomal dominant trait.[1] The presence of von Willebrand's disease is determined by a gene carried on chromosome 12.[2] Occasionally the abnormal gene may appear for the first time in a patient; neither parent will have the abnormality. This occurrence would be called a new "mutation," and the disorder could then be passed on to children in the standard manner.

Rarely, patients have been described with a disorder that appears similar to von Willebrand's disease but does not manifest in the first few years of life. These patients do not have a family history of the disorder and are thought to have acquired the disease because of production of an antibody that decreases the plasma concentration of von Willebrand's factor. These patients are known as having *acquired von Willebrand's disease*.

DIAGNOSIS

If the hair restoration surgeon suspects that a patient has von Willebrand's disease, laboratory tests must be performed to confirm this suspicion. A par-

---

CAUSES OF ABNORMAL INTRAOPERATIVE AND POSTOPERATIVE HEMOSTASIS

Aspirin ingestion
Nonsteroidal antiinflammatory agents
Vitamin E
Oral medications (other than above)
Hemophilia
von Willebrand's disease

> **SUGGESTED WORKUP FOR A PATIENT WITH POSSIBLE VON WILLEBRAND'S DISEASE**
>
> Bleeding time
> Antigenic levels of von Willebrand's factor
> Functional assays for von Willebrand's factor
> Factor VIII levels
> Ristocetin cofactor activity test
> Routine screening studies (i.e., complete blood cell count, platelet count, prothrombin time, and partial thromboplastin time) are often normal in patients with von Willebrand's disease

tial list of the useful tests include bleeding time, antigenic levels of von Willebrand's factor, functional assays for von Willebrand's factor, multimeric structure of von Willebrand's factor, quantitative factor VIII determination, and a ristocetin cofactor activity test.[1] The accompanying box lists the suggested laboratory workup for this disorder.

TREATMENT

Patients with von Willebrand's disease need to take special precautions at the time of any surgical procedure, including hair restoration surgery. Appropriate referral to a hematologist is recommended. Treatment of von Willebrand's disease is possible and is specific for the type of defect present. Some of the medications used to treat this disorder include desmopressin (DDAVP), Humate-P, cryoprecipitate, and platelet concentrates.

CONCLUSION

Abnormal bleeding can be a troublesome and life-threatening complication of hair restoration surgery. Most busy hair transplant surgeons will encounter this problem at some point in their practice. Because von Willebrand's disease is probably the most common hereditary bleeding disorder, this entity should be considered in cases of delayed hemostasis. I have seen two cases of classic von Willebrand's disease and a single case of acquired von Willebrand's disease in my surgical practice.

REFERENCES

1. Coller BS: Von Willebrand disease. In Coleman R and others, editors: *Hemostasis and thrombosis*, ed 2, Philadelphia, 1985, JP Lippincott, pp 69-75.
2. Miller J: Von Willebrand disease, *Hematol Oncol Clin North Am* 4(1):107, 1990.
3. Holmberg L, Nilsson IM: Von Willebrand disease, *Clin Haematol* 14:461, 1985.

11
Selected Topics in Hair Replacement

A. Synthetic Hair Grafting

Shiro Yamada and Kouzo Fukuta

Editor's Note
Although synthetic hair grafting is not available in the United States, there are over 70 franchise operations offering the procedure in southeastern Asia and in Europe. Hair transplant surgeons have a negative opinion of this procedure since they have dealt with the complications of synthetic hair grafting. In its present state, it is doubtful that synthetic hair grafting will ever be available in the United States. However, physicians throughout the world should educate themselves on the various aspects of this technique. We are best equipped to deal with adverse consequences only if we have a sound knowledge of the process. Readers are referred to both the following section on synthetic hair grafting and the subsequent critique by Dr. Marvin I. Lepaw. Finally, the data presented by Drs. Yamada and Fukuta have not been verified in an independent study.

• • •

A hair shaft insertion method using natural hair was first reported in Japan for the surgical repair of baldness of the scalp by Sasagawa[1] in 1930. Since then, no similar report has appeared in the medical journals. We began studies on synthetic hair grafting for the correction of alopecia in 1964. This discussion reviews the developments and summarizes the studies on synthetic hair grafting.

In 1972, we introduced the *N-type method* as the first generation of synthetic hair grafting technology. Since then experimental synthetic hair grafting studies have been conducted on voluntary patients. On June 26, 1975, we presented this new method at the Press Club of the Ministry of Health and Welfare of Japan, after which consultation and treatment were made available to the public. In 1978, the second-generation *P-type method* was introduced and refined into the *Q-type method*, the third-generation technique that is currently in use. During this period, we and cooperating physicians have presented papers, both oral and written, on this subject, on 57 occasions to relevant international and domestic medical societies.[2-11]

Since 1977, more than 10 companies specializing in synthetic hair grafting have appeared in both Japan and the United States (Fig. 11-1). Many of these companies lacked fundamental safety considerations and used synthetic fiber not suitable for grafting into the living human body. As a result, many people who underwent synthetic hair grafting suffered complications (Fig 11-2) and many lawsuits were initiated. At the same time these problems came under the scrutiny of the mass media. Although these experiences brought to light the fact that synthetic hair grafting can be disastrous, our own studies with the P-type method have demonstrated a high safety profile.

The Japanese Ministry of Health and Welfare appointed six university professors, mainly dermatologists, to a research team to investigate the safety and effectiveness of synthetic hair grafting. This research resulted in a general report[12] that convinced the Japanese Ministry of Health and Welfare to allow polyethylene terephthalate (PET) synthetic hair to be available to the general public.

Clinical case reports on patients who had severe complications following synthetic hair grafting and criticisms of various imitators' techniques practiced in the United States were published by physicians in many medical journals.[13-26] In response, the Food and Drug Administration (FDA) held three public hearings in 1979.[27,28] In August 1983, based on these hearings, notice appeared in the U.S. Code of Federal Regulations that prosthetic hair fibers were listed as banned devices.[29]

The number of clinics at which our grafting method is practiced in Japan and abroad currently exceeds 71. The number of patients who have undergone our method of grafting exceeds 80,000 cases over the past 19 years. As a result of our having concentrated on safety in the development of our devices, we have not yet received any reports of severe complications. Earlier we did receive complaints from some patients regarding problems of low fixation rate and durability, but we seldom receive such complaints currently.

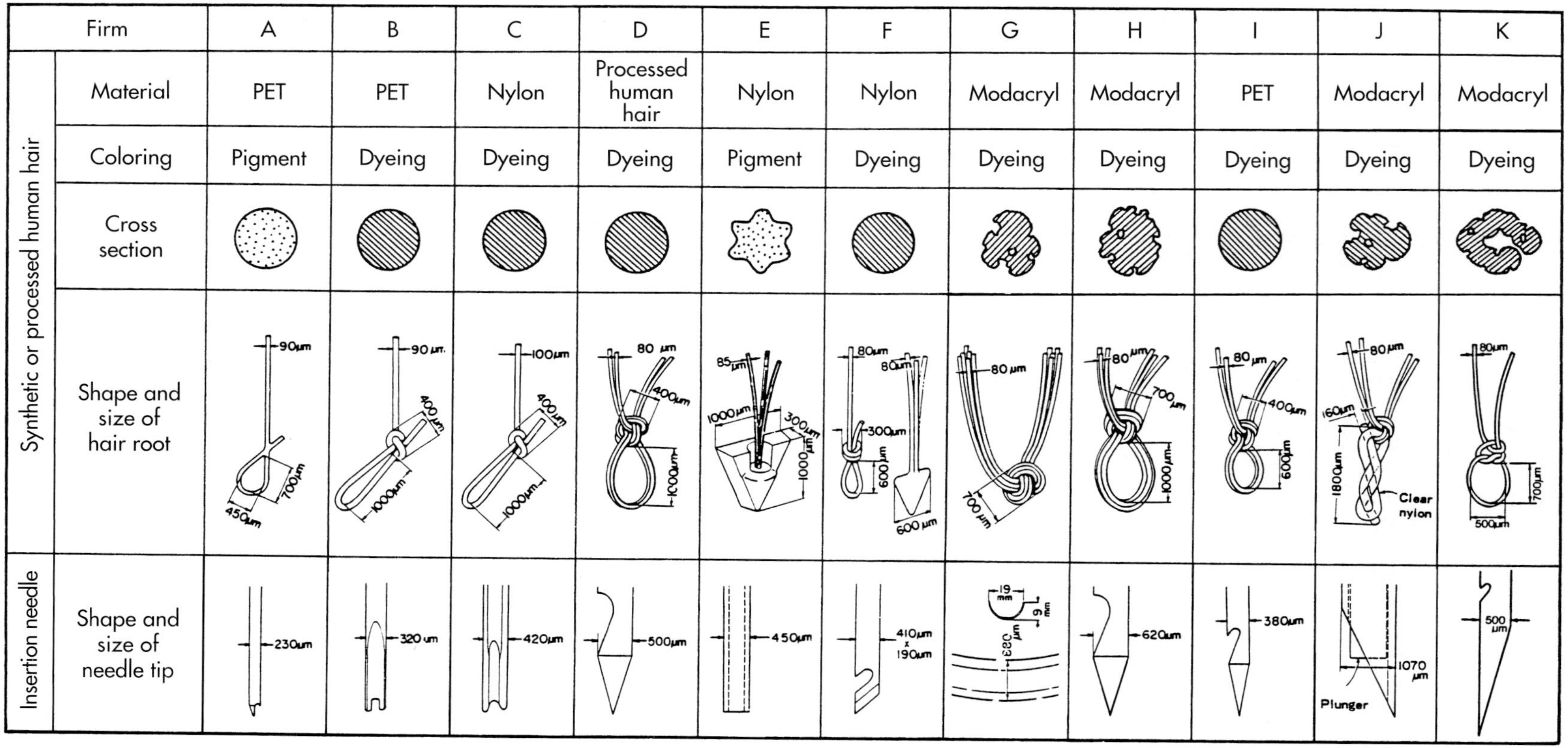

346 Selected Topics in Hair Replacement

Firm		A	B	C	D	E	F	G	H	I	J	K
Synthetic or processed human hair	Material	PET	PET	Nylon	Processed human hair	Nylon	Nylon	Modacryl	Modacryl	PET	Modacryl	Modacryl
	Coloring	Pigment	Dyeing	Dyeing	Dyeing	Pigment	Dyeing	Dyeing	Dyeing	Dyeing	Dyeing	Dyeing
	Cross section											
	Shape and size of hair root											
Insertion needle	Shape and size of needle tip											

FIG. 11-1 Devices and synthetic hair types used for synthetic hair grafting by various companies. A is our method, B to F are those of other Japanese firms, and G to K are those of firms in other countries.

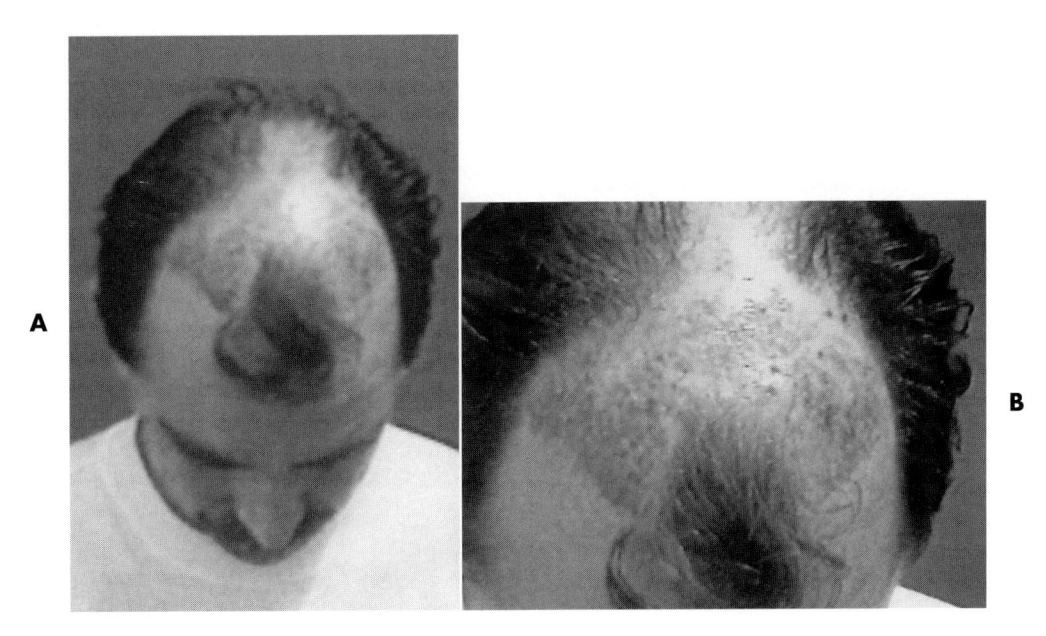

FIG. 11-2 **A,** Patient with a history of non-Nido synthetic hair implants that became infected with resultant scarring. These implants were not produced by Nido. **B,** Closeup view. (Courtesy Dr. Marcelo Gandelman.)

REQUIREMENTS FOR SAFETY AND EFFECTIVENESS OF MATERIALS

A synthetic hair inserted percutaneously into the scalp must remain fixed for a long time; therefore the following minimal requirements are necessary to ensure the safety and effectiveness of the synthetic hair and the grafting device (see boxes).

Synthetic Hair

The first requirement is that the components of the synthetic hair must not dissolve into the human tissue. The synthetic hair we use in our practice consists of polyethylene terephthalate (PET). This material polymerizes completely and is stable without the use of a plasticizer. To use PET as synthetic hair, coloring is necessary, and one of two coloring methods can be used: (1) chemical dyestuffs are added after spinning of uncolored material; (2) coloring pigment compound is mixed with the polymer base before melt-spinning is done. In general, dyeing of the synthetic fibers is achieved with tar dyes. Usually, tar-dispersive dyestuffs use diamino anisol. However, diamino anisol dyestuffs are reported to be carcinogenic by the National Cancer Institute in the United States.[14] Therefore tar-dispersive dyestuffs cannot be used for synthetic hair grafts in the United States.

To circumvent this problem, dyeing is achieved by mixing PET polymer with inorganic pigment,

---

REQUIREMENTS FOR SYNTHETIC HAIR

Must not dissolve
Must be completely removable without fragmentation
Must have disinfectant and antibacterial properties
Must have no residual toxicity or mutagenicity after sterilization
Must have long-term durability
Must be heat stable, even after curling iron use
Must have appearance and tactile properties of natural hair

REQUIREMENTS FOR GRAFTING DEVICE

Must cause minimal tissue destruction
Must have design that prevents inadvertent placement beneath galea
Must be disposable

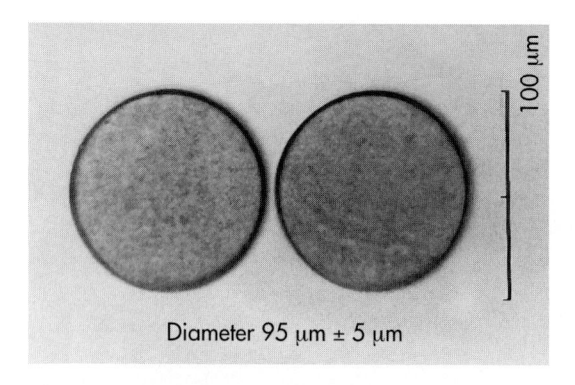

FIG. 11-3 Microscopic cross-sectional view of the PET synthetic hair (QB1 black color) we use in our practice.

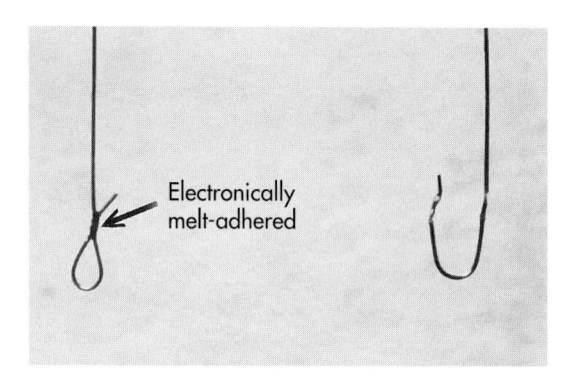

FIG. 11-4 Photographic enlargement of the root portion of the synthetic hair we use *(left)*. If the hair is pulled at a tensile strength of 160 g, the cross-shaped joint separates and the hair is removed as a single filament *(right)*.

TABLE 11-1 Results of Chemical Tests on Nido Synthetic Hairs

ITEM OF TEST	RESULT*
Chemical Test 1	
Residue on ignition	Acceptable
Eluated substance	
Volume of eluant	Acceptable
pH	Acceptable
Heavy metal	Acceptable
Oxidizable substance with	
potassium permanganate	Acceptable
Chemical Test 2	
Residue on ignition	Acceptable
Heavy metals	Acceptable
Eluated substance	
Physical properties	Acceptable
Frothing	Acceptable
pH	Acceptable
Chloride	Acceptable
Sulfate	Acceptable
Phosphate	Acceptable
Ammonium	Acceptable
Lead	Acceptable
Cadmium	Acceptable
Oxidizable substance with	
potassium permanganate	Acceptable
Residue on evaporation	Acceptable
Ultraviolet absorption spectrum	Acceptable

*Results were determined by the Japan Food & Drug Safety Center Laboratory.

namely minute amounts of carbon black powder as a black pigment, ferrous oxide as a yellow pigment, ferric oxide as a brown pigment, and titanic dioxide as a white pigment. These pigments are mixed for the coloring of hairs. For this method the coloring pigment is sealed inside the monofilament and is evenly distributed as shown in Fig. 11-3.

We conducted safety tests for the synthetic hair with the highest content of coloring pigment. These tests were conducted based on the standards for artificial blood vessels and plastic transfusion bags at national institutes in Japan.[30,31] These standards are substantially equivalent to the test of polymers for medical use in implants in the U.S. Pharmacopeia.[32] The results of both tests obtained judgments of "Acceptable" on all items as per Table 11-1. In addition, we conducted a mutagenicity test by Ames method, which functions as screening for carcinogenicity, and a carcinogenicity test using 100 rats as our own test (Table 11-2).

The second requirement of synthetic hair is that it be capable of complete removal, if desired. Our synthetic hair consists of a hair shaft and a root. Fig. 11-4 *(left)* is a photograph through the microscope of the root of the synthetic hair. One end of the monofilament is bent into an α shape, and adhesion at the cross-shaped joint is achieved by electronic melt adhering. The synthetic hair shaft has a tensile strength of 340 g and is constructed such that, if pulled, the cross-shaped joint separates at a strength of about 160 g and complete removal of an intact single filament is accomplished (Fig. 11-4, *right*). If a loop with a knot design were used, this requirement would not be satisfied, and the hair shaft would break off at the portion of the knot, leaving fragments within the skin. The structures of the hair roots of non-Nido systems (see Fig. 11-1) are the probable cause of many of the severe complications.

The third requirement is that the synthetic hair itself must have disinfectant and antibacterial properties. Bacteria constantly invade the scalp tissue from the outside along the percutaneously grafted

TABLE 11-2 Results of Tests on Nido Synthetic Hairs

ITEM OF TEST	TEST ANIMALS AND METHODS	TEST RESULT
Biological Test 1*		
Acute toxicity	10 mice, solution A intravenous injection	Acceptable
	10 mice, solution B intravenous injection	Acceptable
Intradermal reactions	2 rabbits, solution A intradermal injection	Acceptable
	2 rabbits, solution B intradermal injection	Acceptable
Pyrogen	3 rabbits, solution A intravenous injection	Acceptable (0.2, 0, 0° C)
Hemolysis	Defibrinated blood of rabbit, mixed 24 hr	Acceptable
Implantation	2 rabbits, sample and negative control plastic RS intramuscular implantation	Acceptable
Biological Test 2†		
Chronic toxicity	100 rats, 500 days, sample subcutaneous implantation	Negative
Carcinogenicity	100 rats, 500 days, sample subcutaneous implantation	Negative
Mutagenicity Test‡		
Ames test		Negative

*Results were determined by the Japan Food & Drug Safety Center Laboratory.
†Results were determined by the Showa University Laboratory Center.
‡Results were determined by the Japan Food Research Laboratories.

synthetic hair; therefore the danger of infection exists. For this reason an amorphous silver coating of a thickness of 40Å is applied onto a half-inch length of shaft from the α-shaped root of each synthetic hair. As the synthetic hair is inserted and fixed in the scalp, the amorphous silver coating comes in contact with the living tissue. Consequently, positive silver ions are generated and combine with negative chlorine ions in the extracellular fluid. If bacteria are present, the silver ions are taken up and combine with DNA directly in cells, producing a bactericidal action. A shake culture test was conducted in vitro on six kinds of resident bacteria that typically exist on the scalp, and an amorphous silver coating of a thickness of 40Å on the synthetic hair demonstrated a sufficient antibacterial effect. The rate of clinical infection was remarkably reduced by this coating. There is little to no literature on the side effects of silver used in this fashion in humans. We conducted a mutagenicity test on amorphous silver by Ames method with negative results, and no abnormality was recognized from the histopathological studies of biopsy specimens from the operation site. We have seen no detrimental effects from the addition of silver to synthetic hair.

The fourth requirement is that the synthetic hair must have no residual toxicity after sterilization. Sterilization by ethylene oxide gas has the problem of residual toxicity of the gas and therefore is not suitable for the sterilization of a prosthesis. On the other hand, sterilization by γ-rays has the danger that the molecular chains of the synthetic material may be broken by the radiant rays with subsequent deterioration of the strength of the synthetic hair.

We achieve sterilization by an electron beam accelerator. A germ-free status was confirmed by sterility test after applying an electron beam of 8 KGy to the synthetic hairs in a sealed pack. This method does not reduce the strength of the synthetic hairs.

The fifth requirement is that the synthetic hair must have sufficient durability against bending. The synthetic hairs we currently use have a durability of over 1,200,000 times against repeat bending, whereas synthetic hairs of ordinary PET would survive only about 13,000 cycles of repeat bending using an evaluation tester. Synthetic hair breakage has scarcely been reported for hairs actually fixed into the scalp.

The sixth requirement is that synthetic hair must have resistance against heat of over 150° C to endure the use of a hair iron for curling and the use of a hair dryer. In addition to these requirements, the synthetic hair should maintain color tone, gloss, feel, and elasticity similar to natural hair. Moreover, it must be confirmed by a textile test that a synthetic hair will not deteriorate and change in quality physically or chemically.

Grafting Device

The first requirement for a grafting device is that, when a synthetic hair is inserted into the scalp, destruction of the tissue must be minimized. Fig. 11-5 illustrates our grafting device. The insertion needle is projected by applying light force to the push button. The needle, which is made of surgical stainless steel, has a diameter of 0.3 mm, which is the same as that of a 29-gauge injection needle. The structure of the tip of the projected insertion needle makes it possible to catch the loop of a synthetic hair on this thin needle. The needle, despite its thinness, never bends at the time of insertion.

The second requirement is that the insertion needle of a grafting device must have a structure that prevents the needle from passing through the galea aponeurotica when a synthetic hair is being grafted into the scalp. Fig. 11-5 *(bottom)* shows the grafting device in cross section. A spring is built into the push button as a safety measure in order to prevent inadvertent deep placement. Fig. 11-6 shows the action of this safety spring.

The third requirement is that the grafting device must be disposable. The described device is made of plastic and stainless steel and is sterilized by electron beam. It has a mechanism by which a thin insertion needle can slide into the narrow hole of a needle guide composed of plastic.

MATERIALS AND METHOD

The actual synthetic hair and grafting device products are shown in Fig. 11-7. The synthetic hair is available in packs containing 1000 synthetic hairs (Fig. 11-7, *top*). Within each pack the hair is packaged in paper holders containing 20 hairs each (Fig. 11-7, *center*). The grafting devices are available in blister packs containing five units (Fig. 11-7, *bottom*).

Synthetic hairs are available in eight colors ranging from black, brown, gold, and gray to white, and the patients can select their desired hair colors. In case of intermediate colors, a natural look can be obtained if the colors are mixed. The curl of the synthetic hairs is preset. The length of the synthetic hair is 17 cm, but a scale is graduated every 2 cm on the paper holder, and the synthetic hair is cut to an appropriate length with scissors beforehand according to what is needed in the grafted region.

PREOPERATIVE ASSESSMENT

Before an operation, physical examinations and laboratory studies are conducted to determine that a patient is mentally and physically healthy. Contraindications are (1) diabetes, hypertension, and infectious diseases and (2) congenital atrichia, alopecia universalis, and cicatricial alopecia.

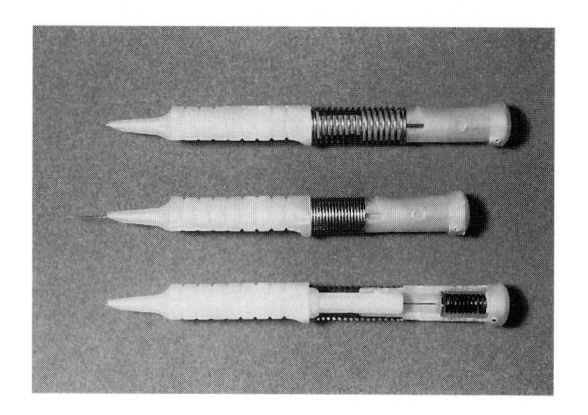

FIG. 11-5 Our grafting device. The device is shown with the insertion needle extended *(center)*. The needle is projected by pressing a push button.

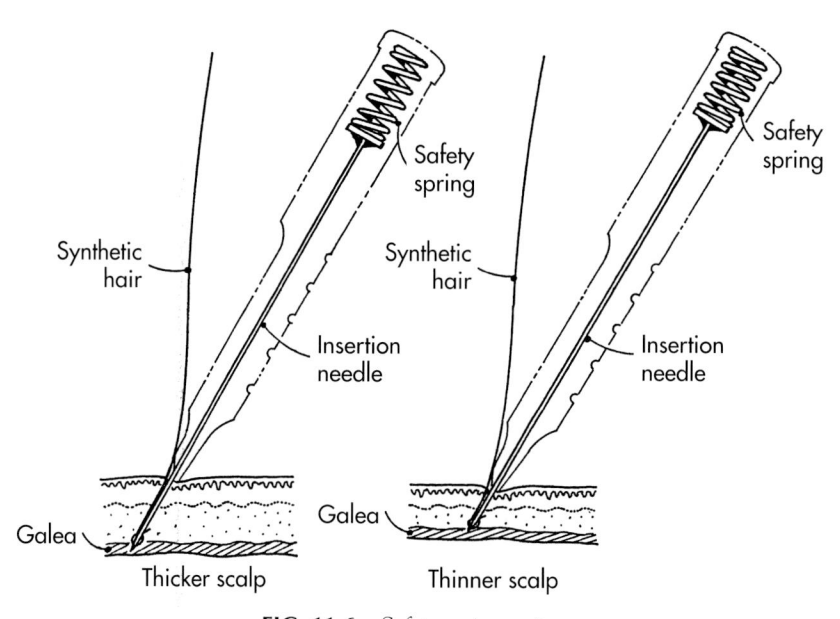

FIG. 11-6 Safety spring action.

Preoperatively the hair and the scalp are washed with shampoo and running water. An antiseptic solution is used as in other surgical operations.

For anesthesia, the injection of 1% lidocaine with epinephrine or the iontophoresis of 8% lidocaine with epinephrine is employed. The latter method is painless and is used in select cases. The addition of a small amount of epinephrine prolongs anesthesia and decreases the amount of bleeding.

Before the procedure, the surgeon must design the hairline. The design should encompass such factors as hair direction, distribution of density, and length of the hairs. It is helpful to employ a hair designer among the staff of a clinic for obtaining the best aesthetic results possible.

TECHNIQUE

The surgeon holds the grafting device with the right hand and the paper holder containing the synthetic hairs with the left hand. As shown in Fig. 11-8, when the push button of the grafting device is depressed, the insertion needle is projected. The needle is passed through the α-shaped loop of a synthetic hair. When the finger is released, the insertion needle retracts with upward tension on the synthetic hair and the α-shaped loop is caught automatically in a small hook at the tip of the needle. While maintaining this state, the grafting device is pressed against the scalp according to the slant of the original natural hair and the push button is depressed completely as shown in Fig. 11-9. The finger is then released from the push button and the grafting device is removed from the scalp, leaving one synthetic hair grafted into the scalp. By repetition of this process the operation is advanced.

It is possible to insert 500 synthetic hairs in 1 hour, and the experienced surgeon can graft up to about 800 hairs. At the initial session, it is necessary to maintain a space of over 3 mm between the synthetic hairs. To increase the density of the grafted synthetic hairs, follow-up grafting is necessary at intervals of 2 to 3 weeks.

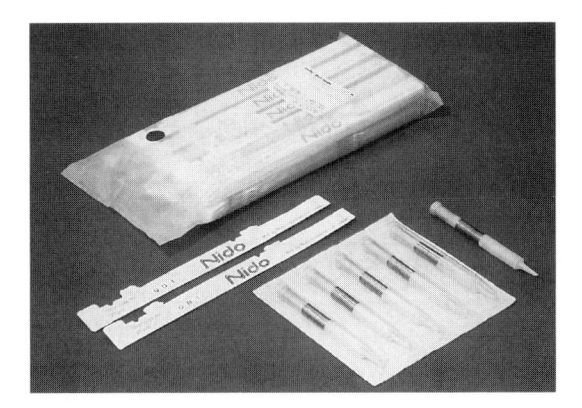

FIG. 11-7 Packaged synthetic hairs and grafting devices.

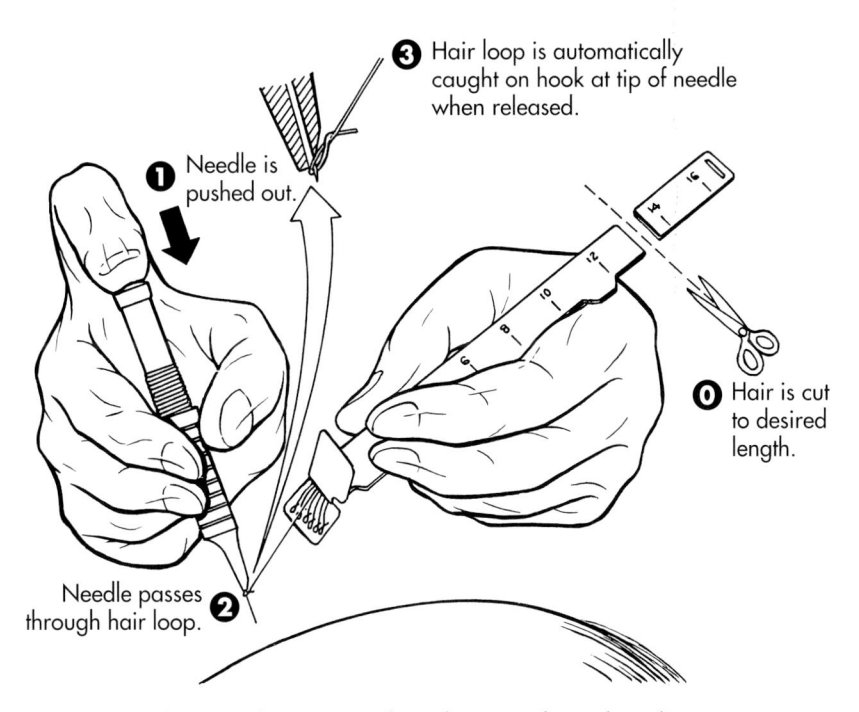

FIG. 11-8 Setting a synthetic hair into the grafting device.

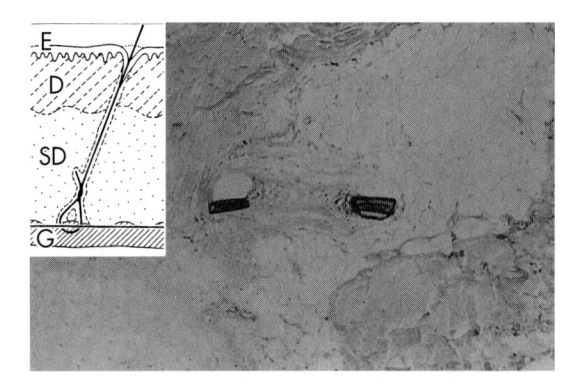

FIG. 11-11 Biopsy specimen at 20 months after grafting (hematoxylin-eosin). E, Epidermis; D, dermis; SD, subcutaneous layer; G, galea aponeurotica.

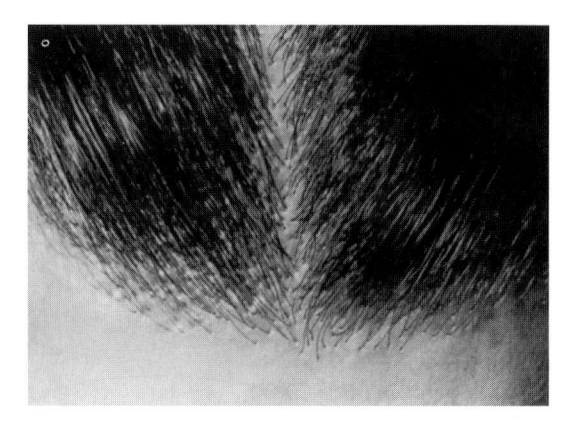

FIG. 11-12 Closeup of hairline grafted with synthetic hair. Larger infundibula are seen at the root of the grafted synthetic hairs. With age, as gray-colored synthetic hairs are grafted on the front edges of the hairline, the hairline maintains a natural appearance.

The epidermis begins to ingrow in a funnel shape along the synthetic hair from about 1 week after grafting, and it is observed by examining biopsy specimens taken with the passage of time that a larger hair infundibulum compared with that occurring in the natural state is seen at 1 month after grafting. These infundibula can be visible and observed as small indentations in the scalp. Fig. 11-12 is a closeup photograph of the scalp in which synthetic hairs were grafted. Dermatopathologists have speculated that the larger hair infundibulum may result from the normal tendency of the epidermis to contract.

We routinely observed the heaviest infiltrates at the level of the middermis at the junction of the epidermal ingrowth along the synthetic hair ends. The degree of this cell infiltration was remarkable at 2 months and the earlier stages, but it decreased at 5 months and was much lower at 20 months. We postulate that this portion may have the most relevance to infection. Fig. 11-13 represents the junction of epidermal ingrowth and fibrous connective tissue. We studied a series of biopsy specimens obliquely sectioned. These were observed by optical and electron microscopy. At 20 months after grafting, the ingrown epidermis and the surface of the synthetic hair were found to be completely opposed without clearance. This phenomenon suggests that the first barrier against the invasion of bacteria from the outside is formed here.

It was observed that a complete basal membrane is formed at the boundary surface between the ingrown epidermis and fibrous connective tissue created around the hair (Fig. 11-14). It is postulated that this structure may function as a second barrier against infection.

Although unproved, the formation of these barriers may contribute to the low infection rate and

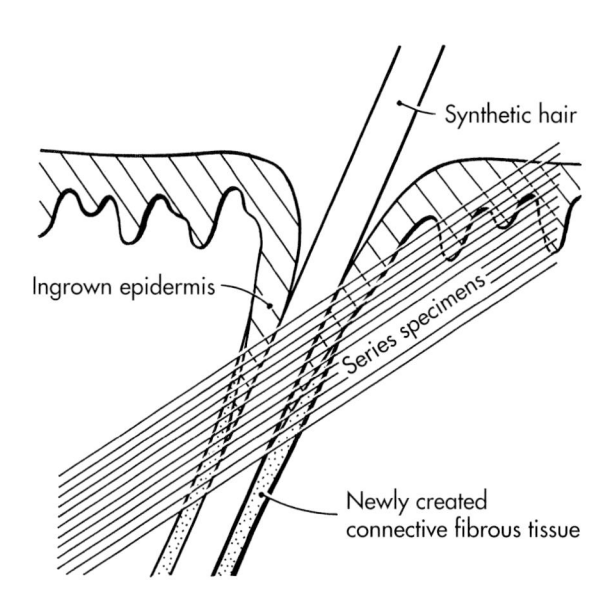

FIG. 11-13 Diagram of a cross section of the scalp depicting the shift from ingrown epidermis along the synthetic hair shaft to fibrous connective tissue.

proliferation of fibrous connective tissue inside the looped root may allow fixation of the grafted synthetic hair for a long period of time.

FIXATION RATES

Taniguchi[9] reported on the statistical study of the fixation rate of the second-generation P-type hairs grafted on 95 patients. The results are presented in Table 11-5. The standard deviations are not small and demonstrate great individual differences in the

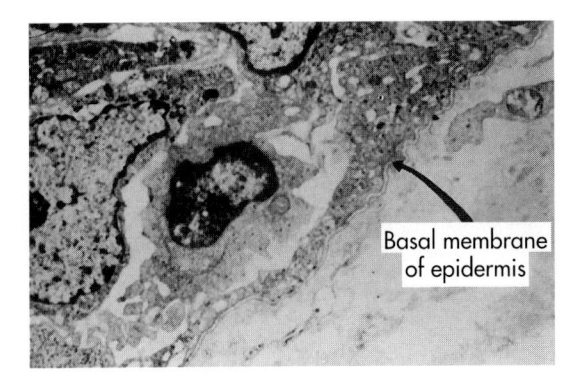

FIG. 11-14 A basal membrane is formed at the boundary surface between the ingrown epidermis and fibrous connective tissue.

TABLE 11-5 Fixation Rate of Second-Generation P-type Hairs (N = 95)

PERIOD AFTER GRAFTING (MO)	AVERAGE FIXATION RATE (%)	STANDARD DEVIATION (%)
6	88.7	6.7
12	78.7	9.4
18	74.6	9

Data from Taniguchi S: *J Jpn Soc Aesthetic Plast Surg* 4:48, 1982.

fixation rate. Subsequent reports from our clinics suggest that the fixation rate of Q-type hairs is higher than that of P-type hairs. When a physician consults with a potential patient, it is important for the physician to inform the patient that not all the grafted hairs will remain fixed, namely, that there are individual differences in the fixation rate.

DISADVANTAGES

The following list states disadvantages of synthetic hair grafting.

1. Not all of the grafted hairs are fixed permanently. Supplementary graftings accompanied by payment are necessary once or twice a year.
2. Synthetic hair is a percutaneous prosthesis. Therefore the danger of infection always exists while the hairs remain in the scalp.
3. Large hair infundibula are created at the base of grafted synthetic hairs on the scalp surface. These infundibula can be recognized easily if they are viewed closely.
4. Discharged sebum and keratin gather in the infundibula and may form into comedo-like substances. For removal of these substances it is effective to use a forceps or a softening liquid before shampooing. We recommend a saturated solution of sodium bicarbonate.
5. Follow-up is necessary. The grafted synthetic hairs must be maintained in the best condition by a hair technician at a clinic. It is necessary to remove the comedo-like substances. There also exists a need for correction of frizzled hairs. We recommend this aftercare treatment take place at 1-month intervals.

ADVANTAGES

The following list states the advantages of synthetic hair grafting.

1. Synthetic hairs can be supplied infinitely.
2. The procedure is relatively simple, allowing the placement of a large number of hairs in a short time.
3. A patient can obtain a natural appearance and can return to social life immediately after surgery.
4. The color tones, length, density, and quantity of hairs can be varied freely, and thermoplastic hairs with curl can produce and maintain a variety of hairstyles.
5. Curling devices can also be used.

CONCLUSION

Our method has been continuously studied and improved for over 20 years. However, the level of our method is still only halfway to our goal. Even if our method reaches our goal, it will be impossible to satisfy all the patients' desires, since synthetic hair never grows and is only a clone hair visually.

However, despite such shortcomings, our method is useful not only for the bald patients who cannot obtain sufficient donor hair for autografts but also for people who desire hair restoration without a great inconvenience to their social lives (Figs. 11-15 and 11-16).

REFERENCES

1. Sasagawa M: Hairshaft implantation method, *Jpn J Dermatol Oncol* 30(5):493, 1930.
2. Fukuta K, Narita I, Jodo T: A new procedure of cosmetic prosthetic surgery, *Jpn J Plast Reconstr Surg* 19:613, 1976.
3. Kobayashi T, Kamiyama G, Akagawa T: A study of synthetic fiber implantation for the baldness, *J Jpn Soc Aesthetic Plast Surg* 1:132, 1979.
4. Kobayashi T, Kamiyama G, Akagawa T: A study of synethetic fiber implantation for baldness. Transactions of the 7th International Congress of Plastic and Reconstructive Surgery, Rio de Janeiro, 1979.
5. Kobayashi T and others: Research and study on the artificial hair implantation, *J Jpn Soc Aesthetic Plast Surg* 3:12, 1981.

FIG. 11-15 A, The author, Dr. Yamada, before synthetic hair grafting at 39 years of age. His baldness was the trigger for his study of synthetic hair grafting. **B,** Dr. Yamada at 67 years of age. He underwent his first synthetic hair grafting 23 years earlier. About 12,000 synthetic hairs are fixed. Dr. Yamada receives supplementary grafting twice a year.

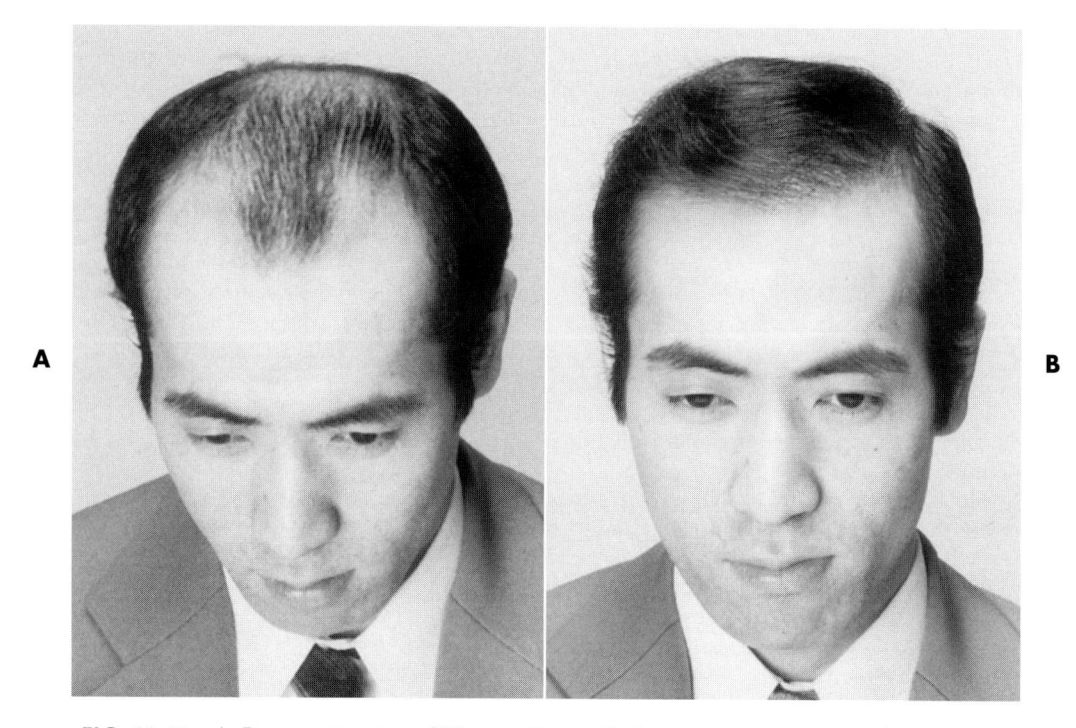

FIG. 11-16 A, Preoperative view of 35-year-old man. **B,** Postoperative view. A total of 4500 synthetic hairs has been grafted.

6. Kobayashi T and others: Research and investigation into synthetic fiber implantation for baldness. Transactions of the 6th Congress of International Society of Aesthetic and Plastic Surgery, Tokyo, 1981.
7. Taniguchi S: Histological findings of the skin following transplantation of plastic hairs, Jpn J Plast Reconstr Surg 20:322, 1977.
8. Taniguchi S: Clinical and histological findings in synthetic hair implantation, J Jpn Soc Aesthetic Plast Surg 2:146, 1980.
9. Taniguchi S: Artificial hair implantation: fixation rate and the histological findings, J Jpn Soc Aesthetic Plast Surg 4:48, 1982.
10. Taniguchi S: A histopathological study of percutaneous implantation of artificial fibers. Transactions of the 8th International Congress of Plastic Surgery, Montreal, 1983.
11. Taniguchi S: A histopathological study of the percutaneous implantation of polyester fibers, Aesthetic Plast Surg 8:67, 1984.
12. Fujita K and others: A study on the effects of artificial hair on humans, The Japanese Ministry of Health and Welfare general report, 1981.
13. DeVries P: Scalped victims left with infection and scars in worst hair fraud ever. Crusade aims to wipe out implants, Med Post (Toronto) pp 1-38, July 1979.
14. DiGregorio VR, Rauscher G: Experience with the complications of synthetic-hair implantations, Plast Reconstr Surg 68:498, 1981.
15. Green J: Synthetic hair implants prove dangerous, useless, FDA Consumer 13:18, 1979.
16. Gonzalez ER, McBride G: Synthetic hair implantations continue: serious complications result, JAMA 241:2687, 1979.
17. Hanke CW, Bergfeld WF: Fiber implantation for pattern baldness, JAMA 241:146, 1979.
18. Hanke CW, Bergfeld WF: Fiber implantation for pattern baldness—review of complication in forty-one patients, J Am Acad Dermatol 4:278, 1981.
19. Hanke CW and others: Hair implant complications, JAMA 245:1344, 1981.
20. Hanke CW, Ceilley RI, Bergfeld WF: Complications of fiber implantation for baldness, Am Fam Physician 24:115, 1981.
21. Lepaw MI: The synthetic fiber implant scam, Int J Dermatol 18:468, 1979.
22. Lepaw MI: Complications of implantation of synthetic fibers into scalps for hair replacement, J Dermatol Surg Oncol 5:201, 1979.
23. Lepaw MI: Scalp injuries from "hair" replacement, Consultant 149:20, 1980.
24. Lepaw MI: Therapy and histopathology of complications from synthetic fiber implants for hair replacement, J Am Acad Dermatol 3:195, 1980.
25. Lepaw MI: Synthetic fibers and processed human hair implants for the correction of male pattern alopecia. In Skin surgery, ed 5, Springfield, Ill., 1982, Charles C Thomas.
26. Lepaw MI: Evaluation of various therapies for damaged scalps due to hair and fiber implants, J Dermatol Surg Oncol 9:460, 1983.
27. Food and Drug Administration: Proceedings of general and plastic surgery device classification panel, Washington, D.C., Jan. 1979.
28. Food and Drug Administration: Proceedings of general and plastic surgery panel, Washington, D.C., March 1979.
29. Food and Drug Administration: Listing of banned devices, prosthetic hair fibers, Code of federal regulations 21:895.101.
30. Ministry of Health and Welfare Japan: Handbook of medical devices, Yakugyo-jihosha, 1980.
31. Ministry of Health and Welfare Japan: Test method of plastic transfusion containers, Jpn Pharmacal X:B-302, 1981.
32. US Pharmacopeia: Biological test-plastics, physico-chemical test-plastics, USP XXI:1235, 1985.

Critique
Marvin I. Lepaw

Caution must be taken in the use of synthetic fiber implants to simulate hair. The following facts and factors should be considered when evaluating an experimental procedure.

Polypropylene terephthalate (PET) in textile form is known as Dacron and is used as a surgical implant in vascular surgery. When used in fiber or suture form, it is known in the United States as Prolene (Ethicon). When used as a percutaneous access device, it has proved to be moderately histocompatible, eliciting a chronic inflammatory reaction predominantly in tissue that is grown into the pores of the fabric.[1]

We are all aware of the less violent foreign body reaction to Prolene in the scalp. However, the wound sutured by this material must be kept fastidiously clean to prevent bacterial contamination. All percutaneous material elicits some sort of foreign body reaction and eventually risks infection.[2] In Halsner's study[3] in Germany in which Nido fibers, instruments, and technique were used, 86% of the patients were unable to comply with the rigid hygiene necessary to prevent infection. The high rate of failure in this European study would translate into serious medical and financial problems, perhaps resulting in numerous malpractice suits in the United States as we witnessed a decade ago. Bouhanna[4] in France graphically illustrated the problems encountered using meticulous photographic technique.

The silver salt used in this new and improved version of the synthetic suture implant technique is silver iodide. In the 1930s Argyrol was a silver iodide solution used as a remedy for nasal congestion. Eventually better remedies plus the increased incidence of argyria resulted in the phasing out of this drug from our medical armamentarium. One wonders if argyria will occur in increasing numbers of people who are having silver-coated simulated hairs implanted and reimplanted on an annual basis.

There is also repeated (annual to biannual) need to replace frayed, broken, or lost fibers that lose their tensile strength through wear and tear from washing, combing, oxidation, sunlight, heat, and aging. In addition, bacteria find their way into the artificial pores created by the insertion of the fibers and cause focal infections. The fibers in these "pores" have to be removed and the areas treated with antibiotics. After healing takes place, the fibers are replaced. The scalp eventually becomes scarred. This scarring was apparent when I recently examined the scalp of one of the authors.

No independent studies over the past 10 years have shown that these fibers are safe. On the contrary, although the reactions and problems are not as severe as those that occur with modified acrylic fibers,[5] there is and always will be the problem of infection and rejection to foreign transepidermal prosthetic devices. The human body is not going to change in this regard without the use of antibiotics and antiinflammatory medications.

The claim of reepithelialization around the fibers needs to be challenged. In a previous study, no further reepithelialization was evident below 3 to 4 mm.[2] One also has to consider the possibility that some of these fibers may break off below or at the skin's surface, making retrieval all but impossible despite the claim of the α-shaped configuration opening when tugged.

Lifetime regular to periodic medical care is required for all the problems encountered, among which are perifollicular pustules, comedo formation, progressive cicatrization, increased scalp induration, and numbness. Added to this medical cost is the lifetime cost of fiber replacement.

Finally, it should be noted that the discussion was written by the president of the Nido Limited Company of Tokyo (a nonphysician) and by a physician in his employ. There is a profound financial interest in selling the fibers, instruments, EC5000 electrocoagulator, and franchises for this technique. The Nido Company holds over 48 patents in 17 countries and supplies and sells all these materials and instruments to over 70 franchise operations in Southeast Asia and Europe.

REFERENCES

1. Yan JY and others: Titanium-coated Dacron velour: a study of interfacial connective tissue formation, *J Biomed Mater Res* 23(2):171-189, 1989.
2. Lepaw MI: Therapy and histopathology of complications from synthetic fiber implants for hair replacement, *J Am Acad Dermatol* 3:195, 1980.
3. Halsner U: Polypropylene fiber implant problems. Presented at the Eighth International Congress on Dermatological Surgery. Barcelona: October 1987.
4. Bouhanna P: Clinical and macrophotographic study of the percutaneous implantation of synthetic hair (Nido SH1). Trends in human hair growth and alopecia research. *Kluwer Acad* 1989.
5. Hanke CW and others: Hair implant complications, JAMA 245:1344, 1981.

B. Hair Follicle Regeneration after Horizontal Resectioning—Implications for Hair Transplantation

Jung-Chul Kim and Yung-Chul Choi*

The hair follicle is composed primarily of epidermal and dermal tissues. A traditional belief is that the vital interaction between these two tissues is in the hair bulb, which plays a central role in hair growth, differentiation, and pigmentation.[1] It is not surprising that many hair transplant surgeons have legitimate concerns about the accidental sectioning of hair bulbs when harvesting donor grafts.[2]

It is noteworthy that the dermal components of the follicle, namely the dermal papilla and the perifollicular sheath, are derived from the same mesenchymal cells.[3] The dermal papilla has long been regarded as the necessary prerequisite for hair growth initiation and maintenance and therefore the source of the hair follicle stem cells. However, there is growing evidence that the perifollicular sheath can be the source of a regenerated dermal papilla after removal of the original papilla. Recent research has shown that stem cells, which initiate hair growth, appear to arise from the region of the "bulge" where the arrector pili muscle inserts into the hair follicle.[4] The lower follicle, namely the impermanent part of the follicle, now appears to be of secondary importance in the regeneration of a damaged follicle.

We have conducted a series of experiments to determine the site of regeneration of the hair follicle. Determination of this site is of great importance in hair transplantation because it indicates the portion of the follicle that must be transplanted for it to survive and regrow.

STUDIES OF REGENERATION OF HAIR FOLLICLE AFTER HORIZONTAL SECTIONING

METHODS. We removed human hair follicles from the occipital scalp by microdissection to study their regenerative activity. Implants were prepared from follicles as follows: (1) the upper one third and lower two thirds of the follicle were obtained by horizontal section just below the sebaceous gland at the base of the infundibulum, (2) the upper and lower halves of the follicle were obtained by horizontal section through the isthmus in the middle portion of the follicle, and (3) the upper two thirds and lower one third of the follicle were obtained by

---

*Edited by David A. Whiting, M.D.

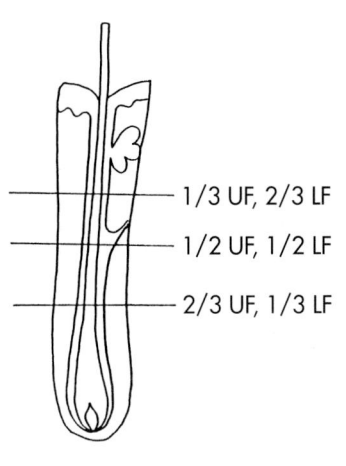

FIG. 11-17 Horizontal sectioning. *LF,* Lower follicle; *UP,* upper follicle; *solid line,* level of cut.

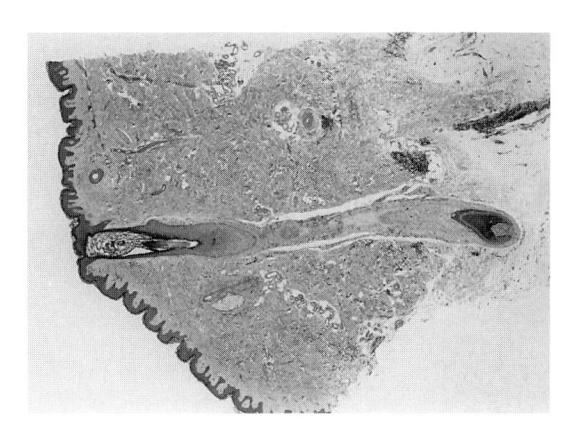

FIG. 11-20 Longitudinal section of a regenerated follicle from a lower-half follicle implant 8 months after transplantation.

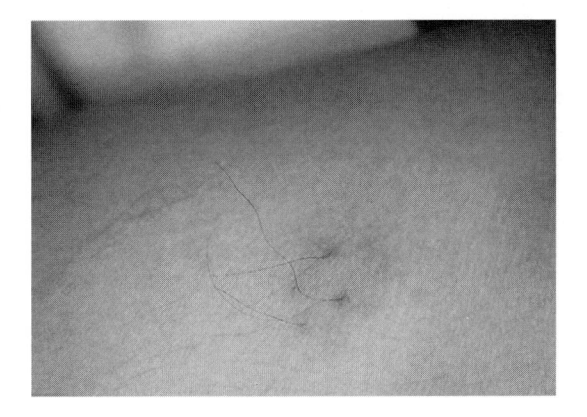

FIG. 11-18 Surface view of the leg 8 months after transplanting an upper-half follicle.

TABLE 11-6 Hair Growth after Horizontal Sectioning

FOLLICULAR SEGMENT	NO. OF TRANSPLANTED HAIR FOLLICLES	NO. OF REGROWN HAIRS (%)
Upper ⅓ follicle	20	0
Lower ⅔ follicle	20	16 (80%)
Upper ½ follicle	20	8 (40%)
Lower ½ follicle	10	2 (20%)
Upper ⅔ follicle	10	6 (60%)
Lower ⅓ follicle	10	0

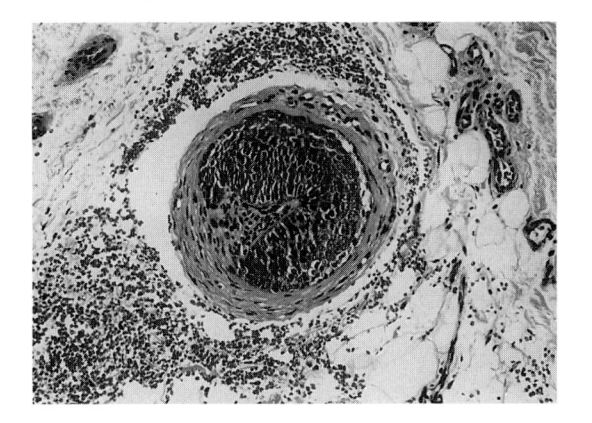

FIG. 11-19 Cross section of the regenerated bulb from an upper-half follicle implant 8 months after transplantation.

horizontal section through the follicle below the level of insertion of the arrector pili muscle, the so-called bulge area (Fig. 11-17). Both upper and lower follicle grafts were transplanted onto the forehead or leg.[5]

RESULTS. When the follicles were transected just below the sebaceous gland, implants of the lower two thirds of the follicle produced normal hair, but implants of the upper one third of the follicle implants were unable to regenerate either a dermal papilla or hair (Table 11-6). When the follicles were transected through the middle portion, the upper-half and lower-half follicle implants both produced new hair growth (Fig. 11-18). Each upper half developed a new small papilla, matrix, and active melanocytes, with the production of a fine hair (Fig. 11-19). Each lower half developed a normal lower follicle and dermal papilla and produced a normal-sized hair (Fig. 11-20); the sebaceous gland did not regenerate until 8 months after grafting. When the follicles were transected at the lower one third, implants of the upper two thirds of the follicle developed a normal dermal papilla and lower follicle and produced a thick hair, but implants of the lower one third of the follicle lacked stem cells and did not produce hair. The thickness of hair growing from any regenerating follicle correlated with the volume of the reconstituted dermal papilla.

CONCLUSION. The midfollicle or isthmus is necessary for the regeneration of a hair follicle.

STUDIES OF PROLIFERATION AND MORPHOLOGY OF FOLLICULAR DERMAL CELLS

First Study

METHODS. To characterize the follicular dermal cells, we cultured the dermal papilla and perifollicular sheath cells of a scalp hair follicle.[6]

RESULTS. When scalp follicle papillae were explanted into the culture, the papilla cells revealed an initial reluctance to divide. Even after several passages, comparison of the growth parameters of papilla cells and skin fibroblasts showed that the papilla cells divided more slowly. At low cell densities, papilla cells assumed a flattened morphologic character with numerous cell processes compared with the more regular, spindle-shaped morphologic appearance of skin fibroblasts. A striking feature of both primary explants and subcultured papilla cells was the consistent way they formed aggregates once a confluent cell density was reached. This appearance contrasted with the regular patchwork patterning of skin fibroblasts. Perifollicular sheath cells from the scalp follicle also displayed a similar flattened morphologic nature and the same aggressive trait as papilla cells.

CONCLUSION. The growth rates of the perifollicular cells were faster than those of the papilla cells but not slower than the dermal fibroblasts.

Second Study

METHODS. We examined the expression of smooth muscle α-actin in hair follicles in situ and in follicular dermal cells in culture by means of immunohistochemistry.[7]

RESULTS. The perifollicular sheath of the follicle was clearly stained with an anti–smooth muscle α-actin antibody, but dermal papilla cells within the follicles were not stained. Smooth muscle α-actin staining of the catagen hair follicle revealed that the perifollicular sheath staining extended into the base of late catagen hair (Fig. 11-21). However, in culture a large percentage of both dermal papilla and perifollicular cells were stained by this antibody. Explant-derived skin fibroblasts were moderately stained by this antibody.

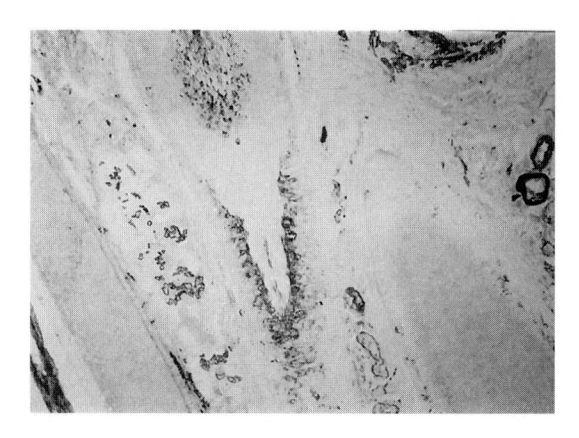

FIG. 11-21 Human catagen hair follicle stained with antibody to smooth muscle α-actin. Dermal sheath staining extended up to the base of the telogen bulb.

CONCLUSION. Because the mesenchymal cells usually express smooth muscle α-actin in the proliferative phase but not in the aggregative phase,[8] dermal papillae seem to be an aggregated form of perifollicular sheath cells.

STUDIES OF SITE OF ANDROGEN ACTION IN HAIR FOLLICLE

METHODS. The cultured dermal papilla and perifollicular sheath cells from human scalp follicles were examined for the presence of androgen receptors and androgen metabolizing enzymes—both characteristics of androgen target cells.

RESULTS. Our studies showed that human papilla and perifollicular sheath cells contained similar mRNA levels of androgen receptor, 5α-reductase type I and type II, 17β-hydroxysteroid dehydrogenase, and aromatase.

CONCLUSION. These results strongly suggest that human papilla and perifollicular sheath cells are targets for androgen action, and confirm their role in modifying follicular behavior.[9]

STUDIES OF SEGREGATION OF KERATINOCYTE COLONY–FORMING CELLS

METHODS. To locate the keratinocyte colony–forming cells, we isolated single hair grafts and transected the middle portions.

RESULTS. When the transient portions were cultured after removing dermal papilla, only perifollicular sheath cells grew. However, when permanent portions were cultured, outgrowing colonies of keratinocytes, surrounded by fibroblasts, were observed.

CONCLUSION. The segregation of keratinocyte colony–forming cells in the upper segment suggests that the upper segment of a follicle may be the reservoir of the stem cells responsible for the long-term growth of the hair follicle.

STUDIES OF EXPRESSION OF CYTOKERATIN 19 IN HAIR FOLLICLE IN SITU

METHODS. We examined the expression of cytokeratin 19, which by means of immunohistochemistry has been associated with regions containing stem cells.

RESULTS. Cytokeratin 19 was present only in the outer root sheath cells of the isthmus. The transient portion of the follicle did not express the antigen.

CONCLUSION. Stem cells are present in the isthmus but not in the lower, impermanent follicle.

STUDIES OF INVOLUTION OF TRANSIENT PORTION OF FOLLICLE DURING STRESS-INDUCED CATAGEN

METHODS. To detemine which segment of a follicle undergoes programmed cell death (apoptosis) during stress-induced catagen, isolated hair follicles were cultured on gelatin-sponge supports. After 2 days of histoculture, follicles were divided into upper and lower segments from which genomic DNA was extracted and analyzed.

RESULTS. Only the lower segment of a follicle undergoes programmed cell death. In contrast DNA from the upper segment of a follicle was intact.

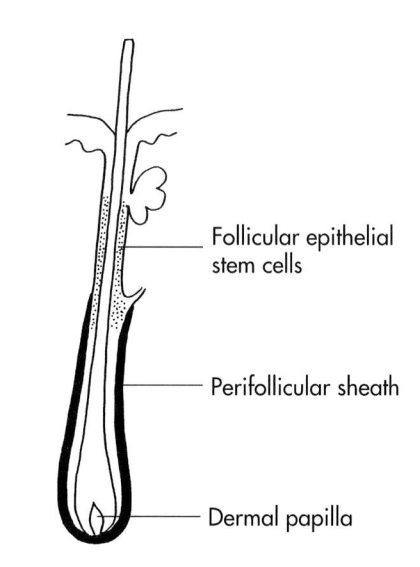

FIG. 11-22 Hypothetical schema showing the location of follicular epithelial stem cells and perifollicular sheath cells, which can reconstitute a new papilla.

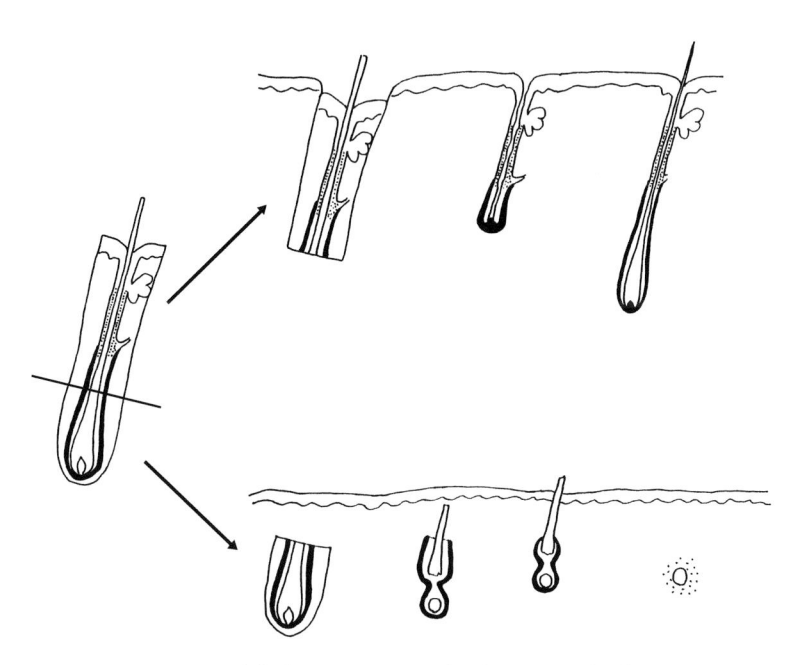

FIG. 11-23 Hair follicle regeneration after lower one-third transection.

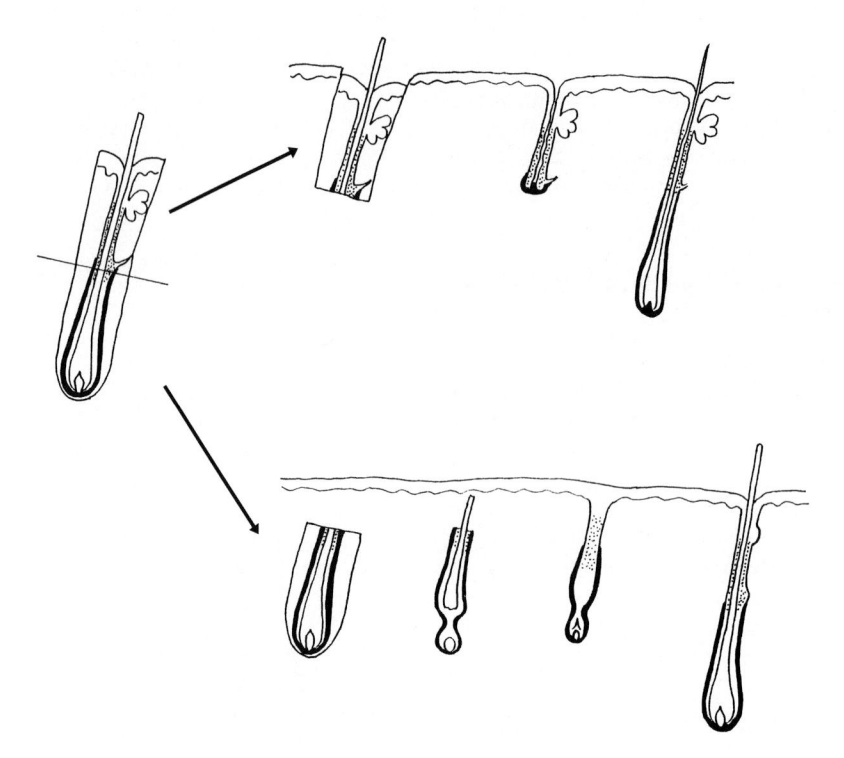

FIG. 11-24 Hair follicle regeneration after one-half transection.

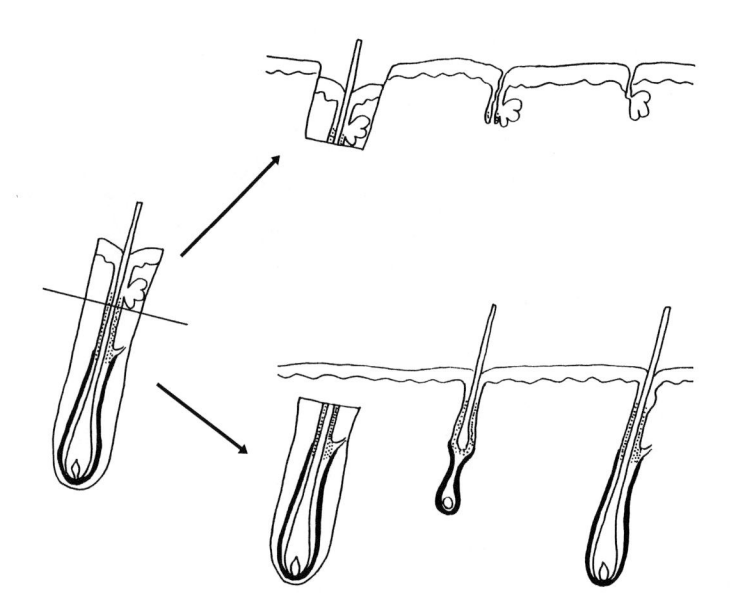

FIG. 11-25 Hair follicle regeneration after upper two-thirds transection.

CONCLUSION. The lower follicular epithelial cells are dispensable.

DISCUSSION

Stem cells initiating hair follicle development have traditionally been thought to reside in the hair bulb matrix.[10] However, the lower segment of the follicle is impermanent and disappears during telogen. It is logical therefore to look for a source of stem cells in the permanent follicle. Recent research by other investigators has suggested that stem cells arise in the area of the bulge at the insertion of the arrector pili muscle.[4] Our experiments suggest that stem cells arise from the perifollicular sheath surrounding the isthmus at the midfollicular level thus arising from not only the bulge area but also the adjacent midfollicular area above it.

CONCLUSION

The midfollicle or isthmus, extending upward from the insertion of the arrector pili muscle to the level of the entry of the sebaceous duct, must be retained intact for regeneration of a new hair follicle.

Regeneration of a new hair follicle appears to depend on the presence of follicular stem cells in the perifollicular sheath around the isthmus (Figs. 11-22 and 11-23). These cells alone are capable of forming a small dermal papilla and subsequently a fine hair. If the dermal papilla from the preceding hair cycle is still present, then a new follicle will form with a normal-sized papilla and subsequent production of a normal-sized hair (Figs. 11-24 and 11-25). Regeneration is not affected by the absence of the lower or impermanent follicle or by the presence of the follicular infundibulum (see Figs. 11-23 and 11-25).

Hair transplant surgeons can be encouraged by the fact that transplanted hairs will regrow despite significant damage to the hair bulb or follicular infundibulum.

REFERENCES

1. Kligman AM: The human hair cycle, *J Invest Dermatol* 33:307-316, 1959.
2. Unger WP, Nordstrom REA: *Hair transplantation*, New York, 1988, Marcel Dekker.
3. Hardy MH: The secret life of the hair follicle, *Trends Genet* 8:55-61, 1992.
4. Miller SJ, Sun T-T, Lavker RM: Hair follicles, stem cells and skin cancer, *J Invest Dermatol* 100:288S-294S, 1993.
5. Choi Y-C, Kim J-C: Single hair transplantation using Choi hair transplanter, *J Dermatol Surg Oncol* 18:945-948, 1992.
6. Jahoda CAB, Oliver RF: Vibrissa dermal papilla cell aggregative behaviour in vivo and in vitro, *J Embryol Exp Morphol* 79:211-224, 1984.
7. Jahoda CAB and others: Smooth muscle alpha-actin is a marker for hair follicle dermis in vivo and in vitro, *J Cell Sci* 99:627-636, 1991.
8. Peled A and others: Expression of alpha–smooth muscle actin in murine bone marrow stromal cells, *Blood* 78:304-309, 1991.
9. Itami S and others: Mechanism of action of androgen in dermal papilla cells, *Ann N Y Acad Sci* 642:385-395, 1991.
10. Van Scott EJ, Ekel TM, Auerbach R: Determination of rate and kinetics of cell division in scalp hair, *J Invest Dermatol* 4:269-273, 1963.

C. Laser Hair Transplantation

1. Principles

Richard E. Fitzpatrick

The combination of the use of slit grafting, micrografting, and minigrafting for hair transplantation plus changes in pulsed carbon-dioxide laser technology have brought these two distinctive fields together in laser hair transplantation. The popularity, success, and sophistication of the use of smaller grafts (one to seven hairs) have steadily and dramatically increased over the last 10 years.[1] Although operative techniques vary, potential problems associated with small-graft hair transplantation always include intraoperative bleeding; graft compression, elevation, or depression; and difficulty with insertion of grafts. The potential use of the carbon-dioxide laser to vaporize tissue in drilling recipient holes has been considered because it may solve one or more of these problems. The most obvious potential benefit is its control of bleeding during surgery. The small vessels encountered in the dermis and superficial subcutaneous fat of the scalp are easily sealed with carbon-dioxide laser vaporization of this tissue since vessels smaller than 0.5 mm in diameter are photocoagulated by the carbon-dioxide laser.[2] Less postoperative pain and edema are thought to occur as well with carbon-dioxide laser surgery than with steel scalpel surgery.[3,4]

The fact that the carbon-dioxide laser can drill a hole in tissue cleanly and blood-free also has the potential advantage of removal of small amounts of bald skin with each recipient hole drilled. Avoidance of compression of grafts and ease of insertion of grafts are made possible by the fact that each hole is created by vaporization of tissue and not by stretching open an incision or puncture wound. Because of the precision achievable with lasers, the incidence of graft elevation or depression may be reduced as well. An important consideration for both the patient and the surgeon is the time required for surgery. By controlling bleeding and improving the surgeon's ability to insert grafts, the carbon-dioxide laser may potentially significantly decrease the operative time required.

Before the development of high-energy, pulsed carbon-dioxide lasers, the use of the carbon-dioxide laser had been impaired by the occurrence of unseen and unwanted residual thermal damage beyond the level of tissue vaporization as a consequence of heat diffusion.[5,6] This damage zone usually extends 100 to 500 µm but may reach as far as 2 mm from the laser impact site when a continuous beam carbon-dioxide laser is used.[7-9] This layer of laser-induced thermal necrosis has been shown to interfere with wound healing and graft survival.[10,11]

When Anderson and Parrish[12,13] developed their concept of selective photothermolysis in describing laser-tissue interaction, they revolutionized the world of cutaneous laser surgery. When these principles are applied to carbon-dioxide laser surgery of the skin, the pulse parameters necessary to control thermal damage become apparent. The most important factor appears to be the pulse duration, which must be less than the thermal relaxation time of the tissue vaporized to prevent thermal diffusion.[12,13] The thermal relaxation time of human skin is thought to be approximately 1 msec.[14] The second factor of importance is the pulse energy. This component is a dosage measurement and correlates with the volume of tissue vaporized in a single pulse. Ideally all the tissue that is intended to be removed should be removed in a single pulse to avoid the potential of thermal diffusion occurring during the delivery of multiple pulses.[14] When conduction (not vaporization) is the only heat transfer mechanism operative, then a pulse frequency as low as 10 Hz may allow significant heat accumulation, and 5 Hz should be considered the upper limit to avoid thermal diffusion when the laser beam is not moved continuously.[15]

The first report of laser hair transplantation was published in August 1994 by Unger and David.[16] Although these authors were enthusiastic about their results and reported decreased bleeding, decreased operative time, and increased hair growth with use of the laser to make recipient slits, they did not report their laser parameters since they believed that ideal settings had not yet been confirmed. Of their 10 patients they reported increased hair yield in four, equal in five, and less in one. They also reported that the resultant crusting from the laser slit grafts was significantly greater and longer lasting than that normally encountered with scalpel slit grafting. This fact is not surprising when the photomicrograph of a laser slit incision is examined. Although the visible thermal necrosis along the walls of the slit is around 50 µm, in the subepidermal region it is closer to 300 µm. It is this area that causes the prolonged crusting and slow healing of the cutaneous surface. They also did not find the laser to be useful in cutting the skin to obtain the donor strip.

I have 20 years' experience in hair transplantation, including 8 years with minigrafting, micrografting, and slit grafting and an additional 15 years' experience in laser surgery. I recently completed a study of eight patients comparing various laser settings of the Ultrapulse carbon-dioxide laser (Coherent Medical Laser, Palo Alto, Calif.) vs. conventional micrografting and minigrafting using 18-gauge and 14-gauge needles to make the recipient sites. Dilators 1 mm and 2 mm in diameter were used to stretch open the puncture wounds and control bleeding in the conventional sites. Round vaporization holes 0.5 mm in diameter and 1.25 mm in diameter and slit rectangles 1 × 3 mm were vaporized using the Ultrapulse carbon-dioxide laser.

Three of the eight patients were treated with the Ultrapulse carbon-dioxide laser as an incisional instrument for the donor area; the remainder were treated with a No. 10 steel scalpel. All grafts were then cut with a No. 10 steel scalpel, and the hairs in each graft were counted. In each patient there were 20 grafts each of five categories: laser micrograft, laser minigraft, laser slit-graft, conventional micrograft, and conventional minigraft. Each patient was examined monthly for a minimum of 6 months. The laser sites were all treated with 450 mJ per pulse, 0.99 sec timed series of pulses × 2 for minigrafting and slit-grafting and 0.8 × 1 for micrografting. The power was varied for groups of two patients at 15 W, 20 W, 30 W, and 50 W. A summary of the results is as follows:

1. In all patients the laser-treated recipient sites had more crusting and slower healing than the non–laser treated recipient sites, with the severity correlating with the power used (Fig. 11-26, A and B).
2. In all patients the conventional micrografts and minigrafts resulted in greater hair yield than the laser micrografts and minigrafts. In some patients there was ≤50% growth of grafts in the laser sites. This finding again correlated with the power used (Fig. 11-26, C).
3. In all patients the conventional micrografts and minigrafts resulted in less scarring and fewer visible signs of surgery when completely healed than the laser micrografts and minigrafts.
4. The operative time for the laser hair transplantation was approximately 50% of that of the conventional grafting because of the lack of bleeding and easier graft placement.

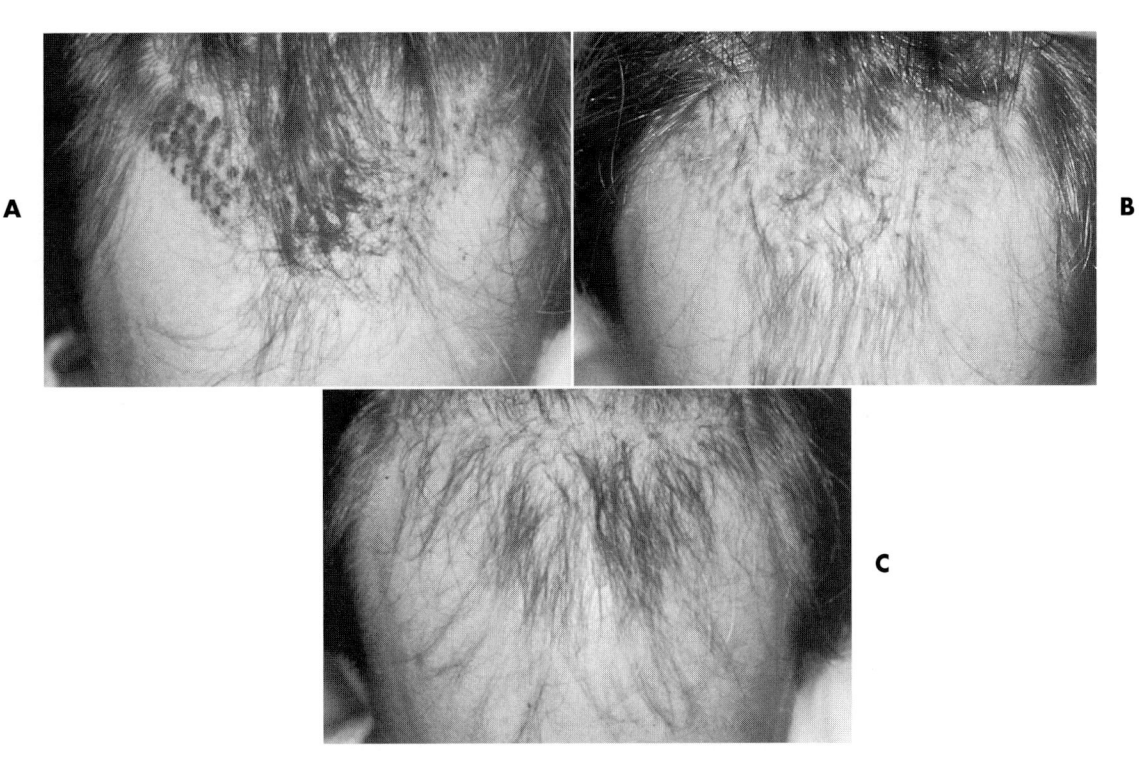

FIG. 11-26 **A,** One-week postoperative view after laser hair transplantation (on right side) and conventional micrografting and minigrafting (on left side). The laser recipient sites reveal more inflammation and crusting than the conventional micrografts and minigrafts. Laser parameters were 450 mJ per pulse and 20 W. **B,** One-month postoperative view. The laser recipient sites are healing more slowly than the conventional recipient sites. **C,** Six-month postoperative view. The laser recipient sites show relatively lighter hair growth than the conventional recipient sites.

5. The laser was not found to be useful in harvesting the donor strip.

The basic problem encountered when trying to vaporize a cylinder of tissue 1.25 mm in diameter or a rectangle 1 × 3 mm is that this amount of tissue is too much to vaporize rapidly with pulses of 450 mJ. Using a repetition rate of 5 Hz results in a very slow and tedious process, and increasing the power results in repetition rates that allow heat accumulation between pulses.

The only feasible method of vaporizing the volume of tissue necessary without causing surrounding thermal necrosis is to make the spot size small enough that a significant depth of tissue is vaporized with each pulse and the beam is moved continuously by hand or by a scanner to form a circular hole or linear slit. This method avoids heat accumulation because each pulse has a new impact site; thus a rapid repetition rate can be used.

The laser system presented in the following section by Villnow and associates does allow for vaporizing a complete cylinder with a single pulse. This system causes minimal tissue damage from heat and permits a rapid repetition rate. However, until the ideal laser parameters and treatment protocols are established, this technique remains an investigative procedure—an exciting and promising one—but investigative nonetheless.

2. Laser-Assisted Hair Transplantation

Malte M. Villnow, Michael Slatkine,
Bernd Strobele, and Douglass Mead

Megasession hair transplantation uses extensive numbers of small grafts in a single session. The average number of implanted grafts in a single session may vary between 300 and 3000 using polished drills and needles.[17] Individual sessions can be lengthy (3 to 5 hours) and tedious. The laser-assisted hair transplantation (LAHT) technique has been successfully used in over 150 patients in Germany. Preliminary results using a similar technique have been obtained independently in the United States.[18] The recipient holes are drilled with the aid of a carbon-dioxide laser flashscanner. The size of the recipient holes varies from 0.8 to 1.5 mm in diameter. The advantage of the carbon-dioxide laser flashscanner for hair transplantation stems from its ability to coagulate blood vessels in recipient sites while keeping the residual necrotic layer thin enough to enable blood to diffuse through it and nourish the graft follicles. In this section we describe the operating principles of the carbon-dioxide laser flashscanner, its tissue interaction, the operating techniques for hair transplantation, and the clinical results.

CARBON-DIOXIDE LASER FLASHSCANNER TECHNOLOGY

The laser used for LAHT is an extremely well-collimated office carbon-dioxide laser operated at 10.6 μm wavelength. The tissue penetration at this wavelength is merely 30 μm. A carbon-dioxide laser consequently products a superficial heating effect. If laser power density is high enough, superficial tissue vaporization will occur. Moreover, if laser heating is fast enough and occurs before absorbed heat diffuses conductively deep into tissue, the superficial vaporization of tissue will be associated with minimal residual thermal necrosis. Also, if laser power density is high enough to instantaneously vaporize tissue, ablation will be char-free and clean. Most well-collimated laser beams generated by carbon-dioxide lasers have a bell-shaped cross section, with high power level at the center and very low power in the peripheries. This laser beam will not allow for drilling holes with char-free "walls" (although the crater bottoms—not walls—may be vaporized without char). A simple way to overcome this deficiency and drill holes with char-free walls is to use a focused beam with a scanner.

The carbon-dioxide laser flashscanner (Sharplan SilkTouch Laser; Sharplan Lasers, Inc., Allendale, N.J.) is a miniature optomechanical beam-focusing scanner compatible with any carbon-dioxide laser. The flashscanner consists of two almost parallel folding mirrors that periodically vibrate and deflect the laser beam (Fig. 11-27). The angular position of the mirrors is precisely controlled by a microprocessor to generate selectable scanning patterns at various speeds on tissue. For LAHT a spiral pattern with *constant* scanning speed ensures homogeneous vaporization of tissue (Fig. 11-28).

The carbon-dioxide laser used in conjunction with the hair transplantation handpiece generates a focused beam of spot size smaller than 0.15 mm diameter on tissue. With a typical laser power level of 30 to 40 W, the optical power density generated

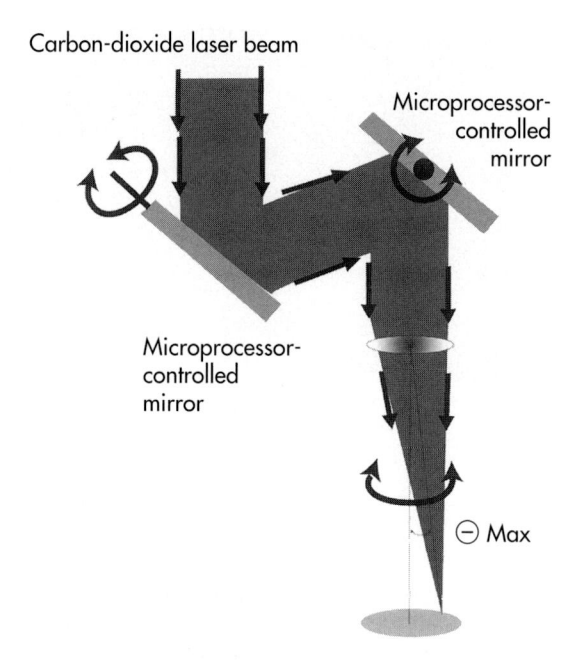

FIG. 11-27 Operating principles of the SilkTouch carbon-dioxide laser flashscanner.

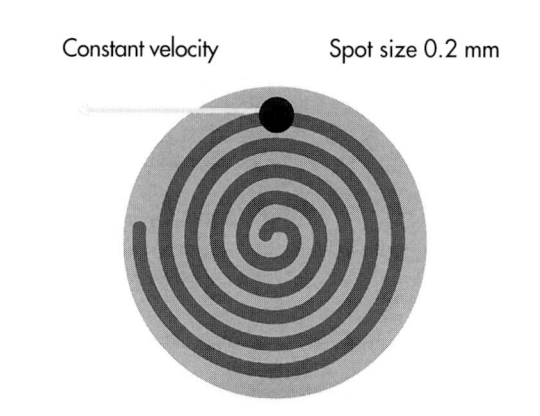

FIG. 11-28 Spiral scan pattern generated by the Silk-Touch carbon-dioxide laser flashscanner on tissue. The small focal beam spot size and fast constant beam velocity are the key to char-free vaporization with only 30 μm thermal necrosis depth on the walls of the recipient sites.

on tissue is more than 700 W/mm^2.[18] This power density is considerably higher than the threshold for vaporization of tissue without char (the threshold for char-free tissue ablation is ~50 W/mm^2).[19] Moreover, the thermal necrosis with this technique at 40 W power level has been measured to be approximately 30 μm, which is adequate for graft acceptance. Thermal necrosis depth would increase at lower power level.

The laser power and time parameters necessary to drill micrograft recipient sites of adequate depth may

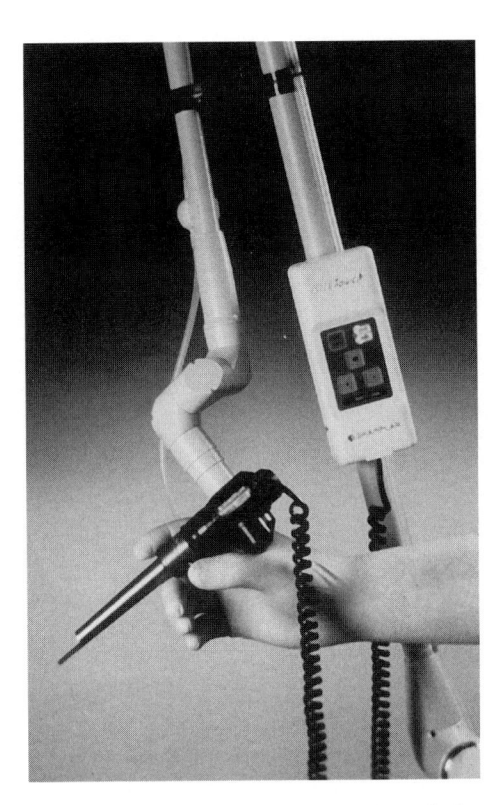

FIG. 11-29 SilkTouch carbon-dioxide laser flashscanner and handpiece for hair transplantation.

SPECIFICATIONS FOR THE SILKTOUCH CARBON-DIOXIDE LASER FLASHSCANNER

Focal length	80 mm
Scanning diameters	0.8-1.4 mm
Scanning duration	0.2 sec
Spot size	0.15 mm
Instantaneous dwelling time	1 msec
Scanning pattern for constant velocity	Spiral

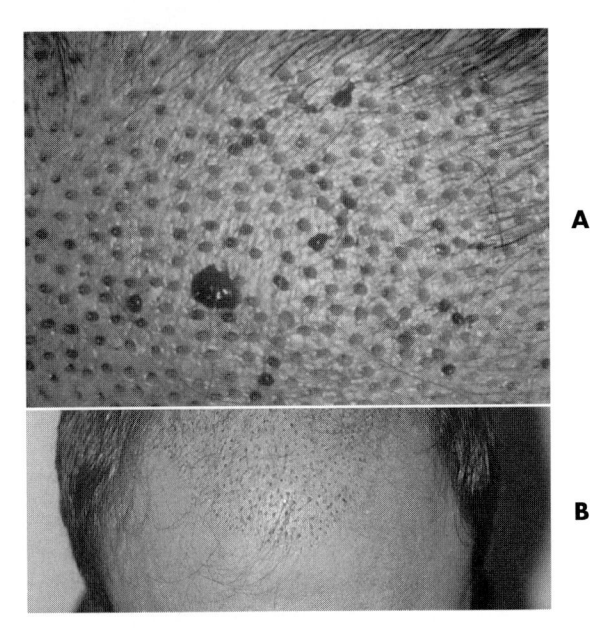

FIG. 11-30 A, Recipient sites vaporized with the SilkTouch laser. A total of 2800 holes was created. Notice the homogeneity and lack of deepithelialization. **B,** Appearance 1 day after surgery.

be estimated on a theoretical basis. The time required for the flashscanner to homogeneously cover a 1 mm round area is set by the flashscan designer to be 0.2 sec (see box). During this time, the 35 W operating laser delivers 7000 mJ to the tissue. Since the typical energy required to completely vaporize tissue is approximately 3000 mJ/mm^2,[19] we expect the laser to drill (vaporize) to a depth of 3 to 4 mm. Table 11-7 presents clinical drilling parameters.

Fig. 11-29 depicts a hair transplantation–focusing handpiece and a typical office laser used with the flashscanner.

OPERATING TECHNIQUE

The initial operating technique is similar to non-laser hair transplantation: removal of a donor strip using the conventional method with a scalpel; preparation of minigrafts, micrografts, and single-hair grafts with a scalpel; and subcutaneous injection of local anesthetic (0.5% lidocaine (Xylocaine) with 1:100,000 epinephrine) to both the donor and recipient sites.

The carbon-dioxide laser is set to single pulse, 0.1 sec at 40 W power level, and the flashscanner is set to its smallest scanning diameter (0.8 to 1 mm). A single test hole is made to verify recipient site depth in the first front line row. If necessary, the pulse duration may be increased to 0.15 sec. Following the first line, the recipient hole diameters are increased to 1.2 mm in the front of the head. Posteriorly, the hole diameters are 1.4 mm and longer pulse durations are used (Table 11-7). Once 5 to 7 mm hole depth has been confirmed, the entire drilling process of all recipient sites is performed before hair grafts are implanted. The field of view should be constantly clear of blood and crust. For each hole, a minimal internal oozing should be observed after recipient site production. Theoretically, this oozing is a sign that the follicle will be nourished by diffusion of fluid and nutrients through the walls of the recipient sites.

368 Selected Topics in Hair Replacement

TABLE 11-7 Laser-Assisted Hair Transplantation Treatment Parameters

LOCATION	SCANNING DIAMETER (MM)	LASER POWER LEVEL (W)	SINGLE PULSE DURATION (SEC)
First line	1	40	0.1
Front of head	1.2	36	0.2
Back of head	1.4	36	0.25

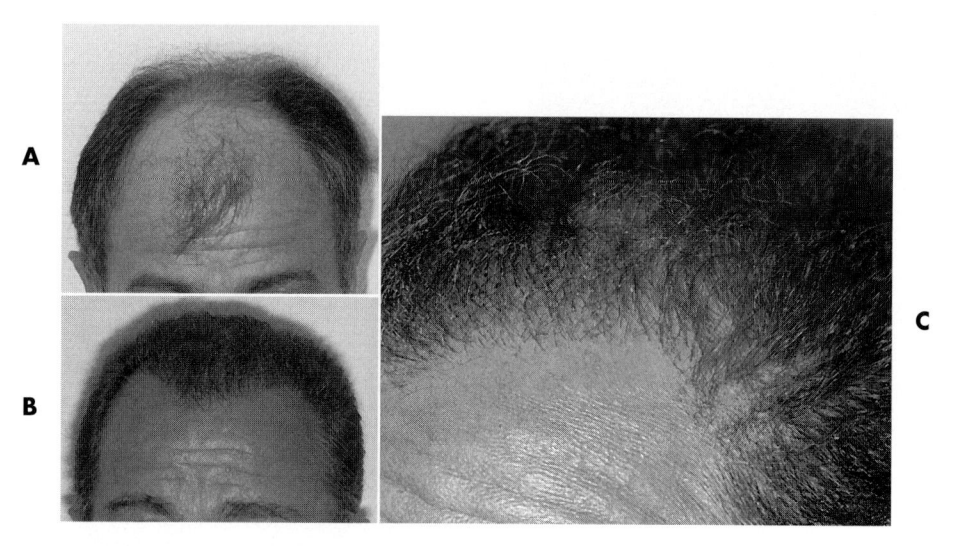

FIG. 11-31 **A,** Preoperative view. **B** and **C,** Postoperative results 4 months after a single session of 1200 grafts.

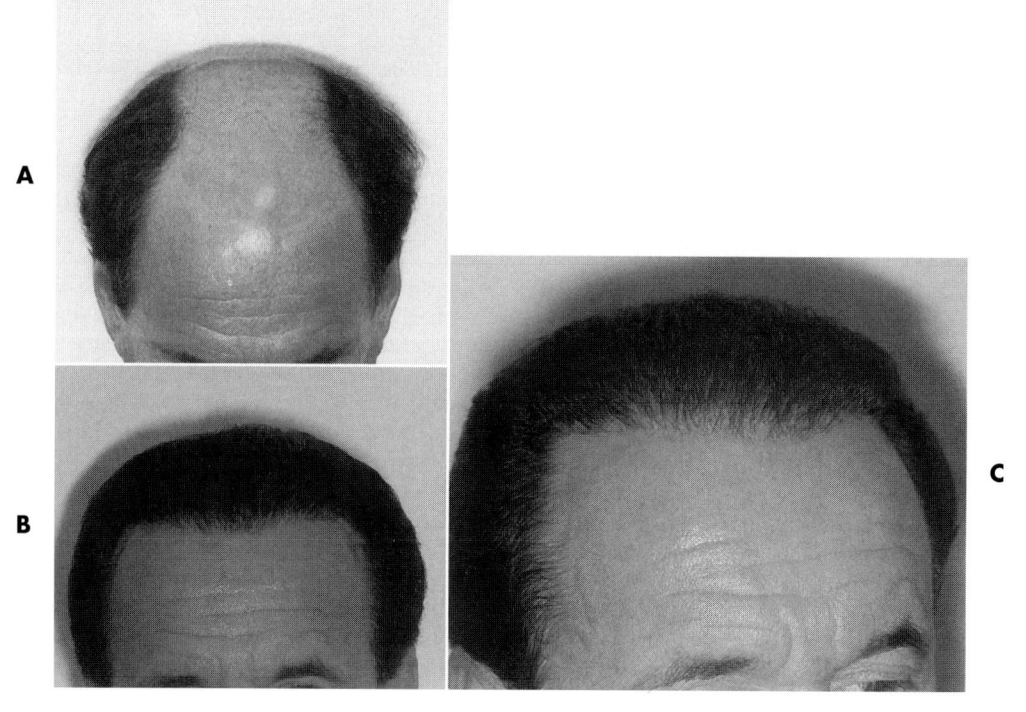

FIG. 11-32 **A,** Preoperative view. **B** and **C,** Postoperative results 4 months after a single session of 2800 grafts.

Following the drilling process, the grafts are simultaneously implanted by three to four clinical assistants in megasessions in which over 2000 grafts are implanted. Postoperative external bleeding does not occur because of wound contraction. There is no requirement for removal of recipient site tissue. After the operation the patient's hair is washed aseptically, and the patient goes home without any dressings.

RESULTS

Over 150 patients have been treated with the carbon-dioxide laser flashscanner with excellent results. We have been able to increase the graft numbers to over 2500 per session. The excellent control of the laser beam and the site visibility enables easy implantation without affecting neighboring hair follicles or previously transplanted hairs. Consequently the laser technique is also suitable for operations requiring grafts to be transplanted among areas of thinning.

Fig. 11-30 shows immediate postoperative results. We observed a lack of char and uniformity of all recipient sites. Fig. 11-31 shows preoperative and 4-month postoperative results after the transplantation of 1200 follicles in a single session. As with nonlaser hair transplants, hair grafts placed in laser-created recipient sites start to grow after 10 weeks. Fig. 11-32 demonstrates a second patient series of results of single-session laser-assisted transplantation.

CONCLUSION

To summarize, laser-assisted hair transplantation with a carbon-dioxide laser flashscanner may improve hair transplantation surgery. The advantages of the carbon-dioxide laser flashscanner are controlled hemostasis, good visibility, reduction of operating time by more than 30%, reduced need for local anesthesia and vasoconstrictors, reduced need for postoperative dressings, and a smooth postoperative skin surface. In the future, laser-assisted hair transplantation may be expected to play a major role in hair restoration surgery.

REFERENCES

1. Buchwach KA: Standard grafts, minigrafts, and micrografts. Their use in hair transplantation, *Facial Plast Surg Clin North Am* 2:149, 1994.
2. Slutzki S, Shafir R, Bornstein LA: Use of the carbon dioxide laser for large excisions with minimal blood loss, *Plast Reconstr Surg* 60:250, 1977.
3. Aschler P and others: Ultrastructural findings in CNS tissue with CO_2 laser. In Kaplan I, editor: *Laser surgery* II, Jerusalem, 1976, Academic Press.
4. Ben-Bassat M, Ben-Bassat J, Kaplan I: An ultrastructural study of the cut edges of skin and mucous membrane specimens excised by carbon dioxide laser. In Kaplan I, editor: *Laser surgery* II, Jerusalem, 1976, Academic Press.
5. Friedman M, Gal D: Keloid scars as a result of CO_2 laser for *Molluscum contagiosum*, *Obstet Gynecol* 70:394, 1987.
6. Shapshay SM and others: Benign lesions of the larynx: should the laser be used? *Laryngoscope* 100:953, 1990.
7. Mihashi S and others: Laser surgery in otolaryngology: interaction of CO_2 laser and soft tissue, *Ann N Y Acad Sci* 267:263, 1976.
8. Hall RR, Hill DW, Beach AD: A carbon dioxide surgical laser, *Ann R Coll Surg Engl* 48:181, 1971.
9. Montgomery TC and others: Comparative gross and histological study of the effects of scalpel, electric knife, and carbon dioxide laser on skin and uterine incisions in dogs, *Lasers Surg Med* 3:9, 1983.
10. Green HA and others: Skin graft take and healing after CO_2 laser and 193 nm excimer laser ablation of graft beds [abstract], *J Invest Dermatol* 92:436, 1989.
11. Fry TL and others: Effects of laser, scalpel and electrosurgical excision on wound contracture and graft "take," *Plast Reconstr Surg* 65:729, 1980.
12. Anderson RR, Parrish JA: Microvasculature can be selectively damaged using dye lasers: a basic theory and experimental evidence in human skin, *Lasers Surg Med* 1:263, 1981.
13. Anderson RR, Parrish, JA: Selective photothermolysis: precise microsurgery by selective absorption of pulsed radiation, *Science* 220:524, 1983.
14. Fitzpatrick RE, Goldman MP: CO_2 laser surgery. In Goldman MP, Fitzpatrick RE, editors: *Cutaneous laser surgery: the art and science of selective photothermolysis*, St Louis, 1994, Mosby, pp 198-257.
15. Brugmans MJP and others: Temperature response of biological materials to pulsed non-ablative CO_2 laser irradiation, *Lasers Surg Med* 11:587, 1991.
16. Unger WP, David LM: Laser hair transplantation, *J Dermatol Surg Oncol* 20:515-521, 1994.
17. Transhair Micro Driller, Dusseldorf, 1993.
18. Grevelink JM, Brennick JB: Hair transplantation facilitated by flashscanner-enhanced carbon dioxide laser, *Operative Tech Otolaryngol Head Neck Surg* 5(4):278-280, 1994.
19. Carruth JAS, McKenzie AL: *Medical lasers—science and clinical practice*, Bristol, 1986, Adam Hilger, pp 58-78.

Editor's Note

The chief advantages of laser surgery as stated by Dr. Villnow and associates are reduced operative time and superior hemostasis. The readers should be aware that Drs. Slatkine, Strobele, and Mead are employed by Sharplan Lasers, Inc., and therefore have a vested interest in this product. This section on laser surgery is presented as preliminary information since no data (specifically, studies documenting graft yield in laser-created recipient sites) are available on the overall efficacy of lasers for hair transplantation. There are many anecdotal reports from hair transplant surgeons (including myself) that hair does grow in a laser-created recipient site. However, the yield may be diminished when compared to that with traditional methods. The preliminary reports of decreased hair growth pertain to cases in which a lower wattage laser was used (i.e., SuperPulsed carbon-dioxide 40 W laser).

ity is made after a 2 or 3 cm cut. The section must be deep enough to reach the subcutaneous fascia without cutting into the galea; No. 15 blades are used. The operator releases the ends and detaches the strips. Two millimeters of fat should extend below the terminus of the hair follicles. Five strips are obtained, linked to one another at each end. The donor site is closed with staples.

PREPARATION OF THE RECIPIENT SITE (Fig. 11-37). The recipient site is prepared using a drilling-aspirator hand engine linked by a catheter to the collector bottle. The rotation of the drilling needle (about 1.3 mm diameter), activated by slight pressure on the treadle, cuts the scalp down to the fatty tissue. Stronger pressure on the treadle initiates the suction. The bald skin fragment is immediately aspirated into the collector bottle. The preparation of the recipient zone is thus accelerated, and it becomes possible to prepare a recipient opening every second.

CUTTING OF THE STRIPS (Fig. 11-38). The assistant does the cutting of the graduated plate while the surgeon prepares the recipient site. The strips are easily separated from one another using a No. 23 blade scalpel by fixing one of the common ends of one strip with the pliers and leaving the other end free. The fat is then trimmed away from the five strips. They are placed flat on the microtome, perpendicular to the severing sides of the blades; the axis of the hair follicle must be strictly parallel to that of the blades. The strips are covered with a silicon sheet 0.5 mm thick, itself covered with a silicon plate 5 mm thick. A rigid metal lid is then placed on top of them. The five strips are cut simultaneously by strong pressure exerted by the press on the lid. When the lid, silicon plate, and silicon sheet are removed, the micrografts remain on the microtome, all in the same direction between the blades.

IMPLANTATION (Fig. 11-39). The patient is placed in a supine position. The assistant stands in front of the microtome. The grafts are wedged between the blades of the microtome, and the assistant points the tip of the collecting needle at the skin of the first graft. The surgeon presses the control treadle, and the graft makes its way through the catheter to the implanting handtool in less then 1 second. The surgeon then activates the piston to propel the graft into the recipient site. The pneumatic expulsion piston must be held in the active position during withdrawal. The procedure is repeated as many times as needed.

INDICATIONS AND CONTRAINDICATIONS

The automated hair transplant system is suitable for sessions during which several hundred grafts have to be implanted. It is appropriate for straight-haired patients who require one to three micrografting sessions and have good hair density in the posterior occipital area.

This technique is contraindicated in patients with frizzy hair because the hair follicles are not perfectly parallel to the blades and thus can be damaged when the strips are cut on the press.

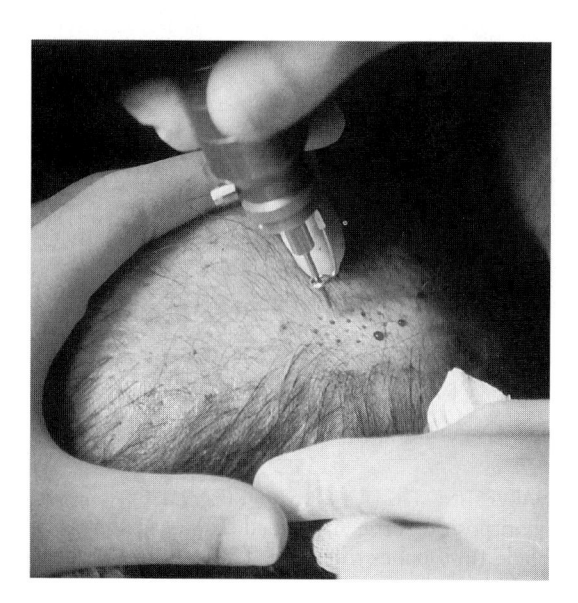

FIG. 11-37 Preparation of the recipient site with the drilling-aspirator hand engine.

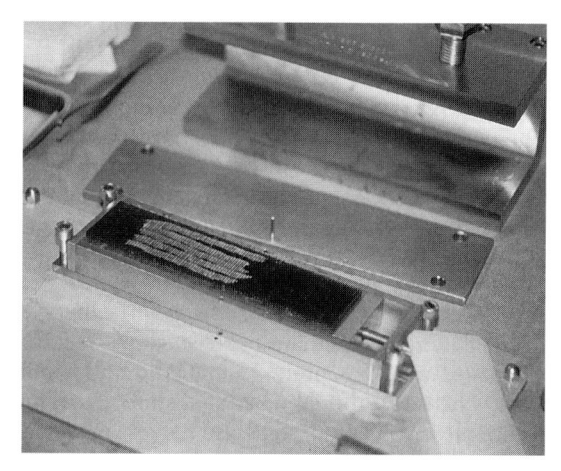

FIG. 11-38 After cutting, the grafts are ready to be aspirated and implanted.

Automated Hair Transplant System: The Boudjema Technique   373

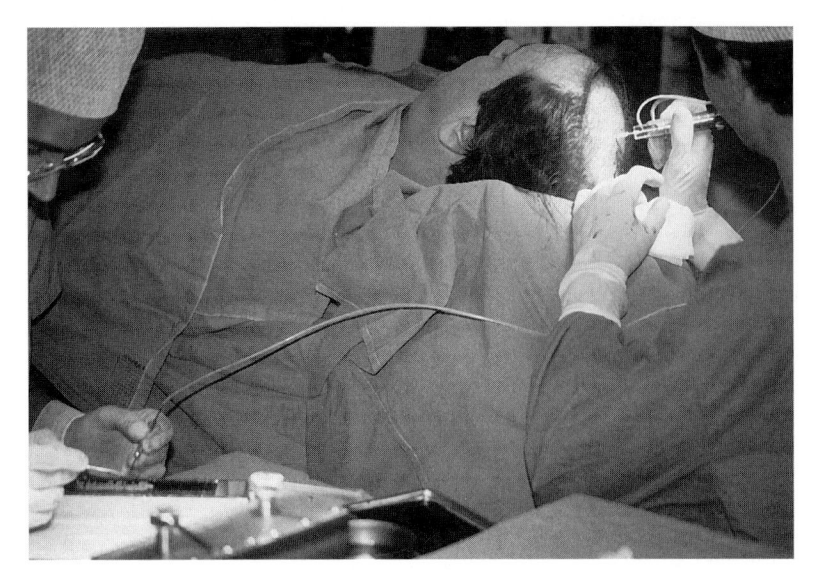

FIG. 11-39   Implantation.

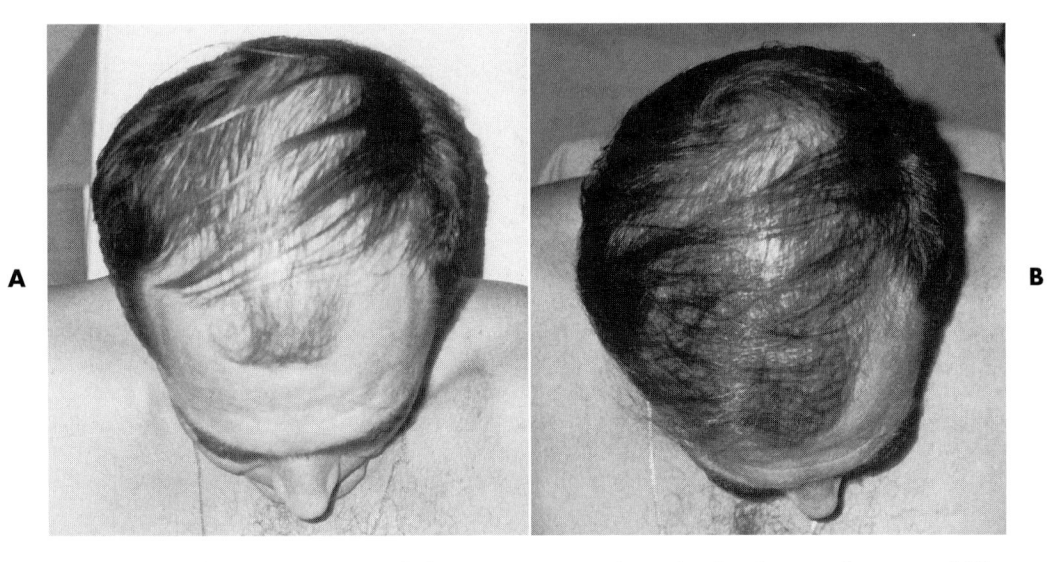

FIG. 11-40   **A,** Preoperative view. **B,** Postoperative view 6 months after the transplantation of 400 grafts in a single session.

ADVANTAGES

There are several advantages to the automated hair transplant system. The first is the rapidity of the procedure (3 to 4 seconds for each graft implanted) and the minimal personnel required. Easy implantation between hairs and fewer manipulations, resulting in better asepsis, make this technique desirable. Another advantage is the absence of conventional instruments that can cause trauma.

SHORTCOMINGS

The use of the automated hair transplant system requires a period of learning. Particularly during the implantation procedure, synchronization between the surgeon and assistant is vital. It is also necessary to rinse and drain the circuits by aspiration of physiological saline solution every 10 or 15 grafts to flush away fat debris and to lubricate the circuits. This is done by dipping the collecting needle in a cup of physiological saline solution. Sterilization of the various instruments requires their dismantling and meticulous cleansing. The diameter of the disposable pipes linking the different handtools must be chosen according to the size of the graft cut on the microtome.

COMPLICATIONS

We have not noticed any complications inherent to the automated hair transplant system except folliculitis similar to that experienced with the manual techniques.

RESULTS

The aesthetic results (Fig. 11-40) are similar to those achieved using exclusively manual techniques. However, the automated hair transplant system technique is twice as rapid. Since the quality of the result depends on hair density, the relevance of the automated hair transplant system is obvious. The aspiration and passage of the grafts through a pipe, which cause friction, do not hinder graft growth.

CONCLUSION

This new automated minigraft and micrograft transplant technique is significantly timesaving in everyday practice without altering aesthetic results. In addition, the reduction in medical staff provides a significant cost saving. Other applications of this technique are under examination (e.g., grafting directly into incisional slits without preparing the recipient zone[7-11]) and should reduce the operating time even more.

REFERENCES

1. Marritt E: Single hair transplantation of hairline refinement: a practical solution, *J Dermatol Surg Oncol* 10:962, 1984.
2. Nordstron REA: For the improvement of the frontal hairline after hair transplantation, *Aesthetic Plast Surg* 5:97-101, 1981.
3. Orentreich N: Autografts in alopecias and other selected dermatological conditions, *Ann N Y Acad Sci* 83:463, 1959.
4. Unger WP, Nordstrom REA: *Hair transplantation,* New York, 1988, Marcel Dekker.
5. Coiffmann F: Use of square scalp grafts for male pattern baldness, *Plast Reconstr Surg* 60:228-232, 1977.
6. Brandy DA: A new instrument for the expedient production of minigrafts, *J Dermatol Surg Oncol* 18:487-492, 1992.
7. Alt TH: Evaluation of donor harvesting techniques in hair transplantation, *J Dermatol Surg Oncol* 10:799-806, 1984.
8. Nelson BR: Hair transplantation in advanced male pattern alopecia: the role of incisional slit grafting, *J Dermatol Surg Oncol* 17:567-573, 1991.
9. Choi Y-C, Kim J-C: Single hair transplantation using the Choi hair transplanter, *J Dermatol Surg Oncol* 18:945-948, 1992.
10. Stough DB: Incisional slit grafting, *J Dermatol Surg Oncol* 17:53-60, 1991.
11. Uebel CO: Capillary microtransplants in the surgery treatment of baldness. In *Actualités de chirurgie esthétique,* Paris, 1992, Masson, pp 60-74.

Editor's Note

This discussion of the automated hair transplant system presented by Drs. Boudjema and Boolauck is remarkable for its engineering and represents the first serious attempt at automated hair transplantation. As the number of grafts per session increases, manpower needs increase as well. An automated hair transplant system is the logical progression of technology. If automation becomes successfully incorporated into hair restoration procedures, Drs. Boudjema and Boolauck will be remembered as the pioneers of this era. Readers should be aware that this system has yet to undergo widespread scrutiny by the hair restoration community.

12
Drug Therapy

A. Drug Therapy for Pattern Baldness

Richard L. DeVillez

Pattern baldness is a natural consequence of a person's genetic makeup and the extent to which the gene is expressed in that individual. The majority of balding individuals are endocrinologically normal, expressing an increased susceptibility of genetically programmed hair follicles to the normal effect of androgens. In approximately 10% of women with pattern hair loss and no signs of clinical hyperandrogenism (e.g., acne, hirsutism), chemical hyperandrogenism is detected.[1-9] Low sex-hormone–binding globulin (SHBG) and elevated free serum testosterone and androstenedione were the most frequent endocrine abnormalities noted.[10-13] Most investigators have found no correlation between hair loss and hormonal values, but a few have noted sideropenia in women with pattern alopecia.[14-17] Pattern baldness in the absence of clinical signs for hyperandrogenism is a progressive process as assessed by historical observation, hair counting using the unit area trichogram, direct hair counts from the patient's balding scalp, or hair counts from a photograph.[18-21] These findings suggest that medication capable of maintaining the existing hair population or restoring some hair growth should be regarded as effective treatment for this condition. Left untreated, androgenic alopecia progressively advances.

MINOXIDIL

Oral minoxidil (Loniten) is a piperidinopyrimidine-derivative vasodilator that possesses trichogenic properties. In vitro studies have shown minoxidil sulfate, the active metabolite, induced vascular relaxation that could be effectively inhibited by drugs that interfere with plasmalemmal potassium permeability.[22] It is proposed that minoxidil sulfate acts like a potassium channel agonist to enhance potassium permeability, resulting in membrane hyperpolarization and causing a reduction in agonist-stimulated calcium influx.[22] The end result is a decrease in cytoplasmic free calcium concentration and relaxation.[22] The relevance of the proposed unique cellular mechanism to its hair growth effect remains to be elucidated.[23]

Topically applied, minoxidil (Rogaine) is a trichogenic agent, but the mechanism by which it or its metabolite, minoxidil sulfate, stimulates hair regrowth in androgenic alopecia has not been determined. It appears that the drug acts at the level of the hair follicle perhaps as a potassium channel agonist or possibly by other mechanisms involving direct stimulation of the hair follicle epithelium or dermal papilla.[24-27] Minoxidil treatment of mouse vibrissae follicles in organ culture resulted in a measurable increase in the incorporation of cysteine into the follicle, normalization of follicular morphology, and proliferation of both matrix and outer root sheath cells.[26] In stumptailed macaques, evidence suggests that the drug reverses the miniaturization process of androgenic alopecia by normalizing the hair follicle cycle, causing an increase in follicular diameter and length of the existing miniaturized follicle.[24] Qualitative evaluation of human transverse biopsy specimens demonstrated hypertrophy of the balding follicle after 15 weeks of treatment with topical minoxidil.[28] The minoxidil-induced hair follicle stimulation does not appear to result from an antiandrogen effect on the follicle epithelium or dermal papilla.[29] Patients who received the drug did not develop abnormal serum androgen concentrations or abnormal urinary excretion of 17-ketosteroids or 17-hydroxysteroids.[30,31] There is evidence that the topical application of minoxidil causes increased scalp blood flow as measured by laser Doppler velocimetry and photopulse plethysmography.[32-34] The role of vasodilation of the scalp blood vessels in promoting hair regrowth in patients remains to be elucidated.

Current evidence suggests that topical minoxidil exerts a direct effect on the hair follicle cells. It affects the dermal papilla, which in turn stimulates the hair matrix cells near the base of the hair follicle.[35] In vitro studies of the follicles of the stumptailed macaque have shown a significant increase in DNA synthesis in follicular and perifollicular cells but not in epidermal keratinocytes following minoxidil therapy.[36] The drug produces a prolonged anagen phase of the vellus and indeterminate hair follicle, which enables these follicles to produce thicker and longer hair, reversing the miniaturization processes of androgenic alopecia.

Clinical Use

Following the reversal of baldness demonstrated in a patient receiving minoxidil for hypertension[37] (Fig. 12-1), topical 2% minoxidil (Rogaine) was evaluated for the treatment of androgenic alopecia in men and women in well-designed clinical trials by domestic[38-45] and international investigators.[46-55] It was the first drug approved by the Food and Drug Administration (FDA) for the treatment of androgenic alopecia in men and women. The large clinical trials enrolled 2326 men and 630 women and used hair count changes from designated balding areas together with patient and physician global evaluations to determine efficacy. Whether determined by direct hair counting from the patient's scalp or by hair counting from a photograph of a permanently marked 1 cm^2 area of the scalp using computer-assisted image analysis, the nonvellus hair counts were significantly higher in those patients treated with minoxidil than in the control patients.[56] Both men and women treated with minoxidil had increased nonvellus hair counts of nearly 20% over baseline (Figs. 12-2 and 12-3). Younger, less bald individuals grew more hair and demonstrated better cosmetic coverage than older, more bald individuals.[57] Women grew slightly more hair than men and demonstrated better cosmetic coverage because hair loss was less.[23] Continued use of 2% minoxidil twice daily is necessary to maintain the regrowth. Patients using less than the prescribed amount or less frequent applications do not have as good results as those who persist with the twice-daily treatment plan.[58,59] Those who stop using topical minoxidil generally experience loss of the regrown hair and additional hair that had been prevented from shedding during the treatment period within 3 to 4 months.[60-62] Restarting drug application will allow recapture of part of the prior growth, but not all, because of a new, more severe hair loss starting point. For those who continue to use topical minoxidil, there seems to be a peak effect at approximately 1 year with a slow decline in regrowth over the subsequent years but substantially better than that seen at the beginning of the treatment.[63,64]

The benefit from using topical minoxidil to avoid the hair loss from transplanted hair autografts has not been adequately evaluated. It seems that some hairs from each graft continue to grow whereas others fall out.[65] Overall many believe

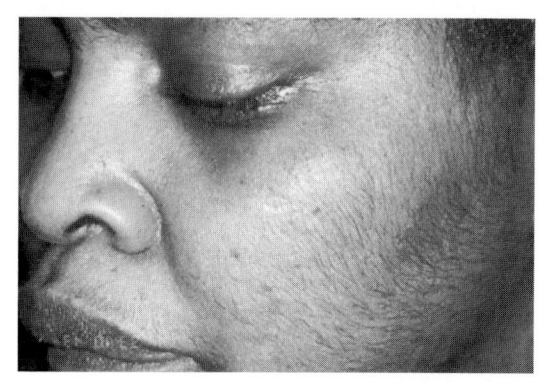

FIG. 12-1 A 40-year-old black woman who required oral minoxidil for control of hypertension. Note the facial hair growth, which can be a side effect of oral minoxidil therapy. (Courtesy Dr. Dow Stough.)

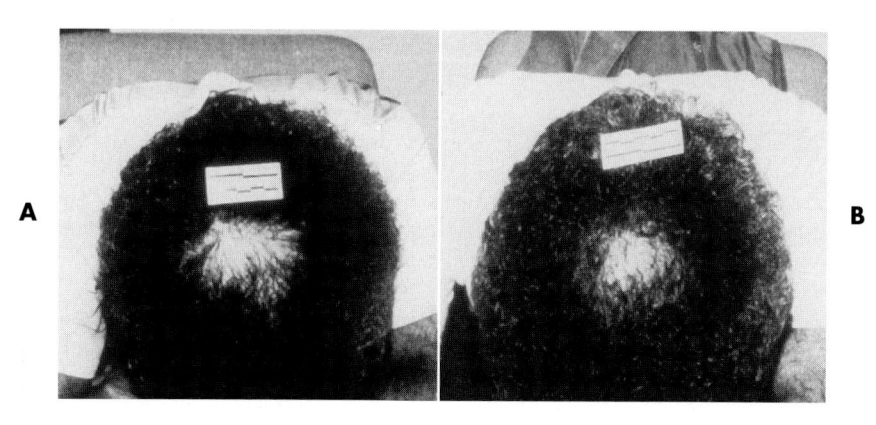

FIG. 12-2 **A,** Male patient with early progressive hair loss. **B,** Result after using 2% topical minoxidil for 1 year.

that using topical minoxidil is an adjunct for better growth from the grafts after hair transplantation surgery. No data are available regarding minoxidil application and the micrograft techniques. Topical minoxidil is not effective in preventing alopecia during chemotherapy.[66]

The combination of topical tretinoin and topical minoxidil demonstrated a marginal but not significant increase in effectiveness compared with minoxidil alone.[67,68] Based on steady-state urinary excretion profiles, the coapplication of topical tretinoin and 2% topical minoxidil resulted in a nearly threshold increase in systemic minoxidil absorption compared with 2% minoxidil alone[69] (see Chapter 12, Part B). Reversal of androgenic alopecia by minoxidil in women was not enhanced by the simultaneous use of intermediate doses of cyproterone acetate.[70]

Topical 2% minoxidil (Rogaine) is a safe drug for treating hair loss. In controlled trials, adverse reactions in those treated with minoxidil did not differ substantially from those experienced by patients receiving the placebo.[71,72] Allergic contact dermatitis occurred in less than 1% of the patients and irritant dermatitis or folliculitis occurred in 3% to 5%.[72,73] Increased hair growth outside the area of drug application (e.g., eyebrows, face, ears, arms, and beard) was reported sporadically, possibly resulting from inadvertent transfer of the topical solution. No relevant hemodynamic effects have been noted in normotensive or hypertensive patients.[72] Although more echocardiographic effects were noted in the patients receiving topical minoxidil by one study group,[74] controlled trials reported that various echocardiographic changes occurred equally in both groups of patients.[72] Following extensive use of the drug to date, there has been no evidence that topical minoxidil is associated with any significant cardiovascular phenomenon.

In the future a more potent version of topical minoxidil is expected. This preparation probably will be a higher concentration of the drug or one with enhanced penetration to improve the level of minoxidil present at the level of the hair follicle. With higher concentration, increased hair growth on the balding scalp would be expected. A twice-daily regimen would still likely be required.

Recommended Dosage

The recommended dosage of 2% topical minoxidil is 1 ml twice daily. One bottle will last 1 month and costs approximately $55. Continuous, uninterrupted use is recommended for optimal results (Fig. 12-4).

PULSE ELECTROTRICHOGENESIS

Electromagnetic and electrostatic current has been effectively used for wound healing and bone regrowth. Electrostatic current has not been associated with tumor induction. A controlled study demonstrated that 60% of subjects noted an increase in hair growth using an electrostatic current device.[75] Over 90% exhibited no further hair loss.[75] A continuation of electrostatic treatment in these groups of patients for an additional year demonstrated a further increase in hair counts and no further hair loss.[76] The subjects sat in a comfortable chair with a hair dryer–type hood over the vertex and frontoparietal areas of the scalp for 12 minutes per week.[75,76] The battery-powered electrostatic field was created within the hood. No patients felt

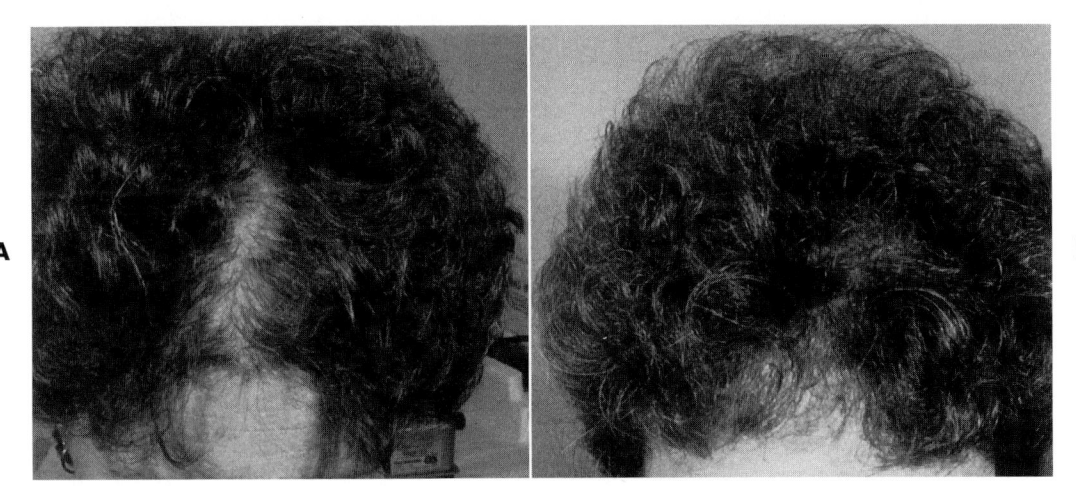

FIG. 12-3 **A,** Female patient with early progressive hair loss. **B,** Result after using 2% topical minoxidil for 1 year.

378 Drug Therapy

any shock sensations, and no other adverse effects were reported.[75,76]

The mechanism for hair growth induction is poorly understood. The positive current is used to prepare the hair for the negative current stimulation for hair regrowth. Throughout the treatment period, pulses of positive current are interjected to continue effective therapy. A larger multicenter trial was conducted and the data, which suggest a positive effect on hair regrowth and cessation of hair loss, have been submitted to the Food and Drug Administration (FDA).

5α-REDUCTASE INHIBITOR

Finasteride (Proscar) is a patented 5α-reductase inhibitor without any androgenic, antiandrogenic, or other steroid hormone effect[77] (Fig. 12-5). Oral finasteride causes suppression of circulating dihydrotestosterone (DHT) without any change in testosterone, cortisol, prolactin, sex-hormone–binding globulin, thyroxine, estradiol, or glucose tolerance.[77-79] Administration of the drug to pregnant women would be expected to cause ambiguous genitalia in any male fetus. Finasteride is playing a major role in the medical management of benign prostatic hypertrophy and holds promise for the prevention of male pattern baldness.[80]

Although no studies have been completed in humans, two studies in stumptailed macaque monkeys have been promising.[81,82] Topical 4-MA (H,N-diethyl-4-methyl-3-oxo-4-aza-5α-androstane-17β-carboxamide), a 5α-reductase inhibitor, was used as a 14 mg/ml solution in DMSO daily on preadolescent stumptailed macaques for 27 months. The

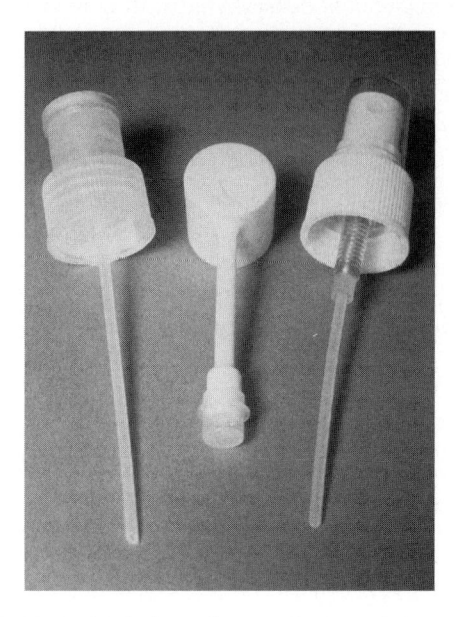

FIG. 12-4 Multiple applicators for topical minoxidil. The extended spray tip *(center)* is the applicator most frequently used by patients, especially women with significant hair remaining.

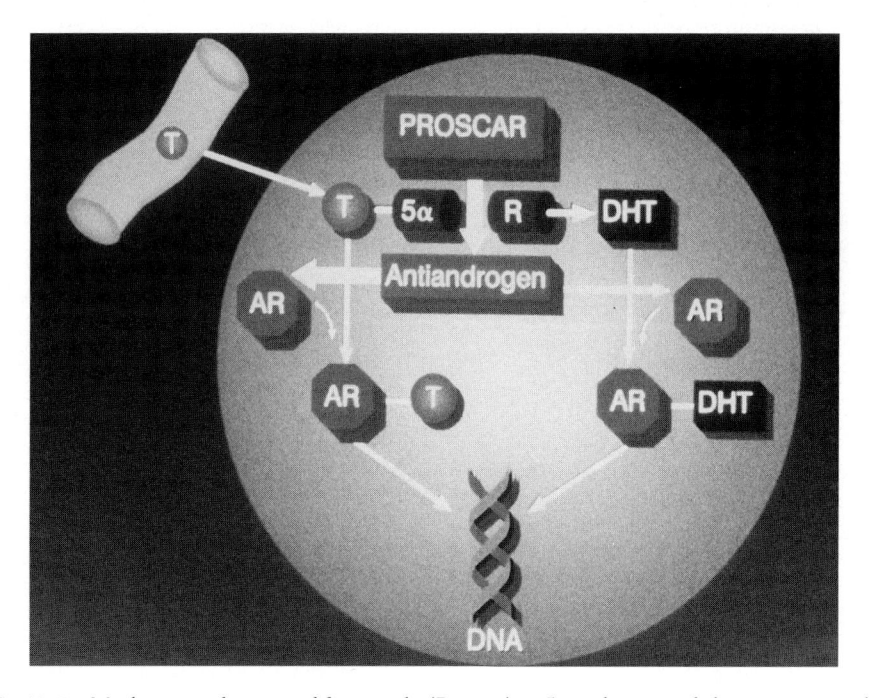

FIG. 12-5 Mechanism of action of finasteride (Proscar), a 5α-reductase inhibitor vs. antiandrogens. 5αR, 5α-reductase; *DHT*, dihydrotestosterone; *T*, testosterone; *AR*, androgen receptor.

control monkeys demonstrated varying degrees of hair loss, whereas the treated monkeys demonstrated prevention of the progression of baldness.[82] A second study was performed in the adult stumptailed macaque using oral finasteride alone and in combination with 2% topical minoxidil.[81] Finasteride alone was effective in preventing further hair loss. The combined use of finasteride and topical minoxidil significantly augmented the effect of either used alone.[81]

The retardation of the conversion of testosterone to dihydrotestosterone by blocking the effect of the 5α-reductase enzyme seems to be a mechanism for stimulating hair growth when used alone and a potential adjunctive therapy with topical minoxidil for the treatment of male pattern baldness.[81]

SYSTEMIC ANTIANDROGENS

Cyproterone Acetate and Ethinyl Estradiol

Women with pattern hair loss have been treated with oral cyproterone acetate and ethinyl estradiol. Cyproterone is antigonadotropic, so estrogens are administered to ensure regular menses and reinforce the antigonadotropic effect.[83] The combination with estrogen is usually delivered in a reverse sequential regimen called *cyclical antiandrogen therapy* (CAT). No large controlled study using CAT for female pattern alopecia has been conducted.[84-86] In one study, 20 women were treated in a CAT regimen using cyproterone acetate and ethinyl estradiol and 20 were left untreated for 1 year.[87] Half of the women in each group had serum ferritin concentrations above 40 µg/L and half had concentrations below 40 µg/L. Based on hair counts, it was determined that those women with serum ferritin concentrations above 40 µg/L treated with the CAT regimen grew more hair than those with a lower serum ferritin and the control patients. There was no correlation between the serum ferritin level and the severity of hair loss, but those women with serum ferritin above 40 µg/L grew more hair.[87] Subsequent studies demonstrated that normal vitamin B_{12} levels were also necessary for an optimal effect.[88]

Current systemic antiandrogen regimens seem effective, but the prospect of long-term therapy, possibly for life, is worrisome, and assessing its value in the long-term treatment of androgenic alopecia is difficult.

Cimetidine

Cimetidine, an H_2 antihistamine approved for the treatment of peptic ulcer disease, is a competitive inhibitor of dihydrotestosterone. In a small clinical trial of 10 women, 300 mg was given five times a day for up to 9 months with good to excellent hair regrowth reported based on serial photography and subjective evaluations.[89] Cimetidine-induced alopecia has also been noted.[90] No large controlled clinical trials have been reported.

Spironolactone

Spironolactone (Aldactone), an aldosterone antagonist that blocks testosterone production in the adrenal gland by depleting microsomal cytochrome P-450 and competitively inhibiting the DHT-receptor at its site of translocation of the complex into the nucleus, has been used for treating female androgenic alopecia.[91] In a study in which six patients with androgenic alopecia were treated with 200 mg spironolactone daily, the patients were pleased with the results after 6 months.[92] The side effects include breast tenderness, irregular menses, and mood swings.[88] Because feminization of a male fetus occurs with spironolactone, the adjunctive administration of oral contraceptive medications is encouraged. No large controlled clinical trials have been performed.

TOPICAL ANTIANDROGENS

Estroprogestational agents have been used for many years in women to treat androgenic alopecia.[93-95] Estrogen increases the production of sex-hormone–binding globulin, which leads to decreased free serum testosterone, whereas progesterone is a competitive inhibitor for 5α-reductase and for binding the cytosol androgen receptor.[94] Studies using topical estrogen, progesterone, or combined estroprogestational agents in women and men have shown minimal improvement in hair regrowth or retarding further hair loss.[96,97] The menstrual irregularities that occur in women and loss of libido or impotence in men have been major problems in the continued use of these preparations for the treatment of pattern baldness.[95-97]

OTHER AGENTS FOR HAIR GROWTH

Tricomin, a peptide-copper complex, was evaluated in a double-blind placebo controlled study of 18 patients with Hamilton type V male pattern baldness.[98] A 2% or a 10% gel formulation was applied twice daily for 6 months and the results compared. The increase in anagen hairs, recorded from a marked reference area by the phototrichogram technique, revealed that patients using the 10% concentration showed an overall trend for hair growth and less hair loss. The mechanism of action is unknown. No adverse effects were reported.

Low-dosage oral retinol, L-cystine, and gelatin were evaluated in a year-long, double-blind study in 47 patients.[99] Patient response was measured using trichograms and hair density measurement before and after treatment. There was modest improvement in the treatment group compared with those receiving the placebo.[99]

A controlled, randomized, double-blind, parallel-group study compared the effects of ViviScall (a food supplement incorporating special marine extracts and a silica compound) with those of a fish extract on 40 young men for 6 months.[100] Nonvellus hair counts were done at baseline, 2, 4, and 6 months. Biopsies of the scalp were performed at baseline and at 6 months. ViviScall was shown to be a moderately to highly effective treatment for androgenic alopecia in young men.[100]

The effects of topical cyclosporine (1%) in olive oil were evaluated in a double-blind study on 20 subjects for 4 months using photographs and hair counts.[101] Two of the 10 patients treated with topical cyclosporine noted significant hair growth; one patient's hair regrowth was cosmetically acceptable. No cutaneous or systemic side effects were noted.[101] An open study involving 11 patients showed similar results without adverse effects.[102]

A randomized, double-blind trial using a Chinese herb extract (Dabao) as a hair restorer was evaluated in 396 men with pattern hair loss.[103] Evaluated with hair counts and photographs, the cosmetic effects in patients using Dabao were judged to be slightly better than those in patients who received a placebo.

Many other small open studies and case reports have demonstrated hair regrowth.[104-109] None have been subjected to rigorous scientific scrutiny.

CONCLUSION

Topical and oral treatments for pattern hair loss in men and women are just that—*treatments*; they are not *cures*. The treatment overrides the effects of the genes and hormones. When the treatment is discontinued, the hair gained is lost and the hair that should have been shed during the treatment period also will fall out. The topical agents developed thus far to treat androgenic alopecia have provided encouraging results, but with continued efforts other new and more effective compounds are certain to be developed in this promising area of dermatological research.

REFERENCES

1. Miller JA and others: Low sex-hormone binding globulin levels in young women with diffuse hair loss, Br J Derm 106(3):331-336, 1982.
2. Kasick JM and others: Adrenal androgenic female-pattern alopecia: sex hormones and the balding woman, Cleve Clin Q 50(2):111-122, 1983.
3. Georgala G, Papasotiriou V, Stavropoulos P: Serum testosterone and sex hormone binding globulin levels in women with androgenetic alopecia, Acta Derm Venereol 66(6):532-534, 1986.
4. Schmidt JB and others: Hypothyroidism and hyperprolactinemia as a possible cause of androgenetic alopecia in the female, Z Hautkr 64(1):9-12, 1989.
5. Noto G and others: Usefulness and limitations of the evaluation of sex-hormone–binding globulin in women with a female pattern of androgen-inducted baldness, G Ital Dermatol Venereol 124(9):389-391, 1989.
6. Montalto J and others: Plasma C19 steroid sulphate levels and indices of androgen bioavailability in female pattern androgenic alopecia, Clin Endrocrinol 32(1):1-12, 1990.
7. Schmidt JB and others: Hormone studies in females with androgenic hair loss, Gynecol Obstet Invest 31(4):235-239, 1991.
8. Schmidt JB: Endokrine konstellation bei der androgenetischen alopezia der frau, Wien Klin Wochenschr 99:21-24, 1987.
9. Georgala S and others: Hormonal status in postmenopausal androgenetic alopecia, Int J Dermatol 31(12):858-859, 1992.
10. Cipriani R and others: Sex hormone–binding globulin and saliva testosterone levels in men with androgenetic alopecia, Br J Dermatol 109(3):249-252, 1983.
11. Pitts RL: Serum elevation of dehydroepiandrosterone sulfate associated with male pattern baldness in young men, J Am Acad Dermatol 16(3, pt 1): 571-573, 1987.
12. Schmidt JB, Lindmaier A, Spona J: Hormonal parameters in androgenetic hair loss in the male, Dermatologica 182(4):214-217, 1991.
13. DeVillez RL, Dunn J: Female androgenic alopecia: the 3α, 17β-androstenediol glucuronide/sex hormone binding globulin ratio as a possible marker for female pattern baldness, Arch Dermatol 122:1011-1015, 1986.
14. Aguilera MC: Diffuse alopecia in women and hyposideremia, Acta Dermo-Sifiliograficas 57(7):169-180, 1966.
15. Dietz O: Studies on masked sideropenia as a cause of diffuse female alopecia, Z Hautker U Geschlkr 41(9):342-346, 1966.
16. Auerbach R: Low iron levels, Arch Dermatol 98(6):681, 1968.
17. Rushton DH and others: Biochemical and trichological characterization of diffuse alopecia in women, Br J Dermatol 123(2):187-197, 1990.
18. Olsen EA and others: Natural history of androgenetic alopecia, Clin Exp Dermatol 15(1):34-36, 1990.
19. Rushton DH and others: Natural progression of male pattern baldness in young men, Clin Exp Dermatol 16(3):188-192, 1991.
20. Jacobs JP, DeVillez RL: Androgenic alopecia, Arch Dermatol 126:1571-1572, 1990.
21. Rushton H, James KC, Mortimer CH: The unit area trichogram in the assessment of androgen-dependent alopecia, Br J Dermatol 109(4):429-437, 1983.
22. Meishiu KD, Cipkus LA: Biochemical mechanisms by which minoxidil sulfate influences mammalian cells, Dermatologica 175(Suppl 2):3-11, 1987.
23. DeVillez RL: The therapeutic use of topical minoxidil, Dermatol Clin 8(2):367-375, 1990.
24. Uno H, Cappas A, Schlagel C: Cyclic dynamics of hair follicles and the effect of minoxidil on the bald scalps of stumptailed macaques, Am J Dermatopathol 7(3):283-297, 1985.
25. Clissold SP, Heel RC: Topical minoxidil: a preliminary review of its pharmacodynamic properties and therapeutic efficacy in alopecia areata and alopecia androgenetica, Drugs 33(2):107-122, 1987.
26. Buhl AE and others: Minoxidil stimulates mouse vibrissae follicles in organ culture, J Invest Dermatol 92:315-320, 1989.
27. Kiesewetter F, Langer P, Schell H: Minoxidil stimulates mouse vibrissae follicles in organ culture, J Invest Dermatol 96(2):295-296, 1991.

28. Novak E and others: Topically applied minoxidil in baldness, *Int J Dermatol* 24(2):82-87, 1985.
29. Nuck BA, Fogelson SL, Lucky AW: Topical minoxidil does not act as an antiandrogen in the flank organ of the golden Syrian hamster, *Arch Dermatol* 123:59-61, 1987.
30. Olsen EA and others: Topical minoxidil in early male pattern baldness, *J Am Acad Dermatol* 13:185-192, 1985.
31. Parker LN, Lifrak ET, Odell WD: Lack of a gonadal or adrenal androgenic mechanism for the hypertrichosis produced by diazoxide, phenytoin and minoxidil, *Biochem Pharmacol* 31:90-93, 1982.
32. Wester RC and others: Minoxidil stimulates cutaneous blood flow in human balding scalps: pharmacodynamics measured by laser Doppler velocimetry and photopulse plethysmography, *J Invest Dermatol* 82(5):515-517, 1984.
33. Bunker CB, Dowd PM: Alterations in scalp blood flow after the epicutaneous application of 3% minoxidil and 0.1% hexyl nicotinate in alopecia, *Br J Dermatol* 117(5):668-669, 1987.
34. DeBoer EM and others: Does topical minoxidil increase skin blood flow? A laser Doppler flowmetry for study, *Acta Derm Venereol* 68(3):271-274, 1988.
35. Headington TJ: Hair follicle biology and topical minoxidil: possible mechanism of action, *Dermatologica* 175(Suppl 2):19-22, 1987.
36. Uno H, Cappas A, Brigham P: Action of topical minoxidil in the bald stumptailed macaque, *J Am Acad Dermatol* 16(3, pt 2):657-668, 1987.
37. Zappacosta AR: Reversal of baldness in patient receiving minoxidil for hypertension, *N Engl J Med* 303(25):1480-1481, 1980.
38. DeVillez RL: Topical minoxidil therapy in hereditary androgenetic alopecia, *Arch Dermatol* 121(2):197-202, 1985.
39. Weiss VC, West DP: Topical minoxidil therapy and hair regrowth, *Arch Dermatol* 121(2):191-192, 1985.
40. Storer JS and others: Topical minoxidil for male pattern baldness, *Am J Med Sci* 291(5):328-333, 1986.
41. Rumsfield JA, West DP, Fiedler-Weiss VC: Topical minoxidil therapy for hair regrowth, *Clin Pharmacol* 6(5):386-392, 1987.
42. DeVillez RL: Androgenetic alopecia treated with topical minoxidil, *J Am Acad Dermatol* 16(3, pt 2):669-672, 1987.
43. Koperski JA, Orenberg EK, Wilkinson DI: Topical minoxidil therapy for androgenetic alopecia: a 30-month study, *Arch Dermatol* 123(11):1483-1487, 1987.
44. Olsen EA: Topical minoxidil in the treatment of androgenetic alopecia in women, *Cutis* 48(3):243-248, 1991.
45. Whiting DA, Jacobson C: Treatment of female androgenetic alopecia with minoxidil 2%, *Int J Dermatol* 31(11):800-804, 1992.
46. Mortimer CH, Rushton H, James KC: Effective medical treatment of common baldness in women, *Clin Exp Dermatol* 9(4):342-350, 1984.
47. Connors TJ and others: Australian trial of topical minoxidil and placebo in early male pattern baldness, *Australias J Dermatol* 31(1):17-25, 1990.
48. Civatte J and others: 2% topical minoxidil solution in male-pattern baldness: preliminary European results, *Dermatologica* 175(Suppl)2:42-49, 1987.
49. DeProst Y: Minoxidil in the local treatment of alopecia areata and of androgenous alopecia, *Ann Dermatol Venereol* 113(5):479-482, 1986.
50. Seidman M and others: Reversal of male pattern baldness by minoxidil: a case report, *Cutis* 28(5):551-553, 1981.
51. Rushton DH and others: Quantitative assessment of 2% topical minoxidil in the treatment of male pattern baldness, *Clin Exp Dermatol* 14(1):40-46, 1989.
52. Braun-Falco O, Bergner T: Androgenetic alopecia in the male: recent developments, *Hautarzt* 40(11):669-678, 1989.
53. Brenner S, Tamir A: Treatment of androgenic alopecia with topical minoxidil, *Harefuah* 121(9):297-302, 1991.
54. Kuan YZ and others: Safety and efficacy of 2% topical minoxidil in the management of male pattern baldness in Chinese, *Chang Keng I Hsueh Chang Gung Med J* 13(2):96-103, 1990.
55. D'Ovidio R and others: A critical review of the results of clinical experimentation with topical minoxidil 2%, *G Ital Dermatol Venereol* 125(4):V-IX, 1990.
56. Mitchell AD, DeVillez R: Minoxidil for male-pattern baldness, *Lancet* 1(8547):1436, 1987.
57. DeVillez RL: Topical minoxidil for androgenetic alopecia: optimizing the chance for success by appropriate patient selection, *Dermatologica* 175(Suppl 2):50-53, 1987.
58. Olsen EA, DeLong ER, Weiner MS: Dose-response study of topical minoxidil in male pattern baldness, *J Am Acad Dermatol* 15(1):30-37, 1986.
59. Shupack JL and others: Dose-response study of topical minoxidil in male pattern alopecia, *J Am Acad Dermatol* 16(3, pt 2):673-676, 1987.
60. Bamford JT: A falling out following minoxodil: telogen effluvium, *J Am Acad Dermatol* 16(1, pt 1):144-146, 1987.
61. Olsen EA, Weiner MS: Topical minoxidil in male pattern baldness: effects of discontinuation of treatment, *J Am Acad Dermatol* 17(1):97-101, 1987.
62. Kidwai BJ, George M: Hair loss with minoxidil withdrawal, *Lancet* 340(8819):609-610, 1992.
63. Katz HI and others: Long-term efficacy of topical minoxidil in male pattern baldness, *J Am Acad Dermatol* 16(3, pt 2):711-718, 1987.
64. Olsen EA and others: Five-year follow-up of men with androgenetic alopecia treated with topical minoxidil, *J Am Acad Dermatol* 22(4):643-646, 1990.
65. Bouhanna P: Topical minoxidil used before and after hair transplantation, *J Dermatol Surg Oncol* 15(1):50-53, 1989.
66. Granai CO and others: The use of minoxidil to attempt to prevent alopecia during chemotherapy for gynecologic malignancies, *Eur J Gynaecol Oncol* 12:129-132, 1991.
67. Bozzano GS, Terezakis N, Galen W: Topical tretinoin for hair growth promotion, *J Am Acad Dermatol* 15:880-883, 1986.
68. London-Wong DM, Hart LL: Minoxidil with tretinoin in baldness, *DICP* 24(1):43-44, 1990.
69. Ferry J and others: Influence of tretinoin on the percutaneous absorption of minoxidil from an aqueous topical solution, *Clin Pharmacol Ther* 47:439-446, 1990.
70. Vermorken AJ: Reversal of androgenic alopecia by minoxidil: lack of effect of simultaneously administered intermediate doses of cyproterone acetate, *Acta Derm Venereol* 63(3):268-269, 1983.
71. Katz HI: Topical minoxidil: review of efficacy and safety, *Cutis* 43(1):94-98, 1989.
72. Spindler JR: The safety of topical minoxidil solution in the treatment of pattern baldness: the results of a 27-center trial, *Clin Dermatol* 6(4):200-212, 1988.
73. van der Willigen AH and others: Topical minoxidil sensitization in androgenic alopecia, *Contact Dermatitis* 17(1):44-45, 1987.
74. Leenen FH, Smith DL, Unger WP: Topical minoxidil: cardiac effects in bald man, *Br J Clin Pharmacol* 26(4):481-485, 1988.
75. Maddin WS, Bell PW, James JH: The biological effects of a pulsed electrostatic field with specific reference to hair: electrotrichogenesis, *Int J Dermatol* 29:446-450, 1990.
76. Maddin WS, Amara I, Sollecito WA: Electrotrichogenesis: further evidence of efficacy and safety on extended use, *Int J Dermatol* 31(12):878-880, 1992.
77. Stoner E: The clinical development of a 5α-reductase inhibitor, finasteride, *J Steroid Biochem Mol Biol* 37:375-378, 1990.

78. Metcalf BW, Levy MA, Holt DA: Inhibitors of steroid 5α-reductase in benign prostatic hyperplasia, male pattern baldness and acne, Trends Pharmacol Sci 10(12):491-495, 1989.
79. Mellin TN, Busch RD, Rasmusson GH: Azasteroids as inhibitors of testosterone 5α-reductase in mammalian skin, J Steroid Biochem Mol Biol 44(2):121-131, 1993.
80. Tenover JS: Prostates, pates, and pimples: the potential medical uses of steroid 5 alpha-reductase inhibitors, Endocrin Metab Clin North Am 20(4):893-909, 1991.
81. Diani AR and others: Hair growth effects of oral administration of finasteride, a steroid 5α-reductase inhibitor, alone and in combination with topical minoxidil in the balding stump tail macaque, J Clin Endocrinol Metab 74:345-350, 1992.
82. Rittmaster RS: Topical antiandrogens in the treatment of male-pattern baldness, Clin Dermatol 6(4):122-128, 1988.
83. Sciaria F and others: Antiandrogens: clinical application, J Steroid Biochem Mol Biol 37:349-362, 1990.
84. Braendle W and others: Effect and side-effect of cyproterone-acetate-treatment, Arch Gynecol 216(4):335-345, 1974.
85. Nardi M and others: Cyproterone acetate—ethinyl estradiol treatment of hirsutism, acne, seborrhea and alopecia, Acta Eur Fertil 6(2):153-165, 1975.
86. Ramsay ID, Rushton DH: Reduced serum vitamin B_{12} levels during oral cyproterone-acetate and ethinyl-oestradiol therapy in women with diffuse androgen-dependent alopecia, Clin Exp Dermatol 15(4):277-281, 1990.
87. Rushton DH, Ramsay ID: The importance of adequate serum ferritin levels during oral cyproterone acetate and ethinyl oestradiol treatment of diffuse androgen-dependent alopecia in women, Clin Endocrinol 36(4):421-427, 1992.
88. Rushton DH: Management of hair loss in women, Dermatol Clin 11(1):47-53, 1993.
89. Aram H: Treatment of female androgenetic alopecia with cimetidine, Int J Dermatol 26(2):128-130, 1987.
90. Tullio CJ, Roberts MA: Cimetidine-induced alopecia, Clin Pharmacol 4(2):145, 1985.
91. Menard RH and others: Studies on the destruction of adrenal and testicular cytochrom P-450 by spironolactone, J Biol Chem 254:1720-1733, 1979.
92. Burke BM, Cunliffe WJ: Oral spironolactone therapy for female patients with acne, hirsutism and androgenic alopecia, Br J Dermatol 112:124-125, 1985.
93. Wustner H, Orfanos CE: Alopecia androgenetica and its local treatment with estrogen and corticosteroid externa, Z Hautkr 49(20):879-888, 1974.
94. Braun-Falco O: Estrogen containing scalp tincture, Dtsch Med Wochenschr 97(4):135, 1972.
95. Dugois P and others: Cutaneous complications of estroprogestative agents: statistical study, Ann Dermatol Syphil 98(5):479-486, 1971.
96. Frieden IJ, Price VH: Androgenetic alopecia. In Thiers BH, Dobson RL, editor: Pathogenesis of skin disease, New York, 1986, Churchill Livingstone, pp 41-55.
97. Van der Willigen AH and others: A preliminary study of the effects of 11 α-hydroxyprogesterone on the hair growth in men suffering from androgenetic alopecia, Acta Derm Venereol Suppl (Stockh) 67:82-85, 1987.
98. Trachy R and others: Hair growth stimulation in male pattern baldness resulting from treatment with a peptide-copper complex PC1031, Int J Dermatol (submitted for publication).
99. Hertel H and others: Low dosage retinol and L-cystine combination improve alopecia of the diffuse type following long-term oral administration, Hautarzt 40(8):490-495, 1989.
100. Lassus A, Eskelinen E: A comparative study of a new food supplement, ViviScall, with fish extract for the treatment of hereditary androgenic alopecia in young males, J Int Med Res 20(6):445-453, 1992.
101. Gilhar A, Pillar T, Etzioni A: Topical cyclosporine in male pattern alopecia, J Am Acad Dermatol 22(2, pt 1):251-253, 1990.
102. Roenigk HH Jr: New topical agents for hair growth, Clin Dermatol 6(4):119-121, 1988.
103. Kessels AG and others: The effectiveness of the hair-restorer "Dabao" in males with alopecia androgenetica: a clinical experiment, J Clin Epidemiol 44(4-5):439-447, 1991.
104. Hauser GA: Placental extract injections in the treatment of loss of hair in women, Int J Tissue React 4(2):159-163, 1982.
105. Shelly WB, Rawnsley HM: Aminogenic alopecia: loss of hair associated with argininosuccinic aciduria, Lancet 2(426):1327-1328, 1965.
106. Munnich A and others: Fatty-acid–responsive alopecia in multiple carboxylase deficiency, Lancet 1(8177):1080-1081, 1980.
107. Charles BM and others: Biotin-responsive alopecia and developmental regression, Lancet 2(8134):118-120, 1979.
108. Fenton DA, English JS, Wilkinson JD: Reversal of male-pattern baldness, hypertrichosis, and accelerated hair and nail growth in patients receiving benoxaprofen, Br Med J 284(6324):1228-1229, 1982.
109. Bazzano GS, Terezakis N, Galen W: Topical tretinoin for hair growth promotion, J Am Acad Dermatol 15(4, pt 2):880-883, 890-893, 1986.

B. Topical Treatment of Pattern Baldness with a Minoxidil/13-cis-Retinoic Acid Solution

Nia Terezakis, Lydia A. Bazzano, and Gail Sansone-Bazzano

Evidence has continued to accumulate demonstrating that certain retinoids can influence the rate of hair growth, can prolong the anagen phase of the hair cycle and shorten the telogen phase as shown in animal models,[1] can induce hair growth independently, and can enhance the effects of minoxidil.

In 1986, we published the results of an initial pilot study[2] demonstrating that tretinoin (retinoic acid) and various combinations of retinoic acid with minoxidil promoted hair growth. There was evidence that the hair growth rate was increased and that the number of hairs per square centimeter was increased with the use of either or both compounds. The combination of tretinoin and minoxidil was more effective than either compound used alone. Since this initial pilot study, subsequent studies have been performed using other retinoids including 13-cis-retinoic acid either alone or in combination with minoxidil. These studies have demonstrated that in certain cases retinoids, when used alone, are also capable of influencing hair growth. The most significant results, however, have been obtained using various combinations of retinoids and minoxidil.

Data to confirm our research have come from other sources as well. A recent study reported by Saksena[3] describes good results in hair regrowth using tretinoin (retinoic acid) in combination with minoxidil and in combination with triamcinolone acetonide. A total of 125 subjects were divided into five equal groups of 25 each. Each group received a different regimen: tretinoin, minoxidil, minoxidil and tretinoin, triamcinolone acetonide, and tretinoin and triaminolone acetonide. The results showed that tretinoin enhanced the trichogenic effect of both minoxidil and triamcinolone acetonide. The best results were obtained with tretinoin and triamcinolone acetonide combined.

A clinical study performed in England by Wilkinson and Binet[4] using a double blind protocol in which 57 subjects were studied demonstrated that the combination of 1% minoxidil and 0.025% tretinoin was more effective than 1% minoxidil alone. The details of this study were presented at the December 1989 meeting of the American Academy of Dermatology. The study subjects were 57 men aged 20 to 50 years with androgenic alopecia. The degree of alopecia was assessed by clinical evaluation and phototrichogram. The subjects were initially randomized into three groups. The reference group was given 2% minoxidil and one comparison group was given 1% minoxidil in combination with 0.025% retinoic acid. A second group was treated with 1.8% minoxidil in combination with 0.025% retinoic acid. The subjects were examined at 6-week intervals. Total hair counts were performed. These hair counts included anagen and telogen hairs, separately, per square centimeter.

Data at 3 months showed that 1% minoxidil plus 0.025% retinoic acid improved hair growth in anagen hair by approximately 35%. In subjects treated with 1.8% minoxidil and 0.025% retinoic acid, the anagen hair counts increased by more than 40%. At 3 months, subjects using 2% minoxidil alone had less than 20% more growth of anagen hairs in the target area. At 7 months there were very clear differences in the group receiving 1.8% minoxidil and 0.025% retinoic acid. This combination was two times more effective in total hair regrowth than was 2% minoxidil.

The results of these studies demonstrated that subjects using the combination of retinoic acid with minoxidil had a greater stimulation of hair growth than those using minoxidil alone. Plasma levels of minoxidil were not elevated during the treatment in the subsample of subjects who were studied.

At the American Academy of Dermatology meeting in 1989, Price and Menefee[5] introduced a new, more accurate method to assess hair growth based on measurements of hair mass. These investigators studied the combination of minoxidil and retinoic acid. The results of their study were summarized as follows (Table 12-1): The percent weight change over the 24-week treatment period identified the minoxidil/tretinoin solution as the treatment with the greatest effect in promoting hair growth. Two percent minoxidil (Rogaine) was the second most effective treatment solution. A 24-week treatment period was sufficient to identify agents that promote hair growth when changes in total hair mass are used to assay hair growth. The most effective compounds showed significant effects in 24 weeks.

TABLE 12-1 Comparison of Treatment Regimens of Male Pattern Baldness Using Averaged Incremental Percent Weight Change over 24 Weeks

TREATMENT	HAIR MASS MEASUREMENT AVERAGED WEIGHT CHANGE (%)
Placebo	11
Minoxidil/tretinoin	60
2% Minoxidil (Rogaine)	46
Normal	20

Price and Menefee[5] stated that once an agent is found to be effective, subjects should be followed for at least 48 weeks to assess how well hair regrowth is maintained. In Price and Menefee's study, the composition of the vehicle was of major importance. Inappropriate compounding can greatly limit the activity and efficacy of the compounds used.

Studies by Lotte and Rougier[6] in France measuring the percutaneous absorption of topically applied minoxidil in combination with retinoic acid in hairless rats were presented in poster form at the 1989 meeting of the American Academy of Dermatology. Their results demonstrated that urinary minoxidil excretion was increased in hairless rats when a solution of 0.031% retinoic acid and 1.5% minoxidil was used in terms of total percutaneous absorption. The result was the same as that found with 2% minoxidil alone. No increase in blood levels of minoxidil was noted, nor were any physiological effects noted.

These results were in part substantiated by studies at the Upjohn Company.[7] These studies showed again that there was an increase in urinary excretion of minoxidil after topical application of 0.05% retinoic acid cream and 2% minoxidil. However, no data to indicate systemic effects from 2% minoxidil on blood pressure were presented nor were any increased blood levels of minoxidil noted. (When this study is compared with the study of Lotte and Rougier, it must be mentioned that the

384 Drug Therapy

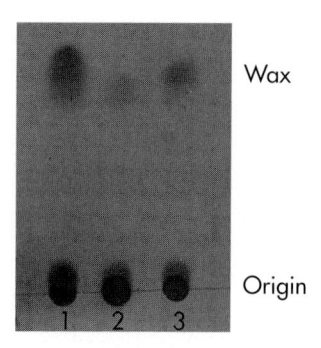

FIG. 12-6 A thin-layer chromatogram showing one subject's wax secretion pattern over a 4-month period. *1*, Baseline wax level; *2*, level 2 months after start of treatment; *3*, level 4 months after start of treatment.

vehicles used were in no way similar, which may have influenced the ultimate result.)

Monti, Motta, and Barbareschi[8] reported an increase in vellus hair growth on photoaged skin treated with topical tretinoin. The abstract was presented at the first meeting of The European Hair Research Society in Brussels November 11, 1989.

AUTHORS' STUDY

Our most recent work has been extended to include other retinoids, particularly 13-*cis*-retinoid acid and minoxidil. Our subjects were treated with 0.025% and 0.05% isotretinoin and 1% and 2% minoxidil (1 ml twice a day applied topically to the scalp) for 6 months. Subjects had the initial scalp sebum se-

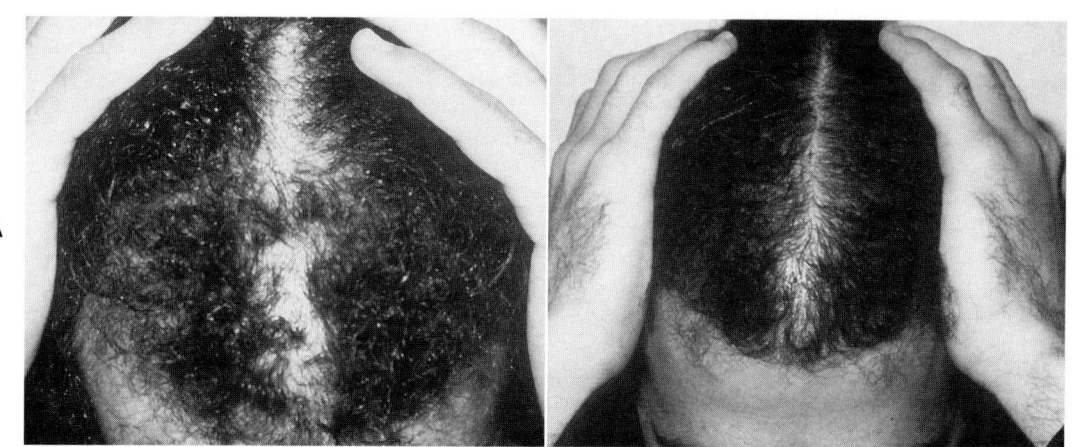

FIG. 12-7 In this 21-year-old man, hair growth in the frontal area filled in after 6 months of treatment with 0.05% 13-*cis*-retinoic acid and 2% minoxidil. **A,** Before treatment. **B,** After treatment.

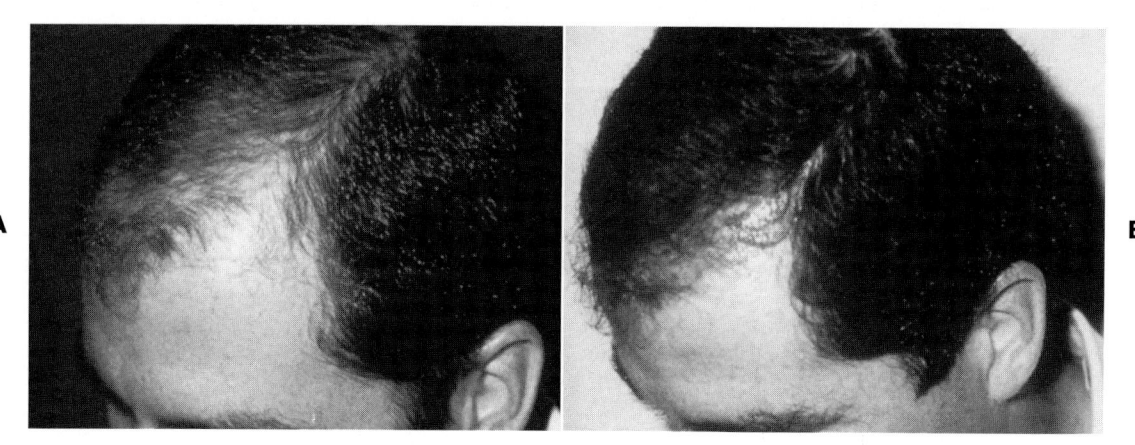

FIG. 12-8 Advanced frontal alopecia in a 32-year-old man. Hair growth in the frontal area filled in after 9 months of treatment with 0.05% 13-*cis*-retinoic acid and 2% minoxidil. **A,** Before treatment. **B,** After treatment.

cretion level determined before entry into the study and two additional sebum secretion levels were obtained during the study. Subjects also agreed to have scalp biopsies both before treatment and after 5 months of treatment. The tissue obtained was used to measure the conversion of ^{3}H-testosterone to ^{3}H-dihydrotestosterone.

Subjects had an initial scalp wash with ethanol to collect scalp sebum after an 8-hour collection period. The subjects underwent three additional scalp sebum collections during the treatment period. Sebum was analyzed for wax esters by thin-layer chromatography.

Hair growth measurements of subjects who were treated with 1% minoxidil and 0.05% isotretinoin were compared with those of patients treated with 1% minoxidil only.

A 1 cm^2 template was used for each patient. Hair counts were performed at baseline and at each clinical visit by means of an individual template. In addition, photographs were taken at each monthly visit, and the diameter of the bald spot at the vertex was measured at each visit.

Results

The results of the effect of 13-*cis*-retinoic acid on scalp sebum production were evaluated via the densitometric determination of wax ester content of sebum. The wax ester content of the scalp sebum decreased in each subject. The mean decrease was 49%, $p = 0.01$.

To determine the effect of 13-*cis*-retinoic acid on the production of dihydrotestosterone (DHT) by the scalp, whole scalp biopsy specimens were incubated with ^{3}H-testosterone before and after 5 months of treatment. In each subject the baseline biopsy showed greater conversion of ^{3}H-testosterone to ^{3}H-DHT than did the biopsy specimens obtained 5 months after treatment with 13-*cis*-retinoic acid. The mean decrease in DHT was 39.4%, $p = 0.01$. Fig. 12-6 shows a thin-layer chromatogram of one subject's wax secretion over a 4-month period.

The photographic results of this pilot study using 2% minoxidil vs. the combination of 2% minoxidil with 0.025% 13-*cis*-retinoic acid (isotretinoin) are shown in Figs. 12-7 and 12-8.

The hair counts in the vertex region were significantly different after 9 months of combination treatment. There was a mean increase of 37% in the hair counts. The minoxidil group on the other hand showed a mean increase in hair counts of only 16%.

DISCUSSION

Recent studies of 13-*cis*-retinoic acid suggest that topical application to facial skin does not result in systemic absorption, which can be measured in the bloodstream. In the case of topical application to the scalp, we must assume that the effect observed—the decrease in sebum production—is an effect of 13-*cis*-retinoic acid on the pilosebaceous unit and specifically on the sebaceous gland itself.

It is known that 13-*cis*-retinoic acid is converted to all-*trans*-retinoic acid in the presence of light, and part of the effect on hair growth can be attributed to all-*trans*-retinoic acid. It is possible that the effect on the diminution in sebum, however, may be attributed to 13-*cis*-retinoic acid.

Studies have shown that a primary site of conversion of testosterone to dihydrotestosterone is in the sebocyte. Although the keratinocytes and fibroblasts also are active, the sebocyte is perhaps, on an activity per weight basis, the principal contributor. If we can assume that sebaceous secretion is an indicator of sebaceous gland activity, then the decrease in sebum must indicate a decrease in activity in the sebocyte.

The effect of 13-*cis*-retinoic acid in combination with minoxidil seems to decrease the amount of androgen conversion to DHT in the scalp skin and to increase the rate of growth of hair. When 1% minoxidil was compared with the combination of 1% minoxidil and 0.05% isotretinoin, the combination was more effective in producing new hair growth and in transforming vellus to terminal hairs.

It has been shown that inhibition of 5α-reductase activity by finasteride in combination with minoxidil topical treatment in the stumptailed macaque can achieve a better effect on promotion of hair regrowth than minoxidil alone.[9] Our results are in keeping with this finding. We suggest that 13-*cis*-retinoic acid can act by reducing the sebaceous gland size and therefore the sebocyte 5α-reductase activity in converting testosterone to dihydrotestosterone.

In conclusion, the data presented herein further confirm the various modes of action and effects of retinoids on hair regrowth.

REFERENCES

1. Bazzano and others: Effect of retinoids on follicular cells, *J Invest Dermatol* 101:138S-142S, 1993.
2. Bazzano, GS, Terezakis N, Galen W: Topical tretinoin for hair growth promotion, *J Am Acad Dermatol* 15:880-883, 890-893, 1986.
3. Saksena M: Enhancement of trichogenic effect of minoxidil and triamcinolone acetonide by tretinoin [abstract]. Presented at the World Congress of Dermatology. New York City, 1992.
4. Wilkinson JW, Binet O: Comparative study of topical minoxidil and minoxidil/retinoic acid combinations in male pattern baldness. Presented at The American Academy of Dermatology Meeting. San Francisco: December 1989.
5. Price V, Menefee E: A comparison study of treatment regimens in male pattern baldness using a quantitative technique. Presented at The American Academy of Dermatology Hair Symposium. San Francisco: December 1989.

6. Lotte C, Rougier A: In vivo percutaneous absorption of minoxidil: influence of tretinoic acid in the formulation. Presented at the American Academy of Dermatology Meeting. San Francisco: December 1989.
7. Ferry JK and others: Influence of tretinoin on percutaneous absorption of minoxidil from an aqueous topical solution, *Clin Pharmacol Ther* 47:439-446, 1990.
8. Monti M, Motta S, Barbareschi M: The increase in vellus hair in photo-aged skin treated with topical tretinoin [abstract]. Presented at the First Meeting of the European Hair Research Society. Brussels: November 11, 1989.
9. Uno H and others: Macaque and rodent models for the screening of drugs for stimulation of hair growth, *J Cutan Pathol.*

13
Hair Care Products

A. The Scientific Basis and Use of Hair Care Products Related to Hair Transplantation

Zoe Kececioglu Draelos

Patients who have undergone surgical hair restoration techniques are anxious to resume their normal hair-grooming procedures and maximize the appearance of existing hair. Although the physician should encourage return to a normal lifestyle quickly to aid the patient in physical and emotional rehabilitation after surgery, cosmetic hair procedures and grooming techniques that might interfere with optimal healing and hair regrowth should be avoided. This discussion focuses on hair-grooming products (i.e., shampoos, conditioners, styling aids) and chemical hair procedures (i.e., permanent waves, dyes) appropriate in the postsurgical period for patients with straight and kinky hair.

Thousands of hair-grooming products manufactured by hundreds of companies are available to consumers worldwide. The specific names of the products and their formulations are subject to frequent change. Furthermore, identical products may be sold in many different packages with different trade names. Consequently, in this discussion the use of proprietary names of specific hair-grooming products has been intentionally avoided. This discussion explains the *type* of hair-grooming products: shampoos, conditioners, hair dyes, hair straighteners, and permanent waves. A determination of the major chemical substances present in each type of hair-grooming product enables the physician to more specifically categorize each product and give general advice and recommendations to patients concerning the use of hair-grooming products.

HAIR-GROOMING PRODUCTS

The postsurgical patient must be counseled on adequate cleansing of the hair to prevent infection as well as on products to improve hair manageability and cosmetic appearance.

Shampoos

Shampoos are intended to remove sebum and dirt from the hair and scalp but are also designed to leave the hair manageable with body and luster.[1] Shampooing assumes the added importance in the postsurgical hair transplant patient of destroying bacteria. Most shampoos on the market today will adequately cleanse the hair and scalp, therefore differences are largely based on cosmetic acceptability.

Shampoos contain detergents, foaming agents, conditioners, thickeners, opacifiers, softeners, sequestering agents, fragrances, preservatives, and specialty additives.[2] Detergents are the primary sebum and dirt removal shampoo components; however, excessive removal of sebum leaves the hair dull, susceptible to static electricity, and difficult to comb.[1] Furthermore, consumers equate cleansing ability with foaming ability, thus demanding shampoos that produce abundant, long-lasting foam. Excessive bubbles are not a technical requirement for good hair cleansing and bacteria removal, but shampoo manufacturers add increased amounts of detergents in addition to foam boosters to obtain the foam that consumers desire. This increased concentration of detergent creates the need for conditioners and other additives in shampoos to improve their cosmetic acceptability.

Shampoo detergents can be chemically classified as anionics, amphoterics, and nonionics (Table 13-1). The anionics are excellent cleansers that may leave the hair harsh, whereas the nonionics produce milder cleansing, leaving the hair more manageable. Amphoteric detergents are unique in that they are nonirritating to the eyes while producing mild cleansing and leaving the hair manageable. Many shampoo formulations combine detergents from the three groups to meet consumer needs.

The most common detergents used in shampoos[3] are (1) sodium laureth sulfate, (2) sodium lauryl sulfate, (3) TEA lauryl sulfate, (4) ammonium laureth

TABLE 13-1 Shampoo Detergents

SURFACTANT TYPE	CHEMICAL CLASS	CHARACTERISTICS
Anionics	Lauryl sulfates, laureth sulfates, sarcosines, sulfosuccinates	Deep cleansing, may leave hair harsh
Amphoterics	Glycinates, propionates, betaines	Nonirritating to eyes, mild cleansing, leave hair manageable
Nonionics	Polysorbate, nonoxynols, polyoxymers	Mild cleansing, leave hair manageable

sulfate, (5) ammonium lauryl sulfate, (6) DEA lauryl sulfate, and (7) sodium olefin sulfonate.

The appropriate shampoo in the postsurgical patient should provide mild, gentle cleansing. Baby shampoos, formulated with amphoteric detergents (cocoamphopropionate, cocoamphocarboxyglycinate, cocoamphoglycinate, cocoamphocarboxypropionate), are well suited for this use because they leave the hair in excellent condition, produce minimal irritation of the skin and eyes, and effect mild cleansing.

To this point, the discussion has focused on shampoo formulation for individuals with straight hair. Shampoo formulation for black and Asian individuals with kinky hair is similar, but several key differences should be mentioned. Individuals with straight hair generally shampoo their hair daily or every other day as sebum renders the straight hair limp and difficult to style. However, individuals with kinky hair shampoo once weekly or once every 2 weeks for several reasons.[4] First, clean kinky hair is dull, frizzy, and difficult to style. Second, kinky hair that has been heat straightened will revert to its normal curly configuration following contact with water. Third, sebum does not coat kinky hair as readily as straight hair.

Shampoos designed for kinky hair therefore must contain milder detergents, pH adjusters, and conditioners. The shampoo must also aid in detangling the hair to reduce grooming trauma and must be known as a conditioning shampoo. Quaternary polymers in shampoos with a pH of approximately 5 will leave kinky hair shiny and aid in detangling.[5] Additional conditioners are added such as humectants, oils, and hydrolyzed proteins. The humectants function to aid in moisture retention, the oils add lubricity to decrease grooming trauma, and the proteins minimally enter the shaft, temporarily improving its physical properties.

Conditioners

After shampooing, the hair ideally should be easy to comb, resistant to static electricity, easy to style, manageable and capable of holding a style. Because detergents do not leave the hair in this condition, conditioning agents are added to the shampoo and may also be applied as a conditioner following shampooing.

FORMULATION. Shampoos and conditioners may contain as many as nine different conditioning agents from the following chemical classes[3]: (1) alkanolamides, (2) glycols, (3) lipids, (4) protein derivatives, (5) quaternaries, (6) surface active agents, and (7) specialty ingredients. Of these, the quaternaries, protein derivatives, and alkanolamides are the most frequently used. These chemical classes are discussed in detail and summarized in Table 13-2.

Quaternary Conditioning Agents. The cationic detergents, also known as *quaternaries, quaternary ammonium compounds,* or *quats,* are conditioning agents found in both shampoos and hair conditioners.[6] They are excellent for smoothing the cuticle, which increases the light reflective abilities of the hair, adding shine and luster. In addition, they are able to electrically neutralize static electricity, thus increasing manageability. These qualities make them an excellent conditioner choice in patients with permanently dyed or permanently waved hair.

Film-Forming Conditioning Agents (Hair Thickeners). Film-forming conditioners apply a thin layer of polymer such as polyvinylpyrrolidone (PVP) over the hair shaft.[7] The polymer fills hair shaft defects, creating a smooth surface to increase shine and luster while eliminating static electricity. The polymer also coats each individual hair shaft, thus "thickening" the hair shaft. For this reason, shampoos and conditioners that contain these substances are called "hair-thickening" products. Consumers may mistakenly believe that these products thicken the hair through new hair growth, which is erroneous. Film-forming conditioners should not be used on fine hair as the added weight of the polymer decreases the ability of the hair to hold a style.

TABLE 13-2 Hair Conditioner Formulations

TYPE	INGREDIENT	ADVANTAGE	HAIR TYPE
Cationic detergent	Quaternary ammonium compounds	Smooths cuticle, decreases static	Chemically processed hair
Film-forming conditioning agent	Polymers	Fills shaft defects, decreases static, adds shine	Dry hair, not fine hair
Protein conditioning agent	Hydrolyzed proteins	Penetrates shaft, temporarily mends split ends	Damaged hair

Protein Conditioning Agents. The most beneficial conditioners in postsurgical patients who have damaged hair are the protein derivatives. These proteins, derived from animal collagen, keratin, or placenta, are hydrolyzed to a particle size (molecular weight 1000 to 10,000) able to enter the hair shaft.[2] Chemical processing of the hair (i.e., permanent dyeing and permanent waving) along with the trauma of grooming, known as *weathering,* remove protein from the hair and damage the protective cuticle. Protein loss results in a hair shaft that fractures more readily, causing hair loss through breakage. Removal of the protective cuticular scales exposes the fragile medulla, which readily splits, a process known as *trichoptilosis* or more commonly *split ends.* Thus hydrolyzed protein conditioners can temporarily strengthen the hair shaft and mend split ends until subsequent shampooing when the product must be reapplied. The source of the protein is not as important as the protein particle size.

PRODUCTS. Hair-conditioning agents may be present in shampoos or in products known as hair conditioners. The use of hair conditioners assumes special importance in hair transplant patients since the newly transplanted hair appears dull, curly, and limp. These products can temporarily add shine and body to the new hair, thus improving its cosmetic appearance.

Hair conditioners are available in three forms[8]: instant conditioners, deep conditioners, leave-in conditioners (Table 13-3).

Instant Conditioning Products. Instant conditioners are so named because they are applied following shampooing, left on the hair for 5 minutes, and subsequently rinsed. These products provide minimal conditioning due to their short contact time with the hair and are basically useful to aid in wet combing and manageability. Their ability to repair damaged hair is somewhat limited.

Deep Conditioning Products. Deep conditioners are left in contact with the hair 20 to 30 minutes and are valuable in caring for hair chemically damaged by permanent waving, chemical straightening, or permanent dyeing procedures. These conditioners should contain hydrolyzed protein, as discussed previously, to temporarily strengthen the hair shaft and repair split ends. These products are sometimes known as protein thickeners. Generally the hair is shampooed to remove this product and then dried and styled.

Leave-In Conditioning Products (Hair-Thickening Products). Leave-in conditioners are applied following towel drying of the hair and are designed to remain on the hair shaft through styling. They are removed with the next shampoo. Products designed for straight hair are known as *blow-drying lotions* or *hair thickeners.* Usually, film-forming conditioning agents, as discussed previously, are the basic ingredient.

Special leave-in conditioners are used by black and Asian individuals with tightly kinked hair to aid in combing, provide additional shine, improve manageability, and enhance styling options (Table 13-4). The traditional leave-in conditioners are pomades. Pomades are oil-based creams containing no water that are applied to finish or retain a hairstyle. The pomade can also contain other substances (e.g., sulfur, selenium sulfide, or tar) designed to treat hair and scalp conditions. If the oily product is a liquid instead of a cream, it is known as a *brilliantine.*

Lighter, less oily leave-in kinky hair conditioners are glycerin-based products. Glycerin does not repel moisture as well as the oily pomades and is therefore not as useful on heat-straightened hair. It functions as a humectant, however, to retain moisture, which is important in chemically straightened hair. For individuals susceptible to pomade acne,[9] however, it is an excellent alternative since the glycerin is noncomedogenic and nonacnegenic. Sometimes these products also contain silicones to improve lubricity and prevent the hair from feeling tacky.

Oil sheen sprays are another form of black hair conditioner because they increase hair lubricity and add a high degree of shine to the styled hair.

TABLE 13-3 Hair Conditioning Products

TYPE	USE	INDICATION
Instant	Apply after shampoo, rinse	Minimally damaged hair, aids wet combing
Deep	Apply for 20-30 minutes, shampoo, rinse	Chemically damaged hair
Leave-in	Apply to towel-dried hair, style	Prevents hair dryer damage, aids in combing and styling

Styling Aids

Styling aids are designed to be applied to the hair following shampooing (Table 13-4). They may be used before drying or after styling. The special leave-in conditioners, previously discussed for individuals with kinky hair, may also be considered styling aids since they perform both functions. This discussion focuses on products designed for straight hair.

Straight-hair styling aids consist of gels, mousses, and sprays. All of them are formulated with polymers designed to add shine and increased hold to the hair.[10] Gels and mousses are usually applied to towel-dried hair before styling, whereas sprays are applied to the finished hairstyle.

These products should not be used in the postsurgical patient until reepithelialization has occurred. Stinging and burning may be experienced on application if used before healing. However, once healing has occurred, these products are extremely valuable to hair transplant patients[11] because (1) they are useful for holding the hair in place, providing camouflage for freshly transplanted areas, and (2) they can be applied to the proximal hair shaft where it exits the scalp to allow the hair to stand away from the scalp, creating the illusion of hair fullness and body.

CHEMICAL HAIR PROCEDURES

Chemical hair procedures are used to alter the structure and color of the hair. Straight hair can be permanently waved, whereas kinky hair can be straightened. Furthermore, dark hair can be lightened and light hair can be darkened. This section discusses the methods and chemicals used to effect these changes.

Permanent Waving

Permanent waving is a method of transforming straight hair to curly hair used by both men and women. The procedure is generally performed by a beautician and takes 1 to 2 hours.

CHEMISTRY. Permanent waving has three processes: chemical softening, rearranging, and fixing. The basic chemistry involves the reduction of the disulfide hair shaft bonds with mercaptans.[12] The process can be chemically characterized as follows[13]:

1. Penetration of the thiol compound (RSH) into the hair shaft.
2. Cleavage of the hair keratin disulfide bond (kSSk) to produce a cysteine residue (kSH) and the mixed disulfide of the thiol compound with the hair keratin (kSSR).

$$kSSk + RSH \rightleftharpoons kSH + kSSR$$

3. Reaction with another thiol molecule to produce a second cysteine residue and the symmetrical disulfide of the thiol waving agent (RSSR).

$$kSSR + RSH \rightleftharpoons kSH + RSSR$$

4. Rearrangement of the hair protein structure to relieve internal stress determined by curler size and hair-wrapping tension.
5. Application of an oxidizing agent to re-form the disulfide cross-links.

$$kSH + HSk \xrightarrow{oxidizing\ agent} kSSk + water$$

APPLICATION PROCEDURE. The application procedure for a permanent wave involves initial shampooing of the hair to remove dirt and sebum, which is the first step in preparing the hair for the chemical treatment (see box). This shampooing allows water to enter the hair's hydrogen bonds, allowing increased flexibility.

The hair is subsequently sectioned into 30 to 50 areas, depending on the length and thickness of the hair, and wound on mandrels or rods. The size of the rod determines the diameter of the curl, with smaller rods producing tighter curls. Sufficient tension must be applied as the hair is wound around the rod to provide the stress required to encourage bond breaking. If too much tension is applied, the hair can be stretched beyond its elastic range, making it so brittle that it will easily fracture.

Tissue paper squares about 5 × 5 cm, known as *end papers,* are applied to the distal hair shafts to

TABLE 13-4 Hair Styling Aids

TYPE	FORMULATION	INDICATION
Spray	Aerosol	Holds finished style
Styling fix or styling spritz	Aerosol	Provides strong hold to finished style
Styling gel	Gel	Applied to towel-dried hair to add body and increase hold
Sculpturing gel	Gel	Applied to towel-dried hair to add body and greatly increase hold
Mousse	Foam	Applied to towel-dried hair or during styling to minimally add body and increase hold
Pomade	Cream	Applied during styling to condition hair
Brilliantine	Liquid	Applied during styling to condition hair

HAIR PERMANENT WAVING PROCEDURE

1. Shampoo hair to remove dirt and sebum.
2. Section hair into 30 to 50 areas.
3. Wind wet hair on rods with appropriate tension while placing end papers on distal hair shafts.
4. Apply waving lotion for 5 to 20 minutes.
5. Perform test curl at the anterior hair line among the transplanted hair.
6. Neutralize hair twice.
7. Dry and style hair.

---

prevent irregular wrapping of the ends around the rod. Failure to use end papers can result in a frizzy appearance of the distal hair shaft.

Next, the waving lotion is applied and left in contact with the hair for 5 to 20 minutes, depending on the condition of the hair. Coarse hair requires a longer processing time than fine hair, and undyed hair requires a longer processing time than permanently dyed or bleached hair.

The beautician should perform a test curl before removing the permanent waving rods to determine if the desired amount of curl has been obtained. This curl is usually placed at the nape of the neck and unwound during the procedure to chart its progress. In most individuals, the hair at the nape of the neck is more resistant to the permanent wave solution, thus if the hair in this region is curled, it can be assumed that the rest of the hair has been adequately curled as well. Unfortunately, easier to curl hair, such as that on the crown and around the face, may be overprocessed, rendering the hair brittle, weak, and frizzy.

For hair transplant patients, the test curl should always be at the anterior hair line among the transplanted hair. This hair generally will curl more readily and is easier to overprocess than the virgin hair at the posterior scalp line.

Once the hair has adequately curled, neutralization is undertaken, and the hair disulfide bonds are subsequently re-formed with the hair in the new curled conformation around the perming rods.[14] The neutralization procedure, chemically characterized as an oxidation step, involves the use of 2% hydrogen peroxide adjusted to an acidic pH.[15] First, two thirds of the neutralizer should thoroughly saturate the hair with the rods in place and be allowed to set for 5 minutes. The rods should then be removed and the remaining one third of the neutralizer should be applied for an additional 5 minutes. The hair should then be carefully rinsed to remove any waving lotion residue.

The newly curled hair is now ready for drying and styling. Most companies recommend avoiding shampooing or manipulating the hair for 1 to 2 days following a waving procedure to ensure long-lasting curls.

A permanent wave is designed to last 3 to 4 months. Even though the curl is designed to be permanent, some relaxation occurs with time as the hair returns to its original conformation. Most of the curl relaxation occurs within the first 2 weeks after processing, a fact that is reassuring to the patient who has had an undesirable result. New hair growth also decreases the curled appearance of the hair.[16]

PERMANENT WAVE TYPES. There are several different types of permanent waves that each require a different waving lotion. The waving lotions consist primarily of a reducing agent in an aqueous solution with an adjusted pH. The most popular reducing agents are the thioglycolates, glycerol thioglycolates, and sulfites. Permanent waves can be simplistically classified into the following groups[17] (Table 13-5): (1) alkaline, (2) buffered

TABLE 13-5 Evaluation of Permanent Waving Products

PERMANENT WAVE TYPE	ADVANTAGES	DISADVANTAGES
Alkaline	Tight, long-lasting curl produced	Harsh on hair (especially bleached or color-treated hair)
Buffered alkaline	Tight, long-lasting curl produced	Less harsh on hair
Exothermic	Produces heat for client comfort	Must be properly mixed
Self-regulated; acid	Limits hair damage, leaves hair soft	Loose curl produced
Sulfite	Less odor	Loose curl produced

alkaline, (3) exothermic, (4) self-regulated, (5) acid, and (6) sulfite.

Alkaline. Alkaline permanents use ammonium thioglycolate or ethanolamine thioglycolate as the reducing agent in the waving lotion. The pH is adjusted to between 9 and 10 since the thioglycolates are not as effective at a lower pH level.[17] These products process rapidly and produce a tight, long-lasting curl but are harsh on the hair. The alkalinity allows hair shaft swelling, which causes problems in individuals with color-treated hair, especially bleached hair. For this reason the concentration of the waving lotion is adjusted, resulting in products designed for fine hair, gray hair, and color-treated hair.

Buffered Alkaline. To reduce the hair swelling resulting from the pH of alkaline permanent waves, a buffering agent such as ammonium bicarbonate is used. These products are known as *buffered alkaline permanents* and result in a tight curl at a pH of 7 to 8.5. They produce a tight, long-lasting curl with less hair damage.

Exothermic. Exothermic permanent waves produce heat as a by-product and increase client comfort because some individuals may feel chilled during the permanent-waving process. The heat is produced when the oxidizing agent, such as hydrogen peroxide, is mixed with the thioglycolate-based waving lotion immediately before scalp application. The reaction of the thioglycolate with the peroxide produces dithiodiglycolate (disulfide of thioglycolate), which limits the extent to which the permanent wave can process. Irreversible hair damage results if the waving lotion is not mixed with the oxidizing agent before application. For this reason exothermic permanent waves are available for professional use only.

Self-Regulated. Self-regulated permanent waves are designed to limit the amount of hair disulfide bond breakage, thus preventing irreversible hair damage. Overprocessing, as a result of leaving the permanent wave solution on the hair longer than recommended, causes extensive hair breakage and acts like a depilatory. Self-regulated permanent waves are designed to form a chemical equilibrium to halt disulfide bond breakage. This equilibrium is accomplished by adding dithioglycolic acid to the thioglycolate-based waving lotion. This type of permanent waving product is recommended for patients with newly transplanted hair.

Acid. Acid permanent waves occur in an acidic environment with a pH of 6.5 to 7.3. They are based on thioglycolate esters such as glycerol monothioglycolate. The lower pH is an advantage since less hair shaft swelling occurs than at higher pH levels, thus hair damage is minimized. These products result in a looser, less long-lasting curl but leave the hair soft. They are ideal for bleached or color-treated hair. It is possible to achieve a tighter curl if the permanent wave is processed with added heat from a hair dryer, but more hair shaft damage results.

The glycerol monothioglycolate in this type of permanent wave is responsible for allergic contact dermatitis in both beauticians and clients.[18] Interestingly enough, the hair may continue to be allergenic even after all products have been thoroughly rinsed from the hair.

Acid permanent waves are the mildest on newly transplanted hair. Once complete healing has occurred and the hair is long enough to wrap around a rod at least once, hair transplant patients may safely undertake this type of permanent wave.

Sulfite. Sulfite permanent waves are mainly marketed for home use. These products differ in that the reducing agent is a sulfite or bisulfite instead of a mercaptan. This difference accounts for the reduced odor, their primary advantage. They require a long processing time at a pH of 6 to 8 and result in loose curls. A conditioning agent must be added to the formulation because the sulfite permanent waves can leave the hair feeling harsh.

Hair Straightening

Whereas permanent waves are designed to curl straight hair in white individuals, there are a variety of techniques for straightening the kinky hair of black and Asian individuals. These hair-straightening techniques can be classified as mechanical, heat, and chemical (Table 13-6). Straightening procedures should be avoided in newly transplanted hair.

MECHANICAL. Mechanical hair-straightening employs heavy cream hair dressings, known as *pomades*, to adhere the hair shaft to the scalp and provide minimal straightening (Table 13-4). They may contain oily substances such as petrolatum, lanolin, mineral oil, castor oil, safflower oil, or olive oil. It is the olive oil–containing pomades that were classically described as causing pomade acne.[9] Pomades actually function best as leave-in conditioners to improve lubricity and add shine as previously discussed, but they are poor hair straighteners.

HEAT. Heat hair-straightening techniques include hot combing and hair pressing. Hot combing is use of a metal comb that is heated to a minimum of 300° F and then drawn through the hair. This action breaks the water–re-formable bonds and allows the hair to be pulled straight.[19] The change is temporary, however, because moisture from perspiration, humidity, or shampooing allows the bonds to reform and the hair returns to its natural kinky state. Thus the results obtained with heat hair-straightening techniques are temporary but can be improved if a pressing oil is added to the hair before hot combing or ironing between hot metal plates. The pressing oil prevents the hair from sticking to the heated device and improves water resistance.

CHEMICAL. Chemical hair straightening, also known as *lanthionization*, breaks disulfide bonds in the hair shaft. The hair is then pulled straight, with disulfide bond re-formation in a new configuration. This process can be accomplished with thioglycolate, lye-based, lye-free, and bisulfite creams.[20]

Thioglycolate straighteners are identical to the permanent wave solutions previously discussed except that they are formulated as thick creams rather than lotions to add weight and aid in holding the hair straight. The best hair straighteners are lye-based and contain up to 3% sodium hydroxide, but they can produce scalp burns and blindness. The newer lye-free straightening products contain guanidine hydroxide but are still strong alkali products.

The mildest hair-straightening products are the ammonium bisulfite creams. Many of the home chemical-straightening products are of this type. They produce the least permanent straightening of all the chemicals discussed. As a general rule, the chemicals that produce the greatest, longest-lasting hair straightening are also the most damaging to the hair shaft.

The same basic application technique is used with all chemical straighteners. It is advised that the hair not be shampooed before the straightening procedure. Petroleum jelly is then applied to the scalp and skin next to the hairline to prevent an irritant contact dermatitis. If this is the first chemical straightening procedure, the straightening cream is applied to the entire hair shaft; if the hair has been previously treated, it is applied only to the new hair growth. The hair is combed or pulled straight for 5 to 20 minutes as the disulfide bonds are broken, depending on the condition of the hair shaft cuticle and the strength of the chemical agent. A neutralizer may then be applied to stop the chemical reaction and the chemical is thoroughly washed from the hair.

It is necessary to recognize that the skill of the beautician in performing the chemical straightening procedure and the quality of the product used are the two most important factors in obtaining a good result without excessive hair breakage. The chemicals should be applied and removed in a minimum of time to prevent scalp burns and irreversible hair damage. Postsurgical hair transplant patients should use nationally marketed hair care products applied by a trained beautician.

TABLE 13-6 Evaluation of Hair Straightening Techniques

METHOD	ADVANTAGES	DISADVANTAGES
Mechanical	Least damaging to hair shaft	Minimal hair straightening
Heat	No chemicals required, can be performed at home	Not water resistant, hot comb alopecia possible
Chemical	Excellent straightening, water resistant, long lasting	Most damaging to hair shaft, can cause chemical burns

HAIR DYEING

Hair dyes can be divided into several types based on their formulation and permanency: gradual, temporary, semipermanent, and permanent (Table 13-7). All permanent and gradual hair dyes are damaging to transplanted hair.

Gradual

Gradual hair dyes, also known as *metallic* or *progressive hair dyes*, require repeated application to produce gradual darkening of the hair shaft. They employ the metal salt, lead acetate, which reacts with sulfur-containing substances in the hair cuticle, giving the hair a characteristic smell. This product will change the hair color from gray to brown over a period of weeks.[21] There is no control over the final color of the hair, only the depth of color, and lightening is not possible. Gradual hair dyes are most popular among men who do not wish to effect a rapid color change and like a product that can be applied in the privacy of their own homes. Gradual dyes cannot be combined with permanent waving or permanent dyeing procedures because unreliable results and hair damage may result.

Gradual dyes are not recommended in the postsurgical hair transplant patient because they render the hair dry and brittle, thus encouraging hair breakage.

Temporary

Temporary hair dyes are named for their ability to be removed with one shampooing. They are formulated with water-soluble acid dyes adapted from the textile industry. Their particle size is too large to penetrate the cuticle, accounting for their temporary nature.[22] They are applied following shampooing in a liquid rinse, gel, mousse, or spray form followed by drying and setting of the hair. These products are generally hypoallergenic and do not produce hair shaft damage.

Temporary dyes can be easily rubbed off the hair shaft, however, and will run onto clothing if the hair gets wet from rain or perspiration. These dyes are appropriate for both men and women with gray hair who wish to remove unwanted tones, add highlights, or subtly color the hair. This product can be used without difficulty in the hair transplant patient.

Semipermanent

Semipermanent hair dyes are removed in four to six shampooings as a result of their intermediate-sized particles that can both enter and exit the hair shaft. The formulation of a typical semipermanent hair dye is: dyes (nitroanilines, nitrophenylenediamines, nitroaminophenols, azos, anthraquinones), alkalizing agent, solvent, surfactant, thickener, fragrance, and water. These products are popular among both men and women for adding shades of brown to the hair or covering less than 30% gray hair. Hair lightening is not possible.[23]

This form of hair dying does not damage the hair shaft and is therefore appropriate in hair transplant patients.

Permanent

Permanent hair dyes are unique in that their color is long lasting and the hair can be dyed both lighter and darker. This tremendous versatility makes this dye type the most popular on the market today, occupying approximately 70% of hair dye sales. Redyeing, of course, is necessary as new growth occurs at the scalp.

This type of hair coloring does not contain dyes but rather colorless dye precursors that chemically react with hydrogen peroxide inside the hair shaft to produce colored molecules. The process entails the use of primary intermediates (p-phenylenediames, p-toluenediamine, p-aminophenols), which undergo oxidation with hydrogen peroxide. These reactive intermediates are then exposed to couplers (e.g., resorcinol, 1-naphthol, m-aminophenol) to result in a wide variety of indoaniliac dyes. These dyes can produce shades from blond to brown to black with highlights of gold to red to orange. Variations in the concentration of hydrogen peroxide and the

TABLE 13-7 Hair Dyes

TYPE	MECHANISM OF ACTION	ADVANTAGES	DISADVANTAGES
Gradual	Aqueous metallic solution	Gradual darker color production	Brittle hair produced, cannot combine with other chemical procedures
Temporary	Textile dye	Easily tones or blends darker hair color	Removal in one shampooing
Semipermanent	Low-molecular-weight textile dye, polymer or vegetable dye	Adds highlights, can darken hair with <30% gray	Removal in four to six shampooings
Permanent	Oxidation coloring	Can lighten or darken hair color, permanent color	Possible allergenicity

chemicals selected for the primary intermediates and couplers produce the color variations.[24]

Permanent dyeing allows shades to be obtained both lighter and darker than the patient's original hair color. Higher concentrations of hydrogen peroxide can bleach melanin, thus the oxidizing step functions both in color production and bleaching. However, hydrogen peroxide alone cannot remove sufficient melanin to lighten dark brown or black hair to blond hair. Boosters, such as ammonium persulfate or potassium sulfate, must be added to achieve great degrees of color lightening. The boosters must be left in contact with the hair for 1 to 2 hours for optimal results. Nevertheless, individuals with dark hair who choose to dye their hair a light blond color will notice the appearance of reddish hues with time. This results from the inability of the peroxide/booster system to completely remove reddish pheomelanin pigments, which are more resistant to removal than brownish eumelanin pigments.

Permanent hair dyes can be used in the hair transplant patient, but complete healing of the scalp must have occurred. Application of the dyes before healing may result in severe stinging and burning. In addition, permanent hair dyes may be allergenic, so patch testing before application is imperative. A higher incidence of allergic reactions may occur in unhealed scalp surgery patients because of the absence of the protective epithelial barrier and direct access of the dye allergen to the dermal vasculature.

Permanent hair dyes are the most damaging to the hair, a fact that the hair transplant patient must understand (see box). This type of hair dye alters the internal hair shaft structure and therefore decreases its strength. Several key points should be remembered to minimize hair shaft damage:

1. If both permanent waving and permanent dyeing are to be performed, the hair should be permanently waved first and permanently dyed second. Ten days should be allowed between the procedures.

2. Lightening or bleaching the hair is more damaging than dyeing the hair to a darker color.
3. Each redyeing procedure further damages the hair shaft, thus the period between redyeing should be as long as possible, and the dye should be concentrated on the new proximal hair growth, not on the previously dyed distal hair shaft.

CONCLUSION

Cosmetic alteration of the hair is important in the hair replacement patient. These individuals value the appearance of their hair and need knowledgeable advice regarding the use of hair cosmetics.

PERMANENT WAVING AND PERMANENT DYEING RECOMMENDATIONS

1. Permanent waving should be performed before permanent dyeing.
2. Permanent dyeing should be performed at least 10 days after the permanent waving procedure.
3. A period of 3 months is recommended before permanent waving or permanent dyeing procedures are repeated in the patient who has recently undergone hair transplantation.

REFERENCES

1. Boullion C: Shampoos and hair conditioners, *Clin Dermatol* 6:83, 1988.
2. Fox C: An introduction to the formulation of shampoos, *Cosmet Toilet* 103:25, 1988.
3. Rieger M: Surfactants in shampoos, *Cosmet Toilet* 103:59, 1988.
4. Brooks G, Lewis A: Treatment regimens for styled black hair, *Cosmet Toilet* 98:59, 1983.
5. Brooks G, Burmeister F: Black hair care ingredients, *Cosmet Toilet* 103:93, 1988.
6. Allardice A, Gummo G: Hair conditioning, *Cosmet Toilet* 108:107, 1993.
7. Finkelstein P: Hair conditioners, *Cutis* 6:542, 1970.
8. Draelos ZK: *Cosmetics in dermatology*, Edinburgh, 1990, Churchill Livingstone, p 87.
9. Plewig G, Fulton JE, Kligman AM: Pomade acne, *Arch Dermatol* 101:580, 1970.
10. Lochhead RY, Hemker WJ, Castaneda JY: Hair care gels, *Cosmet Toilet* 102:89, 1987.
11. Rushton DH, Kingsley P, Berry NL: Treating reduced hair volume in women, *Cosmet Toilet* 108:59, 1993.
12. Brunner MJ: Medical aspects of home cold waving, *Arch Dermatol* 65:316, 1952.
13. Cannell DW: Permanent waving and hair straightening, *Clin Dermatol* 6:73, 1988.
14. Wickett RR: Disulfide bond reduction in permanent waving, *Cosmet Toilet* 106:37, 1991.
15. Heilingotter R: Permanent waving of hair. In de Navarre MG, editor: *The chemistry and manufacture of cosmetics*, Illinois, Allured, 1988, pp 1167-1172.
16. Zviak C: Permanent waving and hair straightening. In Zviak C, editor: *The science of hair care*, New York, 1986, Marcel Dekker, pp 183-209.
17. Lee AE and others: Permanent waves: an overview, *Cosmet Toilet* 103:37, 1988.
18. Morrison LH, Storrs FJ: Persistence of an allergen in hair after glyceryl monothioglycolate–containing permanent wave solutions, *J Am Dermatol* 19:52, 1988.
19. Syed AN: Ethnic hair care, *Cosmet Toilet* 108:99, 1993.
20. Khalil E: Cosmetic and hair treatments for the black consumer, *Cosmet Toilet* 101:51, 1986.
21. Pohl S: The chemistry of hair dyes, *Cosmet Toilet* 103:57, 1988.
22. Corbett JF: Hair coloring, *Clin Dermatol* 6:93, 1988.
23. Corbett JF: Hair coloring processes, *Cosmet Toilet* 106:53, 1991.
24. Zviak C: *The science of hair care*, New York, 1986, Marcel Dekker, p 263.

B. Camouflage Products for Hair Loss

Edward M. Jackson

Dermatologists performing hair replacement procedures are being increasingly called on to recommend hair camouflage products to satisfy their patients' additional needs. Now there are camouflage products for hair loss that can safely be recommended by the physician and used by the patient before, during, and after these procedures. Appearance is so important to patients that the cosmetic industry's most successful program is one based on improving the appearance of chemotherapy patients. This program is now a foundation that is administered by the cosmetic industry trade association, The Cosmetic, Toiletry, and Fragrance Association. This program is called simply the Look Good, Feel Better Foundation.*

Patients continue to ask their physicians for recommendations on products that they can easily and safely use to camouflage hair loss or insufficiency. Until recently there has been little information on such products for physicians to confidently recommend to patients who have hair camouflage needs. The most authoritative source is an article entitled "Primer on cosmetics" published in the *Journal of the American Academy of Dermatology*.[1] However, the information in this source is located in an additional information section that deals with only skin camouflage product manufacturers.

We previously published some basic information,[2] and this discussion is an expansion of that initial treatment of products that camouflage hair loss.

COUVRé ALOPECIA MASKING LOTION

Dermatologists treating hair loss have been aware of an oil-in-water emulsion product that has been available to their patients for over a decade called COUVRé Alopecia Masking Lotion (Fig. 13-1). This standard emulsion with iron oxide pigments is similar to a liquid makeup product and is available in light brown/blond, medium brown, dark brown, black, and gray. COUVRé Alopecia Masking Lotion is very effective in camouflaging hair loss or insufficiency (Figs. 13-2 and 13-3). COUVRé Alope-

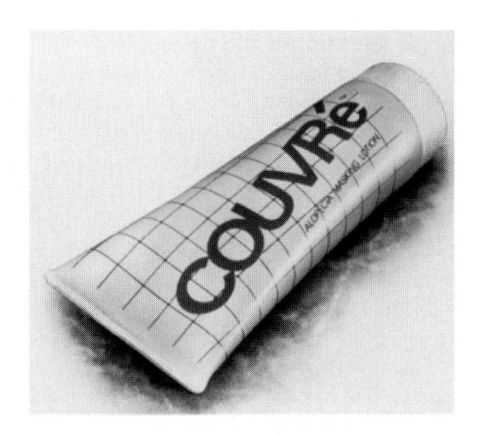

FIG. 13-1 COUVRé Alopecia Masking Lotion.

cia Masking Lotion is available from Spencer Forrest, Inc., 10 Bay Street, Suite 153, Westport, CT 06880, 203-454-2733 or 203-454-2942 (fax).

GLH FORMULA NUMBER 9

A new camouflage hair product called GLH ("for Good Looking Hair") Formula Number 9 (Fig. 13-4) has been featured in an infomercial on cable television. This product is available as (1) an aerosol-spray colored hair thickener in dark brown, medium brown, light brown, auburn, silver black, silver brown, blond, white, and black; (2) a finishing shield aerosol spray that helps to hold the color fast; and (3) a hair cleanser (shampoo) in a squeeze bottle. The colored hair thickener is an aerosolized talc containing iron oxides with a nonchlorofluorocarbon propellant system. The finishing shield aerosol spray is a standard film-forming system, again delivered by a nonchlorofluorocarbon propellant system. The hair cleanser is a gel-like shampoo system with some added natural ingredients such as rosemary and chamomile extract with fragrance and a formaldehyde donor preservative, diazolidinyl urea. The GLH Formula Number 9 products are available from Ronco Hair Products, Inc., P.O. Box 4057, Beverly Hills, CA 90213.

HELPING PATIENTS CHOOSE A CAMOUFLAGE HAIR PRODUCT

Both COUVRé Alopecia Masking Lotion and GLH Formula Number 9 perform the function of camouflaging hair loss and insufficiency and both can be recommended by dermatologists with confidence. However, how well these two different types of products perform this camouflaging function is as much a matter of patient personal preference as it is a matter of patient perception about how well they

---

NOTE: Edward M. Jackson, Ph.D., is president of Jackson Research Associates, Inc., in Sumner, Washington, and a consultant to the consumer products industry. He has no proprietary interest in either COUVRé Alopecia Masking Lotion or GLH Formula Number 9.

*The Look Good, Feel Better Foundation, The Cosmetic, Toiletry, and Fragrance Association, 1101 17th Street NW, Suite 300, Washington, DC 20036, 202-331-1770, 202-331-1969 (fax).

Camouflage Products for Hair Loss **397**

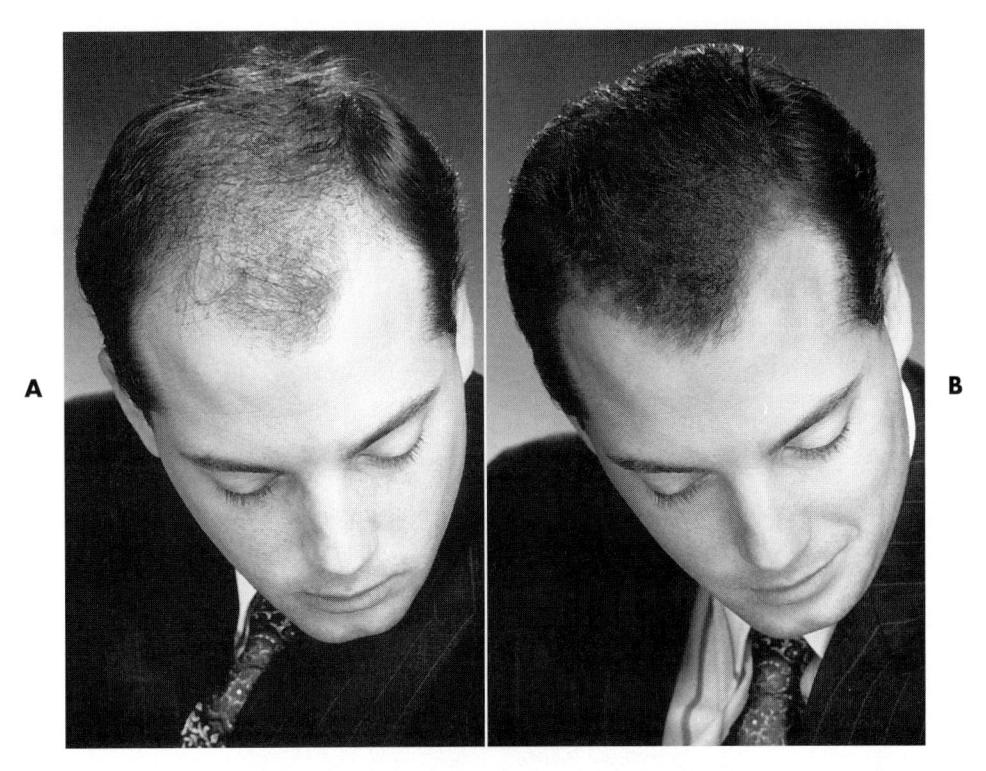

FIG. 13-2 A, Pretreatment view. **B,** Result after the use of COUVRé Alopecia Masking Lotion. (Courtesy Mark H. Kress, Spencer Forrest, Inc.)

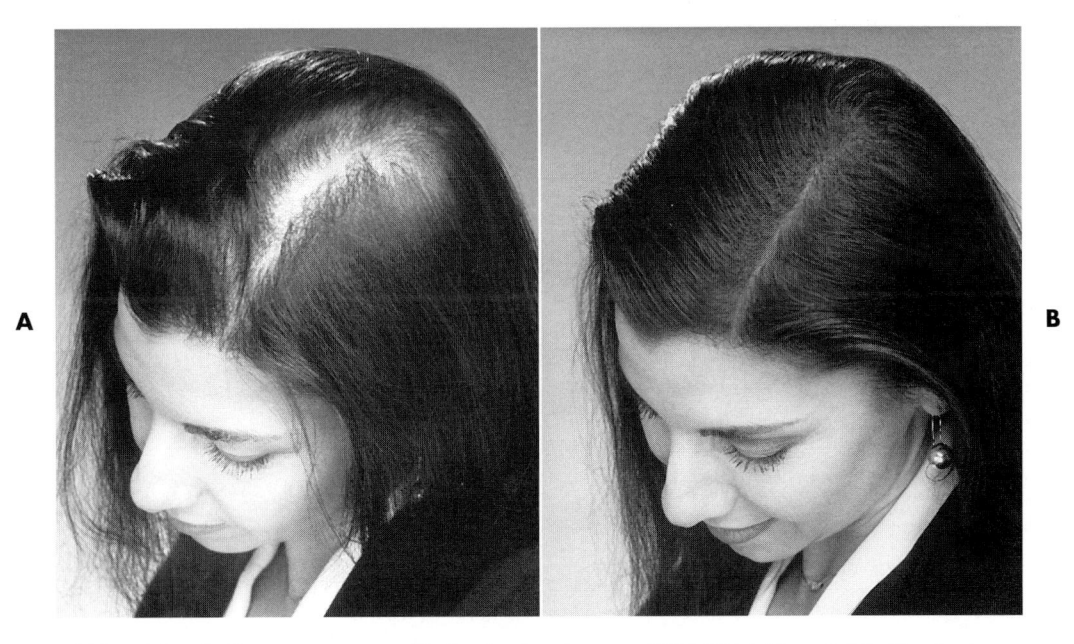

FIG. 13-3 A, Pretreatment view. **B,** Result after the use of COUVRé Alopecia Masking Lotion. (Courtesy Mark H. Kress, Spencer Forrest, Inc.)

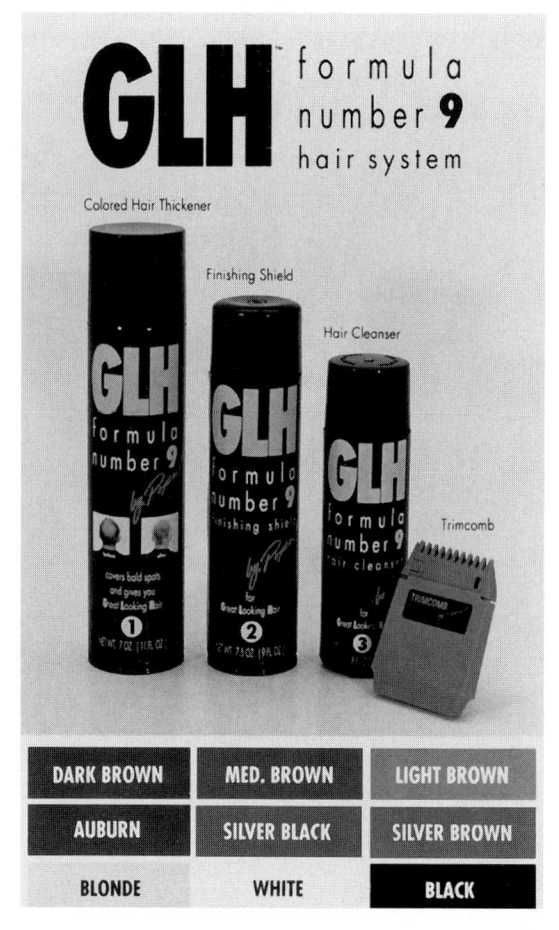

FIG. 13-4 GLH Formula Number 9. (Courtesy Robin Color Laboratories.)

work for the individual. Price, portability, and product form are components in the patient's choice. The patient's preferences can actually influence how well these products are perceived by the patient to effectively camouflage hair loss.

Price has become an increasingly important consideration on the part of both the dermatologist recommending products and the patients who purchase them. The approximate cost of the COUVRé product is $20 a tube for a 4-month supply, which is approximately $80 per year. The GLH Formula Number 9 set of products costs approximately $40 per month, thereby averaging about $480 per year.

CONCLUSION

Providing information on product price, portability, and product form to the patient with hair camouflage needs can help the patient in deciding which product to use to complete his new appearance given in either surgical or medical hair replacement procedures.

REFERENCES

1. Larsen WG and others: Primer on cosmetics, *J Am Acad Dermatol* 27(3):469-484, 1992.
2. Jackson EM: A comparison study of two camouflage products for hair loss, *Cosmet Dermatol* 6(10):46-48, 1993.

14

Nonsurgical Hair Replacement

Michael J. Mahoney

HISTORY

Wigs date back to 3000 BC. Historians are not sure of the materials or construction techniques employed, but their use was extensive. From Egypt came hairgoods of human hair, sheep's wool, and fibers of palm leaves. The Egyptians used dyes to decorate their wigs with stripes, which depicted social standing. Elegancy of style also served to separate the various social classes. However, the first recorded use of wigs to conceal hair loss dates back to Roman times: Hadrian, a Roman emperor, chose to wear a wig because of his lack of hair. History also records that in the mid-1500s Louis XIII of England wore a wig because of hair loss and that many Englishmen with hair loss followed his example.

With the exception of modern times, wigs reached their greatest popularity in the sixteenth, seventeenth, and eighteenth centuries, when powdered wigs were popular for both sexes. The desire to emulate Europe's latest fashions first brought the modern-day wig to the United States in the 1800s and 1900s. The long and curly styles were copied, and white powder along with dyes were used on many wigs. Powdered wigs are still worn today in some judiciary and governmental bodies outside the United States.

Partial hairpieces to disguise male and female pattern hair loss did not gain widespread social acceptance in the current century until the 1920s and 1930s. Sparked by celebrity usage of wigs in the 1930s and 1940s in the motion picture industry, Russian immigrant Max Factor, known more for creating cosmetic makeup, designed wigs and hairpieces for many of Hollywood's leading actors and actresses.

The first Max Factor–designed hairpieces (outside the movie industry) were produced for World War II veterans, many of whom were disfigured by burns and other traumatic injuries. A popular U.S. magazine of the time featured an article on Factor's work, and shortly thereafter thousands of requests for hair additions began to pour into the Max Factor business establishment. This initial spark created an awareness of the availability of such products in the United States. The exposure fueled the imagination of hairdressers, wigmakers, and entrepreneurs to facilitate the demands for such hairgoods in other parts of the country.

During the 1960s and early 1970s, the largest volume of wigs was imported into the United States: an estimated $700 million worth in 1969. Surprisingly, the bulk of these imports were not for people with hair loss but were destined for the fashion industry.

Today we are in the highest volume period of all time for men's hair additions—modern-day hairpieces specifically made for male pattern hair loss—with an estimated half million imported into the United States in 1993 alone.

HAIR ADDITIONS

A hair addition is any external hair-bearing device that is added to existing hair or scalp to give the appearance of a fuller head of hair. Examples include hair weaves, hair extensions, hair units, hair fusion, hair integration, bonding, hairpieces, toupees, wigs, prostheses, and nonsurgical hair replacement. Devices may consist of human hair, synthetics, or a combination.

Confusing to even the nonsurgical hair replacement specialist is the use of sophisticated marketing terms to soften and detract from what may in fact be a hairpiece. The modern-day hairpiece is called a *hair addition* or a *hair replacement* throughout the industry. Universally, the phrase *hairpiece* or *toupee* conjures up a negative image of something unsightly. To combat this negative image advertisers often refer to a system, process, or technique that is claimed to be exclusive to the advertiser. In most cases the only thing exclusive is the copyright or registered trademark of the terminology they are using in the advertising statement. Both the nonsurgical and the surgical hair replacement professions are in the process of eliminating the negative images of the past.

Custom-made products can be produced in any size (Fig. 14-1). The most commonly used hair additions for male and female pattern hair loss are considered "top-of-the-head" hair additions. An average size foundation ranges from 7 to 10 inches in length and 4 to 6 inches in width. Also widely used are partial additions for the crown area and "fillers" worn above the part to fill in a "combover" hairstyle. Crown partial hair additions can range from 2 to 5 inches in width and 2 to 5 inches in length of the foundation. Fillers generally run in size from 1 to 2 inches in width and 3 to 5 inches in length. The largest percentage of partial hair additions are custom made. The balding or thinning area is duplicated in contour and size by designing a template on the client's head. Templates are made from layers of tape over a cellophane material that is then marked and cut as a blueprint for the manufacturer (Fig. 14-2). Other materials such as plaster of paris and fiberglass are also used to build

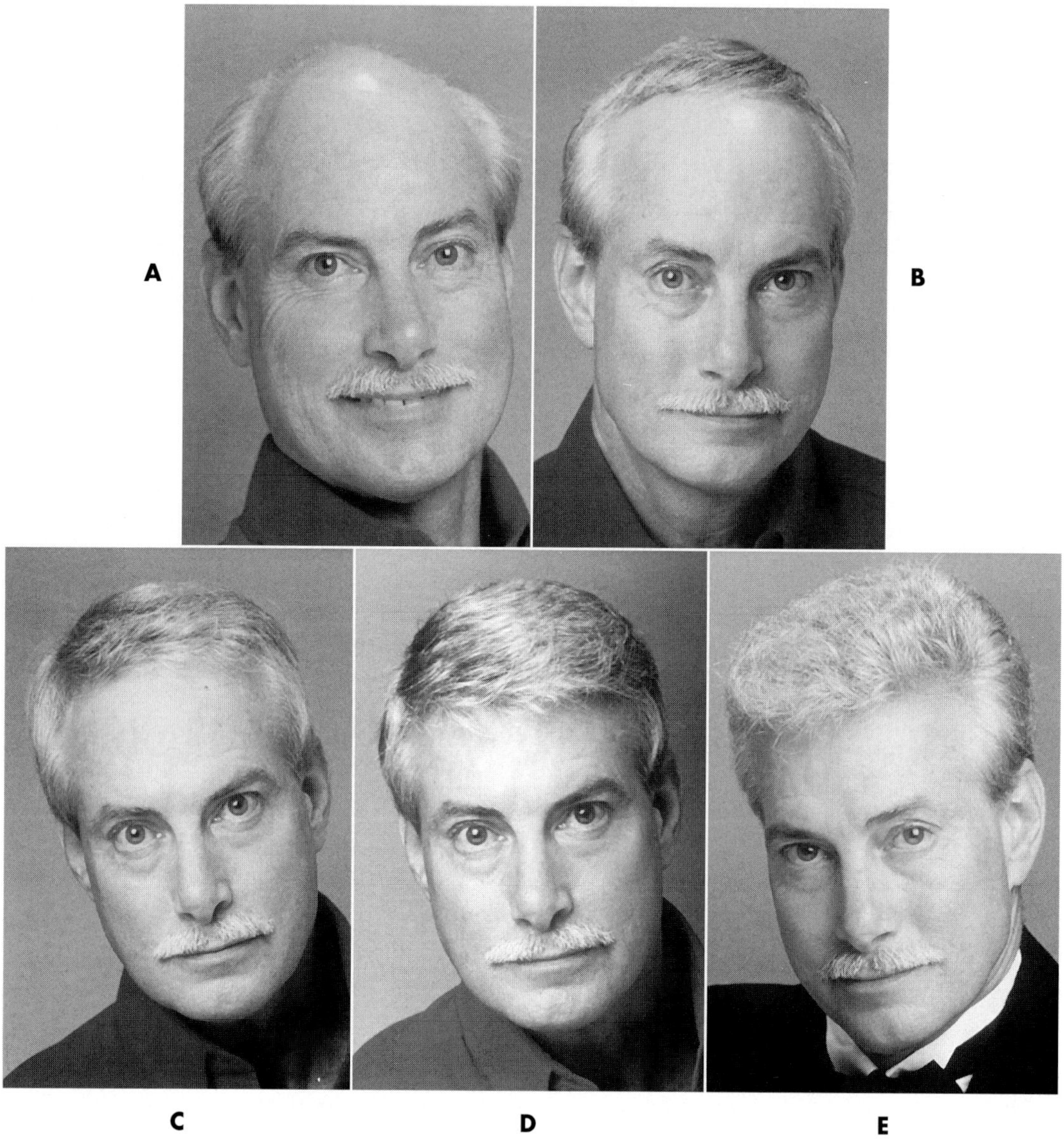

FIG. 14-1 **A,** Subject with Norwood type V alopecia. **B,** Subject after placement of a partial hair addition worn above the part to fill in an abbreviated "combover" hairstyle. **C,** Subject with an intermediate partial hair addition. **D,** Subject with a full top-of-the-head hair addition. The size is approximately 9½ inches × 7 inches. **E,** Subject with a contrasting hairstyle.

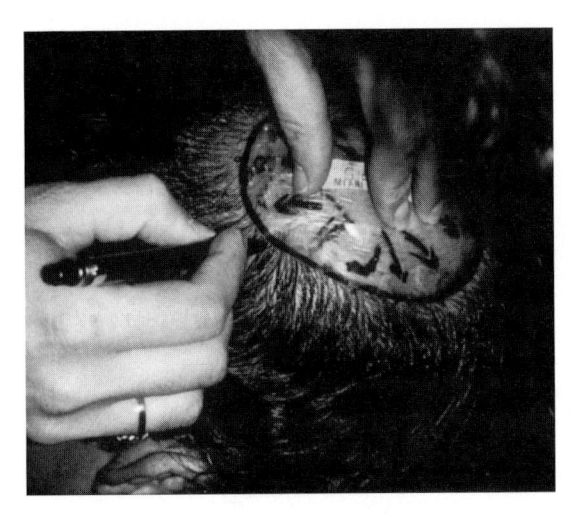

FIG. 14-2 Construction of a template for a custom-made hair addition. Such templates are made from layers of tape over a cellophane material that is marked and cut as a blueprint for the manufacturer.

templates. Hair samples are then cut from the individual's own hair and accompany an extensive order form that has multiple choices for particular factors such as density, percentage of gray, length, choice of materials, and hair direction.

Wigs vs. Partial Hairpieces

A full-cap wig or prosthesis is generally worn by an individual who does not have a hairline to integrate with a partial hair addition. Wigs (i.e., full-cap prosthetics) are rarely designed for male pattern hair loss but instead for those undergoing chemotherapy or those suffering alopecia areata, totalis, or universalis.

It is also possible that in cases involving alopecia areata, the wearer has no choice because of the unpredictability of the condition. (A custom-made partial hairpiece may be ineffective in weeks because of the possible advance of alopecia areata.) Skilled designers avoid the use of full-cap wigs when the client has remaining hair. Even in the case of severe male pattern hair loss such as Norwood type VII, it is still preferable to use the client's existing hair for a hairline.

The wig or full-cap prosthesis should be avoided whenever possible out of consideration for comfort, appearance, and fitting. These products may have a tendency to "ride up" at the occipital region. If the wearer bends forward or backward, the full cap may ride up or the fiber may protrude at an unnatural angle. Usually the partial hair addition for male pattern baldness replaces an average of only 4 inches of the client's frontal hair line. However, the full-cap wig or prosthesis covers approximately 22 to 23 inches of the client's hairline. Because of superior results in appearance and comfort, the client's own hair should be used as much as possible.

Custom-Made vs. "Ready-Made" Hair Additions

Inexperienced specialists and high-volume retailers often market "ready-made" hair additions "off the shelf." Use of these products oftens leads to poor fitting, improper temporal recession design, discomfort, unsatisfactory coloring, improper density, limited styling choices, and limited attachment techniques. The experienced, artistic designer seldom will use off-the-shelf hair prostheses. Only in cases of emergency involving time limitations do most designers use off-the-shelf, ready-made hair additions. A negative feature of the off-the-shelf hair prosthesis is the fact that there are no restrictions set on shelf life. Certain materials such as polyurethane (used in sections such as the part) age, even if not worn. In contrast, the custom-made prosthesis is ensured to have "newly cured" polyurethane and to have top-quality components without any aging defects.

The downside of custom-designed prosthetics is that they usually take 4 to 8 weeks to complete.

COMPONENTS

Modern-day hair additions have evolved from the delicate organic materials used in toupees and hairpieces in the 1930s and 1940s. Silk, cotton, and organic gauze materials have been replaced by polyester, nylon, polyurethanes, and silicone materials for hair addition foundations. The newer synthetic materials eliminate shrinkage and absorption of body oils and perspiration and facilitate 24-hour wear for those with active lifestyles. The simulation of skin provided by polyurethanes and silicone materials along with fine nylon and polyester materials has eliminated overobvious parts and crowns. Most inexpensive hairpieces and wigs are made with machine-made wefts of hairs (rows of hair used mainly in mass-produced wigs) (Fig. 14-3).

As a result of the advent of improved foundation materials and attachment options, modern-day hair additions have improved aesthetically and now accommodate a wider variety of lifestyles.

Fibers

The fibers used in hair additions consist of human hair, synthetic fiber, or combinations of both. In rare cases animal hair such as yak or angora may be used. Human hair generally consists of three basic types: European (the finest texture), Asian (the coarsest, strongest, and most widely available), and Indian (the most popular, combining strength and a medium texture).

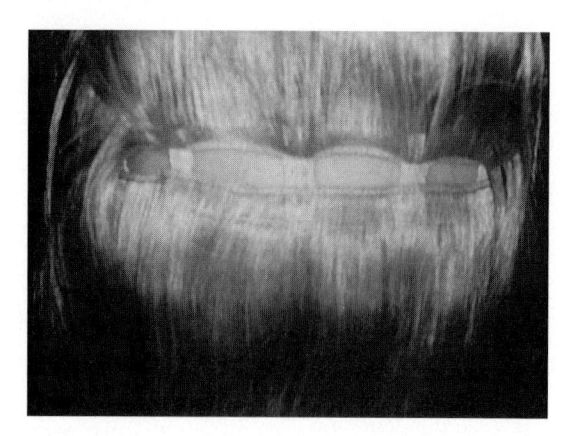

FIG. 14-3 Most inexpensive hairpieces and wigs are made with machine-made wefts of hair with spacing between the wefts.

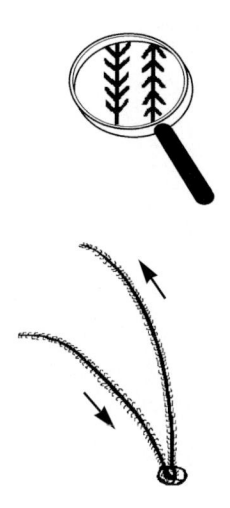

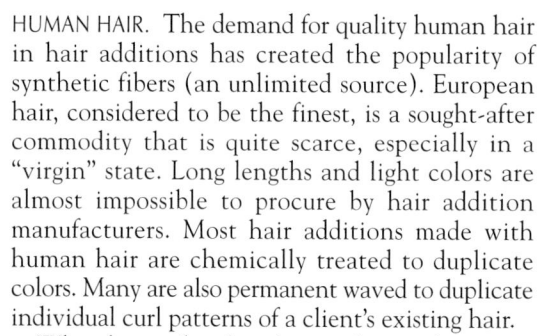

FIG. 14-4 When knotted to a foundation, human hair must be decuticlized to eliminate tangling.

HUMAN HAIR. The demand for quality human hair in hair additions has created the popularity of synthetic fibers (an unlimited source). European hair, considered to be the finest, is a sought-after commodity that is quite scarce, especially in a "virgin" state. Long lengths and light colors are almost impossible to procure by hair addition manufacturers. Most hair additions made with human hair are chemically treated to duplicate colors. Many are also permanent waved to duplicate individual curl patterns of a client's existing hair.

When knotted to foundations, human hair must be decuticlized to eliminate tangling. Otherwise tangling occurs when the individual hair is looped through the foundation and end meets end in opposing directions. If not decuticlized, the cuticle layers lock together, causing severe tangling (Fig. 14-4). Before the decuticlizing process, human hair additions required careful dry cleaning with chemicals such as methanol-based cleaners. After knotting, the opposing ends had to be cut short near the foundation to eliminate tangling. It is estimated that less than 5% of all hair additions today are made with European "virgin" hair (unchemically treated). Other than being rare, "virgin" European human hair is often cost prohibitive; and the procurement, hand sorting, and timely procedure of proper "root turning" to eliminate tangling is a rare and costly art. When available at a reasonable cost, it is the most sought-after fiber by women who wish to wear longer lengths of hair. In contrast, the largest percentage of human hair being used in today's men's hair additions comes from India.

Indian Hair. Indian hair is the most widely available. Religious leaders contact "hair brokers" after the hair is collected during annual rituals. This practice produces a modest source of income for Indian religious groups. Indian women usually cover their hair, thus giving hair addition manufacturers less oxidized hair colors. Rarely do Indians use chemicals such as permanents and colors, a fact that adds to the quality. Collectors of hair purchase either "remys" of hair (bundles of hair that often are not sorted by color and length and most important by the proper direction) or ponytails (which are sorted by color and length and turned in the proper direction).

The hair brokers prefer ponytails and braided lengths that have been cut, thus ensuring synchronization of direction. If the hair is purchased in remys, experienced sorters must go through the tedious task of sorting lengths and colors and placing individual hairs all in the proper direction. The texture and strength of Indian hair accommodates both the chemical processing required in decuticlization and the coloring and permanent waving required for most hair additions.

Asian Hair. Asian hair is ideal for straight, long lengths for individuals who do not require fine-texture hair. Although it may be the strongest hair, it resists curling and styling changes more than the finer textures. With Asian hair, straight styles are preferred.

European Hair. Considered the finest in textures, European hair also can be interpreted as the weakest in strength. It cannot withstand the chemical abuse that the coarser textures can accommodate. European hair is at its best when it is not chemically treated or decuticlized. It is difficult to procure and almost impossible to find in lengths over 22 inches in lighter colors.

Hair of Women in the United States. The hair of most women in the United States is severely damaged. Coloring, perming, teasing, and the excessive use of heat for styling are more popular in our culture than in any other. Add to this the fact that most U.S. women do not wear head coverings; as a result, the hair color is often partially oxidized.

The price paid for hair does not warrant a woman in the United States selling her hair. Although there are exceptions, the United States generally represents the lowest volume contributor of hair used by hair addition manufacturers around the world.

SYNTHETIC FIBERS. The popularity of women's wigs in the 1960s gave birth to the synthetic fiber. It quickly took hold because of its low maintenance and easy access. Over 50% of all men's hair additions now being marketed to the public are made of synthetic fibers. In the 1970s and 1980s it was even more popular, with approximately 60% to 70% of all men's hairpieces being produced with synthetic fiber. Most of the synthetic fibers used today are composed of two polymerized monomers: vinyl chloride and acrylonitrile, which together form modacrylic fiber.

The fibers are manufactured through a metal disk that contains openings that are the width of an average human hair. The openings can be regulated to form varying widths of fiber. The fibers are then stretched and dried. The polymer is colored before or after it has been extruded from the disk. Synthetic fiber has several advantages over human hair:

1. Synthetic fiber hair is lighter in weight and does not add the tension in long lengths that human hair often does.
2. Synthetic fiber has low porosity, causing it to dry faster than human hair.
3. Heat-formed wave and curl patterns hold up far longer in humidity than those in human hair.
4. Synthetic fibers hold their color much longer than human hair.
5. Its source is unlimited and its overall cost is less than human hair.

However, despite the advantages offered by synthetic fibers, human hair for hair additions is gaining in popularity. The recent trend toward human hair is a result of permanent attachment techniques demanded by today's men with more active lifestyles.

Most synthetic fibers cannot withstand the high heat generated by blow dryers and styling devices. Marketing specialists also have found that psychologically men feel more natural with human hair. However, the retail price is usually higher for human hair.

ATTACHMENT OF FIBERS

Just as large grafts were used in the original hair transplants of the 1960s, large knots were used in many of the early hair additions. Yet modern techniques of micrografting and minigrafting used in hair replacement surgery are now reflected in the refined knotting techniques used for attaching hairs to the foundation of hair additions.

The first toupees and hairpieces were made by attaching multiple hairs (an average of four to six) throughout most of the foundation, with single hairs knotted into the hairline. This technique would leave the majority of knots with 8 to 12 ends protruding from the foundation. Similar to large grafts, these larger knots were unattractive under close inspection. Presently in widespread use are hair additions made with one to two hairs per knot, leaving only two to four ends protruding from the foundation.

Individual fibers are attached to foundations in four basic techniques: hand knotted, looped and sealed, punched in, and machine wefted.

Hand Knotted

Hand knotted is the most popular technique. The types of knots used are the single knot (used primarily for synthetic fiber), double knots (used primarily for human hair), and split knots (used to add volume and height).

ADVANTAGES
- The hand-knotting technique is incorporated with the finest "mesh" foundations. The foundations are generally breathable and offer superior ventilation over hard bases such as polyurethane or fiberglass.
- Hand-knotted attachment, when performed by a competent technician, provides strength and a free 360-degree rotation of the direction of the hair. Hair direction can be changed more dramatically with this technique than any other attachment method.

DISADVANTAGES
- When human hair is used, the hair must have the cuticle layers removed to eliminate severe tangling and knots caused by the cuticle layers locking together when protruding ends oppose each other.

Looped and Sealed

The fiber is pulled through the foundation in a loop, without knotting, and then is sealed on the interior foundation of the hair addition.

ADVANTAGE
- The advantage of the looped-and-sealed technique is that it expedites production of the hair addition.

DISADVANTAGES
- The cuticle layers must be removed if human hair is used.
- This technique does not allow directional freedom of the individual hairs, and the hairs may protrude straight up when the technique is not performed by a competent technician. (Competent technicians use V-loops that can be more directional but cannot easily change direction.)
- When materials such as polyurethane are used, the foundation may wear and the hairs may be released.

Punched In

Although not used in the majority of hair additions, the punched-in technique is the most suitable fiber attachment method for today's vacuum-fitted hairpieces and wigs. All have more rigid foundations made with fiberglass, plexiglass, and vinyl. A needle is used to inject individual fibers through the rigid foundation. Individual fibers protruding at the interior of the foundation are folded and then sealed.

ADVANTAGE
- Since this technique leaves individual fibers protruding from the foundation, it gives the most natural appearance under close inspection.

DISADVANTAGE
- The directional insertion of the individual punched hairs cannot be changed easily.

Machine Wefted

Very few machine-wefted partial hair additions are made for men today.

ADVANTAGE
- Those machine-wefted additions that are available are inexpensive.

DISADVANTAGES
- Machine-wefted hair additions are bulky and hair direction is uncontrollable.
- The spacing between wefts appears unnatural, which eliminates partings.

CANDIDATE SELECTION FOR NONSURGICAL HAIR ADDITIONS

Those who are motivated to do something about their hair loss find nonsurgical hair additions the most noncommitting. Unlike surgery, the individual can stop wearing a hair addition at any time. The individual may even have a considerable amount of hair underneath the foundation. With such attachment methods as clips for temporary and removable wear, it is not necessary to shave or remove any hair. Younger men are excellent candidates for hair additions. When the physician cannot yet observe an established pattern of hair loss in an individual in his late teens or early twenties to thirties, a hair addition may be a useful option.

The more we learn, the less competition occurs between the nonmedical hair addition specialists and hair replacement surgeons. There are those individuals who simply will not consider surgery and those who will not consider a hair addition. Nonetheless the two professions interchange clients and patients to a certain degree. The concept of mutual cooperation between hair transplant surgeons and specialists in nonsurgical hair replacement is expounded on by Marritt and Dzubow in Chapter 1, Part F.

A significant number of men will never consider a hair addition since it is not their own hair and they fear the possible embarrassment of losing the hair addition when involved in strenuous activities or sports. Also the "fake" stigma is still prevalent with many men, so hair additions will probably not be totally accepted for some time.

Hair Transplant Patients Who Choose Hair Additions

The hair transplant patient may not be content with the density of hair from the grafts, so may wish to enhance it with a hair addition. The patient may opt for hair transplants in the front to obtain the desired density and then fill in the crown area with a partial hair addition. A patient who has received poor hair transplant results may now believe there is no choice but to cover the poor results with a hair addition.

Hair Addition Clients Who Choose Hair Transplants

The hair addition client may become a hair transplant patient because of his lack of willingness to consistently maintain a hair addition. At a later time the hair addition client may become aware that he is a good candidate for surgery, especially since the results he observes presently are far superior to those in the past.

Overview

The hair addition being the most noncommitting form of hair replacement also offers the most immediate results. It may even act as a blueprint or a realistic example of how important hair may be to the individual before surgical options. Using a hair addition that can be positioned at any starting point may be ideal for assisting the hair transplant physician in establishing a hairline, amount of recession, and a realistic example of the density (thickness) factor. More physicians are currently recruiting nonsurgical hair addition specialists to design small partial hair additions to cosmetically cover patients' scalps while they are undergoing multisessions of hair transplantation.

COST

Ready-Made Wigs

The first classification of hair additions is the full wig (covering the entire scalp). Inexpensive, machine-made, synthetic "ready-made" wigs can be purchased through mail order catalogs, wig salons, and department stores at prices ranging from approximately $59 to $150. These wigs are mostly mass produced with very little hand labor compared with that required for hand-knotted hair additions. Human hair wigs are not as readily available in ready-to-wear wigs. They average approximately $100 to $300 more in cost. Most are produced with Asian hair.

Custom-Made Wigs

Customizing means exact color matching, fitting, and providing all the particular needs an individual may require. Building the hair addition to individual specifications results in a significantly higher cost factor. Specified materials such as human hair and certain foundation materials make the cost difficult to estimate. Depending on the designer and the materials, prices may vary from $750 to $5000. Vacuum wigs range from $1500 to $3500 across the United States.

Partial Hair Additions for Men

Very few partial hair additions for men are machine made or mass produced. It is estimated that fewer than 5% are in the lower price ranges of $250 to $600. (Very few can be found that are hand knotted at these prices. If so, they are generally large, bulky knots containing too many hairs.) Whereas most women look for volume and fullness in a hairstyle, men often seek less hair and a hairstyle that lies much closer to the head. Therefore men require more detailed work in hair additions. The less hair, the more detail is necessary; the more hair, the less detail is needed. The notion that the more hair the hair addition has the more it will cost is in fact just the opposite. The curlier an individual's hair is, the less detail the hair addition requires in workmanship. The straighter the hair, the more detail the hair addition requires. The many variables in producing custom-made hair additions for men create a large range in prices. In quality hair additions the client can expect to invest from $850 to $3500. Other factors in pricing include the experience of the designer and the overhead and advertising expenses of the individual business or chain. A barber or cosmetologist doing hair additions as a sideline may sell a quality hair addition for a substantially lower retail price than a colleague who specializes in hair additions.

The disadvantage relates to the technician's experience. Without the proper design, no matter how talented the cutter is, he/she cannot create a natural-appearing head of hair. It requires approximately 2 to 3 years before hair addition specialists develop the keen aesthetic vision required to produce natural results.

ATTACHMENT

Except for rare allergy problems, most health complications regarding hair additions involve the attachment method. Rarely, a dye or a solvent may not be properly rinsed from a hair addition. In such situations, proper cleansing often will cure the problem of allergic reactions to hair additions. Most hair additions are built of common substances from the clothing and household products industries, substances such as nylon, polyester, polyurethane, cured silicone, and vinyl—none of which commonly causes allergic reactions. Industry specialists would agree that allergic reactions are normally induced by a substance on the fiber and not the fiber itself. Common examples might be scented hair sprays, hair color residues, and cleaning agents.

There are only two basic ways to affix a hair addition: (1) to the scalp and (2) to the existing hair.

Scalp Attachment

ADHESIVES. Adhesives (glues or double-sided adhesive tapes) are generally designed for frequent removal of the hair addition or for application to the frontal area only in semipermanent attachment techniques.

VACUUM-FITTED PROSTHETIC HAIR ADDITIONS. Precise fitting accomplishes a suction fit. This type of attachment is designed to allow for frequent removal of the hair addition.

SURGICAL ATTACHMENT. The tunnel graft procedure is designed for frequent removal of the hair addition (Fig. 14-5). This method involves the formation of skin loops or tunnels that are used to anchor the attachment of a hair addition. In this technique either two or three loops are created surgically using skin grafts from behind the patient's ears. This technique involves raising a bridge of skin at each location and then using a skin graft to complete the tunnel underneath the scalp tissue. The original diameter of each tunnel is 1 cm. Each tunnel is then used as an anchor point for a clip that is attached to the hair addition. Because the hair addition can be removed, the scalp can be properly cleansed and normal hygiene maintained. In addition, the patient is advised to cleanse the skin-lined tunnels periodically with hydrogen peroxide or alcohol as well. When this regimen is followed, infection is rarely a problem.

Complications are rare but do include an attachment clip cutting into the roof of a tunnel or a tunnel being cut or torn open by a sudden pull on the hair addition. This attachment method does provide a fairly secure manner of attaching a hair addition but has the disadvantage of there being two or three tunnel grafts that are quite visible if the hair addition is not worn.

Another type of surgical attachment is the suture technique, which permanently affixes the hair addition to the scalp (Fig. 14-6). In rare cases snaps with opposing inserts sewn into the hair addition are sutured to the scalp for client removal of the hair addition by unsnapping. The suture process of attaching hair additions is no longer readily available because of its discomfort to the patient. Without meticulous hygiene, there is a constant battle against serious infections. The New Jersey Board of Medical Examiners is currently attempting to ban the use of sutures to secure hair additions.

Attachment to Existing Hair

When hair additions are attached to the existing hair in a nonsurgical semipermanent technique, the two main concerns are tension and easy accessibility to the scalp for thorough cleansing.

CLIPS. Small clip devices ranging in size from 2 to 3 cm are sewn underneath the perimeter of the hair addition (Fig. 14-7). They are then combed into the individual's fringe hair (like a barrette) and locked into place. An average of four to five clips are installed on the hair addition. This attachment technique is popular for the man with newly thinning hair who does not wish to remove any hair. This technique also accommodates the client's removal of the hair addition.

WEAVE. The weave, although originally created to include wefts of hair in circular or lateral grid patterns, is now used on the upper portion of the U-shaped fringe of the client's healthy existing hair (Fig. 14-8). Instead of wefts of hair being attached,

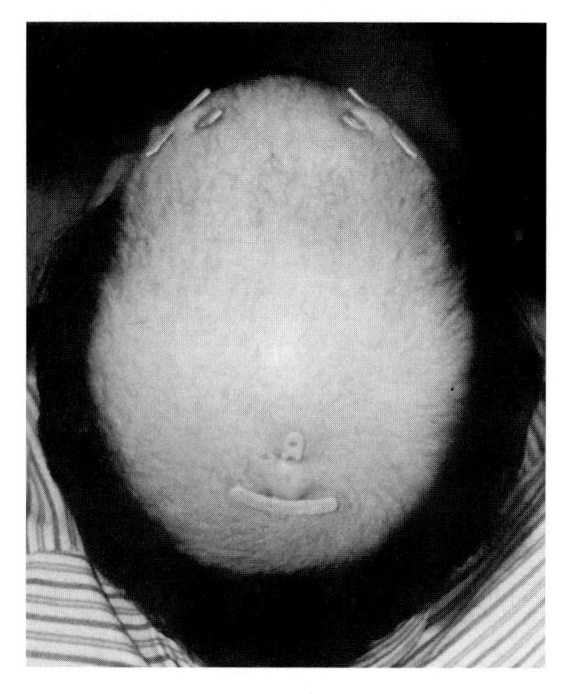

FIG. 14-5 Individual who has undergone the tunnel graft procedure. This method involves the formation of skin loops or tunnels, which are used to anchor the attachment of a hair addition.

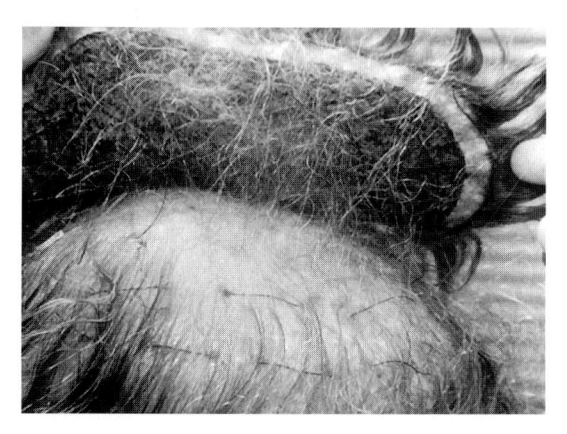

FIG. 14-6 The suture technique requires that the hair addition be attached permanently to the scalp. This method of attachment is less popular than others and is associated with a higher instance of complications.

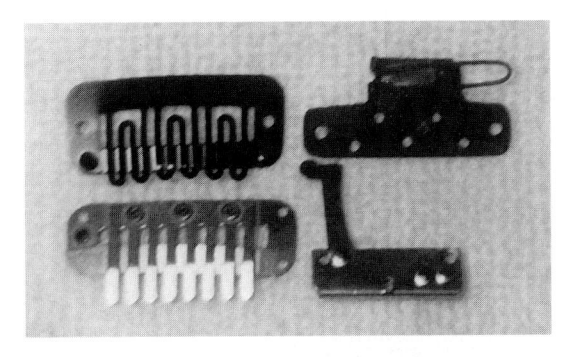

FIG. 14-7 Small clips, ranging in size from 2 to 3 cm, are attached to the perimeter of the hair addition foundation. The individual with this type of attachment can comb and snap the clips into the existing hair and undo them at his leisure.

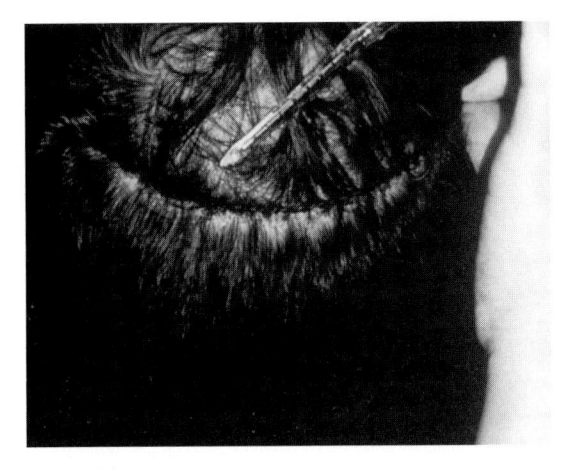

FIG. 14-8 A single braid is interwoven and secured with a monofilament line. The hair addition is then sewn to it. The client must return every 6 to 8 weeks for retightening.

a single braid is interwound and secured with nonshrinking monofilament line around the entire U-shaped pattern, and the hair addition is then sewn to it. As the existing hair grows, the weave becomes looser, generally requiring the client to return on an average of every 5 to 6 weeks for retightening. Since most men do not have adequate hair in the frontal region, an adhesive is used to secure the hair addition to this area.

When the adhesive is removed, this area of the hair addition can be lifted, providing the individual with accessibility to the scalp for proper cleansing and rinsing. If the fringe hair is fine and thin and the weave is done too tightly, the weave may cause excessive tension, resulting in traction alopecia (Fig. 14-9).

For the first-time wearer who does not wish to shave any existing hair (as is necessary in bonding attachment) until he is committed to wearing the hairpiece on a long-term basis, the weave may be a means of wearing the hair addition with a semipermanent attachment method.

BONDING. Bonding is rapidly becoming the most widely used method of semipermanent attachment for hair additions. For marketing purposes only it is known by many different names. This procedure involves cutting the hair in the upper U-shaped fringe area in an approximately ¾-inch wide band (Fig. 14-10, A). The hair in this area is cut to 1 to 3 mm in length. A matching ¾-inch band of vinyl or polyurethane in the outside perimeter of the hair addition is then coated with silicone- or latex-based adhesive (the latter is most commonly used) (Fig. 14-10, B). The hair addition is then applied to the matching area of the already cut hair on the client. The sealant cures to the individual's hair (not scalp), and the hair addition remains in place until, because of hair growth, it becomes loose (normally 3 to 6 weeks). The hair addition is then removed by cutting the individual's hair down to the original 1 to 3 mm length. After the scalp is cleansed and any services necessary are performed, the hair addition is reapplied. This technique, although widely used, should involve precautionary measures such as patch tests. It is also suggested that adhesives not be applied to any abrasions or open wounds in the scalp.

Fusion

This frequently used technique involves the same upper U-shaped fringe hair of the client. Microloops are sewn into the perimeter of the hair addition. Approximately 15 to 25 hairs of the client's own hair are pulled through the loops at matching points of the hair addition's microloops and are

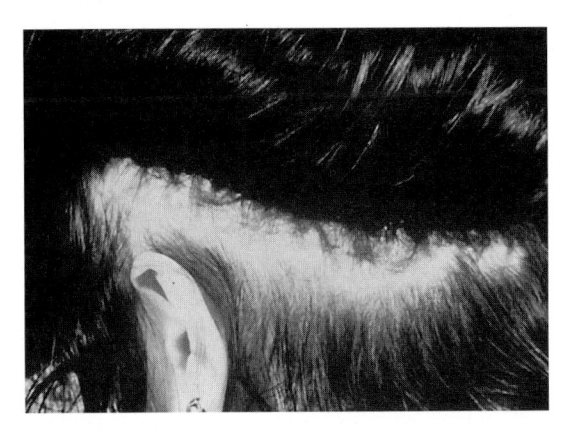

FIG. 14-9 Traction alopecia secondary to a weave placed too tightly.

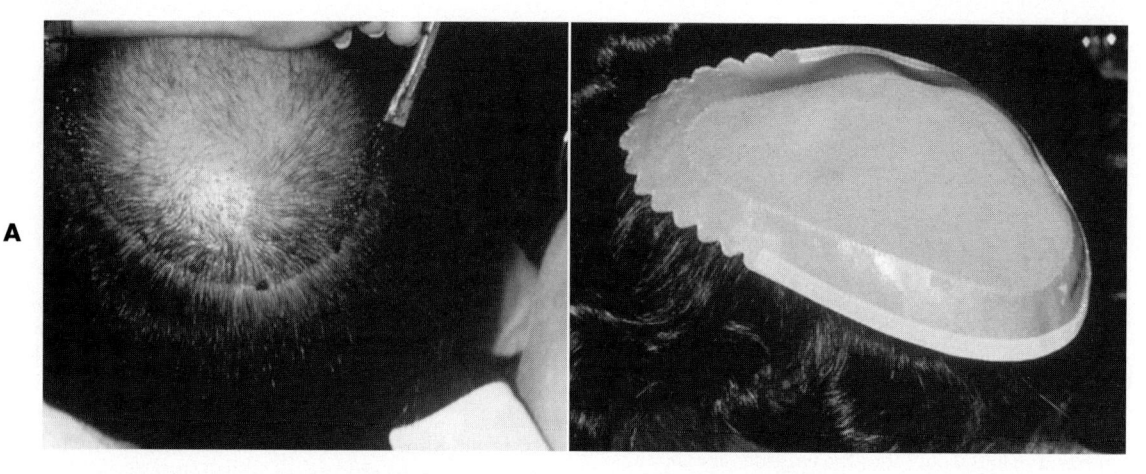

FIG. 14-10 **A,** Bonding is achieved by applying a sealant to a shaved area of the scalp. The hair addition is then applied to this area. Bonding requires reapplication every 4 to 6 weeks. **B,** Following application of the sealant, the base of the hair addition (¼-inch wide perimeter) is affixed to the area where the sealant was applied.

knotted or glued firmly. The glue in this technique is concentrated on the hair only. However, sealant may migrate to the scalp. Therefore a patch test should be done before this technique is performed.

Complications

The aforementioned semipermanent attachment techniques all share some of the same complications if not addressed properly. Traction alopecia can be a factor if any of these attachment techniques are too tight over extended periods of time on hair that is too weak or sparse. If excessively tight attachment is continued for more than 8 weeks, the process can result in scarring alopecia.

Seborrheic dermatitis can occur when the scalp is not cleansed sufficiently. Men must be instructed to meticulously cleanse their scalps underneath the semipermanently attached hair addition. This condition is most common in areas at or near the site of the attachment itself.

SUGGESTIONS

A hair addition should never be considered a one-time investment. Although it is the most immediate and noncommitting form of replacing lost hair, the hair addition requires committed care.

After 30 years of experience in serving clients with hair additions, I have come to the conclusion that there are two categories of clients:

1. Those who wish to simply cover their baldness. These individuals could cover their baldness much more inexpensively with a ball cap. They rarely have their hair addition serviced and are only concerned with covering their hair loss, not with its aesthetics.
2. Those who are seeking to improve their appearance. These individuals would never appear publicly if the hair addition had an unnatural appearance. They invest in appearance and not merely a "cover-up" for their baldness. The result of their dedicated maintenance is undetectability (Figs. 14-11 to 14-13). The individual who wishes to improve his appearance knows that he must invest in two hair additions to be secure and content. He knows that a backup is essential in the case of an unexpected accident to one hair addition. He also knows that many hours can be saved by having service performed on the "second head of hair" without his being present.

COMMON ERRORS IN THE AESTHETICS OF HAIR ADDITIONS

The most common error of specialists and the hair addition wearer is the fear of cutting or thinning too much hair from a hair addition. Since it is a purchased commodity, many believe the value of the hair addition will be lessened by cutting or thinning. Too much density causes a heavy appearance that reduces the natural appearance. Many individuals wearing hear additions never had as much hair even in their early teens!

The second most common error is the placement of the hair addition. Variation of placement by 1 to 2 cm can make the difference between appearing unnatural or appearing natural. An average start-

Nonsurgical Hair Replacement 409

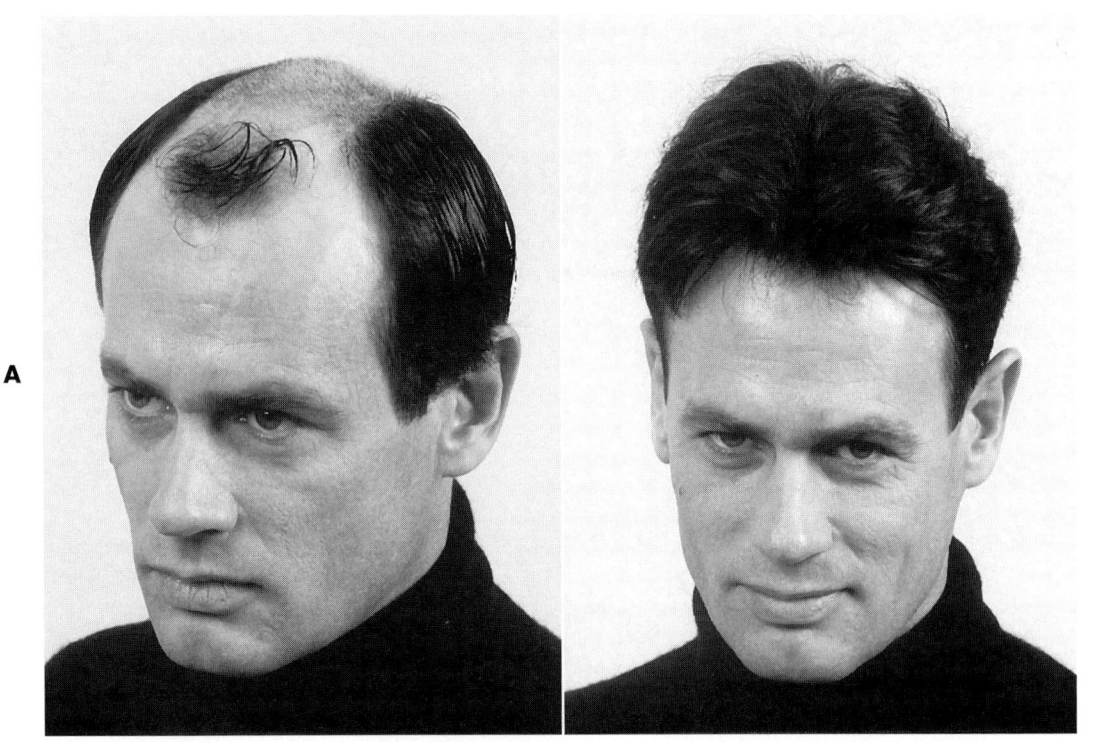

FIG. 14-11 **A,** Subject without hair addition. **B,** Subject with custom-made hair addition in place.

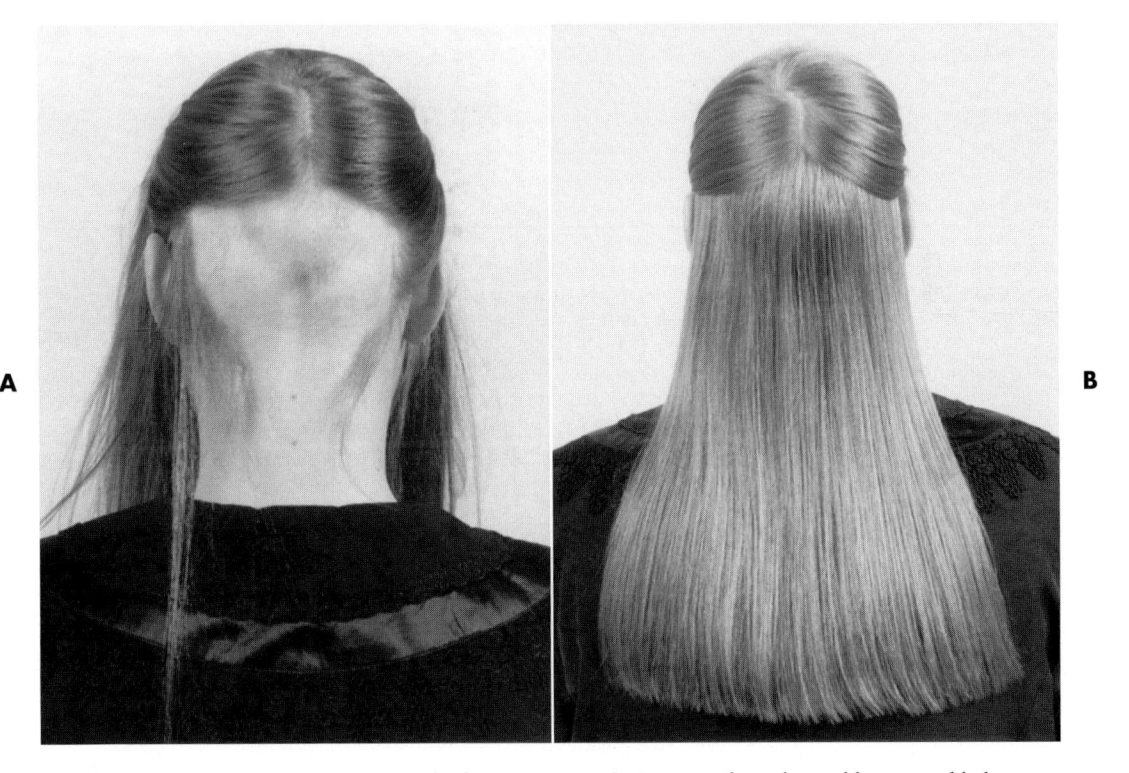

FIG. 14-12 **A,** Female patient with alopecia areata. **B,** Patient after a hair addition is added to the occipital region.

410 Nonsurgical Hair Replacement

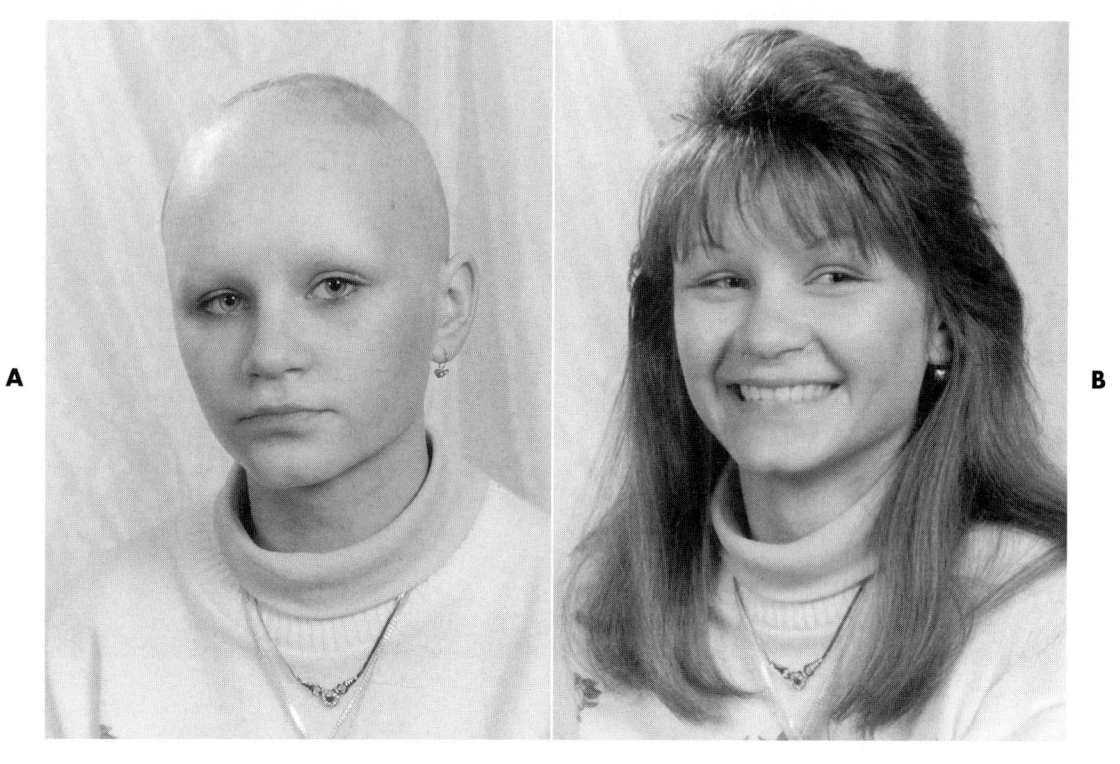

FIG. 14-13 A, Children and young adults are also candidates for hair additions. This patient has alopecia totalis and therefore requires a full-cap prosthesis. **B,** Patient with full-cap prosthesis in place.

TABLE 14-1 Aesthetic Guidelines for Hair Additions

PROBLEM	SOLUTION
Too much hair (density)	Requires proper thinning by skilled professional.
Hairline too low	Instruct client to place hair addition back further (7-8 cm above brow at ages 21-35; 8-10 cm age 50 and up).
Visible line around the perimeter of replacement hair	Color is not correct—human hair can be colored to match. Replacement hair is too dense or cut too blunt—ends must be thin and not cut bluntly to blend into client's own hair.
Hair addition too flat	Length is too long and too dense—proper cutting and thinning are often required to correct this common problem. A small amount of curl also may be necessary.
Client's hair has more gray than hair addition	Gray hair can be added to hair additions by hand-knotting new gray hairs into the foundation.
Obvious hairline	Three factors can lead to unnatural-appearing hairline: (1) length and density, (2) color (often the frontal hairline is too dark on light skin, which can be corrected by highlighting or adding gray, and (3) curl or style (without any curl no hair addition appears natural combed straight back).
Color does not match client's own hair	If the hair addition is human hair, it may be colored, but synthetic fiber cannot be colored and should be replaced.

ing point would be 7 to 8 cm above the brows on a young man 21 to 35 years of age. Many unnaturally place the hair addition 5 to 6 cm above the brows. Often individuals over the age of 50 appear much more natural with a hairline placed 8 to 10 cm above the brows. Since the density of most hair additions has no transition and begins immediately and abruptly, the starting point should always be at least 1 cm behind the normal placement of a hairline. This placement can be upsetting to a young man when he is viewing only the template, and he must be made aware that this point is where the foundation begins, not the hair.

The third most common error is not replacing the hair addition as it loses its natural appearance. The average hair addition lasts approximately 18 months. Those wearing the hair addition semipermanently may need to replace it as often as every 9 to 12 months. At an average cost of $1200 to $1800, this can be a factor in the individual attempting to stretch the time limitation of natural-appearing hair. A good hair addition takes commitment not just in time and maintenance but also financially.

If the client is not instructed properly and the acquired skill and experience of the specialist is lacking, it is virtually impossible to accomplish undetectable results. One should always investigate the procedure and product thoroughly and ask to meet other clients who have undergone the process (Table 14-1). Observing the actual work of the specialist is the most important factor in finding a talented specialist. There are firms that offer a money-back guarantee if for any reason the client is not 100% satisfied. Always ask the question, "What happens if I am not satisfied?" before signing any contracts or making any financial commitment.

words in the English language to describe a service; the U.S. Congress did not want to unduly limit companies in their advertising and promotion.

If a service mark has been awarded to a term, it is protected under the Lanham Act and cannot be used by others in their advertising. The initials ^{SM} appear after a term that has been registered as a service mark. Those initials designate that a service mark has been awarded by the U.S. Department of Commerce Patent and Trademark Office (PTO).

OTHER LIMITATIONS

Simply because someone is the first person to use a mark does not mean it will be registered by the PTO. Even if the inventor of the process being advertised attempts to register a service mark, that does not guarantee that the mark will be awarded. If the applicant is the first and only user of the mark, it will not be registered if the term is merely descriptive.[10] If it is found that the mark is a common descriptive name of the applicant's services, it will no be registered. The mark must distinguish the user's services from the services of others.

If a service mark or trademark becomes a generic term, then no protection is provided. Section 14(c) of the Lanham Act provides for the cancellation of a registered mark if at any time it "becomes the common descriptive name of an article or substance." No matter how much money and effort the user of a generic name has poured into promoting the sale of merchandise and despite the success it has achieved in securing public identification, someone cannot be deprived of the right to call an article by its name.[11]

A mark such as *escalator* loses its protection as a trademark when it becomes a generic term.[12] If the inventor of hair transplants had obtained a service mark on *hair transplants*, that term would now be generic and the inventor would have lost federal protection as a service mark.

It is possible, if sued for "infringement" of a service mark, to file a counterclaim against the plaintiff. Section 37 of the Lanham Act allows for a counterclaim for cancellation of a mark by a defendant who does not own a registered mark. Cancellation of the service mark may be ordered if it is proved that the registered mark has become the "common descriptive name of an article or substance."[13] That happened to Abercrombie & Fitch when they sued Hunting World, Inc., for infringement of the service mark *Safari*. The Court held *Safari* to be a generic term that anyone could use.[11]

REQUIREMENTS

Before a mark can be registered as a service mark, it must be used in some aspect of the promotion of the applicant's services. Actual use of the service mark is the key, not an intent to use the term in the future. The use of the mark is what first establishes the user's rights to the mark. It is not enough for the applicant to be the provider of the services; the applicant must have used the mark to identify the service for which registration is sought.[14]

To be registered as a federal service mark, the mark must be used in interstate commerce, which simply means in commerce between two or more states.

OTHER CONSIDERATIONS

If the PTO refuses to register a service mark because it is "merely descriptive," it may become registered and protected, even if it does not otherwise qualify under the Lanham Act, if it has become "distinctive" of a person's goods or services. A mark that is merely descriptive is not registrable under Section 2(e) but may be registrable under Section 2(f), 15 U.S.C. 1052(f) if secondary meaning is demonstrated. Under 15 U.S.C. 1052(f), if the mark has become distinctive and there is proof of substantially exclusive and continuous use for 5 years before the claim of distinctiveness is made, the mark can be registered *even if* it is "merely descriptive."

A mark that does not meet all the requirements of the principal register may be registered on the supplemental register if it is capable of distinguishing the applicant's goods or services in the future. The court in *In re Bush Bros. & Co.* allowed the applicant to register the mark *DELUXE* on the supplemental register as a trademark for canned pork and beans. The Court held that the term *DELUXE* was capable of becoming distinctive of the source of the applicant's canned pork and beans.[15]

The registration requirements concerning the supplemental register are found in the Lanham Act in Section 23, 15 U.S.C. 1091. Although the protection of the principal register service marks is not available to those on the supplemental register, registration on the supplemental register allows for some protection and is usually advantageous.

Registration on the principal register is not a prerequisite for enforcement of trademark rights; it only makes them easier to enforce. Trademark right is a common law right that exists independent of the statutory process for registration.[16] Registration on the supplemental list confers federal jurisdiction for purposes of enforcement.

PROCESS

Service marks are awarded through the U.S. Department of Commerce Patent and Trademark Office. The cost of the application is $245 for each service mark submitted for registration. The PTO determines if a mark can be registered. A very helpful application booklet can be obtained by writing to the following address: Commissioner of Patents and Trademarks, Washington, DC 20231. General information on service marks can be obtained by calling the PTO at 703-308-HELP.

Before a mark may be registered, it is necessary to ensure that someone else has not already obtained a service mark on the term. There are many different private trademark search companies that can conduct a search. If there is a service mark that is close to the one being applied for, the PTO could reject the application if there would be a "likelihood of confusion" between the marks. The marks do not have to be identical, nor do the services have to be the same.

Tables A-1, A-2, and A-3 list all registered, pending, and abandoned service marks, respectively, on the principal register of the PTO that involve hair transplantation. The lists are current as of April 1994. Hair transplantation service marks are classified by the PTO as services in the category of International Class 42.

TABLE A-1 Registered Service Marks Involving Hair Transplantation

APPROVED AND REGISTERED SERVICE MARKS	REGISTERED OWNER
NU/HART	NU/HART Laboratories, Inc.
Professional Hair Transplant Institute of Mobile "Your own living hair" (with picture)	Michael Lyons
POLYFUSE	Hair Club for Men, Ltd.
HCM	Hair Club for Men, Ltd.
An Investment That Never Stops Growing	Constantine P. Chambers
I'm Not Only The Hair Club President, I'm Also A Client	Hair Club for Men, Ltd.
Hair Club	Hair Club Associates, Ltd.
Simmons	Simmons Hairweaving Tension System, Inc.
Strand-By-Strand	Hair Club Associates, Ltd.
Micrograft	Bosley Medical Group
Hair Club for Men	Hair Club Associates, Ltd.
Mini-Brader	Concept, Inc.

TABLE A-2 Pending Service Mark Applications Involving Hair Transplantation

PENDING SERVICE MARK APPLICATIONS	APPLICANT
Varigrafting	Bosley Medical Institute
Varigraft	Bosley Medical Institute
HRG	Hair Restoration Group, Inc.
Hair Restoration Group	Hair Restoration Group, Inc.
Chambers Dovetail Closure	Constantine P. Chambers
Hats Off Technique	Constantine P. Chambers
HaFo (with picture)	Bergmann GMBH & Co. KG
Feathering Zone Technique (with picture)	Dr. Dowling B. Stough, M.D.
Braids, Weaves & Things	Braids, Weaves & Things, Inc.
National Hair Clinics	National Hair Clinics, Inc.
Hair Club for Kids	Hair Club for Men, Ltd.
Regenix Hair Retention Clinics	Pure Balance, Inc.
Hair Club for Women	Hair Club for Men, Ltd.

TABLE A-3 Abandoned Service Marks Involving Hair Transplantation

ABANDONED SERVICE MARKS	REGISTERED OWNER
Hair Rooting	Men's Hair Now New York, Inc. d/b/a Bioexcell Hair Resource Center
Hair Club for Children	Hair Club for Men, Ltd.
Incision Grafting	Tom Rosanelli, M.D.
Now Available A New and Better Procedure "Line Grafting" (with picture)	Puig Medical Group
Le Metric	Elline's International Hair, Inc.
Bald Area Reduction	Cleveland Hair Clinic, Inc.
Line Grafting (with picture)	Cleveland Hair Clinic, Inc.
The Curbeon Look	Daisy Curbeon

REFERENCES

1. 15 U.S.C. §1053 (1982).
2. 15 U.S.C. §1127 (1982) and Suppl III (1985).
3. *In re* Canadian Pacific, Ltd. 754 F.2d 994, 224 USPQ 973.
4. *In re* Bright Crest, Ltd. 204 USPQ 591 (TTAB 1979).
5. *In re* Bed & Breakfast Registry 791 F.2d 157, 229 USPQ 818 (Fed. Cir. 1986).
6. *In re* Northland Aluminum Products, Inc., 777 F.2d 1566, 1559, 227 USPQ 961, 963 (Fed. Cir. 1985).
7. *In re* Metpath, Inc., 223 USPQ 88 (TTAB 1984).
8. *In re* Gyulay 820 F.2d 1216 (Fed. Cir. 1987).
9. Stix Products, Inc. v. United Merchants Manufacturers, Inc., 295 F. Suppl 479, 488 (S.D. W.Y. 1988).
10. *In re* National Shooting Sports Foundation, Inc., 219 USPQ 1018 (TTAB 1983).
11. Abercrombie & Fitch Co. v. Hunting Worth, Inc., 537 F.2d 4 (2d Cir. 1976).
12. Haughton Elevator Co. v. Seeberger 85 U.S.P.Q. 80 (1950).
13. 15 U.S.C. §1064(3), §1065(4).
14. *In re* Universal Oil Products Co. 476 F.2d 653, 177 USPQ 456 (CCPA 1973).
15. *In re* Bush Bros. & Co. 884 F.2d 569 (Fed. Cir. 1989).
16. California Cooler, Inc. v. Loretto Winery Ltd., 774 F.2d 1451 (1985).

APPENDIX B

Surgical Products for Hair Transplantation

Mark R. Avram, Francisco Jimenez, and Dow B. Stough

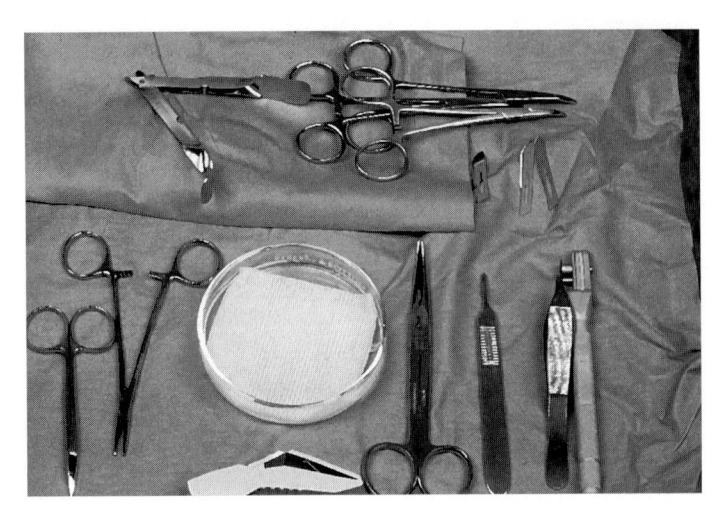

FIG. B-1

STERILE SURGICAL TRAY FOR EXCISING DONOR STRIP (FIG. B-1)

1. Multiple bladeholder with straight 2 mm spacers (Van Sickle Co., G. Tiemann & Co., Byron) Bladeholders, $98; spacers, $6 each
   Fig. B-2

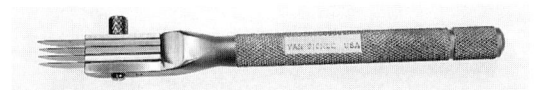

FIG. B-2

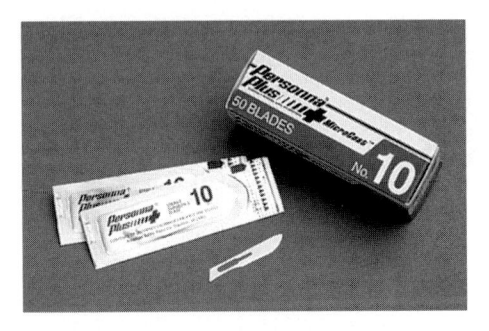

FIG. B-3

2. No. 10 Personna Plus blades, $27.50 for box of 50
   Fig. B-3
3. No. 3 scalpel handle, $12
   Fig. B-1
4. Specialized strip scissors (Van Sickle Co.), $120
   Fig. B-4
5. Three small micro-mosquito 4¾" hemostats, $50 each
   Fig. B-1

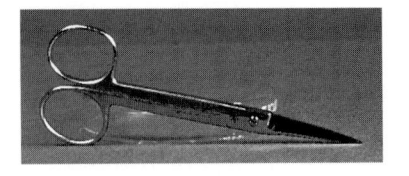

FIG. B-4

417

418 Appendix B

6. Adson's forceps with teeth, $45
   Fig. B-1
7. Needle holder, $60
   Fig. B-1
8. 3M Precise DS-25 staples (3M Medical Division), $106.75 for box of 10
   Fig. B-5
9. Staple remover, $2.80
   Fig. B-1
10. Petri dishes with gauze and chilled saline solution at 4° C
    Fig. B-1

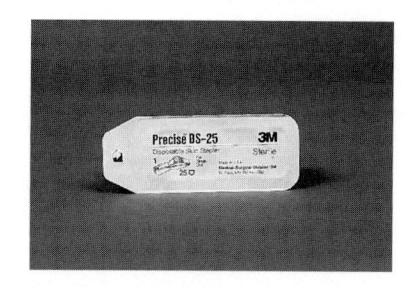

FIG. B-5

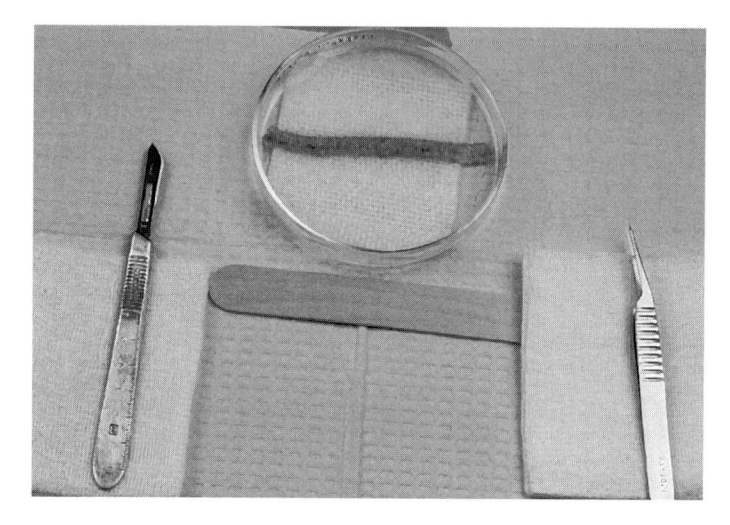

FIG. B-6

SURGICAL TRAY FOR CUTTING GRAFTS
(FIG. B-6)

1. Jeweler's forceps (Van Sickle microdilator forceps, Snowden Pencer microvascular jeweler's forceps), $86 to $100
   Fig. B-7

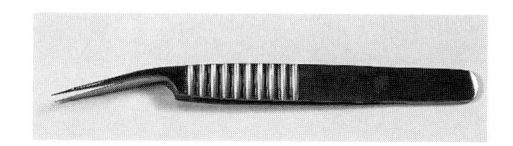

FIG. B-7

2. No. 3 scalpel handle with No. 10 blade
3. Plastic 13" × 10" cutting board
4. Tongue blade
5. Petri dish with chilled saline solution
6. Nu-Gauze 3" × 3" sponge (Johnson & Johnson) for base of petri dish
   Fig. B-6

SURGICAL TRAY FOR PREPARING RECIPIENT SITE

1. Hand engine
   Model 25D (Robbins Instruments, Inc.; Bell), $1300
   Fig. B-8

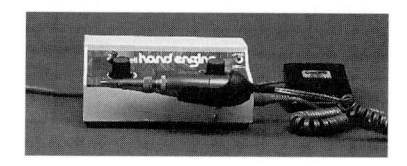

FIG. B-8

AEU-12 Electrimax (Aseptico), $975
Fig. B-9

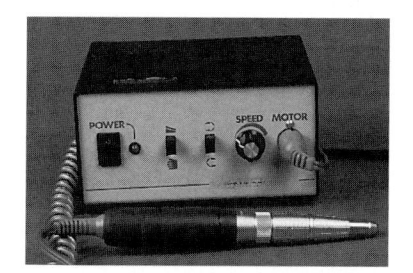

FIG. B-9

Exelna II Mobile Unit, #403601 (Bell), $850
Fig. B-10

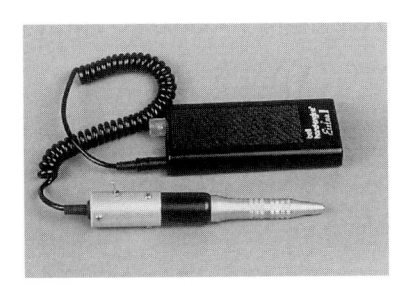

FIG. B-10

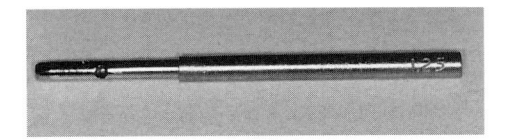

FIG. B-11

2. Hair transplant punches, 1 mm, 1.25 mm, 1.5 mm (G. Tiemann & Co.; Robbins Instruments, Inc.; Benn Instrument Co.), $15 to $40 per punch
   Fig. B-11
3. Instrument for single-hair recipient site
   Fig. B-12 *From left to right:* Beaver No. 6100 blade (Swann-Morton Ltd.); Yeh needle (Accuderm, Inc.); 18-gauge NoKor needle (Becton-Dickinson); standard 18-gauge needle

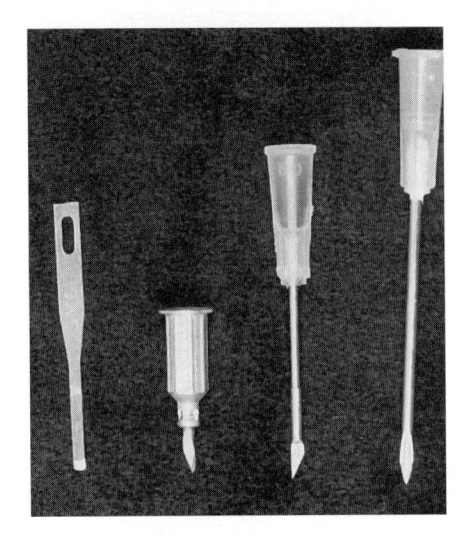

FIG. B-12

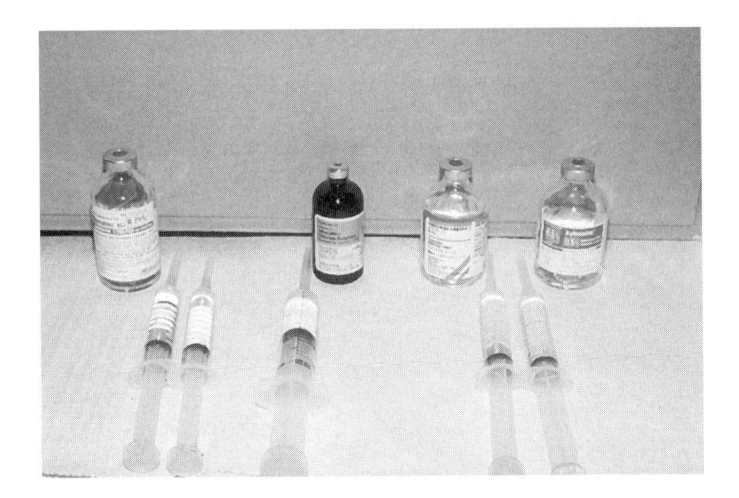

FIG. B-13

TRAY FOR GRAFT IMPLANTATION

1. Jeweler's forceps
2. Petri dish

SYRINGES AND ANESTHETIC (FIG. B-13)

1. 0.5% lidocaine with 1:200,000 epinephrine (Fig. B-14); one or two 10 ml syringes for donor site and two 10 ml syringes for recipient site

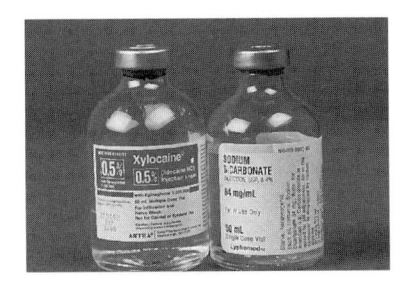

FIG. B-14

2. 20 ml saline solution for donor site
3. 12 ml saline solution containing 0.1 ml 1:1000 epinephrine (1:120,000 total epinephrine concentrate) for recipient site
Fig. B-15

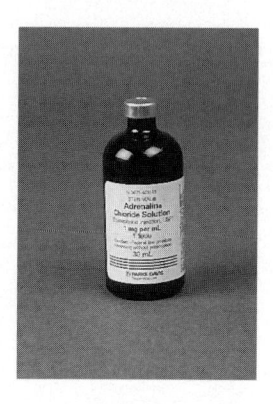

FIG. B-15

OTHER SUPPLIES

1. Prōn Pillō (Robbins Instruments, Inc.), $96
Fig. B-16

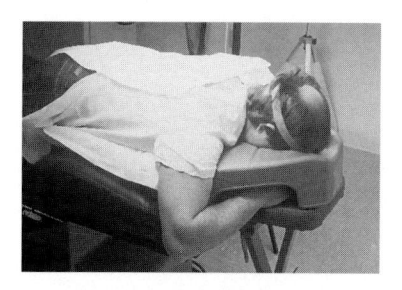

FIG. B-16

2. Mustache trimmer (Whal, Inc.)
Fig. B-17

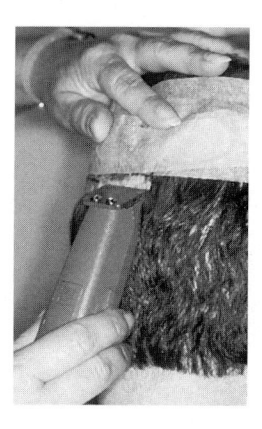

FIG. B-17

3. 3% Hydrogen peroxide (a 1:1 mixture with water is placed in a spray bottle for dampening the scalp during the surgical procedure)
Fig. B-18

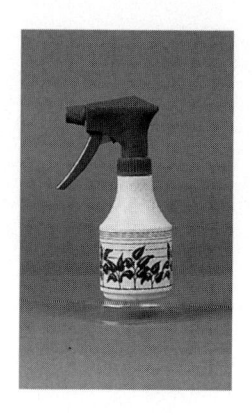

FIG. B-18

4. Adhesive tape remover (Detachol, Ferndale Laboratories, Inc.), $5.05 per 4 oz bottle
5. Trichoscope (Welch-Allen, Inc.)
Fig. B-19

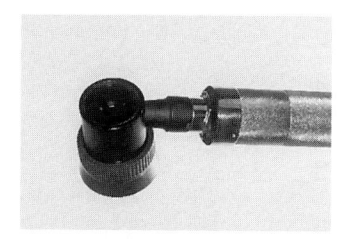

FIG. B-19

6. Postoperative dressings
Telfa nonadhesive 3″ × 8″ dressing (Kendall), $10 to $16 per box of 100
Micropore 1-inch tape (3M), $15 per box of 12
Reston 20 × 30 cm foam (3M), $25 per bag
Tubular cotton-blend 6″ stockinette dressing (De Busk, Inc.), $12 per roll
Fig. B-20

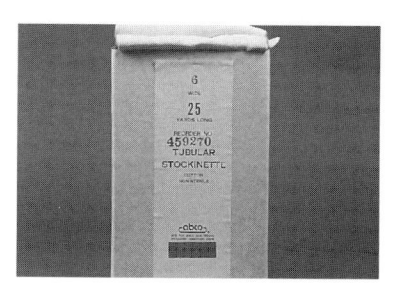

FIG. B-20

Conforming gauze 3" × 131" bandage (Kling) (Johnson & Johnson), $6.30 per bag
Gauze 4" × 4" sponges
7. Emergency kit (Bayan International Co.) Fig. B-21
8. Pulse oximeter (Nelcor, Inc.)

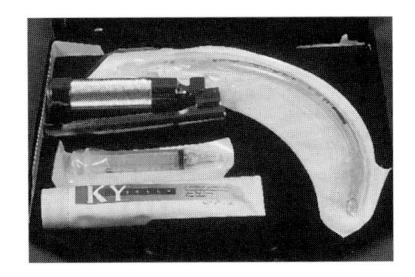

FIG. B-21

APPENDIX D

Determination of Hairline Placement

Sajjad Khan and Dow B. Stough

Re-creation of an aesthetically pleasing permanent hairline is the most challenging aspect of hair restoration surgery, and careful planning is key to achieving optimal results. The hairline should restore symmetry, harmony, and proportion of the face without being perceived as artificial or unnatural to the observing eye. From a frontal view the hairline should look soft and oval, and from a profile view it should look horizontal with gentle but well-defined frontotemporal angles. The hairline should never be placed lower than the superior border of the upper third of the face (Fig. D-1). In blacks and Hispanics, the general appearance of the hairline is more round, with slight blunting of the frontotemporal triangles.

HAIRLINE PLANNING

A transplanted hairline cannot be altered easily without leaving detectable scars; therefore the hair transplant surgeon has limited flexibility after the initial grafting sessions. After marking the hairline, the surgeon should view the proposed hairline from the front, back, and profile. The hairline should be viewed in mirrors as well. Guidelines for hairline planning are based on reference points: the frontal midpoint (A), midpupillary point (B), apex of the frontotemporal triangles at the lateral canthal level (C), and temporal peaks (D) (Fig. D-2).

Frontal Midpoint

The frontal midpoint should never be placed lower than the superior border of the upper third of the face because the normal adult male hairline is above this level—at least 7 cm from the glabella. Mistakes are often made in marking the midglabellar reference point. A horizontal line through the eyebrows identifies the midglabellar point. To determine the border of the upper third of the face, the glabella-to-chin distance is determined and

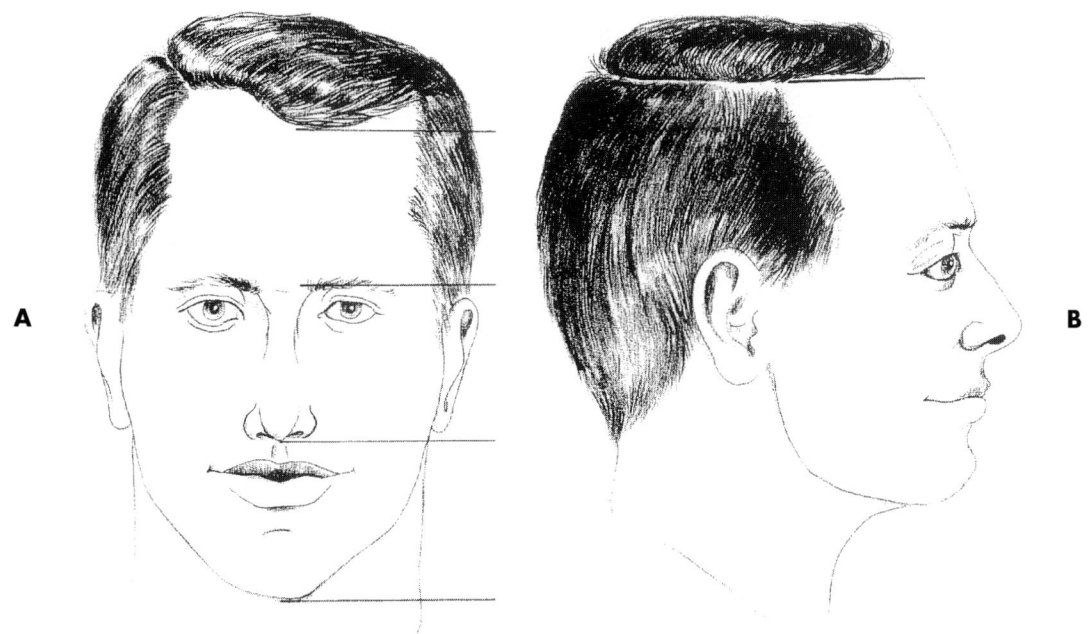

FIG. D-1

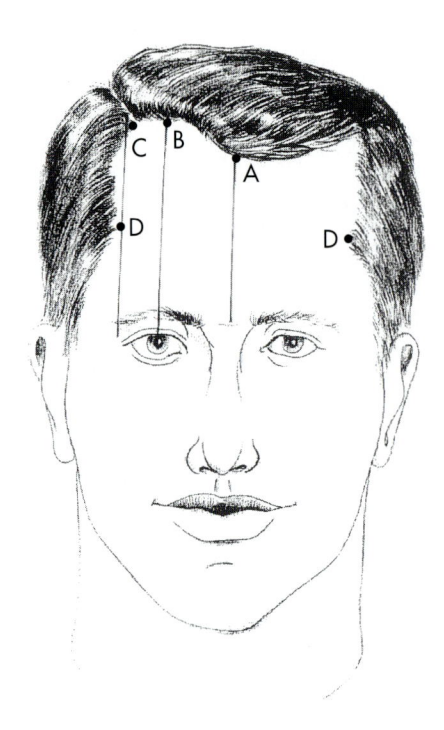

FIG. D-2

then divided in half. In men the average glabella-to-chin distance is 13 to 15 cm. A transplanted hairline is placed slightly higher than the upper third of the face. The midpoint is thus placed 8 to 9 cm above the glabella for minimum to moderate hair loss or potential hair loss. The midpoint is placed 9 to 11 cm from the midglabellar point for moderate to extensive hair loss or potential hair loss. A receding temporal hairline and the presence of a forelock can also affect the placement of the midpoint. The midpoint can be placed 1 cm higher than planned if the temporal peak recedes completely as occurs in moderate to extensive baldness.

In a patient with a family history of long-term forelock retention and a thick, retained forelock at a relatively low level, the midpoint is placed in the posterior segment of the thick, retained forelock 8 to 9 cm from the glabella. If the patient presents with a thin, retained forelock at a very low level (i.e., 4 to 6 cm), the surgeon should not consider placement of any grafts anteriorly or within this forelock.

If the patient is viewed in a profile view and a horizontal line is drawn forward from the apex of the frontotemporal triangle, the anterior point of this line provides an estimate for frontal midpoint placement. After all the criteria have been evaluated, if the marked midpoint lies on the flat surface of the top of the scalp, it requires very little adjustment. Most but not all adult hairlines fall on the relatively flat surface of the scalp. Surgeons should try to place the hairline on the flat portions of the scalp as opposed to the vertical forehead areas (Fig. D-3).

Midpupillary Point

To mark the midpupillary point on the brow, as the patient looks straight ahead, a vertical line is placed through the pupil. This vertical line is intersected with a tangential line on the flat surface of the scalp. The intersection of these two lines is called the midpupillary point (point B in Fig. D-2).

Apex of Frontotemporal Triangle

The apex of the frontotemporal triangle is formed where the posterior part of the frontal hairline meets the superior part of the temporal hairline.

The lateral canthus is a reference point for marking the apex of the frontotemporal triangle. The lateral canthus point is marked on the eyebrow, and then a vertical line is extended from this point. This vertical line (A in Fig. D-4) is intersected at a 90-degree angle with a horizontal line toward the scalp (B). The intersection of these two lines is the apex of the frontotemporal triangle (point C in Fig. D-4).

The depth of the apex is the distance from the frontal midpoint to the apex point (range 4 to 7 cm). If the temporal peaks recede, then the apex of the frontotemporal triangle should lie 1 to 2 cm behind a pretragal vertical line that is drawn at the anterior part of the sideburns. The apex should not fall behind the pretragal vertical line (D in Fig. D-4). If the apex is completely lost and hair restoration is required, the extent and planning of grafting will depend directly on the remaining donor area and individual potential for hair loss.

If the superior portion of the temporal hairline recedes and the frontotemporal triangle is lost, two options exist: (1) do nothing and allow an isolated anterior forelock to remain and bald alleys to develop[1] and (2) extend the temporal hairline superiorly to meet the frontal hairline at the outer canthal level, which will create a natural part at the frontotemporal triangle. The hair naturally parts at the apex of the frontotemporal triangle in most individuals. Parting at this level creates curves that are aesthetically pleasing to the eye and provide symmetry, harmony, and proportion to the face with a natural elliptical appearance.

GUIDELINES FOR FRONTAL HAIRLINE PLACEMENT

The frontal hairline should look oval from the front view and horizontal from the profile view and should preferably be placed on the flat surface of the scalp. The frontal hairline is drawn by uniting midpoint (A), midpupillary point (B), and apex point of the frontotemporal triangle (C) (Fig. D-5). The

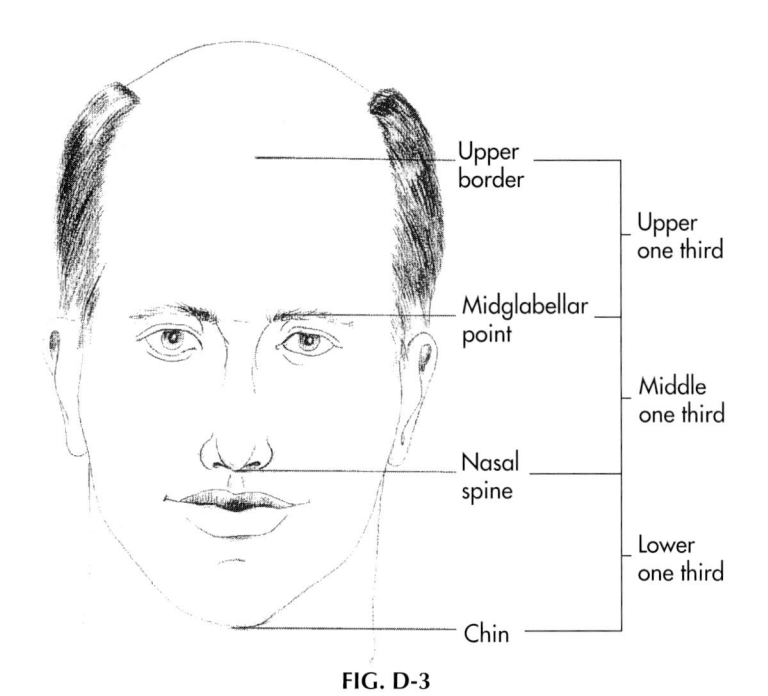

Determination of Hairline Placement 427

FIG. D-3

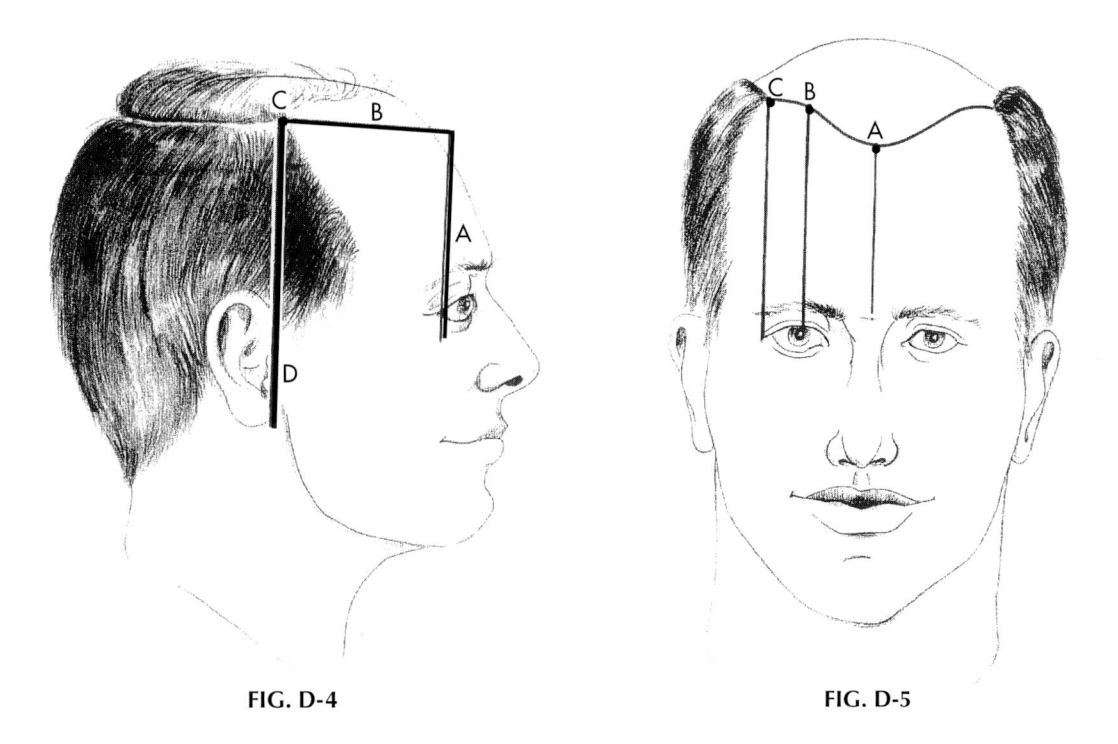

FIG. D-4

FIG. D-5

frontal hairline is not a straight line or wall; it should have gentle concavities near the midpupillary point. Thus, after the aforementioned points are joined, some modification is necessary.

GUIDELINES FOR TEMPORAL HAIRLINE PLACEMENT

The temporal hairline extends from the anterior part of the sideburn to the apex of the frontotemporal triangle. Ideally it has a temporal peak 2 to 3 cm above a line drawn vertically from the lateral part of the eyebrows. The temporal peaks will thin and recede with time. Temporal peaks recede completely in moderate and severe baldness. In patients with mild to moderate hair loss, a temporal hairline recedes posteriorly. If the apex lies on the vertical canthal plane and is not deeper than 7 cm, then no effort should be made to restore the temporal hairline. In patients with extensive hair loss, the temporal hairline recedes not only posteriorly but also inferiorly and the apex is completely lost. Restoration of the temporal hairline in these patients requires placing the apex of the frontotemporal triangle as explained earlier. Again, no effort is made to restore the temporal peaks and the temporal hairline is brought up to connect with the apex (point C in Fig. D-6). If reconstructed, it should slant back and upward to meet the apex and create the frontotemporal triangle and should be 1 to 2 cm deep from its anterior part (point D in Fig. D-6). Temporal hairline reconstitution depends on the density of the donor area and it may not be created if the donor area is scanty; an isolated frontal forelock can be created in such cases.[1]

GUIDELINES FOR FRONTOTEMPORAL TRIANGLE RESTORATION

The frontotemporal triangle is formed by the junction of the frontal and temporal hairlines as they meet at the apex of the frontotemporal triangle, which lies at the outer lateral canthal plane. In adult men, the frontal hairline recedes superiorly (arrow 1 in Fig. D-7) and the temporal hairline posteriorly (arrow 3 in Fig. D-7). The depth of this triangle from midpoint of the frontal hairline to the apex of the frontotemporal triangle varies from 4 to 7 cm.

With mild to moderate baldness, the frontal hairline is lost. The temporal hairline recedes posteriorly and the apex of the frontotemporal hairline recedes along the lateral canthal plane.

To restore the frontotemporal triangle in mild to moderate baldness, the frontal hairline should be placed as described earlier. If the apex of the frontotemporal triangle lies in front of the pretragal vertical line on the canthal plane, then the frontal hairline should simply connect with the apex. If the apex is displaced on the canthal plane behind the

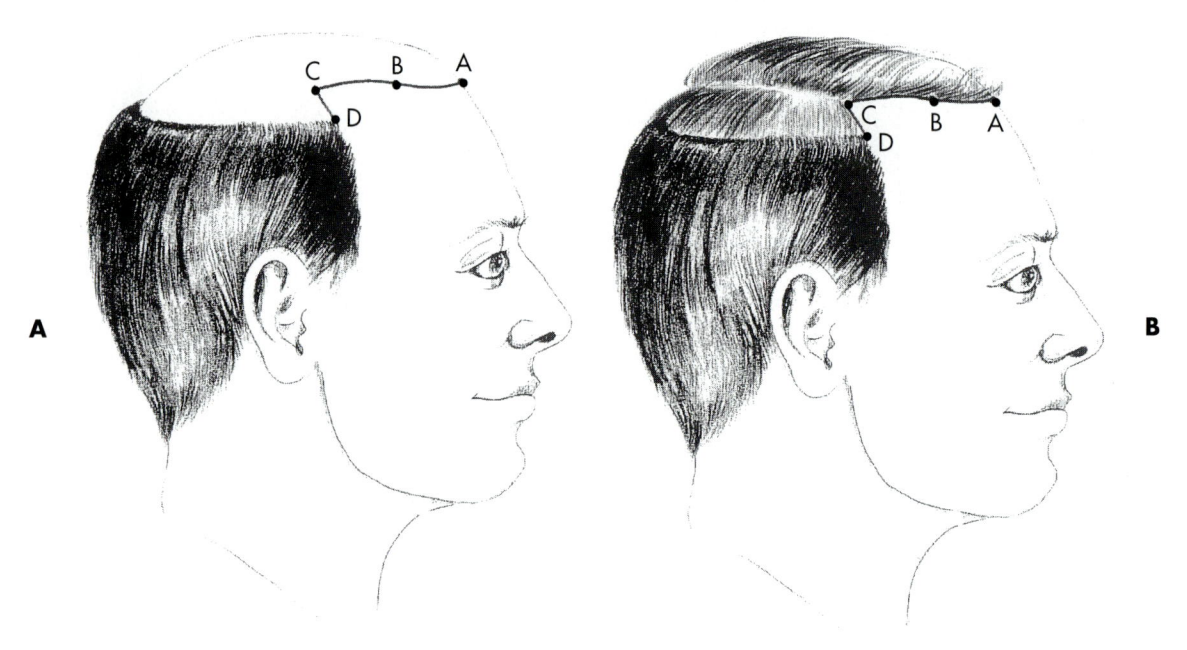

FIG. D-6

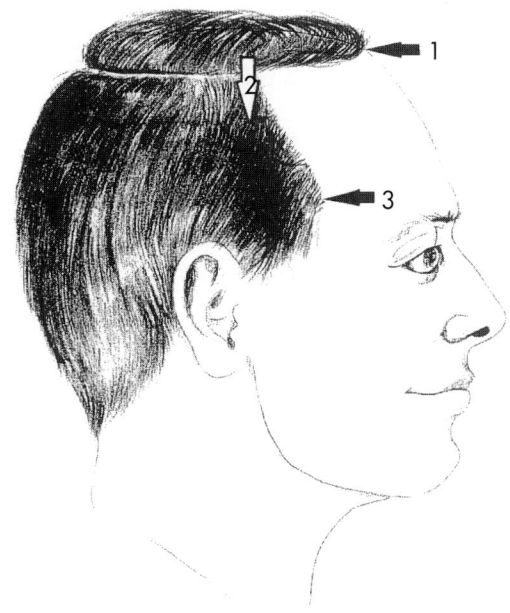

FIG. D-7

pretragal vertical line, then efforts are made to restore the apex as well because an apex more than 7 cm deep gives an unnatural appearance as a result of the long distance to the anterior frontal hairline.

In patients with extensive baldness, the frontal hairline is lost. The temporal hairline recedes posteriorly as well as inferiorly (arrow 2 in Fig. D-7), and the apex of the frontotemporal triangle is lost. The temporal hairline part of the triangle is restored and the temporal hairline is moved anteriorly and brought up and back to unite with the frontal hairline at the apex of the frontotemporal triangle.

TRANSITION ZONE

After the hairline is marked, it is restored using only micrografts and the transition zone is built with gradually increasing density. From front to back, this transition from nonhairy areas to hairy areas with gradually increasing density avoids unpleasant abruptness. When single- and two-hair grafts are implanted, adjacent recipient sites are made in a slightly interrupted manner rather than in lines.

CONCLUSION

The hairline is a permanent part of hair transplant surgery that cannot be altered easily. The re-created hairline should appear oval from front view and horizontal from profile view, with slight, gentle, inward curves near the midpupillary points. A transplanted hairline is preferably placed on the flat surface of the scalp as opposed to the vertical forehead plane. The apex of the frontotemporal triangle falls on the outer vertical canthal plane, which is used as the part line. A transition zone prevents the creation of an "abrupt" hairline, which commonly occurred with older standard round grafts. The dimensions provided are general guidelines that require tailoring based on the individual patient.

REFERENCE

1. Marritt E, Leonard L: A redefinition of male pattern baldness and its treatment implications, *Dermatol Surg* 21:123-135, 1995.

APPENDIX E

Overview of the Surgical Procedure

Mark R. Avram and Francisco Jimenez

We have found the following summary of the surgical procedure to be most helpful for those physicians who have never seen a transplant procedure, are training new staff, or are considering entering this field.

1. When the patient arrives for his hair transplantation session, all laboratory work including hepatitis A, B, and C and HIV tests are reviewed. Written consents (previously read and signed by the patient before taking diazepam) are reviewed. The patient is asked if he has taken diazepam (Valium) and an oral antibiotic 1 hour before surgery as prescribed.
2. Before each session a series of photographs is taken to provide objective documentation to follow the progress after each hair transplantation session.
3. The patient is brought into the operating room and asked to put on a comfortable cotton surgical gown. The surgeon estimates the number of single-hair grafts, 1 mm grafts, and 1.25 mm grafts that are going to be transplanted. The appropriate donor site is located and the area is shaved with a mustache trimmer, leaving a few millimeters of hair growth over the strip of the area to be excised. The hair surrounding the donor area is taped down, away from the surgical site.
4. A Trichoscope is used to estimate the patient's hair density. With this information, the surgeon calculates the length of strip needed to obtain the number of grafts desired.
5. The patient is placed on his stomach on the operating table with the head on a Prōn Pillō. The donor area is cleaned with alcohol and anesthetized with 10 to 20 ml of 0.5% lidocaine with 1:200,000 epinephrine. Ten to 20 ml of saline solution is infiltrated to obtain dermal turgor.
6. The strip is harvested using a triple-bladed knife. Bleeding vessels are coagulated or sutured as needed. The donor site is closed using staples.
7. A pressure bandage is placed over the donor area. The patient rests for approximately 15 to 20 minutes while two technicians of the team begin cutting the desired size and number of grafts from the donor strip. The grafts are placed in cold saline solution in petri dishes.
8. Nitrous oxide is available and offered to the patient. Bilateral supraorbital blocks are performed. After standard surgical preparation, approximately 10 to 20 ml of 0.5% lidocaine with 1:200,000 epinephrine is injected into the recipient site. In addition, a mixture of 12 ml of normal saline solution and 1 ml 1:1000 epinephrine is added for hemostasis.
9. Graft recipient sites are made using 1 mm and 1.25 mm hair transplant punches and a hand engine. The single-hair graft recipient sites are made using an 18-gauge NoKor needle, No. 6100 Beaver blade, or Yeh needle.
10. The hair grafts are placed into the recipient sites by two technicians using jeweler's forceps.
11. After the transplant session is completed, a pressure dressing is applied over both the donor area and the recipient area overnight. Polysporin ointment is placed over the donor area strip site with a nonadherent dressing (Telfa pad) covering the entire area, and Reston foam is placed over the dressing to minimize the pressure over the donor site. After the Reston foam is applied, gauze is placed over the area, followed by a Kling dressing and Micropore tape to secure the dressing to the patient's scalp. A 6-inch stockinette is placed over the dressing to apply additional pressure to the scalp overnight. The patient is given detailed wound care instructions in addition to pain medications (oxycodone hydrochloride 5 mg and acetaminophen 500 mg) and antibiotics (first-generation cephalosporin, cephradin [Velosef] 500 mg, to be taken 6 hours postoperatively). The patient is given the staff's home telephone numbers and instructed to contact the staff at any time with any questions.
12. The hair transplant procedure as outlined takes approximately 3 hours.

APPENDIX F

Medical Questionnaire for Hair Replacement Surgery

Name: _____ Telephone: (H) _____

(W) _____

Address: _____

City: _____ State: _____ Zip Code: _____

Age: _____ Date of Birth: _____ Occupation: _____

IT IS EXPRESSLY UNDERSTOOD THAT THE INFORMATION CONTAINED HEREIN SHALL NOT BE RELEASED WITHOUT THE WRITTEN PERMISSION OF THE PATIENT.

Health History   *Remarks*

1. Are you generally in good health?   Yes _____ No _____ _____

2. Are you presently under a physician's care?   Yes _____ No _____ _____

3. Have you had prior hair transplants?   Yes _____ No _____ _____

   If yes, where? _____

4. Do you or have you ever had:

	Yes	*No*	*Remarks*
a) Heart disease	_____	_____	_____
b) Hypertension	_____	_____	_____
c) Liver disease	_____	_____	_____
d) Kidney disease	_____	_____	_____
e) Lung disease	_____	_____	_____
f) Fainting spells	_____	_____	_____
g) Convulsions	_____	_____	_____
h) Venereal disease	_____	_____	_____
i) Diabetes	_____	_____	_____
j) Dizziness	_____	_____	_____

	Yes	No	Remarks

5. Have you ever had any type of bleeding disorder (i.e., easy bruising, abnormal nosebleeds, profuse bleeding when cut)? _____ _____ _____

6. Do cuts on your skin heal normally? _____ _____ _____

7. Do you have any tendency toward keloid formation (raised, ridged scars)? _____ _____ _____

8. Do you require additional anesthetics (lidocaine, Xylocaine, Marcaine, etc.) at a dentist's office? _____ _____ _____

9. Have you EVER had any allergic reaction to anesthetics? _____ _____ _____

10. Have you had any allergic response or adverse reactions to substances placed on your skin? _____ _____ _____

11. Do you regularly take aspirin and/or vitamin E? _____ _____ _____

12. Do you have any allergic response or adverse reactions to medications or drugs? _____ _____ _____

13. Describe and list the medications and drugs you currently take:
_____

14. Name, address, and telephone number of personal physicians:
_____

15. Name and address of pharmacy you use most often:
_____

Additional Information or Explanation:
_____

I attest that the above information is accurate and that I have fully answered all of the questions to the best of my knowledge.

_____   _____
Patient Signature   *Date*

APPENDIX G

Consent for Hair Transplantation

You have the right, as a patient, to be informed about your condition and the recommended surgical, medical, or diagnostic procedure to be used so that you may make the decision whether or not to undergo the procedure after knowing the risks and hazards involved.

1. I, _____, do hereby consent and agree to have hair replacement surgery performed on me, and any other medical services that, during the procedure, become medically reasonable and necessary.
2. I am aware that good results will depend in part on my completing the necessary number of operations, which has been estimated to me to be _____. However, because many variables exist, I have not been promised or guaranteed good results. I also understand that the quality and amount of my preexisting hair is a major factor in the ultimate results. I understand that I will not have hair of the same thickness as I had before the onset of my hair loss.
3. Before consenting to cosmetic surgery, I state that I have read and discussed with my physician the following literature, which has been supplied to me:
   1. Brochure
   2. List of complications
   3. Preoperative instructions
4. I fully understand the results that I may reasonably expect. An explanation of this procedure has been given to me. I do understand that I will not have a full head of hair after the procedure is complete.
5. A hair transplant may not look natural on those with dark hair and light skin.
6. The minimum amount of operations has been explained to me to be _____. I understand that more operations may be recommended at a later date.
7. I understand there will be scarring associated with this procedure. I understand that hair transplants are not perfect.
8. I am aware that complications may occur. The more common complications and a partial list of rare complications of this surgery have been explained to me, and I have reviewed a list of them, which I initialed and dated. A copy of that list is attached to this request. Unforeseen, rare complications such as unanticipated reaction to medicine and anesthetics, uncommon infections, and unusual healing responses (wide scars) are a possibility. Every unforeseen complication may not have been discussed with me in detail, but I understand that such risks do exist.
9. I consent to and authorize the administration of such local anesthetics and nitrous oxide as may be considered necessary by those performing the surgery on me.
10. I consent to and authorize the performance of cosmetic surgery by Dr. _____, his/her associate doctors, and hair assistant technicians.
11. I believe I have been well informed. I understand that although good results are hoped for and expected, cosmetic surgery results cannot be guaranteed because of the nature of the human body and the healing process. There are also risks of reasonable errors in judgment and implementation, which are possible in any surgical procedure.
12. The pros and cons and alternatives to hair transplants have been explained to me. I have the option of doing nothing at all, wearing a hairpiece or wig, using prescription medication, or receiving a hair transplant. A combination of the above is also possible. I am informed on all options.
13. It has been explained to me that the amount and location of future hair loss on the scalp, including the sides or back area, cannot at this time be predicted. I do understand it is possible to lose my existing hair at any time in the future. I do understand this hair loss may affect the appearance of the grafted area. Hair transplants may not be permanent. They are usually

very long lasting but rarely have been noted to fall out after 1 to 10 years. In the majority of men some thinning of all areas occurs. Most men do not lose all of their hair in the donor area (back of head) with age. A very small percentage of men (less than 10%) do lose a majority of their donor hair and this could affect the final result.
14. This consent was read and signed while I was not under the influence of medications that cause drowsiness.
15. I certify that this form has been fully explained to me, that I have read it or have had it read to me, that the blank spaces have been filled in, and that I understand all of its contents.

A thorough understanding of the above paragraph is required before a patient consents to hair restoration surgery. I have had opportunities to ask questions on this subject.

Date _____ Time _____ a.m./p.m.

_____
Patient/Other Legally Responsible Person

_____
Witness

_____
Patient's Name (Printed)

_____
Address

_____
City, State, Zip Code

_____
Home Telephone Number

_____
Work Telephone Number

Date _____ Patient _____

Date _____ Patient _____

MORE COMMON COMPLICATIONS

Please Initial

1. Nausea and vomiting from pain medication _____
2. Bleeding (less than 5%) _____
3. Infection (less than 1%) _____
4. Excessive swelling _____
5. Temporary headache _____
6. Temporary numbness of scalp _____
7. Scarring around grafts _____
8. Poor growth of grafts _____
9. Reactions to medications (less than 1%) _____
10. Fainting (less than 1%) _____
11. Occasional small ingrown hair, causing a cyst (less than 10%) _____

RARE COMPLICATIONS (PARTIAL LIST ONLY)

Please Initial

1. Keloid formation _____
2. Complete failure of growth of transplanted hair _____
3. Persistent scalp pain _____
4. Total loss of donor hair _____
5. Permanent numbness of scalp _____
6. Noticeable scarring of donor area _____
7. Unnatural growth of transplanted hair _____
8. Loss of transplanted hair _____
9. Allergic reactions or other medication-related problems _____

I have read and understand all of the possible complications listed above.

Signature _____ Date _____

Witness _____ Date _____

APPENDIX H

Patient Instructions for Hair Replacement Surgery

BEFORE SURGERY

1. A blood test, including HIV and hepatitis A, B, and C, is required before the procedure.
   If you are an established patient with the clinic but it has been 1 year or more since your last HIV and hepatitis panel, you will need to have the tests repeated before your next visit to the clinic.
2. Do not take vitamin E, all other vitamins, or aspirin for 1 week before the procedure. This restriction includes all products containing aspirin.
3. Do not consume alcoholic beverages for 48 hours before the procedure.
4. Discontinue the use of Rogaine 1 month before the procedure.
5. The night before and the morning of the procedure, shampoo the scalp and hair with Hibiclens, avoiding the eyes and ears.
6. Please advise us if you have recently had a temperature of 101° F or higher.
7. Take the prescribed antibiotics 1 hour before surgery and 6 hours postoperatively.
8. Take diazepam (Valium) (10 mg) 40 minutes before arriving at the clinic. *Do not drive yourself to the clinic if you have taken Valium.*
9. Eat a *light* breakfast before coming to the office. *This is important.*
10. Bring with you any medications left over from previous visits.

FIRST 48 HOURS POSTOPERATIVELY

1. Eat something after leaving the clinic.
2. Take care when getting in and out of the car while your scalp is still numb. Bumping your head may dislodge some grafts.
3. You will feel drowsy for some time after the operation so you *must not drive* yourself home.
4. On reaching home, you should not lie flat but rest and sleep with head on several pillows.
5. Take it easy for the remainder of the day. *Do not get hot. Do not* do any heavy lifting or strenuous exercise for at least 5 days. *Do not* lean over to tie your shoes or pick up objects from the floor for the first 48 hours because this may provoke bleeding.
6. On rare occasions spotting of some blood from either the donor or recipient areas may occur. If bleeding occurs, apply tissue or a clean towel over the bleeding area. Exert light pressure with the palm of your hand for a minimum of 10 minutes without interruption. If bleeding persists, please call the office, cellular phone, or numeric pager.
7. To avoid excessive bleeding, *do not* drink any alcoholic beverages for 2 days following hair transplant procedures. Also avoid use of marijuana and other nonprescribed chemical substances for 1 week following surgery.
8. Take pain medication at the first signs of discomfort. *Do not wait until you have pain.* Take this medication with food.
9. Take a diazepam (Valium) tablet and one pain tablet approximately 20 minutes before retiring for the night.
10. Take the prescribed antibiotics 6 hours after surgery.
11. Sleep with your head elevated on two or three pillows.
12. Until the graft recipient sites have healed, keep the areas clean by applying half-strength hydrogen peroxide (50% water, 50% hydrogen peroxide) before shampooing. After your daily shampoo (we suggest using baby shampoo), apply Polysporin ointment to each graft. Use a cotton swab to apply the Polysporin to the grafts. *Do not* use Hibiclens after the hair transplantation.
13. *Do not* pick or scratch at crusts (scabs) at any time. Crusts will form over the transplant sites and solidify during the first few days. These crusts will naturally fall off within 2 weeks.

14. Remove any dressing on the day following the operation. The donor area (on the back of the head) should be soaked in a bathtub and the scalp gently washed. *Do not touch grafts (on the top and the crown of the head) for 5 days.* However, you may pour shampoo and water over them and then rinse. An electric hair blow dryer may be used.
15. Apply ice packs to the forehead area 3 to 4 days postoperatively if postoperative edema (swelling) of the forehead and eyes develops. *Do not apply ice to grafts.* This edema is not serious and resolves spontaneously.
16. If a graft does get knocked out, place it in a large tumbler of cold water with a ½ teaspoon of salt and place it in the refrigerator. Apply firm pressure to the bleeding area. Arrangements can be made to reinsert the graft.
17. Wait at least 1 week postoperatively before wearing a hairpiece. Discuss your particular hairpiece and the possible effect of its use on hair growth with your surgeon.
18. Please call the office the day after surgery. If it is a weekend, please call the pager number. Please make arrangements to visit the office for a follow-up visit in 1 or 2 weeks' time.

WITHIN THE FIRST 3 WEEKS

1. No special treatment is required for the grafts, but it is suggested that you wash the scalp daily with shampoo until the crusts have separated. Normal scalp washing may then be resumed.
2. The donor area will be closed with either dissolvable sutures or sutures/staples that require removal after 7 days. We will provide you with a staple remover. Please contact the office the day after the surgery to clarify if you should remove the staples.
3. After hair grafts are placed in the frontal region of the scalp, you may expect some swelling around the eyes. On rare occasions one or two "black eyes" may develop. The swelling usually develops on the third day after the operation and subsides after the next 2 or 3 days. The swelling is a natural response to the operation and no treatment is necessary. If desired, treatment may be administered as described above.
4. Exercising must not be done for the first four days postoperatively. After 4 days you may engage in exercise activities that involve mild exertion with no body contact. These activities include slow jogging, bicycling, and very mild weight lifting. After 10 days you may perform vigorous exercise such as fast running or moderate weight lifting provided that extreme strain such as heavy weight lifting or body contact does not occur. After 3 weeks any degree of exercise or reasonable training will not be harmful to your hair transplants.
5. Infection in the grafts is rare, but if you should develop redness, pus, swelling, or tenderness around any of the grafts, please call the office. Antibiotics are rarely necessary.
6. Occasionally some tender swelling may be detected in the region behind the ears. This swelling is caused by enlarged lymph nodes that will subside in a few days.
7. Crusts will form over each graft within 1 to 2 days. These generally come away after 1 to 2 weeks, taking many of the old graft hairs with them. After the first 10 days you may assist the process by gently rubbing but do not force their removal. Crusts must be off the scalp by 3 weeks. *You will see long hair on either side of the crusts. This is normal—do not worry.*

WITHIN THE FIRST 12 MONTHS

1. After the graft hairs have been lost, there will be a period of several weeks when the hair transplants are bare and dormant. The new hair will begin to appear after approximately 12 weeks. At first only a few hairs will be seen, and these hairs will grow at the normal rate of 1 cm per month. The number of new hairs will continue to increase for up to 12 months.
2. With second and subsequent operations, the onset of growth of the new hairs may be delayed and on rare occasions may not commence until 18 weeks postoperatively.
3. Often the new hair is a little darker and coarser than the preexisting hair. The new hair may also have a slight crinkle and look "frizzy" and "curly," but the texture virtually always returns to normal with continued growth after 6 to 18 months.
4. You may notice some persistent numbness in the donor and newly grafted regions. This sensation will gradually improve over several months as the cut nerve fibers regenerate.

If you require any further advice or information, please do not hesitate to telephone.

APPENDIX I

Hair Transplant Forum International

Dow B. Stough

The *Hair Transplant Forum International* is an informal newsletter circulated among hair transplant surgeons throughout the world. This newsletter allows for the rapid communication of ideas and techniques. Due to the slow review process involved in publishing articles in established medical journals, the *Hair Transplant Forum International* is the only publication in which a rapid informational exchange is offered. Most hair transplant surgeons find this publication very interesting. The editorial comments and nonreviewed opinions offer insight into major controversies in the field today. The editor has no financial interest in this publication but highly recommends this newsletter to all hair transplant surgeons.

Hair Transplant Forum International
1211 North Shartel Ave., Ste. 403
Physicians and Surgeons Building
Oklahoma City, OK 73103
405-235-1418

Index

A

Acid, retinoic, 382-385
Acid permanent wave, 392
Acquired progressive kinking of hair, 319-320
Addition, hair, 399-411; *see also* Hair replacement, nonsurgical
Adhesive for hair addition, 405
Advancement flap, frontoparietal, 269
Adverse drug reaction, 70, 88-89
    as emergency, 334, 337-340
    midazolam and, 101
Advertising, legal issues of, 54-55
Aesthetics, 162-169; *see also* Hairline
    failure of, 34
    of hair addition, 408-411
    in women, 211
African-American patient
    alopecia in, 17
    hair replacement in, 205-207
Age
    alopecia with, 15, 17
    young, 62-67
Alkaline permanent wave, 392
Allergy
    drug, 70, 87-88
    symptoms and treatment of, 335
Alopecia
    androgens in, 10-12
    classification of, 13-20
        in females, 18-20
        in males, 13-18
    drug therapy for, 375-385; *see also* Minoxidil
    in female, 210-216
        classification of, 18-20
        psychosocial effect of, 2
        treatment of, 210-216
    flaps for; *see* Flap
    history of hair replacement for, 59-61
    in male transsexual, 207-210
    masking products for, 396-398
    number of grafts and, 159
    pathology of, 10
    pathophysiology of, 8-10
    physical changes with, 162-163
    progression of, 304-305
        behind flap, 330
    psychological effect of, 1-7
    reevaluation of treatment of, 30-32
    senile, 17
    in transsexual, 209
Anagen, 222
    pathophysiology of, 10

Anaphylactoid reaction, 338-340
    symptoms and treatment of, 335
Anaphylaxis, 338-340
    chlorhexidine gluconate and, 69
    symptoms and treatment of, 335
Androgen
    alopecia and, 13
    hair follicle and, 360
Androgenic hair loss; *see* Alopecia
Anesthesia, 81-111
    Asian patient and, 204
    for automated hair replacement, 371
    buffered lidocaine for, 96
    for female patient, 213
    importance of, 81
    instrumentation for, 111-112
    local
        administration of, 83-87
        adverse reactions to, 88-89
        dosage of, 82, 83
        duration of action of, 82-83
        historical development of, 81-82
        monitored anesthesia and, 102
        side effects of, 87-88
    malignant hyperthermia and, 336, 337-338
    monitored, 97-103
        local anesthesia with, 102
        maintenance of, 102-103
        perioperative, 98-99
        postoperative recovery from, 103
        preoperative considerations in, 97-98
        propofol and midazolam for, 99-101
        sedation in, 101-102
    nerve block, 89-93
    nitrous oxide and, 104-105
    postoperative pain control and, 105-107
    punctiform technique and, 173
    scalp reduction and, 114-115, 240-241
    scalp-lifting and, 286
    single-hair transplantation and, 189
    toxicity of, 335, 337, 338
    tumescent, 93-96
Anesthesia outlets in surgical suite, 80
Angioedema, 336, 340-342
Angiogenesis, 220
Anterior auricular muscle, 23
    innervation of, 25
Antiandrogen, 379
Antibiotic, drug interactions with, 334
Antibiotic prophylaxis, 68-73

Antibiotic prophylaxis—cont'd
    endocarditis and, 71-73
    guidelines for, 69-71
    host risk factors and, 68
    preoperative skin preparation and, 68-69
    prosthetic joints and, 73
    scalp microbiology and, 68
Aponeurosis of scalp, 21
Appearance, unnatural, 312; *see also* Aesthetics; Hairline
Argon beam coagulator, 115, 116
Arterial oxygen saturation, 99
Arteriovenous malformation, 326-327
Artery
    anatomy of, 23-24
    scalp-lift and, 269, 276-277
Asian hair, 402
Asian patient, 201-205
    complications in, 205
    donor harvesting in, 203-204
    hair and skin color in, 202, 402
    hairline and, 202
    preoperative evaluation of, 202-203
    recipient site in, 204-205
    scarring in, 202
    technique for, 203
Assistant
    improperly trained, 315-316
    surgical, 186
        scalp-lifting and, 286-287
Astemizole, 334
Atropine, 337
Attachment of hair addition, 405-408
Auricular artery, 24
Auricular muscle, 25
Auricular region of scalp, 23
Auriculotemporal nerve, 25
Autofocus, of camera, 47
Autograft, history of, 59-61
Automated hair transplantation, 370-374
Automatic camera, 45-46

B

Background, photographic, 48-49
Bacteremia, 71-72
Baldness; *see* Alopecia
Bandage, postoperative, 109-110, 224-227
Barbiturate, 338
Behavioral coping, 5-6
Benzodiazepines, 338
Beta-adrenergic blocking agent, 87, 334, 337

441

Betamethasone, 107
Bilateral occipitoparietal flap, 267-268, 271
Bilateral occipitoparietal scalp-lift, 267-268, 271, 272
Bioelastic silicone sheeting, 280
Biological creep, 245
Biomechanical properties of skin, 255-256
Biopsy
 epidermoid cyst and, 321-323
 synthetic hair replacement and, 352-353
Bitemporal flap
 Brandy, 268-269
 modified, 269
Bitemporal hair loss in female, 214
Black patient
 alopecia in, 17
 hair restoration in, 205-207
Bleeding
 in donor area, 136
 scalp reduction and, 115
 small-graft transplantation and, 156
Bleeding disorder, 342-343
Blood supply
 to scalp, 23-25
 tissue expansion and, 253
Bonding, of hair addition, 407
Boudjema technique, 370-374
Brandy bitemporal scalp-lift, 268-269, 272
Browlift, 235-236
Buffered alkaline permanent wave, 392
Buffered lidocaine, 96
Bupivacaine, 240

C

C1 inhibitor deficiency, 340-341
Camera for patient photography, 42, 44-48
Camouflage products for hair loss, 396-398
Capsule, tissue expansion and, 253
Carbon dioxide, drug toxicity and, 88
Carbon-dioxide laser, 363-369
Cardiac arrest, 335
Cardiovascular system
 cardiac drug interactions and, 87
 endocarditis prophylaxis and, 71-72
 midazolam and, 100, 101
Catagen, 222
 stress-induced, 361
Cautery, scarring caused by, 326
Cefadroxil, prophylactic, 71
Celestone Soluspan, 107
Cell
 keratinocyte colony–forming, 360-361
 tissue expansion and, 257
 wound healing and, 219, 220
Central nervous system
 anesthetic toxicity and, 87
 midazolam and, 100, 101
Cephalosporin, prophylactic, 70-71
Cervical plexus, 25
Chemical dye for coloring hair, 347-348
Chemical hair procedures, 390-393
Chemotherapy, hair loss in flap from, 330
Chinese patient, alopecia in, 17

Chlorhexidine gluconate, 68-69
Chlorpromazine, for hiccups, 333
Choi hair transplanter, 125-127
Cimetidine, 379
Circumferential scalp reduction, 279-280
13-*cis*-retinoic acid, 382-385
Clamp, tension, for rapid intraoperative tissue expansion, 259-266
Classification
 of alopecia, 13-20
  in females, 18-20, 212
  in males, 13-18
 of scalp laxity, 241
 standard graft, 76-77
Clip, for attachment of hair addition, 406
Coagulation disorder, 342-343
Coagulator, argon beam, 115, 116
Cobblestoning, 153, 311-312, 315
Cocaine, as anesthetic, 81
Collagen, inflammation and, 219
Colony-forming cell, keratinocyte, 360-361
Color, skin and hair, 151
 in Asian patient, 202
 mismatch of, 312
Communication, physician-patient, 26-30
Complications, 299-343
 alopecia progression and, 304-305
 angioedema and, 340-342
 arteriovenous malformation as, 326-327
 in Asian patient, 205
 of automated hair replacement, 373
 in black patient, 206-207
 compression as, 313
 dense, coarse hair and, 301
 donor harvest and, 309-310
 emergency, 334-340
 epidermoid cyst as, 320-323
 of hair addition, 408
 hair shaft and, 316-320
 hair-bearing flaps and, 327-331
 hairline placement and, 299-300, 306-309
 of harvesting donor hair, 137-138
 hiccups as, 331-334
 initial consultation and, 306
 linear strip grafting and, 303
 of new techniques, 312-313
 of old techniques, 310-312
 patient selection and, 299, 306
 poor hair growth as, 314-316
 responsibility of physician and, 299
 of scalp extension, 247
 of scalp reduction, 241-242
 scalp-lifting and, 295
 scarring as, 323-326
 synthetic hair replacement and, 352
 vellus thinning as, 301-302
 vertex and, 302
 von Willebrand's disease and, 342-343
 wall effect as, 301
Compression
 as complication, 313
 strip harvesting with micrografting and, 181
Conditioner, 388-389

Confidentiality, 50
Consent, informed, 56-57
 for female patient, 212
 form for, 435-436
Consultation, 26-30
 legal issues of, 55-56
Contraction, scar, 153
Contracture, wound, 220
Coping, with alopecia, 5-6
Cortisone, edema and, 107-108
COUVRé masking lotion, 396, 397
Cowlick, 160-161
Creep, 32
 definition of, 245
 tissue expansion and, 256
Crown, problems with, 308-309
Crusting, postoperative, 108
Curly hair
 in black patient, 205
 transplantation effects on, 317, 318
Current, electromagnetic and electrostatic, 377-378
Custom-made hair addition, 401
Cuticle, transplantation effects on, 317-319
Cycle, hair, 222
Cyclosporine, 380
Cyproterone acetate, 379
Cyst, epidermoid, 320-323
Cytokeratin, 361
Cytokine, wound healing and, 220-221

D

Debridement, scalp, 424
Dehiscence, wound, of donor site, 137
Delayed scalp extension, 245, 246
Density, hair, 139-140, 141
 inadequate, 312
 naturalness vs., 147
Depigmentation, 153
Dermal cell, follicular, 360
Dermatitis, 137-138
Dermis
 tissue expansion and, 253
 wound healing and, 220
Detergent, for hair, 387-388
Diazepam, 337
Diffuse alopecia, unpatterned, 17
Dihydrotestosterone, alopecia and, 10
Dilator, strip harvesting with micrografting and, 185
Dissection
 single-hair, 197-199
 surgical planes of, 288-289, 290, 291
 vertical strip, 195-199
Donor site, 131-149; *see also* Harvesting of donor hair
 anesthesia of, 94
 in Asian patient, 203-204
 automated hair replacement and, 371
 in black patient, 206
 bleeding in, 136
 closure of, 136-137
 complications in, 137-138
 density of, 152-153
 detectable, 331
 dressing for, 223
 elliptical harvesting in, 142-147
 estimation of graft requirements in, 138-142

Donor site—cont'd
  female patient and, 213
  harvesting methods for, 131, 133-135
  incisions in, 135
  infiltration of, 136
  instruments for, 112, 117-121
  micrograft survival in, 147-149
  poor-quality, 314
  problem areas in, 132-133
  punctiform technique and, 173-174
  scalp-lift and, 274
  scarring of, 324-326
  strip release in, 135-136
  surgical tray for, 417-418
Donutting, 314-315
Dressing, postoperative, 109-110, 221-227
Drug interaction/reaction, 334, 337
  adverse, 70, 88-89
  anesthetic and, 87
  as emergency, 337-340
Drug therapy, 375-385
  antiandrogen, 379
  antibiotic prophylaxis and, 68-73; see also Anesthesia
  cyclosporine, 380
  L-cystine, 379
  minoxidil, 375-377; see also Minoxidil
  pulse electrotrichogenesis and, 377-378
  5α-reductase inhibitor, 378-379
  retinoic acid, 382-385
  retinol, 379-380
  tricomin, 379
  ViviScall, 380
Duralastic strip, 280
Dye, chemical, 347-348
Dyeing, hair, 394-395

E
Edema
  buffered lidocaine and, 96
  postoperative, 107-108
  scalp reduction and, 241-242
Electric knife, 128-129
Electrical outlets in surgical suite, 80
Electrocoagulation, 115
  scarring caused by, 326
Electrotrichogenesis, 377-378
Elliptical harvesting of donor hair, 135, 142-147
Emergency situations, 334-340
EMLA, 83-84, 85, 86
Endocarditis, 71-73
Endocrine disorder, 13
Epicranius muscle
  anatomy of, 21
  innervation of, 25
Epidermal growth factor, 221
  alopecia and, 12
Epidermis
  removal of, 184
  synthetic hair replacement and, 354
  tissue expansion and, 252-253
Epidermoid cyst, 320-323
Epinephrine
  anesthesia and, 82
  angioedema and, 341
  Asian patient and, 204

Epinephrine—cont'd
  beta-blocker and, 336
  drug interaction with, 87
  malignant hyperthermia and, 339
  reaction to, 88
Epithelialization, 220
Equipment; see Instrumentation
Erythropoiesis, 334
Ester anesthetic, 81-82
Ethinyl estradiol, 379
European hair, 402-403
Exothermic permanent wave, 392
Expansion, scalp; see Scalp reduction, scalp expansion in
Exposure, of camera, 47, 49
Extension, scalp, 33, 245, 246-250
Eye injury, 69
Eyebrow transplantation, 216-218
Eyelash transplantation, 218

F
Face lift, in male transsexual, 209-210
Family, influence on patient, 64-65
Fascia, 22-23
Fat, tissue expansion and, 253
Female, gender change to, 207-210
Female patient, hair damage in, 403
Female pattern baldness, 210-216
  anesthesia and, 212
  classification of, 18-20
  diagnosis of, 210-211
  donor site and, 212
  evaluation of, 211
  informed consent for treatment of, 211
  pathophysiology of, 8, 9
  psychological effect of, 2, 4
  recipient site and, 212-213
  technical considerations in, 213-216
Fiber, of hair addition, 401-403
Fibroblast
  synthetic hair replacement and, 353
  tissue expansion and, 253-254
Fibroblast growth factor, 220-221
Film, photographic, 48-49
Film-forming conditioning agent, 388
Finasteride, 378-379
Fistula, arteriovenous, 326-327
Fixation rate in synthetic hair replacement, 354-355
Flap
  in Asian patient, 203
  bilateral occipitoparietal, 267-268, 271, 272
  bitemporal
    Brandy, 268-269, 272
    modified, 269
  complications of, 327-331
  in female patient, 212
  Frechet, 239-240, 243-245
  frontoparietal advancement, 269
Flash, photographic, 45-47
Flora, of scalp, 68
Focusing screen, of camera, 47
Follicle, hair
  in black patient, 205
  epidermoid cyst and, 321, 323
  in female patient, 213-214
  pathophysiology of alopecia and, 9
  poor growth after transplantation and, 314

Follicle, hair—cont'd
  regeneration of, 358-363
  synthetic hair replacement and, 353
Folliculitis
  after transplantation, 314
  in black patient, 206-207
  as donor site complication, 137
Foltene, 202
Foreign body reaction, 322, 323
Forelock, frontal
  classification of, 17
  management of, 160
  treatment approach for, 40-41
Frechet extender, 246-249
Frechet flap, 243-245
  scalp reduction and, 239-240
Frontal forelock
  classification of, 17
  management of, 160
  treatment approach for, 40-41
Frontal hairline; see Hairline
Frontal nerve, 90
Frontoparietal advancement flap, 269
Frontotemporal gulf, 306-308
Frontotemporal triangle, 426, 428-429
Full-cap prosthesis, 401
Fusion, of hair addition, 407-408

G
Galea
  anatomy of, 21-22, 23
  tissue expansion and, 259-260
Gender change, 207-210
Genetics
  of alopecia, 15
  predictability of baldness and, 31-32
GLH Formula Number 9, 396, 398
Grading of graft, 182-184
Graft; see also Donor site
  in black patient, 206
  complications of, 314-316
  definition of, 76-77
  epidermoid cyst and, 320-323
  estimation of, 138-142
  eyebrow, 217-218
  hair growth in, 108-109
  improper direction and angulation of, 312
  instrumentation for, 112-113
  NoKor microslit, 122-125
  number needed, 141
  punctiform technique and, 174-175
  requirements of, 222-223
  scalp reduction and, 236-237, 239-240
  single-hair, 187-195; see also Single-hair transplantation
  strip harvesting with micrografting and, 182-184
  surgical tray for, 418, 419
  synthetic hair, 345-358; see also Synthetic hair grafting
  test, 65
  vertical strip dissection for, 195-199
Graft sectioning table, 78-79
Gray hair, color mismatch in, 312
Grooming products, 387-390
Growth factor, wound healing and, 220-221
Growth of hair, 108-109
  hairpiece affecting, 315

Growth of hair—cont'd
  patterns of, 153
  poor, after transplantation, 314-316
Guanidine hydroxide, 393

H

Hair
  of Asian patient, 202
  attachment of hair addition to, 406-407
  bulk of, 152
  change in texture of, 316-320
  character and strength of, 152
  cycle of, 222
  dense, coarse, 301
  density of, 139-140, 141
    appearance of, 151-153
    inadequate, 312
  of female patient, 212
  growth of, 108-109, 153
    hairpiece affecting, 315
    poor, after transplantation, 314-316
  ingrown
    in black patient, 206-207
    in suture line, 138
  permanent for, 391-392
  progressive kinking of, 319-320
  straighteners for, 393
  synthetic, 345-358; see also Synthetic hair grafting
Hair addition, 399-411; see also Hair replacement, nonsurgical
Hair care products, 387-393
Hair follicle; see Follicle, hair
Hair loss; see Alopecia
Hair Loss Effects Questionnaire, 3
Hair replacement; see also Donor site
  in Asian patient, 201-205
  automated, 370-374
  in black patient, 205-210
  complications of, 299-343; see also Complications
  consultation about, 26-30
  in eyebrow, 216-218
  in eyelashes, 218
  in female, 210-216
  hair addition and, 404-405
  hair shaft sequelae of, 316-320
  history of, 59-61
  instrumentation for, 111-129; see also Instrumentation
  laser, 363-369
  nonsurgical, 399-411
    aesthetics of, 408-411
    attachment of, 405-408
    attachment of fibers in, 403-404
    components of, 401-403
    cost of, 405
    history of, 399
    patient selection for, 404-405
    types of, 399-401
  overview of, 431
  single-hair, 187-195
    instrumentation for, 125-127
  small-graft, 151-199; see also Small-graft hair transplantation
  synthetic, 345-358; see also Synthetic hair grafting

Hair replacement—cont'd
  trademarks and service marks involving, 413-416
  in younger patient
    patient selection for, 62-63
    psychological approach to, 63-65
    technical approach to, 65-67
Hair shaft, 316-320
Hair Transplant Forum International, 439
Hairline
  in Asian patient, 202
  in male transsexual, 208-209
  patient's view of, 29-30
  placement of, 170-172
    determination of, 425-429
    flaps and, 329-331
    improper, 299-301, 306-309
  rule of, 66-67
  scalp reduction and, 229, 236-237
  scalp-lift and, 274
  side, 161
  single-hair transplantation and, 187
  small-graft transplantation and, 160
  strip harvesting and, 304
    with micrografting, 179, 185
Hairpiece; see also Hair replacement, nonsurgical
  poor hair growth and, 315
  postoperative use of, 108
Hair-shaper blade, 196
Halo formation, 34, 35-38
Haloperidol, for hiccups, 333
Hand engine harvesting, 133-135
Hand-knotted hair addition, 403
Harvesting of donor hair
  in Asian patient, 203-204
  for automated hair replacement, 371
  bleeding and, 136
  closure and, 136-137
  complications of, 137-138
  elliptical, 135, 142-147
  estimation of graft requirements in, 138-142
  in female patient, 213
  inappropriate techniques of, 309-313
  incisions for, 135
  infiltration and, 136
  instruments for, 117-121
  methods of, 133-135
  micrograft survival in, 147-149
  strip, 134, 135
    definition of, 77
    length of, 140, 142
    micrografting with, 177-186
    multibladed knife for, 117-121
    strip release in, 135-136
Healing, wound, 219-227
  dressings and, 221-227
  inflammatory phase in, 219
  proliferative phase in, 220-221
  small-graft transplantation and, 153
  tissue remodeling phase in, 221
Heart disease
  cardiac arrest and, 335
  drug interactions in, 87
  endocarditis prophylaxis and, 71-72
Heat hair straightening, 393
Heating, of synthetic hair, 349

Hemostasis
  scalp reduction and, 114-115
  scalp-lifting and, 289, 293
Hemostatic scalpel, scarring caused by, 325, 326
Hereditary disorder
  angioedema as, 336, 340
  von Willebrand's disease as, 342-343
"Hermes' wing" hairstyle, 164
Hiccups after scalp surgery, 332-334
Histiocyte, synthetic hair replacement and, 353
Horizontal resectioning, 358-363
Hua Laan Chon Kan, 195
Human hair, in hairpiece, 402
Hyperkalemia, 339
Hypertension, minoxidil for, 376
Hyperthermia, malignant, 336, 337-338
Hypertrophic scarring, 206-207, 324
Hyperventilation, drug toxicity and, 88
Hypoglycemia, 336

I

Implantation, automated, 372-373
Incision
  for Frechet flap, 244
  for harvesting, 135
    strip, 185
  for scalp reduction, 230-235, 242
  scalp-lifting and
    ligation of occipital artery and, 269
    planning of, 286
Indian hair, 402
Infarction, myocardial, 335
Infection
  antibiotic prophylaxis for, 68-73
  in Asian patient, 204
  nerve block and, 92
  scalp reduction and, 241
  synthetic hair and, 349, 352
Infiltration
  for anesthesia, 84
  of donor area, 136
  synthetic hair replacement and, 353, 354
Inflammation
  synthetic hair replacement and, 353
  wound healing and, 219
Informed consent, 56-57
  for female patient, 212
  form for, 435-436
Ingrown hair
  in black patient, 206-207
  in suture line, 138
Inhaler, for nitrous oxide, 104
Injector, needleless, 84
Innervation of scalp, 25
Instructions, postoperative, for hair replacement surgery, 437-438
Instrumentation, 111-129, 417-421
  hair transplantation and, 111-114
  harvesting donor tissue and, 117-121
  manufacturers of, 417-421
  NoKor microslit grafting and, 121-125
  retraction-sectioning and, 127-129
  scalp reduction and, 114-117
  scalp-lifting and, 293

Instrumentation—cont'd
   single-hair transplantation and, 125-127
   tissue expansion and, 260-261
Interaction, drug, 87, 334, 337
Intraoperative period
   anesthesia maintenance in, 102-103
   photography during, 50
   scalp extension in, 249-250, 255-257
   tissue expansion in, 258
      tension clamps for, 259-266
Intravenous sedation, 101-102
Inverted-Y posterior incision, 234

J
Japanese patient, 17
Joint infection, prosthetic, 73

K
Keloid, 324
   in donor site, 138, 331
Keratinocyte, 220
Keratinocyte colony–forming cell, 360-361
Ketorolac, 334
Kinked hair, 316-319
Knife
   electric, 128-129
   multibladed, 117-121
      graft estimation when using, 138-142
      single-hair transplantation and, 189
      technique for, 135

L
Landmarks of scalp, 20
Lanham Act, 413, 414
Lanthionization, 393
Laser hair transplantation, 363-369
Law, trademark and service mark, 413-416
Legal issues
   advertising as, 54-55
   informed consent as, 56-57, 212
   trademark and service marks as, 413-416
Lens, of camera, 47-48
Lidocaine
   dosage of, 82, 83
   instrumentation for, 112-113
   postoperative edema and, 96
   scalp reduction and, 240-241
   scalp-lifting and, 286
   technique for, 85-86
Lifting, scalp; *see* Scalp-lifting
Ligation, of occipital artery, in scalp-lift, 269, 276-277
Lighting
   for photography, 48
   for surgical suite, 78
Linear hand engine harvesting, 134
Linear scar harvesting, 131
Linear strip grafting, 303, 304
Local anesthesia, 81-89; *see also* Anesthesia, local
Loniten; *see* Minoxidil
Looped-and-sealed hair addition, 404
Loose areolar layer of scalp, 22

Low forelock, management of, 160
Ludwig classification of female baldness, 18-20, 211, 212, 214
Lye-based hair straightener, 393
Lymphocyte, inflammation and, 219

M
Machine-wefted hair addition, 404
Macrolide antibiotic, 334
Male pattern baldness; *see* Alopecia
Male transsexual, 207-210
Malformation, arteriovenous, 326-327
Malignant hyperthermia, 336, 337-338
Manual camera, 45-46
Manufacturers, instrument, 417-421
Marzola lateral scalp-lift, 266-267
Masking lotion, for alopecia, 396, 397
Massage, scalp, 285
Mechanical creep, 245
Mechanical hair straightening, 393
Medicolegal issues, 54-57
Megatransplant session, 154-159, 162
   laser, 365
Metallic hair dye, 394
Microbiology, 68-73
Micrograft; *see also* Small-graft hair transplantation
   in Asian patient, 203
   definition of, 76, 77
   elliptical donor harvesting and, 145
   flap posterior to, 329-330
   scalp-lift and, 274
   strip harvesting with, 177-186
   survival of, 147-149
Micro-Pen, 128-129
Microslit grafting, NoKor, 122-125
Microtome, 370-371
Midazolam, 99-102
   anesthesia and, 84-85
Middle temporal artery, 24
Midfrontal forelock, alopecia with, 17
Midline transplantation, for Red Sea syndrome, 35
Minigraft; *see also* Small-graft hair transplantation
   definition of, 76, 77
   elliptical donor harvesting and, 145
   scalp-lifting and, 269-279
Minoxidil
   for Asian patient, 202
   postoperative use of, 109
   punctiform technique and, 174
   retinoic acid with, 382-385
   topical, 376-377
Modified bitemporal flap, 269
Monitored anesthesia, 97-103; *see also* Anesthesia, monitored
Monitoring, cardiovascular, 114-115
Monoamine oxidase inhibitor, 87
Motor nerves of scalp, 25
Multibladed knife
   elliptical harvesting and, 143
   graft estimation when using, 138-142
   single-hair transplantation and, 189
   technique for, 135
   types of, 117-121, 417
Muscle
   auricular, 23

Muscle—cont'd
   epicranius, 21
   innervation of, 25
   occipital, 290
   tissue expansion and, 253
   trapezius, 291
Myocardial infarction, 335

N
Naturalness vs. density debate, 147
Necrosis
   central, 314-315
   prevention of, 285-286
   scalp-lifting and, 269, 277, 295
   shotgun harvesting and, 133
Needle
   NoKor, 122-125, 419
   for synthetic hair, 350
Needleless injector for anesthesia, 84
Nerve block, 87, 89-93
   scalp reduction and, 241
Nervous system
   anatomy of, 25
   anesthetic toxicity and, 87
   of scalp, 21
Neuralgia
   in donor site, 138
   postoperative, 106-107
Neuromuscular blocking agent, 338
Nitrous oxide, 104-105
   scalp reduction and, 240, 241
NoKor microslit grafting, 122-125
Nonsurgical hair replacement, 399-411; *see also* Hair replacement, nonsurgical
Nonvolumetric expansion, 245
Norwood classification system of male pattern baldness, 15-17

O
Occipital artery
   anatomy of, 25
   scalp-lifting procedure and, 269, 276-277
Occipital muscle transection, 290
Occipital zone, harvesting in, 132, 133
Occipitoparietal scalp-lift, 267-268, 271, 272
Office surgery, 97
Opioid, 338
Oriental patient, 17
Otoscope, for hair density determination, 139
Overdose, anesthetic, 87
Oximetry, perioperative, 98-99
Oxygen, drug toxicity and, 88

P
Pain control, postoperative, 105-107
Parents, influence on patient, 64
Paresthesia, 92
   scalp-lifting and, 295
Parietal zone, harvesting in, 133
Partial hairpiece, 401
Partial scalp reduction, 35; *see also* Scalp reduction
Patent and Trademark Office, 414
Patient instructions, postoperative, 437-438

Pattern baldness; see Alopecia
Peninsula effect, 330-331
Pericranium, 22
Peripheral scarring, 311
Permanent hair dye, 394-395
Permanent wave, 390-391
Phenothiazine, 87
Photography, 41-54
   background for, 49
   baseline exposure values in, 49
   camera systems for, 42, 44-47
   confidentiality and, 50
   do's and don'ts in, 50, 51-53
   equipment for, 44-49
   special situations in, 50
   standard views in, 42, 43-44
Phrenic nerve, hiccups and, 333
Physical changes with baldness, 162-163
Pierce closure, 133
Pinched appearance, 313
Pitting, as complication, 313
Planes of dissection, 288-289, 290, 291
Platelet-derived growth factor, 221
Platelets, inflammation and, 219
Plexus, cervical, 25
Plugginess, 153
   as complication, 313
   treatment of, 161
Polyethylene terephthalate, 347, 357
Pomade, 393
Popping, as complication, 313
Posterior auricular artery, 24
Posterior auricular muscle, 23
Posterior Y-plasty, 261
Postoperative period
   pain control in, 105-107
   patient instructions for, 437-438
   recovery from anesthesia and, 103
Potassium, 339
Preoperative care
   antibiotic prophylaxis and, 68-69
   for Asian patient, 202-203
   monitored anesthesia and, 97-98
   scalp-lifting and, 285-286, 294
   synthetic hair replacement and, 350-351
Preservative, saline, 315
Progression of alopecia, 304-305
   behind flap, 330
Progressive hair dye, 394
Progressive kinking of hair, 319-320
Prolene suture, 112
Prolonged scalp extension, 246-249
Prophylaxis, antibiotic, 68-73
Propofol, 99-102
Propranolol, 87
Proscar, 378-379
Prosthetic hair addition, 399-411; see also Hair replacement, nonsurgical
Prosthetic joint infection, 73
Pruritus, 138
Pseudofolliculitis barbae, 206-207
Psychological effects of alopecia, 1-7, 162-166
Pulse electrotrichogenesis, 377-378
Pulse oximetry, perioperative, 98-99
Pump, tissue expander, 257, 258

Punched-in technique for hair addition, 404
Punctiform technique, 172-177

Q

Quaternary conditioning agent, 388
Questionnaire
   hair loss effects, 3
   medical, for hair replacement surgery, 433-434

R

Ready-made hair addition, 401
Recipient site
   anesthesia of, 94
   in Asian patient, 204-205
   automated hair replacement and, 371
   dressing for, 223
   in female patient, 213-214
   instrumentation for, 112-113
   in single-hair transplantation, 190
   surgical tray for, 418
Recruitment, tissue, 254-255, 257-258
"Red Sea" syndrome, 35
5α-Reductase, alopecia and, 10, 12
5α-Reductase inhibitor, 378-379
Reduction, scalp; see Scalp reduction
Refined donor harvesting, 131
Regeneration of hair follicle, 358-363
Registered trademark or service mark, 413-416
Relaxation, stress, tissue expansion and, 256
Replacement, hair; see Hair replacement
Resectioning, horizontal, 358-363
Respiratory system, midazolam and, 100-101
Restoration, hair; see Hair replacement
Retinoic acid with minoxidil, 382-385
Retinol, 379-380
Retraction-sectioning technique, 127-129
Retroauricular zone, 132
Ridging, 311
Ring flash unit for photography, 48
Rogaine; see Minoxidil
Rule of thirds, 66-67, 429-431

S

Sagittal scalp reduction, 232-235
Saline infiltration, of donor area, 136
Saline preservative, 315
Scalp
   anatomy of, 20-23
   attachment of hair addition and, 405-406
   in female patient, 214, 216
   microbiology of, 68
   multiple surgeries and, 156
   nerve block of, 89-93
   postoperative dressing for, 109-110, 221-227
   surgical planes of, 288-289, 290-291
Scalp Debridement Unit, 424
Scalp expansion, 33; see also Scalp reduction
   terminology for, 245-246

Scalp extension, 33, 245, 246-250
   circumferential scalp reduction and, 279-280
   intraoperative, 249-250
   prolonged, 246-249
Scalp reduction, 229-266
   anesthesia for, 240-241
   approaches to, 33-40
   in Asian patient, 203
   browlift with, 235-236
   circumferential, 279-280
   complications of, 241-242
   in female patient, 212
   Frechet flap in, 243-245
   grafting after, 239-240
   hairline grafting preceding, 236-237
   incisions for, 230-235, 242
   instrumentation for, 114-117
   misconceptions about, 32-33
   partial, 35
   patient selection for, 229-230
   scalp expansion in
      biology of, 251-255
      definitions of, 245-246
      intraoperative, 255-257
      techniques of, 257-258
      tension clamps for, 259-266
   scalp extension in
      intraoperative, 249-250
      prolonged, 246-249
   scalp-lifting vs., 284
   terminology in, 245-246
   undermining in, 237-239
Scalpel
   for automated transplant, 370
   hemostatic, scarring caused by, 325, 326
Scalp-lifting, 266-298
   anatomy and, 288-292
   anesthesia for, 286
   complications of, 295
   future of, 295, 298
   hemostasis and, 289, 293
   history of, 33, 266
   incision for, 286
   instrumentation for, 114-117, 293
   planning of, 283-285
   preoperative expansion for, 285-286
   scalp reduction vs., 284
   small-graft hair transplantation with, 266-282
      bilateral occipitoparietal flap in, 267-268
      Brandy bitemporal flap in, 268-269
      circumferential scalp reduction and, 279-280
      frontoparietal advancement flap in, 269
      ligation of occipital artery in, 269
      Marzola lateral lift and, 266-267
      minigrafting and, 269-270
      modified bitemporal flap in, 269
      results of, 280
      three-step approach to, 270-279
   stretchback and, 293, 295
   surgical assistants in, 286-287
   undermining and, 293, 296
Scar
   in Asian patient, 202

Scar—cont'd
  in black patient, 206
  as complication, 323-326
  harvesting of grafts and, 309
  hemostatic scalpel causing, 325, 326
  peripheral, 311
  scalp extension and, 247
  scalp reduction and, 230-235
  scalp-lifting and, 274, 295
  small-graft transplantation and, 153
  synthetic hair replacement and, 357
  widening of, 137
Scrub, surgical, 69
Seborrheic dermatitis, 137
Sectioning, 127-129
  horizontal, 358-363
Sedation
  anesthesia and, 84-85
  intravenous, 101-102
Seizure, 336
  as drug reaction, 88
Seldane, 334
Self-image, alopecia and, 2-4
Self-regulated permanent wave, 392
Semipermanent hair dye, 394
Senile alopecia, 17
Sensory nerves of scalp, 25
Service mark law, 413-416
Sexual development, alopecia and, 13
Shaft, hair, synthetic, 348
Shampoo, 387-388
  chlorhexidine gluconate, 68-69
Shaw hemostatic scalpel, scarring caused by, 325, 326
Sheeting, bioelastic silicone, 280
Shotgun hand engine harvesting, 133-135
Side hairline, 161
Silicone sheeting, bioelastic, 280
Silver, for synthetic hair, 349, 357
Single-hair transplantation, 187-195
  discussion about, 190-192
  dissection and, 197-199
  for eyebrow, 217-218
  for eyelashes, 218
  frontal hairline in, 187
  instrumentation for, 125-127
  long-term consequences of, 192, 194
  obtaining grafts for, 188-189
  origins of, 187
  procedure for, 189
  requirements for, 192
  technique of, 189-190
Skin
  color of, 151
    in Asian patient, 202
  donor, amount needed, 158
  preoperative preparation of, 68-69
  of scalp, 20
  stretched, 251-259; see also Scalp expansion
    anatomy of, 251-255
    expansion techniques and, 257-258
    intraoperative expansion and, 255-257
Slot formation, scalp extension and, 247-248

Small-graft hair transplantation, 151-199
  artistic craftsmanship in, 162-170
  hairline placement in, 170-172
  master plan for, 159-161
  megatransplant sessions in, 154-159
  punctiform technique of, 172-177
  quantifiable aspects of, 151-154
  scalp-lifting procedure with, 266-282; see also Scalp-lifting
  single-hair, 187-195
  strip harvesting and, 177-186
    background of, 178-181
    compression and, 181
    definition of, 177-178
    dilators in, 185
    donor site closure and, 182
    graft grading in, 182-184
    graft insertion in, 185-186
    graft preparation for, 184
    hairline and, 185
    limited depth incisions in, 185
    removal of epidermis in, 184
    session size for, 181
    strip harvesting and, 181-182
    vertical strip dissection and, 195-199
Social image, hair loss and, 1-7
Sodium bicarbonate
  edema and, 96
  local anesthetic and, 82
Sodium chloride, tumescent anesthesia and, 95
Sodium hydroxide, 393
Spacer sizing, 190
Spinal nerve, hiccups and, 333
Spironolactone, 379
Spouse, influence on patient, 64
Staphylococcal infection
  in Asian patient, 204
  endocardial, 72
  synthetic hair and, 352
Staple, 136-137
  single-hair transplantation and, 189
  strip harvesting with micrografting and, 182
Stereoscope, 143-144, 145
Sterilization of synthetic hair, 349
Straightening, hair, 393
Streptococcal infection, endocardial, 72
Stress relaxation, 32
  tissue expansion and, 256
Stress-induced catagen, 361
Stretchback
  causes of, 241
  scalp extension and, 247, 256-257
Stretched skin, 251-259; see also Scalp expansion
  anatomy of, 251-255
  expansion techniques and, 257-258
  intraoperative expansion and, 255-257
Strip grafting, linear, 303, 304
Strip harvesting of donor hair, 134, 135-136
  definition of, 77
  in female patient, 213
  length of, 140, 142
  micrografting with, 177-186
  multibladed knife for, 117-121

Strip harvesting of donor hair—cont'd
  vertical, 195-199
Studio setup for photography, 44-45
Styling aid, 390
Subcutaneous layer of scalp, 20-21
Subgaleal region, 25
Sulfite permanent wave, 392
Superficial musculoaponeurosis, 23
Superficial temporal artery, 24
Superior auricular muscle, 23
  innervation of, 25
Supplies, operative, 417-421
Supraorbital artery, 23-24
Supraorbital nerve, 25, 90
Supratrochlear artery, 23-24
Supratrochlear nerve, 25
  anatomy of, 90
Sure-Closure device, 249-250
Surgical assistant, 186
  scalp-lifting and, 286-287
Surgical attachment of hair addition, 406
Surgical products, manufacturers of, 417-421
Surgical scrub, 69
Surgical suite, 78-80
Suture
  donor site closure with, 136-137
  scalp reduction and, 237
  scalp-lifting and, 293, 295
  types of, 112
Syncope, 336
  as drug reaction, 88
Synthetic fiber, for hair addition, 403
Synthetic hair grafting, 345-358
  advantages and disadvantages of, 355
  complications of, 352
  critique of, 357-358
  fixation rates for, 354-355
  histopathological studies of, 352-354
  history of, 345
  materials used for, 350
  preoperative assessment of, 350-351
  safety and effectiveness of, 347-350
  technique of, 351-352
  types of, 346
Systemic antiandrogen, 379

T
Table, graft sectioning, 78, 80
Telogen, 222
Telogen defluvium, 313
Temporal artery, 24
Temporal fascia, 22-23
Temporal hairline, 427
Temporalis muscle, 25
Temporary hair dye, 394
Temporoparietal fascia, 23
Temporoparietal flap
  design for, 331
  problems with, 327-331
Temporoparietooccipital flap
  design for, 330
  problems with, 327-331
Tension clamps for tissue expansion, 259-266
Terfenadine, 334
Terminology, graft size, 76-77

Test graft, 65
Thickener, hair, 388
Thinning of hair
  diffuse, unpatterned, 301-302
  in female patient, 214-216
Thioglycolate, 393
30-30-30-30 scalp massage, 285
Tight scalp, scalp extension and, 248
Tissue expander pump, 257, 258
Tissue expansion; *see also* Scalp expansion
  chronic, 257-258
  immediate, 258
  tension clamps for, 259-266
  terminology of, 245
Tissue remodeling, 221
"Toothbrush" look, 313
Topical anesthetic, 83-84
Topical antiandrogen, 379
Topical minoxidil; *see* Minoxidil
Toradol, 334
Toupe; *see* Hair replacement, nonsurgical
Towel clamp, for tissue expansion, 260-261
Toxicity, drug, 88-89
  anesthetic, 87, 337, 338
Trademark law, 413-416
Transforming growth factors, 221
  alopecia and, 12
Transplantation, hair; *see* Hair replacement
Transsexual male, 207-210

Trapezius muscle, 291
Triangle, frontotemporal, 426, 428-429
Triazolam, 334
Trichoscope, 139
Tricomin, 379-380
Trigeminal nerve, 25
Tumescent anesthesia, 86-87, 93-96
  instrumentation for, 112-113

U

Ultra-closeup photography, 50
Ultrapulse carbon-dioxide laser, 364
Undermining
  in scalp reduction, 237-239
  scalp-lifting and, 293, 296
  in tissue expansion, 257-258
Unnatural appearance, 312
Unpatterned, diffuse alopecia, 17

V

Vacuum-fitted prosthetic hair addition, 405-406
Vagus nerve, hiccups and, 333
Vascular system
  anatomy of, 23-25
  scalp-lift and, 269, 276-277
  tissue expansion and, 253
Vasovagal syncope, 336
Vertex
  problems with, 302, 303, 308-309
  strip harvesting with micrografting and, 180
Vertical strip dissection, 195-199

View, photographic, 42, 43-44
Viscoelastic properties of skin, 255-256
Volumetric expansion, 245
Von Willebrand's disease, 342-343

W

Wall effect of hairline, 301
Wave, permanent, 390-391
Weaving, of hair addition, 406-407
Wig, 401; *see also* Hair replacement, nonsurgical
Wound closure, tension clamps in, 264-265
Wound dehiscence, of donor site, 137
Wound healing, 219-227
  dressings and, 221-227
  inflammatory phase in, 219
  proliferative phase in, 220-221
  tissue remodeling phase in, 221

Y

Y incision, 234
Younger patient
  psychological approach to, 63-65
  selection of, 62-63
  technical approach to, 65-67
Y-plasty, posterior, 261

Z

Zigzag scalp reduction, 230-235
Z-plasty, 231
Zygomaticofacial nerve, 25